W9-DDA-925

CURRENT MANAGEMENT OF HYPERTENSIVE AND VASCULAR DISEASES

MEDICAL TITLES IN THE CURRENT THERAPY SERIES

CURRENT MANAGEMENT

OF HYPERTENSIVE

AND VASCULAR DISEASES

JOHN P. COOKE, M.D., Ph.D., F.A.C.C.

Assistant Professor of Medicine
Director, Section of Vascular Medicine
Division of Cardiovascular Medicine
Falk Cardiovascular Research Institute
Stanford University Medical Center
Stanford, California

EDWARD D. FROHLICH, M.D., F.A.C.C.

Alton Ochsner Distinguished Scientist
Vice President for Academic Affairs
Alton Ochsner Medical Foundation
New Orleans, Louisiana

B.C. Decker
An Imprint of Mosby–Year Book

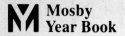

Mosby
Year Book

Dedicated to Publishing Excellence

Publisher: George Stamathis
Senior Managing Editor: Lynne Gery
Project Supervisor: Amy Gewirtzman

Printed in the United States of America

Mosby–Year Book, Inc.
11830 Westline Industrial Drive
St. Louis, MO 63146

Library of Congress Cataloging-in-Publication Data
Current management of hypertensive and vascular diseases / [edited by]
    Edward D. Frohlich, John P. Cooke.
        p.   cm. — (Current therapy series)
    Includes bibliographical references and index.
    ISBN 1-55664-356-X : $79.50
    1. Blood-vessels—Diseases—Treatment.   2.   Hypertension-
-Treatment.   I. Frohlich, Edward D., 1931-   . II. Cooke, John P.
III. Series.
    [DNLM: 1. Hypertension—therapy.   2.   Vascular Diseases—therapy.
WG   340   C97657]
RC691.C95   1992
616.1´306—dc20
DNLM/DLC   91-38258
for Library of Congress   CIP

92 93 94 95 96 GW/MY/MY 9 8 7 6 5 4 3 2 1

CONTRIBUTORS

J. MICHAEL BACHARACH, M.D., M.P.H.

Fellow in Cardiovascular Diseases, Mayo Clinic, Rochester, Minnesota

HERBERT BENSON, M.D.

Associate Professor of Medicine, Harvard Medical School, and President, Mind/Body Medical Institute, New England Deaconess Hospital, Harvard Medical School; Chief, Division of Behavioral Medicine, New England Deaconess Hospital, Boston, Massachusetts

JOHNNY BIRBE

Senior Medical Student, University of Barcelona Medical School, Barcelona, Spain

DAVID H. BLANKENHORN, M.D.

Professor of Medicine and Director of Atherosclerosis Research Institute, University of Southern California School of Medicine, Los Angeles, California

FRANCISCO L. CANALES, M.D

Clinical Instructor in Surgery, Harvard Medical School; Associate, Plastic and Reconstructive Surgery, Beth Israel Hospital, Boston, Massachusetts

VICTOR L. CARPINIELLO, M.D.

Associate Clinical Professor of Urology, University of Pennsylvania School of Medicine, Philadelphia, Pennsylvania

KENNETH J. CHERRY Jr., M.D.

Associate Professor, Mayo Medical School, Rochester, Minnesota

JAMES H. CHESEBRO, M.D.

Consultant in Cardiovascular Diseases and Internal Medicine, and Professor of Medicine, Mayo Medical School, Mayo Clinic and Foundation, Rochester, Minnesota

JAY D. COFFMAN, M.D.

Professor of Medicine, Boston University School of Medicine; Chief, Peripheral Vascular Section, University Hospital, Boston University Medical Center, Boston, Massachusetts

RICHARD A. COHEN, M.D.

Professor of Medicine and Physiology, and Director, Vascular Biology Unit, Department of Medicine, Boston University School of Medicine, Boston, Massachusetts

JOHN P. COOKE, M.D., Ph.D., F.A.C.C.

Assistant Professor of Medicine, Director, Section of Vascular Medicine, Division of Cardiovascular Medicine, Falk Cardiovascular Research Institute, Stanford University Medical Center, Stanford, California

GREGORY S. COUPER, M.D.

Instructor, Department of Surgery, Division of Cardiac Surgery, Harvard Medical School, Boston, Massachusetts

FILIPPO CREA, M.D., F.A.C.C., F.E.S.C.

Lecturer in Cardiovascular Sciences, University of London, Royal Postgraduate Medical School; Honorary Senior Registrar, Hammersmith Hospital, London, England

ROBERT G. DLUHY, M.D.

Associate Director, Endocrinology and Hypertension, Brigham and Women's Hospital, Boston, Massachusetts

MAGRUDER C. DONALDSON, M.D.

Assistant Professor of Surgery, Harvard Medical School; Associate Surgeon, Brigham and Women's Hospital, Boston, Massachusetts

DAVID J. DRISCOLL, M.D.

Professor of Pediatrics, Mayo Medical School; Head, Section of Pediatric Cardiology, Mayo Clinic and Foundation, Rochester, Minnesota

TIM A. FISCHELL, M.D.

Assistant Professor of Medicine, Stanford University School of Medicine, Stanford, California

WILLIAM K. FREEMAN, M.D., F.A.C.C.

Assistant Professor of Medicine, Mayo Medical School; Consultant, Division of Cardiovascular Diseases, Mayo Clinic and Foundation, Rochester, Minnesota

RICHARD FRIEDMAN, Ph.D.

Associate Professor of Psychiatry and Psychology, State University of New York at Stony Brook School of Medicine, Stony Brook, New York; Research Director, Mind/Body Medical Institute, New England Deaconess Hospital, Harvard Medical School, Boston, Massachusetts

EDWARD D. FROHLICH, M.D., F.A.C.C.

Alton Ochsner Distinguished Scientist and Vice President for Academic Affairs, Alton Ochsner Medical Foundation, New Orleans, Louisiana

HEATHER J. FURNAS, M.D.

Clinical Instructor in Surgery, Harvard Medical School; Associate in Plastic and Reconstructive Surgery, Beth Israel Hospital, Boston, Massachusetts

VALENTIN FUSTER, M.D.

Hilda A. and Arthur M. Master Professor of Medicine, and Chief, Division of Cardiology, Mount Sinai School of Medicine and Medical Center, New York, New York

BERNARD J. GERSH, M.B.Ch.B., D.Phil., F.R.C.P. (UK)

Professor of Medicine, Mayo Medical School; Consultant in Cardiovascular Diseases and Internal Medicine, Mayo Clinic, Rochester, Minnesota

SAMUEL Z. GOLDHABER, M.D.

Associate Professor of Medicine, Harvard Medical School; Staff Cardiologist, Brigham and Women's Hospital, Boston, Massachusetts

ROBERT A. GRAOR, M.D.

Staff, Department of Vascular Medicine and Cardiology, Cleveland Clinic Foundation, Cleveland, Ohio

BRUCE H. GRAY, D.O.

Department of Vascular Medicine and Cardiology, Cleveland Clinic Foundation, Cleveland, Ohio

JOHN W. HALLETT Jr., M.D.

Associate Professor of Surgery, Mayo Medical School, Rochester, Minnesota

MELANIE E. HARGARTEN, M.S.

Program Coordinator, Cardiovascular Rehabilitation Center, University Hospital, Denver, Colorado

JOHN A. HEIT, M.D.

Assistant Professor of Medicine, Mayo Medical School; Consultant, Division of Cardiovascular Diseases, Mayo Clinic, Rochester, Minnesota

WILLIAM R. HIATT, M.D.

Associate Professor, University of Colorado School of Medicine; Chief, Section of Vascular Medicine, University Hospital, Denver, Colorado

JACK HIRSH, M.D.

Professor of Medicine, McMaster University Faculty of Medicine; Director, Hamilton Civic Hospitals Research Centre, Hamilton, Ontario, Canada

HOWARD N. HODIS, M.D.

Assistant Professor of Medicine, and Member, Atherosclerosis Research Institute, University of Southern California School of Medicine, Los Angeles, California

LARRY H. HOLLIER, M.D., F.A.C.S.

Clinical Professor of Surgery, Louisiana State University Medical Center and Tulane University Medical Center; Chairman, Department of Surgery, Ochsner Clinic and Alton Ochsner Medical Foundation, New Orleans, Louisiana

GENE G. HUNDER, M.D.

Professor of Medicine, Mayo Medical School, Rochester, Minnesota

JULIE R. INGELFINGER, M.D.

Associate Professor of Pediatrics, Harvard Medical School; Co-Chief, Pediatric Nephrology, Massachusetts General Hospital, Boston, Massachusetts

K. CRAIG KENT, M.D.

Assistant Professor of Surgery, Harvard Medical School; Associate in Surgery, Beth Israel Hospital, Boston, Massachusetts

ALEXANDER S. KHOURY, M.D.

Hypertension Fellow, University of Texas Southwestern Medical Center, Dallas, Texas

JULES Y. T. LAM, M.D.

Assistant Professor of Medicine, University of Montreal Faculty of Medicine; Cardiologist, Montreal Heart Institute, Montreal, Quebec, Canada

J. MICHAEL LAZARUS, M.D.

Associate Professor of Medicine, Harvard Medical School; Physician and Director of Clinical Services, Nephrology Division, Brigham and Women's Hospital, Boston, Massachusetts

J. T. LIE, M.D.

Professor of Pathology, Mayo Medical School and Mayo Graduate School of Medicine; Consultant in Pathology and Cardiovascular Diseases, Mayo Clinic and Foundation, Rochester, Minnesota

THOMAS F. LÜSCHER, M.D.

Assistant Professor of Medicine, University of Basel; Consultant and Head, Division of Clinical Pharmacology, University Hospitals, Basel, Switzerland

ATTILIO MASERI, M.D., F.R.C.P., F.A.C.C.

Sir John McMichael Professor of Cardiovascular Medicine, University of London, Royal Postgraduate Medical School; Director of Cardiology, Hammersmith Hospital, London, England

IRENE MEISSNER, M.D.

Assistant Professor of Neurology, Mayo Medical School and Mayo Graduate School of Medicine; Staff Consultant in Neurology, Mayo Clinic and Mayo Foundation, Rochester, Minnesota

FRANZ H. MESSERLI, M.D., F.A.C.C., F.A.C.P.

Director, Hemodynamics Laboratory, Section of Hypertensive Disease, Ochsner Clinic; Professor of Medicine, Tulane School of Medicine, New Orleans, Louisiana

D. CRAIG MILLER, M.D.

Professor of Cardiovascular Surgery, Stanford University School of Medicine, Stanford, California

WAYNE L. MILLER, M.D., Ph.D.

Assistant Professor of Medicine, Mayo Graduate School of Medicine; Senior Associate Consultant, Division of Cardiovascular Diseases and Internal Medicine, Rochester, Minnesota

WILLIAM M. MOORE Jr., M.D.

Fellow in Vascular Surgery, Alton Ochsner Medical Foundation, New Orleans, Louisiana

DAVID NAIDE, M.D.

Associate Professor of Medicine, Cardiovascular Institute, Hahnemann University School of Medicine, Philadelphia, Pennsylvania

THOMAS C. NASLUND, M.D.

Fellow in Vascular Surgery, Ochsner Medical Center, New Orleans, Louisiana

JANE W. NEWBURGER, M.D., M.P.H.

Professor of Pediatrics, Harvard Medical School; Senior Associate, Department of Cardiology, Children's Hospital, Boston, Massachusetts

JEFFREY W. OLIN, D.O.

Head, Section of Atherosclerosis and Lipids, Department of Vascular Medicine, Cleveland Clinic Foundation, Cleveland, Ohio

MALCOLM O. PERRY, M.D.

The H. William Scott Jr., Professor of Surgery, Vanderbilt University School of Medicine, Nashville, Tennessee

JOSEPH F. POLAK, M.D.

Associate Professor of Radiology, Harvard Medical School; Director, Noninvasive Vascular Imaging, Brigham and Women's Hospital, Boston, Massachusetts

REED E. PYERITZ, M.D., Ph.D.

Professor of Medicine and Pediatrics, The Johns Hopkins University School of Medicine; Clinical Director, Center for Medical Genetics, The Johns Hopkins Hospital, Baltimore, Maryland

C. VENKATA S. RAM, M.D.

Professor of Internal Medicine, University of Texas Southwestern Medical Center; Director, Hypertension Clinics, Parkland Memorial Hospital and St. Paul Medical Center, Dallas, Texas

RICHARD N. RE, M.D.

Vice President and Director, Division of Research, Alton Ochsner Medical Foundation, New Orleans, Louisiana

JUDITH G. REGENSTEINER, Ph.D.

Assistant Professor of Medicine, Vascular Section, University of Colorado Health Sciences Center, Denver, Colorado

THOM W. ROOKE, M.D.

Assistant Professor of Medicine, Mayo Medical School; Stanley J. Sarnoff Fellow in Cardiovascular Research, Division of Cardiovascular Diseases, Mayo Clinic, Rochester, Minnesota

EUGENE ROSSITCH Jr., M.D.

Chief Resident, Neurosurgery, Duke University Medical Center, Durham, North Carolina

MOHAMED H. SAYEGH, M.D.

Instructor in Medicine, Harvard Medical School; Associate Physician, Renal Division, Department of Medicine, Brigham and Women's Hospital, Boston, Massachusetts

ANDREW I. SCHAFER, M.D.

Professor and Vice-Chairman, Department of Medicine, Baylor College of Medicine; Chief, Medical Service, Houston Veterans Affairs Medical Center, Houston, Texas

ALEXANDER SCHIRGER, M.D.

Professor of Medicine, Mayo Medical School, Hypertension, Cardiovascular Diseases, Internal Medicine, Rochester, Minnesota

GARY L. SCHWARTZ, M.D.

Assistant Professor of Medicine, Mayo Medical School, Rochester, Minnesota

ANDREW P. SELWYN, M.D.

Associate Professor of Medicine, Harvard Medical School; Physician, Brigham and Women's Hospital, Boston, Massachusetts

ROGER F. J. SHEPHERD, M.D.

Consultant in Cardiovascular Diseases, Mayo Clinic, Rochester, Minnesota

SHELDON G. SHEPS, M.D.

Professor of Medicine, Mayo Graduate School of Medicine; Divisions of Hypertension and Cardiovascular Diseases, Mayo Clinic, Rochester, Minnesota

YASUSHI F. SHIBUTANI, M.D.

Instructor of Urology, University of Pennsylvania School of Medicine, Philadelphia, Pennsylvania

ALAN SINGER, M.D.

Fellow, Division of Cardiovascular Medicine, Stanford University School of Medicine, Stanford, California

CAREN G. SOLOMON, M.D.

Fellow in Endocrinology, Brigham and Women's Hospital, Boston, Massachusetts

DILEK K. SOWERS, M.D., F.A.C.E.P.

Staff Physician, Emergency Room, Bon Secours Hospital, Grosse Pointe, Michigan

JAMES R. SOWERS, M.D.

Professor of Medicine, Wayne State University School of Medicine; Director, Division of Endocrinology, Metabolism and Hypertension, Department of Internal Medicine, Harper Hospital, Detroit, Michigan

PETER C. SPITTELL, M.D.

Senior Clinical Fellow, Cardiovascular Diseases, and Special Clinical Fellow, Vascular Medicine, Mayo Clinic, Rochester, Minnesota

EILEEN M. STUART, R.N., M.S., C.C.R.N.

Lecturer in Nursing, Boston College, and Senior Scientist, Mind/Body Institute, New England Deaconess Hospital, Harvard Medical School; Director, Cardiovascular Program, Division of Behavioral Medicine, New England Deaconess Hospital, Boston, Massachusetts

ROBERT P. SUNDEL, M.D.

Instructor in Pediatrics, Harvard Medical School; Director of Rheumatology, Children's Hospital, Boston, Massachusetts

JERRY W. SWANSON, M.D.

Assistant Professor of Neurology, Mayo Medical School; Consultant Neurologist, Mayo Clinic, Rochester, Minnesota

SASKIA R. J. THIADENS, R.N.

Director, Aurora Lymphedema Clinic, and President, National Lymphedema Network, San Francisco, California

JOSEPH UPTON, M.D.

Clinical Associate Professor of Surgery (Plastic Surgery), Harvard Medical School, Boston, Massachusetts

DAVID D. WATERS, M.D.

Director, Research Center, Montreal Heart Institute, Montreal, Quebec, Canada

ANTHONY D. WHITTEMORE, M.D.

Associate Professor of Surgery, Harvard Medical School; Chief, Division of Vascular Surgery, Brigham and Women's Hospital, Boston, Massachusetts

ALAN C. YEUNG, M.D.

Instructor in Medicine, Harvard Medical School; Associate Physician, Brigham and Women's Hospital, Boston, Massachusetts

MICHAEL B. ZEMEL, Ph.D.

Professor of Nutrition, Physiology and Medicine, and Head, Department of Nutrition, University of Tennessee School of Medicine, Knoxville, Tennessee

PAULA C. ZEMEL, Ph.D.

Assistant Professor of Nutrition and Public Health, University of Tennessee School of Medicine, Knoxville, Tennessee

A new field of medicine is evolving. Vascular medicine is beginning to take form as a small, but growing, cadre of internists develop special skills in the management of vascular diseases. What areas does this new field encompass? As defined by the National Institutes of Health, vascular medicine is that discipline which has as its objectives "the clinical characterization of all vascular diseases (arterial, venous, lymphatic, cerebral, coronary, aortic, renal, and peripheral), the pathogeneses of these diseases (including atherosclerosis, lipid metabolic disorders, systemic and pulmonary hypertension, lymphedema, thrombosis, vasculitis, and vasospastic disorders), as well as the diagnostic, therapeutic, and preventive approaches to these diseases."

Vascular diseases are the greatest causes of morbidity and mortality in this country. Coronary artery disease, cerebrovascular disease, and pulmonary embolism alone account for about one-third of the deaths annually in the United States. It is largely for this reason that the National Heart, Lung and Blood Institute (NHLBI) of the National Institutes of Health has funded two centers of vascular medicine in 1991 (at Stanford University Medical Center and at Harvard University's Brigham and Women's Hospital) and plans to fund more in the future, for the purpose of enhancing research, education, and clinical care in this important area of medical practice.

Hypertension affects a sizeable proportion of our population (one in five white and two in five black individuals). It is a major risk factor for premature atherosclerosis, and it accelerates development of coronary heart disease and myocardial infarction. In addition, it is a major predisposing factor for chronic renal failure, especially for end-stage renal disease in the patient with diabetes mellitus. In at least 90 percent of patients with hypertension, the elevated arterial pressure is related to changes in vascular reactivity or structure of the resistance vessels. Thus, because hypertension is a vascular disease in and of itself, and because it is so prevalent, the first two sections of this book are devoted to its treatment.

Despite the significance of vascular disease as a major health problem, none of the conventional areas of medical training has been devoted exclusively to its study. As a result, the care of these patients has been fragmented among many specialized areas of medicine. For example, the patient with intermittent claudication more than likely has significant coronary and/or carotid disease and may also have hypertension, hyperlipidemia, diabetes mellitus, or a history of tobacco use. Ideal management of these patients requires an integrated, multidisciplinary interaction among internists, radiologists, and surgeons with special expertise in vascular medicine. One of the goals of the NHLBI initiative is to forge such collaboration at centers for vascular medicine. This overall integrated approach surely will result in improved medical care of these patients. This multidisciplinary collaborative approach will also provide a rich educational environment for a new breed of internists who will receive comprehensive training in all aspects of vascular disease. Moreover, these programs will serve as national models of excellence for the ideal management of vascular disease. It is of particular significance at this time that such individuals with vascular medicine training and orientation of practice are now eligible for full Fellowship in the American College of Cardiology.

Further, multiple technological forces are driving the emergence of this new field. Advances in imaging technology are among these factors. Refinements in duplex ultrasonography and magnetic resonance imaging have advanced our ability to characterize diseases of blood vessels noninvasively. Tools with even greater precision, such as radiolabeled monoclonal antibodies, will permit visualization of atherosclerotic plaques and are under development. Advances in invasive imaging continue to make an important impact on the diagnosis and treatment of vascular diseases. Quantitative angiography has improved our ability to document reversal or regression of atherosclerotic plaque in response to new therapeutic strategies. It has also been of great utility in studies of vascular reactivity and in our understanding of how the endothelium modulates blood vessel tone. Angioscopy has provided new insights into the pathophysiology of ischemic syndromes. By directly visualizing the lumen of the coronary artery, investigators have shown that unstable angina is associated with fresh thrombus superimposed on an ulcerated lesion, whereas stable angina is induced by a hemodynamically significant, but stable, plaque. Intravascular ultrasonography, still in its infancy, has already extended our knowledge of post-transplant atherosclerosis, plaque morphology, and vascular injury after angioplasty.

Equally impressive has been the proliferation of new interventional techniques that enable innovative treatment of vascular disease. Catheter techniques such as balloon angioplasty, atherectomy, and vascular stenting are expanding what we can do for patients with a variety of arterial and venous diseases.

Pharmacologic agents for treatment of hypertension and hyperlipidemias continue to become more specific and effective, extending our ability to tailor medical treatment programs for individual patients while introducing a new element of complexity in management. Improved drug treatment of hyperlipidemias promises to retard atherosclerosis and even induce regression of occlusive lesions. Meanwhile, the focus of antihypertensive therapy has shifted from merely reducing arterial pressure to other ramifications of therapy in these patients. New antihypertensive compounds will be associated with fewer adverse metabolic side effects than encountered with earlier agents. These agents will prevent or modify the effects of hypertensive disease on target organs such as thickening of the vessel wall, reversing left ventricular hypertrophy, reducing left ventricular compliance, and even preventing end-stage renal disease.

Progress in antiplatelet, antithrombotic, and thrombolytic therapy has already altered our approach to arterial occlusive disease and venous thrombosis. A variety of antithrombotic agents and thrombolytic substances under development will soon be added to our therapeutic armamentarium, which will also include calcium channel antagonists and potassium channel agonists with greater vasoselectivity. On the more distant horizon, gene therapy provides great promise to revolutionize medicine, much as did the advent of antibiotics and anesthesia in the not-too-distant past. All manner of diseases may potentially be palliated or cured with gene therapy. In many cases recipient cells for the transcript will be the endothelium of the blood vessel, since these are the cells that have the greatest access to the luminal contents and comprise an enormous surface area.

The field of vascular medicine is also expanding as a result of the great strides being made in vascular biology. Over the last ten years, it has become apparent that the blood vessel is a complex organ that modulates its own tone, growth, and interaction with circulating blood elements. The endothelium and smooth muscle of the blood vessel wall synthesize and release a large number of vasoactive factors, modulators of blood fluidity, and local mediators of vessel growth. Disturbances of this system in pathophysiologic states are being elucidated at a frenetic pace. As these basic insights are applied to vascular medicine, the field will continue to expand, and the benefits to our patients will be immense.

This textbook has been conceived to bring the practicing clinician up to date on the latest concepts in the management of the hypertensive and vascular diseases. This is a rapidly changing field, so an effort has been made to concentrate on the practical application of new advances in vascular medicine. To this end, respected and expert clinicians from diverse fields impacting on vascular medicine bring their experience to bear on this rapidly developing field of cardiovascular medicine. In summary, this volume is produced in the spirit of the recent NHLBI initiative: to synthesize a multidisciplinary collaboration that will improve the overall care of the patient with highly complex problems long ignored in the traditional subspecialty textbooks.

John P. Cooke
Edward D. Frohlich

CONTENTS

CURRENT MANAGEMENT
OF HYPERTENSIVE
AND VASCULAR DISEASES

ESSENTIAL HYPERTENSION

NONPHARMACOLOGIC ADJUNCTS TO THERAPY

RICHARD FRIEDMAN, Ph.D.
EILEEN M. STUART, R.N., M.S., C.C.R.N.
HERBERT BENSON, M.D.

The purpose of this chapter is to present the rationale for nonpharmacologic treatment of hypertension, the practical issues concerning implementation, the actual techniques, and the comprehensive treatment program developed by the authors and their colleagues.

The efficacy of nonpharmacologic treatment of hypertension has been well established. Borderline hypertensive patients exposed to these interventions can exhibit reductions in blood pressure of sufficient magnitude to obviate the need for drugs. Medicated hypertensive patients who add nonpharmacologic treatments to their regimens can maximize blood pressure control on a minimum of antihypertensive drugs. Meta-analyses of the accumulated results have given a clear indication of therapeutic efficacy. There is endorsement from both the World Health Organization (WHO) and the Joint Committee for the Detection, Evaluation and Treatment of Hypertension for nonpharmacologic treatment. Furthermore, there is general consensus that nonpharmacologic therapies should be considered routinely in the treatment of mild hypertension and adjunctively in cases of moderate or severe hypertension. The advantages of such approaches are the reduction in adverse pharmacologic side effects as well as medication costs. The magnitude of blood pressure reductions varies widely according to the type of nonpharmacologic interventions applied and the characteristics of the treated population. Nonetheless, some summary statements may be made concerning the magnitude of the effects. Systolic blood pressure reductions of 10 to 15 mm Hg and diastolic blood pressure reductions of 6 to 10 mm Hg are typically observed in nonpharmacologic intervention programs. As many as 20 to 25 percent of patients with mild hypertension can become normotensive with nonpharmacologic interventions.

There are three emerging trends concerning the nonpharmacologic treatment of hypertension. First is the shift in emphasis away from the issue of efficacy toward that of practicality. Nonpharmacologic treatment has been shown to be effective, but questions regarding implementation require attention. The second trend relates to the profiling of patients before therapy. It is important to determine which nonpharmacologic approach is best for a particular patient. Definitive protocols have not yet been developed but can be addressed. The third trend is the shift in emphasis from reduction of the blood pressure value alone to the more comprehensive approach of cardiovascular risk factor reduction. The major clinical trials that emphasized blood pressure reduction in isolation from other risk factors did not demonstrate an accompanying decrease in overall cardiovascular mortality. Therefore, nonpharmacologic treatment programs for hypertension are evolving into comprehensive risk factor intervention programs. Of course, the primary reason for reducing blood pressure is to reduce cardiovascular risk. Nonpharmacologic treatment programs not only reduce this risk by lowering blood pressure, but also can reduce other cardiovascular risk factors at the same time.

IMPLEMENTATION

Most clinicians treating hypertension now consider nonpharmacologic treatments to be effective, but the practical issues regarding patient motivation, monitoring, and the engineering of behavioral change can appear formidable. A legitimate concern of many clinicians is whether such interventions can be successfully and practically accomplished. Many clinicians are not comfortable instituting and monitoring the behavioral changes required. Whereas most clinicians support, at least in theory, nonpharmacologic treatment of mild hypertension, particularly for patients whose diastolic pressures are between 90 and 94 mm Hg, very little time is usually spent counseling patients about the behavioral interventions required. The reasons for this are threefold. First, an overwhelming majority of physicians consider that their training did not adequately prepare them for counseling patients on how to bring about the important behavioral changes required. Consequently, the use of nonpharmacologic treatment approaches for hypertension may be more inhibited by physicians' discomfort with teaching behavioral change than by the ability of the interventions to bring about the desired goal. Second, most physicians report little confidence in the effectiveness of their recommendations for nondrug approaches to hypertension control. Third, most report that there is little time in an office visit to bring about behavioral change. To address these issues, physicians need to consider referring hypertensive patients for nonpharmacologic treatment to centers or practitioners who routinely engage in this type of endeavor and who can devote the time to approach this concept effectively.

It is also important for clinicians to recognize their bias toward the practicality of changing behavior. Adherence to nonpharmacologic intervention strategies is not uniform. Although adherence to both nonpharmacologic and pharmacologic regimens represents a challenge to the practitioner, this is hardly a reason to abandon either form of treatment.

Physicians need not become behavioral change experts to endorse the usefulness of nonpharmacologic therapy or to use these approaches in treating their patients. The first step for the physician is to endorse the value of nonpharmacologic therapy and of behavioral change. This can be a major issue because many physicians are still committed to aggressive pharmacotherapy. A second step involves the endorsement of the patient's participation in a program specifically designed to bring about the desired changes. The third step is a willingness to reinforce the changes once the program is completed when the patient returns for follow-up care.

These are very realistic goals for a physician to accomplish within the context of a brief office visit. It is not always practical or cost effective for physicians to establish programs within their office to bring about the behavioral change required for successful nonpharmacologic interventions. It is, however, crucial to motivate and refer patients appropriately.

Patients who are suitable candidates for nonpharmacologic intervention may be at a variety of stages regarding their readiness to change. It is imperative for the clinician to assess patients' readiness to change and to intervene in the most effective manner. Prochaska and DiClemente have described four stages of change: (1) precontemplation, (2) contemplation, (3) action, and (4) maintenance. It is important for the clinician to understand which stage the patient is in and then to prepare the patient to take action. A belief that multiple risk factor reduction is an effective treatment strategy, communicating to patients the belief that they can successfully change their adverse life style behaviors, referral to an effective clinical program, and support to maintain the changes are the crucial contributions of the practicing physician. However, some patients do not want to approach their medical problems from a nonpharmacologic behavioral perspective. Some cannot easily accept the rationale for reducing medical symptoms by behavioral strategies; others may see the cost in personal terms as outweighing the benefits. For a variety of reasons, patients may be unwilling or unmotivated to make the required behavioral changes. A referral to a Behavioral Medicine clinician may be appropriate in these circumstances.

INTERVENTIONS

There are some well-established, therapeutic interventions: weight reduction, sodium restriction, reduction of alcohol consumption, exercise, elicitation of the relaxation response and stress management, and smoking cessation. The procedures by which these nonpharmacologic interventions can be coordinated into an effective treatment program are described later.

A fundamental question concerning the use of nonpharmacologic treatment strategies for hypertension concerns therapeutic efficacy for any particular individual as opposed to the aggregate. The literature certainly indicates that these interventions work. Nonpharmacologic therapies can produce persistent, clinically significant reductions in blood pressure of the same magnitude as those resulting from drug therapy. Hence, the issue of clinical efficacy is not in question.

One remaining problem is the heterogeneity of response to nonpharmacologic interventions. An obvious example is that of weight reduction. An obese patient can significantly reduce blood pressure with weight loss, but a thin hypertensive patient is unlikely to benefit from this strategy. Owing to differences in underlying pathophysiologies, some hypertensive patients may be more or less likely to profit from exercise training, sodium restriction, or elicitation of the relaxation response. The diagnostic process and prescription of nonpharmacologic therapies lacks precise sensitivity and specificity. Although the presence or absence of relevant characteristics such as obesity and smoking is easily determined, other factors are less easily observed: e.g., sodium sensitivity and exercise conditioning. Therefore, careful attention needs to be paid to assessing the risk profile as specifically as possible and intervening in the most efficacious manner. As with any intervention strategy, each intervention should not be expected to be universally effective.

NONPHARMACOLOGIC INTERVENTION STRATEGIES

We recommend a comprehensive nonpharmacologic treatment program as being more effective than unidimensional interventions, for two reasons. First, we lack precise diagnostic methods; second, we believe that the interventions work synergistically. Each of the nonpharmacologic components of our program is described briefly before presentation of the comprehensive program.

Weight Reduction

Weight reduction for obese hypertensive patients should be the first treatment strategy for mild hypertension and a complementary strategy for all obese patients requiring drugs. Weight reduction intervention is recommended for patients who are more than 10 to 20 percent above ideal body weight. The specifics of the intervention do not differ greatly from those usually applied to obese patients. There is nutritional guidance and education concerning the caloric content and fat concentrations of food as well as the caloric requirements of the patient. Patients need to be told of the healthy eating choices available and to develop an increased awareness of behavioral dietary habits. This requires careful attention to monitoring food intake and behavioral habits on a consistent basis. Patients should learn that foods lower in calories also tend to be lower in saturated fat and sodium, thereby maximizing their cardiovascular benefits. It is important to impress on patients that dietary change requires dedication and commitment. Monitoring progress on a regular basis is necessary to achieve optimal adherence. Dietitians are important collaborators in achieving these ends.

Realistic expectations concerning weight loss are necessary. The short-term goal is weight loss of between 1 and 1.5 pounds each week. The long-term goal is to achieve and maintain body weight within 10 percent of the ideal.

Advice to "lose weight" or "cut back," no matter how well intentioned, is not likely to yield positive results. Most weight loss programs succeed in the short term but fail in the long run. Those programs that are based on behavior modification principles, and include exercise and psychological factors such as elicitation of the relaxation response and stress management, work better than approaches that do not include these components. In our experience, patients do best when referred to programs offering a comprehensive approach to weight loss as part of the overall risk profile. The referral process for this intervention and for all other nonpharmacologic therapy is a crucial aspect of treatment. Physicians should enthusiastically indicate that weight loss and the other changes result in reduced blood pressure and lowered cardiovascular risk, and should convey their belief that the patient can succeed. Long-term maintenance is enhanced with appropriate follow-up support.

Sodium Restriction

Although sodium restriction as a treatment for elevated blood pressure has been suggested for many years, its use is still controversial. Arguments concerning the appropriateness of sodium restriction involve consideration of the "sodium-sensitive" patient. If it were possible to establish easily which hypertensive patients were sodium sensitive and apply sodium restriction to these, there would be less argument over its use, but at this time there is no consensus on such a diagnostic methodology. Consequently, sodium restriction is usually appropriate for hypertensive patients, and unlikely to result in adverse side effects. Some specific populations are beginning to emerge. For example, elderly patients with isolated systolic hypertension exhibit sig-

nificant blood pressure reductions with sodium restriction. Therefore, sodium restriction is appropriate in this group.

Most agree that, for sodium restriction to be therapeutically effective, daily consumption needs to be reduced to or below 2,000 mg. Some patients find this difficult, although in our experience it is a realistic and attainable goal. To place this goal in perspective, 2,000 mg per day is ten times above the necessary metabolic requirements. However, the average American ingests between 8,000 and 9,000 mg of sodium per day. Therefore, to restrict oneself to 2,000 mg requires some physiologic and psychological adjustment. Sodium restriction pays dividends in a variety of ways. When patients become more aware of their sodium ingestion, they have a tendency to restrict their total caloric intake as well, thereby facilitating weight loss. They also tend to eat less prepared and "junk" food. A reduction in the consumption of saturated fats results in additional reduction of total cardiovascular risk.

Reduction of Alcohol Intake

Alcohol consumption is associated with elevated blood pressure, and its reduction is associated with reduced blood pressure. Most authorities advocate that alcohol consumption in hypertensive patients be reduced to less than 2 oz per day. When made aware of the relationship between alcohol and elevated blood pressure, most patients can make appropriate adjustments.

Exercise

Regular physical exercise at an appropriate frequency, intensity, type, and duration has a positive effect on overall cardiovascular risk profile. Therefore, an appropriate exercise plan should be instituted for hypertensive patients. A symptom-limited, graded exercise tolerance test should be performed before initiating an exercise prescription in sedentary patients who are over age 40 or have identified cardiac risk factors. Patients who express a desire for structure or support tend to do better exercising with group support. The exercise prescription need only be at a moderate work load; in fact, this is preferable. The target heart rate should be calculated at 60 to 70 percent of the actual maximal heart rate obtained on the exercise tolerance test. The prescription should be for aerobic exercise three to five times a week for 20 to 60 minutes in a moderate range. Twenty minutes is the minimal time to achieve an aerobic conditioning effect; the longer time contributes more to weight reduction and modification of other risk factors. Moderate exercise yields about the same blood pressure–lowering benefits as vigorous exercise. We focus our monitoring on ratings of perceived exertion—the Borg scale—rather than on target heart rate.

As is the case for sodium restriction, the institution of an exercise program for the treatment of hypertension has multiple benefits. Individuals who begin regular exercise have a tendency to lose weight, and consequently other cardiovascular risk factors are reduced. Another important asset is that a regular exercise program can result in a reduction of psychological stress. Regular exercise can reduce negative psychological symptomatology, thereby setting the stage for more effective behavioral change.

Relaxation Response and Stress Management

There have been no definitive clinical investigations establishing that stress or increased sympathetic tone causes hypertension. Nonetheless, there is ample evidence that reducing stress and eliciting the relaxation response has a salubrious effect on blood pressure and other cardiovascular risk factors. In our experience, regular elicitation of the relaxation response and stress management are important aspects of nonpharmacologic intervention. We believe these approaches to be less well understood, and therefore less used, than the other nonpharmacologic approaches. Therefore, the rationale for their use will be described in more detail than that for the other interventions.

The relaxation response is an integrated physiologic response that is opposite to the fight-or-flight response. Acute elicitation of the relaxation response is characterized by decreased oxygen consumption, heart rate, blood pressure, respiratory rate, minute ventilation, and arterial blood lactate. There is an increase in slower brain wave activity. Its regular elicitation results in sustained blood pressure reduction. The most likely explanation for the effects observed are reduced responsiveness to plasma norepinephrine.

Numerous reports in the literature support the antihypertensive efficacy of elicitation of the relaxation response, but the evidence for its long-term effects in lowering blood pressure is less clear-cut. The specific indications for prescribing the intervention are also not clear. Several recent reports suggest that patients with high levels of adrenergic drive or of anger or anxiety may profit more from elicitation of the relaxation response than patients with lower levels of these. As more sensitive assessment tools are being evaluated, we have found that most patients can benefit from this intervention without adverse side effects.

There are many techniques to elicit the physiology of the relaxation response, including progressive muscle relaxation, meditation, autogenic training, yoga, and biofeedback. Two components are needed to elicit the response: mental focusing on a repetitive word, phrase, sound, prayer, or image; and the adoption of a passive attitude to intrusive thoughts. Patients are instructed to elicit the relaxation response by using a technique comfortable to them, and to do so once or twice daily for 20 minutes.

If the rationale for use of the relaxation response is presented appropriately, it can be accomplished by most patients and is an effective intervention in lowering blood pressure. Not only does the relaxation response reduce blood pressure in many hypertensive patients, but it also has a positive psychological effect on most of them. This latter effect, in our opinion, is important for the success of nonpharmacologic therapy.

All humans experience stress. For some, even mild stress is associated with elevations in blood pressure. The distinguishing characteristic between those who have hypertension and those who do not is not necessarily that hypertensive patients have more stress in their lives or handle their stress differently from normotensive patients. Rather, in patients predisposed to hypertension, stress may be associated with increased physiologic arousal and subsequently increased blood pressure. Hence, the need to learn stress management skills becomes important.

Asking patients to make the other life style changes such as dietary restrictions, exercise programs, and smoking cessation is likely to result in stress. Daily elicitation of the relaxation response can reduce stress and set the stage for more effective behavioral change. We emphasize to patients that including relaxation response training as part of their nonpharmacologic treatment does not necessarily imply that stress was a causative factor in hypertension. For some patients, this etiologic relationship is appropriate, but the rationale for elicitation of the relaxation response does not hinge only on its stress-alleviating effects. The relaxation response decreases responsivity to plasma norepinephrine and also reduces anxiety, which in turn facilitates behavioral change, because anxiety can impede learning.

Many patients observe that stress is a major issue in their blood pressure elevations and contributes to other detrimental life style behaviors such as smoking, overeating, and lack of exercise. For these, stress management is an integral part of treatment. For other patients, the suggestion that stress may play some role in their blood pressure elevations is not appropriate or may be seen as threatening. In this case, the elicitation of the relaxation response and stress reduction may be seen as facilitating other behavioral change such as cessation of smoking or weight reduction. If the rationale for elicitation of the relaxation response and stress management training is presented in a practical, nonthreatening manner, the vast majority of hypertensive patients accept the usefulness of these measures and respond positively.

Home monitoring of blood pressure is another stress management strategy that tends to desensitize patients to blood pressure measurement and enhances feelings of self-control.

Tobacco

There have been no definitive investigations establishing that cigarette smoking causes hypertension. Nonetheless, there is ample evidence that cessation of smoking is associated with a reduction in cardiovascular risk. The cardiovascular risks associated with hypertension coupled with smoking are high. An individual with hypertension who smokes has an increased risk of myocardial infarction and stroke three to five times greater than that of a hypertensive patient who does not smoke. Consequently, it is crucial to impress on hypertensive patients the necessity of stopping smoking. The direct relationship between smoking and blood pressure in this case becomes less important than the relationship among multiple cardiovascular risk factors.

The need to engineer smoking cessation as part of a nonpharmacologic treatment program in hypertension highlights the need to consider patients from a multidimensional perspective. In addition to smoking being one of several risk factors, the behaviors associated with risk factors are interrelated. Smoking cessation approaches for hypertensive patients are no different from those in other similar programs. Exhortation on the part of physicians is often unsuccessful. Again, as is the case for weight loss, referral to a multifactorial, nonpharmacologic treatment program or a smoking cessation program may be useful.

Other Dietary Considerations

Recently it has been suggested that the addition of potassium, calcium, and magnesium to the diet of hypertensive patients might be beneficial. These strategies are not yet considered routine parts of nonpharmacologic treatment and are recommended only when specific deficits are identified. An additional dietary concern is the specific issue of restriction of saturated fat in the diet to lower cholesterol. Since the primary reason for reducing blood pressure is to reduce cardiovascular risk, a reduction in saturated fat, although not directly associated with a reduction in blood pressure, is an important component of nonpharmacologic treatment. The synergistic effects of hypertension and high cholesterol are significant. In our program, the goal is to reduce cholesterol to less than 200 mg per deciliter, to reduce low-density lipoprotein (LDL) to less than 140 mg per deciliter, to increase high-density lipoprotein (HDL) to greater than 40 mg per deciliter, and to reduce the total cholesterol-to-HDL ratio in females to less than 3.5 and in males to less than 4.5.

"White-Coat" Hypertension

Another perspective on nonpharmacologic treatment approaches concerns the "white-coat" effect. For some patients, the situation-specific stimuli associated with clinical blood pressure measurements are anxiety-inducing and stressful, thus producing artificially high measurements. This in turn can lead to a misdiagnosis of hypertension and unnecessary treatment. As many as 20% of mild essential hypertensives may be misclassified owing to this effect. The stimuli associated with the measurement procedures cannot easily be eliminated, but repeated measurements over time is the standard strategy used to eliminate these anxiety-induced effects. Also, ambulatory monitoring is one strategy that can often be used to circumvent the "white-coat" effect. Furthermore, physician referral for treatment to behavioral specialists is an option. In this case, the nonpharmacologic treatment is more focused on the relaxation response and desensitization to the measurement procedure itself, and special attention can be given to the home blood pressure readings obtained by the patient.

MULTIFACTORIAL NONPHARMACOLOGIC TREATMENT PROGRAM

Throughout this chapter, we have indicated the usefulness of nonpharmacologic antihypertensive therapy in a specialized group format. The 13-session program developed by the authors and their colleagues at the New England Deaconess Hospital incorporates the components described above and is outlined in the Appendix to this chapter.

RECOMMENDATIONS

In our experience, it is both practical and effective to approach nonpharmacologic treatment of high blood pressure as part of a comprehensive strategy to reduce the overall cardiovascular risk profile. This goal is best accomplished when approached in collaboration with the practicing physician who can identify patients at risk, refer them for treatment, engender the expectancy that they can succeed in the difficult process of changing behavior, and provide ongoing monitoring and support to maintain behavioral change and prevent relapse.

Acknowledgment. Supported by grant HL 22727 from the Public Health Service, a grant from the American Heart Association, Suffolk County, N.Y. Affiliate, and the Fetzer Institute. The authors thank Vivian Stabiner, Nancy McKinnon, and Sarah Reiff for their help in the preparation of this chapter.

SUGGESTED READINGS

Caudill M, Friedman R, Benson H. Relaxation therapy in the control of blood pressure. In: Blaufox MD, Langford H, eds. Nonpharmacologic therapy of hypertension. Bibl Cardiol 1987; 41: 106–119.

Kaplan NM. Clinical hypertension 5th ed. Treatment of hypertension: non-drug therapy. Baltimore: Williams & Wilkins; 1990:163–181.

The 1988 report of the joint national committee on detection, evaluation and treatment of high blood pressure. U.S. Department of Health and Human Services. Arch Intern Med 1988; 148: 1023–1038.

THE NEW ENGLAND DEACONESS HOSPITAL
COORDINATED NONPHARMACOLOGIC PROGRAM

Each session is held weekly and lasts 2 hours. Between 10 and 15 patients are treated in each group. Each 2-hour session follows the following format: 15 minutes of mutual data collection, 30 minutes of supervised exercise, 15 minutes of elicitation of the relaxation response, and 60 minutes of lecture/discussion.

Preprogram screening

Rule out secondary causes of hypertension and perform a baseline physical examination. Establish motivation for attending and readiness to change, and set mutual goals.

Session 1
Knowledge
Skills

- Pathophysiology of hypertension
- Instruction in diaphragmatic breathing

Session 2
Knowledge
Skills

- Physiology of the relaxation response (RR)
- Self-monitoring of blood pressure (BP)
- Diaphragmatic breathing

Session 3
Knowledge
Skills

- Instruction in low-sodium and weight-reducing diet
- Self-monitoring of BP, daily elicitation of the RR
- Three-day food record to calculate sodium content and calories in diet

Session 4
Knowledge
Skills

- Instruction in low-cholesterol diet
- Daily: self-monitor BP, elicit the RR, and follow 2,000-mg sodium diet and recommended calories
- Three-day food record to calculate cholesterol content in food and behaviors associated with eating

Session 5
Knowledge
Skills

- Cardiovascular benefits of exercise
- Daily: self-monitor BP; elicit the RR; and follow recommended sodium, calorie, and cholesterol diet

Session 6
Knowledge

Skills

- Individualize prescriptions for RR practice, exercise, and diet and a review of medical progress to date
- Daily: self-monitor BP; elicit the RR; and follow recommended sodium, calorie, and cholesterol diet
- Exercise within prescribed intensity 20 minutes three to five times per week

The above skills are practiced daily and continue to be monitored for the remainder of the program. For the sake of brevity they will not be repeated under skills for sessions 7 through 13.

Session 7
Knowledge
Skills

- Behavior change theory
- As in Session 6, but also identify past pattern of successful and unsuccessful behavior change
- Establish goals and make a plan to accomplish these goals

Session 8
Knowledge
Skills

- Stress pathophysiology and stress buffers
- As in Session 6, but also identify physiologic response to stress
- Begin to *stop* and *take a breath* when encountering a stressor

Session 9
Knowledge
Skills

- Benefits of Hatha Yoga in eliciting the RR
- As in Session 6, but also practice in Hatha Yoga with emphasis on mindfulness of physical body and mental quieting
- Recognize that emotions can influence the body and the effect of positive emotions on health
- Practice positive affirmations each day

Session 10
Knowledge
Skills

- Cognitive restructuring theory and automatic thoughts
- As in Session 6, but also *stop; take a breath;* and *reflect* on those automatic, unconscious, fleeting thoughts that influence behavior

Session 11
Knowledge

Skills

- Cognitive restructuring theory
- Beliefs, attitudes, and assumptions that cause difficulty
- As in Session 6, but also *stop; take a breath;* and *reflect* on the beliefs, attitudes, and assumptions that underlie automatic thoughts and response to stress

Session 12
Knowledge
Skills

- Cognitive restructuring theory and alternative coping styles
- As in Session 6, but also *stop; take a breath;* and *reflect* on the beliefs, attitudes, and assumptions that underlie automatic thoughts and influence responses to stress, and choose how to respond (cope)

Session 13
Knowledge
Skills

- Creative thinking
- As in Session 6, but also *stop, take a breath, reflect,* and *choose* how to respond based on a wide range of *possibilities*

Attitudes

Throughout the 13 sessions the knowledge-based content and skills are designed to engender attitudes of mindfulness, openness, flexibility, positivity, and self-appreciation. As described by Kobassa, patients begin to view new experiences as a challenge rather than a threat, with a sense of control rather than helplessness, and with a feeling of commitment rather than alienation.

Postprogram interview

- Review progress in the program
- Set goals for maintaining progress and continued growth and health
- In patients with mild hypertension, these nonpharmacologic approaches should be applied 3 to 6 months before drug therapy is instituted.
- In patients already on antihypertensive pharmacologic agents, no adjustments should be made for the first 4 to 5 weeks unless the patient is symptomatic. At 4 to 5 weeks when the behavioral changes have started to become part of the patient's life style, gradual decrements in medication can begin.
- The decision to decrease medication should take into account home as well as office blood pressure recordings and behavioral change.

INITIAL PHARMACOLOGIC THERAPY

EDWARD D. FROHLICH, M.D., F.A.C.C.

Prospective clinical trials have demonstrated the efficacy, safety, and feasibility of antihypertensive therapy not only by maintaining reduction and control of arterial pressure but by preventing and reversing many of the complications of hypertensive cardiovascular disease. Initially, these studies demonstrated reduction of the uniformly dismal mortality rate of malignant hypertension. Subsequently, antihypertensive therapy was shown to be efficacious in patients with elevated diastolic pressure first above 129 mm Hg, then 115 to 129 mm Hg, then 105 to 114 mm Hg, and still more recently in excess of 90 mm Hg. However, at present doubt remains in the minds of some authorities as to whether a subset of patients with mild hypertension (i.e., 90 to 94 mm Hg) should be treated with drugs or whether only nonpharmacologic modes of treatment might be more effective.

It was through these prospective clinical trials that a formalized schema for the treatment of hypertension was initially developed. This therapeutic algorithm, the "stepped care" approach, recommended the introduction of a single pharmacologic agent; if arterial pressures were not controlled with that first-step therapeutic choice (i.e., a thiazide-related diuretic), a second antihypertensive agent (i.e., an adrenergic inhibitor) would be added. Similarly, if pressure still remained uncontrolled with the foregoing two agents, a third, and if necessary a fourth agent would be added (Fig. 1).

This stepped-care approach was rational in its formulation, sound physiologically, and pragmatic in its use. It was rational for several reasons. First, most patients with hypertension demonstrated at least some reduction in pressure with the thiazide. Second, with coexistent dietary sodium restriction, over 60 to 70 percent of patients with mild to moderate hypertension would be afforded control of diastolic pressure (< 90 mm Hg). Third, the earlier studies had clearly demonstrated a potentiating and synergistic effect of the thiazides when used with other antihypertensive agents, thereby enhancing their effectiveness and permitting the use of lower doses of other agents (including the thiazides themselves), thereby diminishing their adverse effects. Finally, arterial pressure reduction with the other drugs (e.g., the earlier adrenergic inhibiting compounds and direct-acting vascular smooth muscle vasodilators) was associated with fluid retention. This intravascular volume expansion could be prevented by the diuretic, thereby permitting the use of lower doses of the other agents (preventing this "pseudotolerance" phenomenon). More recently, this effect has not been experienced with the newer agents, allowing for their use as "first-step" agents.

Alternative Agents for Initial Therapy. As indicated, recent clinical experience has taught us that certain new classes of antihypertensive drugs may produce a prolonged reduction and control of arterial pressure without associated volume expansion. Thus, the exclusive use of a diuretic as a first-step agent is no longer necessary today. In this respect, beta-adrenergic receptor blocking drugs, other adrenergic inhibiting compounds, angiotensin converting enzyme (ACE) inhibitors, and the calcium antagonists all are effective in controlling arterial pressure over prolonged periods without the need for previous or concomitant use of a diuretic. However, if any one class of antihypertensive agents fails to control arterial pressure, another agent from a different class of drugs may be substituted or added to the first selection. Thus, the question is not whether stepped care is empirical and outmoded. The concept remains sound and still obtains results in good medical practice: it has evolved as do all dynamic thinking and processes. Therefore, the question is not whether we employ stepped care, but, more reasonably, what should the initial step of therapy be?

FIRST-STEP OPTIONS

It goes without saying that a sound basis of treatment for all patients with hypertension is a practical implementation of nonpharmacologic therapeutic modalities (see the chapter *Nonpharmacologic Adjuncts to Therapy*). These include reduction of body weight to levels as close to the "ideal" as is possible (less than 115 percent of ideal body weight), restriction of daily dietary sodium intake to less than 100 mmol (approximately 2 to 3 g of sodium or approximately 5 g of salt), avoidance of all tobacco products, and moderation in the use of alcohol (to less than 1 oz of distilled spirits or their equivalent daily). In addition, dietary restriction of foods high in cholesterol and animal fats and a prudent exercise program are excellent health measures.

Currently, there are six classes of antihypertensive drugs that may be considered among the therapeutic options for selection as a first step of therapy: diuretics, beta-adrenergic receptor blocking drugs, peripherally acting adrenergic blocking drugs, centrally acting adrenergic inhibiting compounds, ACE inhibitors, and calcium antagonists. The direct-acting vascular smooth muscle relaxants (e.g., hydralazine, minoxidil) are not reasonable options for initial therapy because of their high incidence of pseudotolerance or intravascular volume expansion. Other possibilities for initial therapy in the future might include dopaminergic compounds, serotonin inhibitors, prostaglandin-related drugs, renin inhibitors, angiotensin II receptor antagonists, potassium channel agonists, agents that augment the biologic life of the atrial natriuretic peptide, and others.

It should be apparent from the following discussion that some classes of agents may come closer than others to what would be considered the ideal antihypertensive agent for initial therapy (Table 1). It seems equally

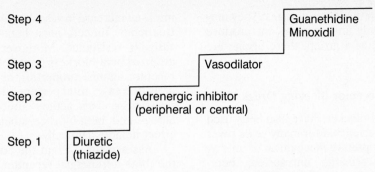

Figure 1 Original concept of stepped care treatment of hypertension.

Table 1 Characteristics of an Ideal Antihypertensive Agent for Initial Therapy

1. Efficacious as monotherapy
2. Well tolerated (i.e., low incidence of side effects)
3. Convenient (i.e., one daily administration)
4. Dosage easy to titrate
5. Augments action of other antihypertensive agents
6. Low incidence of pseudotolerance
7. Inexpensive
8. Controls pressure in a clinically identifiable segment of the hypertensive population

obvious that if a compound is selected for initial therapy, it should be efficacious in controlling pressure as a monotherapeutic agent. It should control arterial pressure in a significant number of patients with hypertension who can be identified by their clinical and laboratory characteristics. The drug selected should be well tolerated, with a low incidence of side effects. It would be most convenient if the medication could be administered only once daily; also, if the dosage needs to be increased to provide better control of pressure, dose titration should be easy without producing unwanted symptoms and side effects. Moreover, if the agent is inadequate to control pressure, it should also be able to augment the antihypertensive action of added agents without producing pseudotolerance (i.e., expansion of intravascular volume). Finally, the ideal agent should be relatively inexpensive.

The following discussion concerns the characteristics of each group of antihypertensive agents, with an assessment of that class of compounds as an ideal first-step option.

Diuretics

Rationale. The justification of diuretic agents and their track record over 30 years are well established. These agents reduce pressure by contracting extracellular fluid volume, presumably through their natriuretic effect, but this action alone does not fully explain their antihypertensive action. Initially, they reduce cardiac output, but as intravascular volume and cardiac output return toward pretreatment levels, total peripheral resistance falls. They also attenuate the pressor effects of endogenous circulating pressor substances, alter neural function, and induce naturally occurring vasodilator systems.

It could be reasoned that as monotherapeutic agents these drugs would be of greatest value in patients whose hypertension is more volume dependent. Indeed, patients with a variety of forms of essential hypertension have been shown to be relatively more volume dependent: blacks, women, the elderly, and patients with suppressed plasma renin activity. Furthermore, patients with certain secondary forms of hypertension may be more responsive to diuretics: women receiving oral contraceptives, patients with steroidal hypertension (including primary aldosteronism), and patients with renal parenchymal disease (even if their renal excretory function is normal).

Most of these patients respond to hydrochlorothiazide (or equivalent diuretic congeners) in doses of 12.5 to 50 mg once daily. Occasionally, it may be necessary to increase the dose to 100 mg. To protect against hypokalemia, it is wise to control dietary sodium intake, to use potassium supplements, or to add potassium-retaining agents (e.g., spironolactone, triamterene, or amiloride). Other metabolic side effects include hyperuricemia, hyperglycemia, hypercholesterolemia, and a slight rise in serum creatinine levels.

In some patients with renal parenchymal disease in whom renal function is significantly impaired, an agent that acts at the loop of Henle is indicated and more effective than a thiazide. In contrast to the thiazides, these "loop" agents demonstrate a linear dose-response relationship, and as long as there are functioning nephrons to respond to them, a response may be expected. Patients with volume-dependent secondary forms of hypertension may respond better to agents that specifically inhibit the mechanism responsible for the hypertension. For example, spironolactone may be more reasonable and appropriate for the patient with primary aldosteronism.

Assessment. It is apparent, then, that the thiazide class of diuretics (including their congeners) provides as close to an ideal type of first-step agents as we have. They have stood the test of time as effective monotherapy for a large percentage of the hypertensive population, and they are well tolerated with a relatively low incidence of side effects, particularly in the lower dosages. They may be administered once daily and they do not produce pseudotolerance. Finally, as a group, these agents are inexpensive.

Beta-Adrenergic Receptor Blocking Drugs

Rationale. The beta-blockers have also been used for initial therapy for hypertension for many years (over 25 years). Although their precise mechanism of antihypertensive action still remains unresolved, beta-adrenergic receptor inhibition not only inhibits adrenergically mediated functions, but also suppresses the renal release of renin and participation of the renin-angiotensin system.

Patients who respond better to beta-adrenergic receptor blocking drugs generally are younger, white, and male, with a hyperdynamic circulation or higher plasma renin activity. Clinically, these patients may also demonstrate greater lability of arterial pressure, a faster heart rate, increased force of cardiac contraction, and postural hypertension and may present symptoms of cardiac awareness. The beta-adrenergic receptor blocking drugs have also been found to be effective in other diseases and have been used for long-term treatment of patients with previous myocardial infarction, angina pectoris, cardiac dysrhythmias, migraine headaches, and even glaucoma (for the latter, in the form of eyedrops). Therefore, if these diseases coexist in a patient with hypertension, the beta-blocking drugs may obviate the need for a second antihypertensive agent. Clearly, it is a more rational and feasible approach to administer one agent than two or more. This simplicity of therapy favors overall adherence to a treatment program, is more cost effective, and lessens the risks of side effects and problems related to drug-drug interactions.

A variety of beta-blocking drugs are available for clinical use (acebutolol, atenolol, metoprolol, nadolol, pindolol, propranolol, and timolol). Others with more innovative actions may be released shortly. Each may be associated with its own side effects, and no one agent is identical to the others. It therefore seems reasonable that if, for example, maximal dosages of a lipid-soluble agent achieve suboptimal control of pressure, switching to a more water-soluble agent may provide adequate control without the need to discontinue the entire therapeutic class. Why some patients develop side effects with one beta-blocker but not with another is not known, but this clinical reality should be kept in mind. These agents are contraindicated in patients with a history of asthma, chronic obstructive lung disease, heart block, or cardiac failure, and relatively contraindicated in patients with a history of depression, insulin-dependent diabetes mellitus (IDDM), peripheral arterial insufficiency, or hyperlipidemia. The beta-blockers all reduce arterial pressure associated with a decline in cardiac output and heart rate (although those compounds with intrinsic sympathomimetic activity reduce these cardiac actions less); consequently, calculated total peripheral resistance increases. This, however, does not imply an increase in vascular resistance in all organs with treatment. Indeed, most beta-blockers decrease renal vascular resistance. Moreover, a recently introduced group of beta-blockers (e.g., celiprolol) possesses beta$_2$-receptor agonist properties, and consequently immediately decreases total peripheral as well as organ vascular resistances. This action, although different from the alpha- and beta-blocker labetalol, has the same net effect hemodynamically.

Assessment. From the above, it also appears that the beta-adrenergic receptor blocking drugs closely approach the ideal for a first-step agent. The hypertensive population who are likely to respond to this form of therapy may be predicted with some degree of clinical confidence, particularly when one excludes patients in whom these drugs are contraindicated. Excluding such patients, these agents can usually be administered once daily with a low incidence of side effects and with easy dose titration. Their action will be augmented by a diuretic, and pseudotolerance has not been a major problem, particularly in individuals with mild to moderately severe hypertension. Although these drugs may cost more than the diuretics, this may be offset by the lack of need for potassium-retaining, uricosuric, or hypoglycemic agents (e.g., with diuretics).

Peripherally Acting Adrenergic Inhibiting Agents

Rationale. These drugs reduce arterial pressure through a variety of mechanisms that suppress adrenergic stimulation of vascular smooth muscle. Ganglionic blocking agents have all but disappeared from clinical use, although trimethaphan (an intravenously administered agent) is still occasionally used in certain hypertensive emergencies. Reserpine is still available and acts by depleting the neurohumoral transmitter norepinephrine from the postganglionic nerve ending. It also depletes catecholamines and serotonin from neurons in the central nervous system, which explains its side effect of depression. Guanethidine, another agent that has been available for many years, also depletes catecholamines from the postganglionic nerve ending but has no effect on the central nervous system neurons. Its use has generally been reserved for patients with more severe hypertension, with relatively few side effects. Probably because of this, another agent very similar to guanethidine (guanadrel) has been introduced for use in patients with hypertension of mild to moderate severity.

Another subgroup of the peripherally acting adrenergic agents inhibits the postsynaptic alpha$_1$-adrenergic receptor sites on vascular smooth muscle membranes, thereby reducing vascular resistance. Not infrequently, after the first dose of these agents, the patient may develop symptomatic orthostatic hypotension, which may occasionally persist. Nevertheless, some physicians have used these compounds (e.g., prazosin, terazosin, indoramin) as their initial step, particularly in younger patients with hypertension and a history of depression, asthma, chronic lung disease, hyperlipidemia, and IDDM. Urapidil is another compound that, in addition to having this peripheral postsynaptic alpha$_1$-adrenergic receptor inhibiting effect, also stimulates central postsynaptic adrenoreceptors, thereby providing a dual action in reducing pressure.

Assessment. Although some of these agents (e.g., prazosin) have been prescribed as initial therapy, they may require the addition of a diuretic to prevent pseudotolerance. This may also serve to provoke orthostatic hypotension. The dose range of reserpine is rather narrow, and increased doses could provoke side effects (e.g., nasal stuffiness, depression). These agents cost more than hydrochlorothiazide or propranolol but are relatively inexpensive.

Centrally Acting Adrenergic Inhibitors

Rationale. These drugs lower arterial pressure by stimulating specific postsynaptic alpha-receptor sites in specific nuclei of the brain (e.g., nucleus tractus solitarii). They diminish adrenergic outflow from the brain directed toward the cardiovascular and renal systems. Compounds such as clonidine and guanabenz stimulate these alpha-receptors directly, but methyldopa must be converted intraneuronally to its metabolite, alpha-methyl-norepinephrine, which in turn exerts the central alpha-adrenergic agonistic effect.

They all reduce arterial pressure through a fall in total peripheral resistance without decreasing cardiac output or blood flow to the vital organs. For these reasons, these compounds may be administered as a first option of therapy in older patients, individuals with impaired renal function, and patients in whom other forms of treatment may be contraindicated. However, in some patients the prolonged reduction of arterial pressure may be associated with an expanded intravascular volume, thereby requiring the addition of small doses of a diuretic agent. Finally, the prototype of an agent that rapidly reduces cardiac mass is methyldopa. However, studies have not yet shown that reduction of cardiac mass with pharmacologic agents also reduces the inherent risk associated with left ventricular hypertrophy.

Assessment. These compounds have usually been employed as second-step agents because an associated expansion of intravascular volume and pseudotolerance may occur with prolonged use. In recent years, reports have demonstrated their efficacy in once-daily dosing in selected populations (e.g., elderly patients) with good control of pressure. Although these agents cost more than diuretics, they are relatively inexpensive. However, their side effect profile may be greater than that of diuretics or beta-blockers.

Angiotensin Converting Enzyme Inhibitors

Rationale. This class of antihypertensive drugs acts by inhibiting the ACE (an aminopeptidase) that cleaves the terminal two peptides from the decapeptide angiotensin I and forms the vasoactive octapeptide angiotensin II. These agents are particularly effective in patients whose hypertension is dependent on angiotensin II (e.g., essential hypertensive patients with cardiac failure or with a high plasma renin activity, and patients with renal arterial disease) who have been unresponsive to other forms of therapy. Since their initial introduction, these drugs have also been shown to be effective in patients with mild to moderately severe hypertension, those with normal or low plasma renin activity, and anephric patients. The mechanism in this latter and larger group of patients is most likely related to the presence of tissue renin-angiotensin systems in vascular and myocardial muscle cells.

A small initial dose of the agent, followed by observation for a few hours in the office, will provide insight into the effectiveness of the drug. If necessary, the antihypertensive action can be enhanced by addition of a diuretic agent. At present several ACE inhibitors are available (e.g., captopril, enalapril, lisinopril), and many more are in clinical trials. They may produce proteinuria and leukopenia, and frequent laboratory studies should be obtained during the first 3 months of therapy to alert the clinician and patient to their existence (particularly in patients with renal disease or those receiving immunosuppressive therapy). Less severe side effects include rash, ageusia, and a chronic cough; these are reversible by withdrawal of therapy.

Assessment. Good control of arterial pressure with the ACE inhibitors is usually experienced. There seems to be a very low incidence of side effects with these compounds. Pseudotolerance has not been a problem, and further control of pressure can be expected with the addition of a diuretic. These agents are more expensive than hydrochlorothiazide or propranolol, but the lack of metabolic side effects offsets the additional cost.

Calcium Antagonists

Rationale. Calcium antagonists have also been used to treat hypertension for many years. They lower arterial pressure through a vasodilating mechanism of inhibiting the entry of calcium ions into vascular smooth muscle, thereby reducing total peripheral and organ vascular resistances. Some of these agents (e.g., diltiazem, nitrendipine) increase renal blood flow without increasing glomerular filtration rate. This action is similar to that of the ACE inhibitors, through preferential dilatation of the afferent glomerular arteriole. These compounds have also been used for angina pectoris and coronary artery spasm, and therefore may be used to reduce arterial pressure in hypertensive patients with coronary arterial insufficiency who may have demonstrated suboptimal control of pressure with a beta-adrenergic receptor blocking drug. Moreover, they may be of particular value for older patients with coronary artery disease who may have diabetes mellitus and impaired sexual function associated with other antihypertensive therapy.

Several calcium antagonists are currently available. Verapamil has an action both to dilate vessels and to

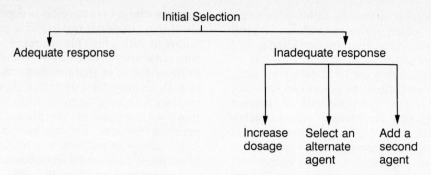

Figure 2 Algorithm for the stepped care approach to treatment of hypertension.

slow cardiac rate; the latter action is not shared with nifedipine. Nifedipine reduces arterial pressure and induces a reflex stimulation of heart rate, particularly in its capsule formulation; this side effect occurs less frequently in its long-acting formulation. Diltiazem possesses both effects, although there is a lesser cardiac slowing than with verapamil. Nicardipine and isradipine are also available, and many other compounds are available in other countries or are on trial.

Assessment. These drugs appear to be fairly well tolerated and there is a low incidence of side effects. Their dosage may be increased easily without side effects, and they may be prescribed as monotherapeutic agents with a low incidence of pseudotolerance, possibly because they have an intrinsic natriuretic effect. Some of these compounds must be given more than once daily, although others have a sustained action for once-daily administration. However, this may still require divided dosing in some patients. Although they cost more than the thiazides, this may be offset by the fact that they do not require additional therapy for metabolic side effects.

THE SECOND STEP

If, after selection of one of the above options for the initial therapy, optimal pressure control is not achieved, it is reasonable to add a second agent. This may permit the use of lower doses of the first agent. It may even be wise to withdraw the first agent in favor of the second, once pressure is controlled (Fig. 2). For example, this might be elected if a beta-adrenergic receptor blocking drug had been added to the initial choice of a diuretic. Alternatively, a diuretic may be safely added in lower doses to any of the other options for initial therapy.

THE THIRD STEP

If neither of the first two agents selected is effective in optimally controlling arterial pressure, any one of the vasodilators, adrenergic inhibitors, ACE inhibitors, or calcium antagonists can be added to either or both of the first two choices. For example, hydralazine, a vasodilator, may be added to the diuretic and beta-blocking drug. Alternatively, the beta-blocker can be discontinued, and methyldopa or captopril may be added. However, more potent agents, including minoxidil or guanethidine, may be substituted for hydralazine or another adrenergic inhibitor, respectively. However, most patients with hypertension (85 to 95 percent) achieve control of pressure with just two agents; patients with hypertension refractory to therapy should be evaluated for secondary forms of hypertension (see the chapters *Renovascular Hypertension, Endocrine Hypertension,* and *Renal Parenchymal Disease and Hypertension*).

REMARKS

A vast array of antihypertensive drugs is available for the initial step in the treatment of patients with hypertension. Therefore, after fully evaluating the patient, the physician should exercise clinical judgment to select the agent whose mode of action may be most suited to the pathophysiologic mechanism responsible for elevating the pressure in that patient, and least likely to aggravate any coexisting medical disorders. With control of arterial pressure, cardiovascular morbidity and mortality will be reduced, and with the selection of more specific forms of therapy, the treatment program can be best tailored to the individual patient, with fewer side effects.

SUGGESTED READING

Frohlich ED. Hypertension. In: Rakel RE, ed. Conn's current therapy 1989. Philadelphia: WB Saunders, 1989:225.

Frohlich ED. Life quality: A major consideration in healthcare delivery—especially with hypertensive diseases. Cardiovasc Drugs Ther 1989; 3:821–823.

Frohlich ED. LVH, cardiac diseases and hypertension: recent experiences. J Am Coll Cardiol 1989; 14:1587–1594.

Frohlich ED: Hypertension. In: Abrams WB, Berkow R, eds. Cardiovascular disorders. The Merck manual of geriatrics. NJ: Merck Sharp & Dohme, 1990:336.

Frohlich ED (chairman), Gifford R Jr, Horan M, et al. Nonpharmacologic approaches to the control of high blood pressure. Report of

the Subcommittee on Nonpharmacologic Therapy of the Joint National Committee on Detection, Evaluation, and Treatment of High Blood Pressure, 1984. Hypertension 1986; 8:444–467.
The Joint National Committee on Detection, Evaluation, and Treat-

ment of High Blood Pressure (member). The 1988 Report. Arch Intern Med 1988; 6148:1023–1038.
Perry HM Jr. Multicenter hypertension trials: Past, present, and future. Curr Opinion Cardiol 1990; 5:615–625.

HYPERTENSION IN THE ELDERLY*

FRANZ H. MESSERLI, M.D., F.A.C.C., F.A.C.P.

Systolic pressure and, to a lesser degree, diastolic pressure increase with age in westernized populations, and each year more and more elderly patients fulfill (arbitrarily set) criteria of hypertension. The National Health Survey in the United States has shown that the prevalence of hypertension may reach 50 percent in patients over 65 years of age. Since life expectancy has increased from approximately 47 years at the turn of the century to 73 years today, and probably will continue to increase, we can expect up to 25 million hypertensive elderly patients in the United States in the near future (more than 10 percent of the total population).

Several misconceptions may contribute to widespread confusion regarding the definition, evaluation, treatment, and prognosis of essential hypertension in patients older than 65 years. First, arterial pressure increases with age in most westernized populations, and an elevated pressure is therefore thought to be a normal finding in the elderly. Second, the function and blood flow of vital organs diminish with age, and an elevated pressure is regarded as a physiologic compensatory process serving to restore or maintain adequate blood flow. Third, elderly patients with essential hypertension often have systolic hypertension only, and many physicians believe that a diastolic pressure elevation is a harbinger of heart attack, stroke, and death.

Should we then consider hypertension in the elderly as an adaptive process serving to maintain perfusion of vital organs? Unfortunately, there is nothing adaptive or benign about hypertension in the elderly. The Veterans Administration Cooperative Study has shown that 63 percent of those over age 60 with untreated hypertension

will suffer a cerebrovascular accident, congestive heart failure, myocardial infarction, or a dissecting aneurysm within 5 years. Further studies from the Framingham cohort, the United States, Belgium, and Scandinavia corroborate these findings. Even patients with isolated systolic hypertension have a drastically higher mortality rate from all cardiovascular and renal diseases than those without hypertension.

Can we therefore expect that correction of hypertension will improve both length and quality of life in our senior citizens? Surprisingly, findings from several studies are contradictory in this regard and do not permit definite conclusions, although recently the European Working Party for Hypertension in the Elderly showed a distinct improvement in morbidity and mortality rates in patients receiving therapy.

Until more conclusive data become available, it seems reasonable to use an empiric approach and to lower blood pressure in moderation by using the drugs that not only lower arterial pressure but also specifically correct certain hemodynamic, fluid volume, and endocrine abnormalities in elderly hypertensive patients without compromising quality of life.

NONPHARMACOLOGIC MODALITIES

Nonspecific measures such as sodium restriction, weight loss, and, if feasible, mild aerobic exercise should be encouraged in overweight, inactive, elderly patients. An excess of adipose tissue expands intravascular volume and also burdens the left ventricle with a high preload. This may further impair left ventricular function and thereby accelerate the decline of its performance. The Framingham Study has indicated that obese hypertensive patients are at particularly high risk of developing congestive heart failure. Similarly, elderly patients are more susceptible to the effects of fluid and salt overload; an excessive salt load (particularly when combined with alcohol, as often happens at birthday parties, and on holidays) may temporarily overload the extracellular fluid volume space by more than 2,000 ml and thereby give rise to congestive heart failure and acute pulmonary edema. Such a dismal course of events is particularly apt to happen in an elderly patient whose heart was poorly compensated in the first place.

It must be remembered, however, that for various reasons the elderly patient's compliance with dietary measures is notoriously poor. First, the elderly person tends to have a very established, rigid daily schedule and

*Portions of this chapter were reproduced or adapted from a chapter by Franz H. Messerli entitled, "Essential Hypertension in the Elderly" in *Cardiovascular Disease in the Elderly,* 2nd ed., Franz H. Messerli, ed., Boston: Martinus Nijhoff Publishing, 1988:85–108; and from a chapter entitled "Management of Hypertension in the Elderly" by Franz H. Messerli, Ehud Grossman, and Schmuel Oren, in *Hypertension and the Elderly,* London: Science Press, 1988:37–48. All portions of these chapters have been reproduced or adapted with permission.

Table 1 Reasons for Noncompliance with Prescribed Drug Treatment

1. Poor transportation facilities
2. Long waiting times in doctor's office
3. Poor doctor-patient relationship
4. Complicated treatment schedules
5. Side effects to treatment
6. Mental confusion: inability to cope with complex drug regimen
7. Cost (?)

Modified from Messerli FH, Grossman E, Oren S. Management of hypertension in the elderly. In: Messerli FH, Swales JD, eds. Hypertension in the elderly. London: Science Press, 1988:39.

life style and may be reluctant to consider any changes. Second, it is cumbersome, time-consuming, and expensive to prepare fresh (unprocessed and therefore low-salt) meals three times a day, whereas canned food and TV dinners (high sodium) are much more convenient to prepare. Third, because the taste buds of elderly people lack sensitivity, these patients have a habit of adding more salt to overcome lack of taste. Fourth, dietary salt restrictions in the elderly usually have little antihypertensive effect (and thus impress neither patient nor physician), although a low sodium intake may prevent diuretic-induced hypokalemia. Finally, it may be next to impossible to follow a daily exercise program because of concomitant problems such as osteoarthritis, peripheral vascular disease, parkinsonism, depression, lack of appropriate facilities, or even fear of being assaulted (Table 1). Clearly, it is tedious and time-consuming to motivate elderly patients to change their life style and dietary habits and to encourage them to participate in a regular physical fitness program. However, the cardiovascular benefits from such nonspecific measures often outweigh the frustration they create.

ANTIHYPERTENSIVE MEDICATION

The elderly hypertensive patient is characterized hemodynamically by a lower cardiac output, higher systolic and lower diastolic pressure, and higher total peripheral resistance than younger patients with similar elevations of mean arterial pressure. Therefore, an antihypertensive agent should lower arterial pressure by lowering total peripheral resistance. Apart from reducing total peripheral resistance, an ideal antihypertensive agent should also maintain or increase systemic and regional (target organ) blood flow and preserve cardiac performance, prevent fluid and salt retention, and avoid reflexive stimulation of the sympathetic adrenergic or renin-angiotensin system. Moreover, the drug should prevent impairment of target organ function (left ventricular hypertrophy [LVH], nephrosclerosis) or, when impaired function is manifest, permit it to improve. Because of specific hemodynamic, fluid volume, and endocrine findings, the elderly patient is particularly susceptible to adverse effects of antihypertensive drugs, and inappropriate treatment has been shown to lead to

transient ischemic episodes and even fatal neurologic events.

Diuretics

Over the past three decades, diuretics have been the cornerstone of treatment for hypertension, especially in the elderly. Indeed, most patients' arterial pressure responds well to small doses of diuretics. However, diuretics have a tendency to produce volume depletion, which may cause orthostatic hypotension in elderly patients whose intravascular volume is contracted. Furthermore, the ability to dilute the urine and excrete a waterload is often impaired in the elderly, and thiazides may rapidly induce severe hyponatremia. Thiazides may cause hypokalemia, hyperglycemia, hyperuricemia, hypomagnesemia, and hypercalcemia. Hypokalemia may lead to life-threatening cardiac arrhythmias, especially in patients with LVH. Therefore, serum potassium levels should be monitored closely, especially during the first few months of therapy.

In cases of even mild hypokalemia, corrective measures are advocated. Kaplan and associates emphasized the benefit of maintaining potassium balance, which not only prevents hypokalemia but also improves blood pressure control. Concomitant use of a potassium-sparing diuretic or angiotensin converting enzyme (ACE) inhibitor may also prevent life-threatening hypokalemia and improve patient compliance. However, with potassium-sparing diuretics such as amiloride hydrochloride, spironolactone, or triamterene, there is a risk of hyperkalemia, particularly if the patient has renal insufficiency, diabetes mellitus, or hyporeninemic hypoaldosteronism or is receiving a nonsteroidal anti-inflammatory drug (NSAID), ACE inhibitor, or potassium supplement. Moreover, elderly patients are more susceptible to developing dehydration, prerenal azotemia, and urinary incontinence from diuretic use.

Data from the Framingham Study indicate that the presence of LVH carries an ominous prognosis regardless of levels of arterial pressure. In contrast to some antihypertensive agents such as methyldopa, calcium antagonists, and ACE inhibitors, diuretics do little to reverse or prevent LVH and do not lower the risk of sudden death or coronary artery disease. In a study of drug-induced illnesses requiring hospitalization, diuretics accounted for 6 percent of adverse reactions. I therefore do not recommend thiazide diuretics as first-line antihypertensive agents for uncomplicated essential hypertension in the geriatric population.

Beta-Blockers

Although the antihypertensive mechanism of beta-blockers is not yet clearly defined, most of these agents exert their antihypertensive effect by lowering cardiac output while increasing, or at best not changing, total peripheral resistance. Since the cardiac reserve and/or cardiac output of an elderly person is reduced and the total peripheral resistance is higher, beta-blockers are, with some exceptions, poor choices as first-line treatment. Moreover, there is some evidence that responsiveness to beta-blocking drugs is reduced in the elderly, and that elderly people are more susceptible to adverse central nervous system effects than younger patients.

Beta-blockers are contraindicated in patients with bradydysrhythmias, congestive heart failure, or bronchospasm, and they are relatively contraindicated in peripheral vascular disease and diabetes mellitus. Labetalol, which in addition exerts alpha-blockade, has been given to patients with peripheral vascular disease and even to patients with congestive heart failure without having a demonstrably negative inotropic effect. It has been suggested that pindolol, perhaps because of its intrinsic sympathomimetic activity, exerts its antihypertensive effect by lowering total peripheral resistance while maintaining systemic and renal blood flow. These hemodynamic properties make both agents acceptable choices for treatment of hypertension in the elderly.

Beta-blockers are still recommended for certain patients with angina pectoris, hyperkinetic heart syndrome, and hypertension, or as supplements to arteriolar vasodilators and perhaps certain calcium channel blockers. However, the metabolic clearance rate of beta-blockers may be decreased in the elderly, and receptor sensitivity is diminished. Therefore, the drug effects in any individual patient are less predictable, and when beta-blockers are initiated the principle "starting low and going slow" is appropriate.

Antiadrenergic Drugs

Agents such as methyldopa, clonidine, and reserpine lower arterial pressure by predominantly decreasing total peripheral resistance without reducing renal blood flow, and by only minimally changing cardiac function. They are useful in the management of hypertension in the elderly. Methyldopa has proved effective in reducing both blood pressure and left ventricular mass, an effect that is often independent of the effect on arterial blood pressure. This agent, therefore, may be a good choice for the elderly hypertensive patient who is not in congestive heart failure. Methyldopa is known, on rare occasions, to cause orthostatic hypotension, Coombs-positive hemolytic anemia, liver dysfunction, and (because of its central effect) depression. Elderly patients are more likely to develop orthostatic hypotension and, therefore, should have their blood pressure measured in both standing and sitting positions.

Clonidine can cause constipation and dry mouth, both of which may be intolerable in the elderly. It also has some negative inotropic effect that is undesirable in patients with a low cardiac output or latent congestive heart failure. Moreoever, rebound hypertension has been described after abrupt withdrawal from clonidine (and other antiadrenergic agents) owing to sympathetic overshoot. Elderly patients are more likely to forget to take their drugs than younger patients, and so clonidine

by mouth should be administered cautiously. A new transcutaneous form of clonidine seems to be considerably better tolerated than the oral medication. Transcutaneous clonidine not only has fewer and less severe side effects than the oral form but also improves compliance, since it can be applied once a week and does not lead to rebound hypertension. Its only drawbacks are occasional skin reactions. Transcutaneous clonidine has been a good agent for treatment of geriatric hypertension in our hands.

Although in the past so-called pseudoresistance was occasionally encountered in patients who were placed on antiadrenergic agents (fluid and sodium retention antagonizing the antihypertensive effect), this rarely presents a problem with the small doses currently given to elderly patients. In contrast to previous work from the Cleveland Clinic, Campese and associates observed no fluid and sodium retention in a group of patients who received antiadrenergic medication under metabolic ward conditions. My experience has shown that most elderly hypertensive patients tolerate small doses of antiadrenergic agents very well, particularly when they adhere to a moderately strict low-sodium diet.

Postsynaptic Alpha₁-Blockers

Prazosin, terazosin, and doxazosin lower arterial pressure by decreasing total peripheral resistance while maintaining systemic and regional blood flows. These agents have been used successfully for the treatment of congestive heart failure, at least over the short term. Postsynaptic alpha₁-blockers are often useful in the management of hypertension in the elderly. Their main drawback is orthostatic hypotension that occasionally occurs after the first dose and with subsequent increments. Because the elderly patient is prone to orthostatic hypotension, these agents have to be used very carefully; however, they may be good choices in patients who have latent congestive heart failure.

Direct Arteriolar Vasodilators

Hydralazine and minoxidil cannot be used as monotherapy because they produce palpitations, shortness of breath, and headaches and may even precipitate angina pectoris or acute myocardial infarction in susceptible patients. These untoward effects can be mitigated or abolished by the addition of a beta-blocker or other antiadrenergic agents. Arteriolar vasodilators have the advantage of not producing orthostatic hypotension since they affect only the arterioles and have no effect on the capacitance vessels. Hydralazine should be used in a dosage less than 200 mg per day; higher doses have been associated with lupus erythematosus. Salt and water retention due to stimulation of the renin-angiotensin-aldosterone system occurs but is much more common with minoxidil. This can be overcome by adding a loop diuretic such as furosemide. Thus, arteriolar vasodilators are most often used in combination with diuretics as well as beta-blockers and are therefore third-line agents.

Calcium Antagonists

Calcium antagonists have been successfully used to treat acute hypertensive crisis and as first-line agents for long-term antihypertensive therapy. They lower arterial pressure by reducing total peripheral resistance while maintaining or even improving blood flow to vital organs. Although they all lower arterial pressure by the same mechanism (class effect), the hemodynamic effect of one agent may differ from that of another. This hemodynamic heterogeneity can be demonstrated by examining the negative inotropic and chronotropic properties of the drugs, which are probably most pronounced with verapamil (in the isolated myocyte) and probably least pronounced with some of the newer agents such as isradipine and felodipine. These in vitro observations notwithstanding, I was unable to document any negative inotropic effects of verapamil with oral dosing over 3 months in patients with mild essential hypertension.

Calcium antagonists have been shown to be effective as first-line antihypertensive agents in elderly patients. They can be given to patients with chronic obstructive pulmonary disease, diabetes mellitus, or peripheral vascular disease as well as those with coronary artery disease. In contrast to other vasodilators, they do not cause sodium and water retention but instead have a mild natriuretic effect. They certainly are the agents of choice in patients with concomitant angina pectoris. Their antihypertensive effect appears to be a function of pretreatment levels of arterial pressure, and therefore the risk of hypotension is low. Adverse effects are uncommon. The dihydropyridine calcium antagonists cause headache, flushing, ankle edema, and gingival hypertrophy. These adverse effects are most common at the start of treatment and tend to disappear with prolonged therapy. Verapamil and diltiazem may cause headaches and constipation, which again are usually mild and tolerable. All calcium antagonists should be used with caution, if at all, in patients with congestive heart failure. My current approach is to start a patient on 120 to 180 mg of verapamil SR once a day, 90 mg of diltiazem SR twice a day, 2.5 mg of isradipine twice a day, or 30 mg of long-acting nifedipine once a day, and to increase the dosage very gradually (Table 2).

Angiotensin Converting Enzyme (ACE) Inhibitors

ACE inhibitors have been shown to lower arterial pressure predominantly by decreasing peripheral resistance concomitantly with dilatation of the capacitance vessels, while maintaining systemic and regional blood flow. Because of this hemodynamic effect, ACE inhibitors are excellent agents for the treatment of congestive heart failure, and therefore clearly the drugs of choice in geriatric patients suffering from both hypertension and congestive heart failure. Indeed, the Consensus study has clearly documented that the average survival of patients with class IV congestive heart failure can be significantly prolonged by using an ACE inhibitor such as enalapril. Also, there is recent evidence indicating that ACE inhibitors may improve the patient's quality of life.

Table 2   Recommended Regimen for Elderly Hypertensive Patients

Drug	Initial Dose	Special Concern (Side Effects)
Methyldopa	250 mg bid	Orthostasis, liver damage, hemolysis, depression
Clonidine	0.1 mg bid	Constipation, dry mouth, negative inotropic effect, rebound hypertension
Transdermal clonidine	2.5 mg	Skin reaction
Prazosin	1 mg bid	Orthostatic hypotension
Verapamil SR	120 mg qd	Constipation; should not be used with beta-blockers
Diltiazem SR	90 mg bid	Headache
Long-acting nifedipine	30 mg qd	Flushing, headache, leg edema, gingival hypertrophy
Isradipine	2.5 mg bid	Leg edema, palpitations
Captopril	6.25 mg bid	Rash, fever, agranulocytosis, proteinuria, renal deterioration, unexplained cough, hyperkalemia
Enalapril	5 mg qd	Rash, fever, agranulocytosis, renal deterioration, unexplained cough, hyperkalemia
Lisinopril	5-10 mg qd	Same as Enalapril

Modified from Messerli FH, Grossman E, Oren S. Management of hypertension in the elderly. In: Messerli FH, Swales JD, eds. Hypertension in the elderly. London: Science Press, 1988:44.

This effect may well be connected with the improvement of blood flow to vital organs, a more relevant goal of antihypertensive therapy than simply lowering arterial pressure. Side effects are rare and consist of cough, rash, fever, leukopenia, and proteinuria. Since elderly patients very often have low plasma renin activity, low doses of a diuretic may have to be added to stimulate the renin-angiotensin-aldosterone cascade and make the blood pressure more amenable to the effect of the ACE inhibitor. However, I always start with an ACE inhibitor first, and only if the patient's response is insufficient add 12.5 to 25 mg of hydrochlorothiazide. The combination of potassium-sparing diuretics with ACE inhibitors should be avoided because it may lead to significant hyperkalemia.

PREVENTION OR REVERSAL OF TARGET ORGAN DAMAGE

The major target organs affected by long-standing arterial hypertension are the brain, heart, and kidneys. Thus, LVH, coronary artery disease, congestive heart failure, nephrosclerosis, and cerebrovascular disease are common sequelae of long-standing, untreated hypertension. It must be emphasized that target organ disease often has a natural history and prognosis of its own, independent of arterial pressure. Thus, LVH increases the risk of sudden death and acute myocardial infarction five to six times over similar blood pressure elevations without LVH. Patients with LVH have 40 to 50 times more premature ventricular contractions and often higher-grade arrhythmias than patients without LVH or normotensive subjects. These observations therefore indicate that the process of LVH per se increases ventricular ectopic activity and may herald sudden death.

Given these observations, antihypertensive therapy should not only lower arterial pressure but also prevent or even improve target organ damage. Although a variety of antihypertensive agents reduce left ventricular mass and maintain or improve renal blood flow (ACE inhibitors and calcium antagonists), little is known of the effect of these agents on long-term morbidity and mortality. The recent observation that ectopic ventricular activity can be reduced concomitantly with left ventricular mass and arterial pressure by calcium antagonism in patients with essential hypertension and mild LVH (whereas no improvement in ectopy or in left ventricular mass was seen with diuretics) permits us to speculate that these agents may become useful in the future for the prevention of morbidity and mortality associated with target organ disease.

DRUG INTERACTIONS

Not infrequently, elderly patients have concomitant disease requiring other long-term medications. Some of these drugs may either potentiate or antagonize the antihypertensive effect, and in some cases may even produce hypertension de novo in a previously normotensive patient. Certain antihypertensive agents may also change blood levels of other drugs. Tricyclic antidepressants are known to elevate blood pressure in susceptible patients and can antagonize the antihypertensive effect of antiadrenergic drugs such as reserpine, guanethidine, and methyldopa. Since antiadrenergic agents and beta-blockers tend to aggravate depression, which is common in elderly patients, one should be careful when prescribing tricyclic antidepressants to these patients.

Levodopa may produce transient hypotension or, less often, hypertension. Sympathomimetics found in antitussive and decongestant over-the-counter agents often substantially elevate arterial pressure. Steroids, widely used in immunologic disorders, collagen disease, arthritis, and bronchial asthma, can cause hypertension. NSAIDs commonly used in degenerative joint disease and rheumatoid arthritis may hamper diuresis and

directly increase blood pressure by mineralocorticoid-like activity or prostaglandin synthetase inhibition. Either licorice abuse or carbenoxolone sodium used for gastric ulcer may produce hypertension that resembles hyperaldosteronism. Cyclosporine A, an immunosuppressive agent, can elevate blood pressure to hypertensive levels. Verapamil can elevate digoxin blood levels. Beta-blockers may attenuate the hypoglycemic effect of insulin; mutatis mutandis, they also may predispose to the development of insulin resistance and hyperglycemia in diabetics.

COMBINATION THERAPY

Like monotherapy, combination therapy of hypertension in the elderly has to take into account specific clinical and pathophysiologic features of the geriatric population. I often add a low dose of a diuretic, e.g., 12.5 mg hydrochlorothiazide daily, to therapy for patients who retain fluid while taking antiadrenergic drugs or who do not respond sufficiently to ACE inhibitors. A low-dose diuretic stimulates the activity of the renin-angiotensin system and makes arterial pressure more amenable to the effects of the ACE inhibitor. Patients should be advised to restrict their dietary sodium intake, because a high salt diet can easily override the beneficial effects of a low-dose diuretic. In patients with a tendency toward congestive heart failure or renal impairment, the addition of a loop diuretic may be preferable to a thiazide diuretic. A combination that has been very well tolerated in my experience is that of an ACE inhibitor with a calcium antagonist. This combination is remarkably free of adverse effects, it improves or maintains the blood flow and function of target organs, and it has a rather powerful antihypertensive effect.

SUGGESTED READING

Gavras H, Gavras I, eds. Hypertension in the elderly. Boston: John Wright, 1983.
Kaplan NM, Carnegie A, Raskin P, et al. Potassium supplementation in hypertensive patients with diuretic induced hypokalemia. N Engl J Med 1985; 312:746–749.
Messerli FH. Hypertension in the elderly. In: Messerli FH, ed. Cardiovascular disease in the elderly. 2nd ed. Boston: Martinus Nijhoff, 1984:65–81.
Messerli FH, Grossman E, Oren S. Management of hypertension in the elderly. In: Messerli FH, Swales JD, eds. Hypertension in the elderly. London: Science Press, 1988:37.

HYPERTENSION IN CHILDREN

JULIE R. INGELFINGER, M.D.

Essential hypertension in children is becoming increasingly recognized, even in the first 5 years of life. Such a diagnosis is generally achieved by exclusion, and the younger the child the more aggressive should be the evaluation to rule out definable causes prior to making a diagnosis of primary or essential hypertension. In this chapter I consider the management of the child with apparent essential hypertension.

The main goal in the management of a child with elevated blood pressure after ruling out obvious secondary causes is to bring the blood pressure level to within the normal range for age through the use of the least amount of intervention possible. While hypertension without any known cause has been reported with increasing frequency even within the first year of life, any child under the age of 5 years with marked hypertension deserves a complete evaluation including measurement of renal function, imaging of the kidneys (and the renal vessels) as well as screening for endocrine and central nervous system abnormalities (see the section *Secondary Hypertension*). An older child with mild-to-moderate hypertension may be managed initially without a full diagnostic evaluation, but a child of any age with severe hypertension should have a full evaluation. Thus, the approach to a child with mild, moderate, or severe hypertension depends on the child's age as well as the degree of hypertension. Once definable causes of hypertension have been ruled out, therapy will depend both on the amount of blood pressure elevation as well as assessment of the child within his or her family, i.e., how the child and family interact and how this might affect compliance with suggested therapy.

A word about blood pressure measurement in children is important, as not only do the technique used and size of the cuff (and its inner bladder) play a role, but the state of the patient may be harder to assess than in adults. Data sets concerning normative blood pressure vary greatly in childhood and are believed in large degree to reflect the emotional state of the children. Studies in which the children had had an opportunity to become used to the team of individuals taking the measurements have, in general, lower mean, diastolic, and systolic blood pressure curves. Pediatric blood pressure cuffs are available in several sizes, which should be chosen on the basis of each child's size rather than chronologic age (Table 1). A child should have baseline blood pressure measured in as nonthreatening a situation as possible. If blood pressure is found to be severely elevated, appropriate measures and a search for definable causes must be undertaken. (Note that in this chapter it is assumed that evaluation for definable causes of hypertension has already been "negative"; nonetheless, severe blood pressure elevation in a child with "essential hyperten-

Table 1 Blood Pressure Cuff Sizes

Cuff Category	Bladder Width (cm)	Bladder Length (cm)
Neonate	2.5–4.0	5.0–9.0
Infant	4.0–6.0	11.5–18.0
Child	7.5–9.0	17.0–19.0
Adult	11.5–13.0	22.0–26.0
Large adult	14.0–15.0	30.5–33.0
Thigh	18.0–19.0	36.0–38.0

From Task Force on Blood Pressure Control in Children – National Heart, Lung, and Blood Institute: Report of the Second Task Force on Blood Pressure Control in Children. Pediatrics 79:1, 1987; reproduced by permission of *Pediatrics*.

sion" should alert the clinician involved to rethink the situation.) If blood pressure is found to be less elevated, however, repeated measures should be performed at subsequent times, keeping in mind the time of day, the child's state, activity, postural position, and so forth. With 24-hour ambulatory blood pressure monitoring devices available, it may be helpful to obtain such recordings prior to beginning costly evaluations and lengthy and expensive treatment plans.

THERAPEUTIC ALTERNATIVES

Several modalities for lowering blood pressure in children with essential hypertension have been used, including dietary manipulation, exercise, stress reduction, and pharmacotherapy. Because many children with early essential hypertension come from families with known primary hypertension, a nonpharmacologic approach should be administered initially. Severe hypertension, however, should always first be controlled with the use of drugs.

Dietary Therapy

Weight Control. A first consideration in dietary management is whether the child's weight and height are appropriate for age. An overweight child should be encouraged to diet for several reasons. From the point of view of blood pressure control, weight loss will not only help the child become more active but will also help to lower the blood pressure through a combination of cardiovascular and hormonal changes that take place with weight loss. Weight reduction in early childhood should always involve the entire family, and a therapeutic alliance with the patient is essential in the adolescent period. Realistic weight goals are important, and the effectiveness of the weight reduction program is enhanced by frequent visits combined with ongoing consultations with a nutritionist, as well as with a social worker, psychologist, or psychiatrist for emotional support. A comprehensive program should not only include an individualized diet prescription but a concomitant program of prescribed graded exercise. Obtaining and maintaining food records are helpful, because the nature of the child's eating pattern will become more evident and lead to strategies of the most appropriate interventions. Stimulus-control methods such as limiting the availability of high-calorie foods in the home, eating only in the kitchen or dining room only at scheduled times, and avoiding activities such as television watching with food will be helpful. Often the entire family is overweight and needs to be on a weight reduction diet, and working with the whole family toward weight reduction in several family members is most effective. Providing food lists with calorie content and making adjustments so that favorite foods are allowed can also be helpful. For the adolescent, peer weight loss groups may be more successful than individual diet plans, and lifestyle packages that include dietary practice together with a prescribed exercise program plus nutritional and psychological counseling will result in a more permanent weight loss.

Sodium Sensitivity. Dietary therapy should also be aimed at determining whether the hypertensive child is sodium sensitive. As with adults, the reduction of sodium in a child's diet can be very difficult to achieve once the child is accustomed to a high-salt appetite. Again, the approach to successful dietary sodium reduction for a child with hypertension must also involve the family. Most efficacious is a sodium "allowance" in which a moderately reduced intake of sodium chloride is the aim, with some favorite high-salt foods allowed, while the total intake of sodium is fixed. In order to accomplish successful dietary sodium reduction for young children the family should be given lists of low-sodium foods and spices that are allowed as well as high-sodium–containing foods to avoid. The use of these lists as well as cookbooks such as the American Heart Association's low-salt cookbook provide a good starting point for a no-added-salt diet. Nevertheless, compliance with salt reduction, especially in adolescents, may be fraught with difficulties. In such an instance a therapeutic trial of diuretics may provide similar information (See section on diuretics). Often it is helpful to discern whether any first-degree relatives with hypertension appear to respond to a decreased salt diet. If any do, this response would suggest a salt sensitivity. Furthermore, enlisting the help of the involved adult in the child's evaluation and subsequent therapy will likely be helpful.

Additional Dietary Considerations. Two major considerations are important in prescribing dietary therapy in the first decade of life. One is the fact that the child with hypertension, like any child, is growing. Thus, *severe* restriction of *any* component of the diet is likely to affect growth adversely. A second consideration is that good nutrition is sadly lacking in a vast proportion of the general pediatric and adolescent population. Thus, general nutritional support and advice is certainly indicated in the child with hypertension. Various dietary manipulations in addition to calorie and sodium restriction have been advocated for the therapy for hypertension including high-potassium diet, high-calcium and magnesium diet, and relatively low starch and sugar intake. With the exception of achieving ideal weight and lowering salt in the diet, there are no large-scale studies to support dietary manipulation as efficacious in the treatment of the child with early primary hypertension. In part this lack of support exists because such studies have not yet been done, but in part it is also believed that a growing child has greater requirements per kilogram than an adult. Suffice it to say that it makes good sense to have at least adequate potassium, calcium, and magnesium intake. There would be no harm in pushing intake of these substances as long as the child has normal renal function and does not have hypercalciuria.

Exercise

American children in general have a woeful propensity to be sedentary television watchers and Nintendo players. Although exercise alone will not normalize blood pressure, an analysis of a large amount of data suggests that dynamic exercise is a very helpful adjunct to the control of blood pressure. For the very young child, exercise should include exercise classes or family-supervised aerobic activities. Physical education should be prescribed for the hypertensive school-age child once blood pressure is controlled satisfactorily. However, a hypertensive child is often a sedentary child who sits in a corner if not urged to participate in sports. It is therefore necessary to specify and prescribe a graded series of exercises starting with walking for 10 to 15 minutes a day and progressing to 30 to 45 minutes of aerobic exercise a day with activities such as walking, running, biking, or swimming. A teenager should be asked to do 30 to 60 minutes of daily exercise. If a child is completely unconditioned, it is necessary to write out the exercise prescription specifically, starting with 10 minutes per day and working up from there. The combined cooperation of the patient's school, family, and friends is often helpful. For an overweight teenager, weight loss combined with aerobic exercise may be especially helpful.

The child or teenage athlete presents a different problem. In this situation it is critical to adhere to a program of blood pressure reduction that does not exclude participation in sports. Formal exercise testing should be done to decide whether pharmacologic therapy is indicated. If exercise testing results in a systolic blood pressure increase to more than 210 mm Hg or a rise in diastolic pressure, pharmacotherapy should be initiated. (In teenagers with normal blood pressure, it is not unusual for systolic blood pressure to reach 190 to 200 mm Hg at the peak of dynamic exericse. In both normal and hypertensive children, diastolic pressure generally stays the same or falls at the peak of dynamic exercise.) If pharmacotherapy is indicated, recent experience suggests that the athletic child or teenager does best on agents such as converting enzyme inhibitors, which do not interfere with cardiac output or cause volume depletion.

Both dynamic and isometric exercise appear to

result in lowered *resting* blood pressures in "trained" children. Whereas dynamic exercise appears to cause no increase in diastolic pressure during *peak* effort, isometric exercise does. Although healthcare professionals generally encourage dynamic exercise, many committed teenage athletes may do isometric exercises such as weight lifting whether or not it is "allowed." Although few data are available, it would appear that once blood pressure is reasonably controlled, isometric exercise is not harmful. In fact, some evidence suggests that resting blood pressure may be even lower in athletes who do isometric exercise than in those who do dynamic exercise only.

In the patient with marked hypertension, it is obviously necessary to establish blood pressure control prior to starting an exercise program. Generally, this testing need not delay the exercise program for more than 1 to 2 weeks. It is also worthwhile to question whether hypertension in an athlete may be caused or aggravated by the purposeful ingestion of steroids, as several surveys have suggested that a surprising percentage of high school football players and wrestlers (15 to 20 percent) may take these drugs.

Stress Reduction Therapy

While it is often the case that hypertension is discovered in a young child during a time of family stress, alleviation of the stressful situation may take some time. It is difficult to get a very young child to be able to understand and cooperate with stress reduction techniques. However, a child of 8 to 10 years may well be able to participate in exercises involving relaxation techniques or biofeedback. However, before prescribing such therapy it is important to assess the child's interest as well as the family's attitude. Several things have become evident to me after more than a decade of assessing youngsters and their families for stress reduction prescriptions. First, the whole family has to think that stress reduction is a worthwhile project, or it will not work. Second, emphasizing the performance of these techniques in a simple, straightforward manner is imperative. Third, an adolescent patient has to be very interested in stress reduction or it will not only be counterproductive as a technique but may be destructive to the physician-patient relationship. However, for a child or teenager and his or her family who are interested, either biofeedback or relaxation techniques are helpful in the control of blood pressure. The assessment used in my unit is one of trying relaxation techniques in the clinic if the patient and his or her family appear to be interested. We teach the patient to do relaxation techniques and monitor blood pressure with a Dinamap, recording blood pressure changes. If the patient expresses the wish to continue with relaxation techniques and exercises after such an instruction session, we have them monitor blood pressure at home before and after applying the prescribed technique. This type of approach can be a successful adjunct to blood pressure control, but long experience has suggested that only about one in three pediatric patients are at all seriously interested in these techniques.

Drug Therapy

The principles involved in hypotensive therapy for children are in many ways similar to those used in the treatment of hypertension in adults. However, the pharmacokinetic mechanisms of numerous drugs may differ in the young child, and many hypotensive agents are not approved by the Food and Drug Administration (FDA) for use in early childhood. Data from long-term follow-up studies of infants, children, and adolescents treated for prolonged periods with hypotensive agents are simply not available for most classes of medication. The doses of hypotensive agents in many instances are obtained empirically. Even with all of these caveats there are still several practical pointers that may be worthwhile. (Drug dosages of oral hypotensive agents used in childhood are listed in Table 2.)

Particular considerations in choosing a specific drug for pediatric therapy may include family history, the child's activity level, and the child's other medical history. Often a child will respond well to a hypotensive agent that a parent or grandparent has received for the treatment of primary hypertension. Although this finding may reflect the fact that patients with salt-sensitive hypertension may respond well to the use of diuretic agents while patients with vasospastic hypotension may respond well to converting enzyme inhibitors, it may also reflect the fact that a parent is comfortable with a drug with which he or she is familiar. If the parent can say "Well, Dad does fine on Dyazide" or "Grandma did well on captopril," he or she is much more likely to be positive about having his or her child receive that medication.

Activity and conditioning ought to be considered in giving a child a particular antihypertensive agent. An athletic child may well feel unable to compete while taking a beta blocker, because cardiac output may become relatively decreased. Similarly, someone who engages in a summer sport may feel "washed out" while taking a diuretic agent. Because little is known about the effects of hypotensive agents on growth and development, school function, personality development, and long-term health status, one should be very careful to explain both expectable side effects and unknown factors to parents and to older children and teenagers. Although one may be concerned that adherence to a particular regimen will be problematic after such talks, experience dictates that a straightforward approach in this regard is extremely important in the pediatric age group.

Diuretics

Diuretic treatment may be especially efficacious in the child or teenager with a family history of salt-sensitive essential hypertension. Diuretics may also be helpful in assessing the presence or absence of salt sensitivity in an older child or adolescent who is judged unlikely to be able to comply with a salt-restricted diet.

Table 2 Oral Hypotensive Agents*

Generic Name (Trade Name)	Pediatric Dosage	How Supplied
Diuretic		
Chlorothiazide (Diuril)	20–30 mg/kg/day	Tablet, 250 or 500 mg; liquid, 250 mg/5 ml
Hydrochlorothiazide (HydroDIURIL, Esidrix)	2–3 mg/kg/day	25, 50, or 100 mg tabs
Chlorthalidone (Hygroton)	25–50 mg/day in adult; ? in child	25 or 50 mg tabs
Amiloride (Midamor)	5 mg/day in adult; ? in child	5 mg tabs
Furosemide (Lasix)	1 mg/kg/dose; 2–3 mg/kg/day	20, 40, 80 mg tabs; oral solution, 10 mg/ml
Ethacrynic acid (Edecrin)	1 mg/kg/dose; 2–3 mg/kg/day	25, 50 mg tabs
Bumetanide (Bumex)	0.5–2 mg in adult; ? in child	0.5, 1 mg tabs PO
Spironolactone (Aldactone)	3.3 mg/kg/day for edema; ? for hypertension	25, 50, 100 mg tabs
Triamterene (Dyrenium)	100 mg in adult; ? in child	50, 100 mg tabs
Acetazolamide (Diamox)	5 mg/kg/day	125, 150 mg tabs
Vasodilator		
Hydralazine (Apresoline)	0.1–3.0 mg/kg	10, 25, 50 mg tabs q4–6h
Minoxidil (Loniten)	0.2 mg/kg to start; maximum 30–40 mg	2.5, 10 mg once or twice daily
Central alpha-stimulator		
Clonidine (Catapres)	0.05–2.4 mg b.i.d.	0.1, 0.2 mg q8–12h; patches, 1 × /wk 0.1 or 0.2 mg
Guanabenz	4 mg b.i.d. to start in adult ? in child	4,8 mg b.i.d.
Beta-Blocker		
Propranolol (Inderal)	0.5 mg/kg/day to start	10, 40 mg q6–12h
Propranolol-LA (Inderal LA)	For older child	80 mg/day
Metoprolol (Lopressor)	2 mg/kg/day	50, 100 mg q12h
Nadolol (Corgard)	40 mg/day in adult; ? in child	40, 80, 120, 160 mg
Atenolol (Tenormin)	50 mg/day in adult; ? in child	50, 100 mg once daily
Timolol (Blocadren)	0.3 mg/kg/day in adult; ? in child	10 mg q12h
Pindolol (Visken)	0.3 mg/kg/day in adult; ? in child	5–10 mg q8–12h
Acebutolol (Sectral)	200 mg b.i.d. in adult; ? in child	200 mg q12h
Peripheral α-alpha-blocker		
Prazosin (Minipress)	1 mg t.i.d. in adult; ? in child	1, 2, 5 mg q8h
Phenoxybenzamine (Dibenzyline)	Individualized starting dose, 2–5 mg; range 20–100 mg/day	100 mg cap q12h
Combined alpha/beta-blocker		
Labetalol (Normodyne, Trandate)	100 mg b.i.d. in adult; ? in child	100, 200, 300 mg; up to 600 mg b.i.d.

*Note that additional oral agents including newer ACE inhibitors and calcium channel blockers have been released, but the experience in children and adolescents is very limited, thus this is only a partial listing. The optimal doses for children are not known even for those agents that are listed.

Table continues on following page

Table 2 Oral Hypotensive Agents—cont'd

Generic Name (Trade Name)	Pediatric Dosage	How Supplied
False transmitter		
Methyldopa (Aldomet)	10 mg/kg/day	125, 150 mg tab or 25 mg/5 ml oral suspension
Angiotensin-converting enzyme (ACE) inhibitor		
Captopril (Capoten)	0.51 mg/kg/day	25, 50, 100 mg q6–12h
Enalapril (Vasotec)	? in child	5, 10, 20 mg once daily
Lisinopril (Prinavil)	? in child	5, 10, 20 mg once daily
Central Inhibitor		
Reserpine (Sandril, Serpasil, Reserpoid)	0.02 mg/kg/day	0.1, 0.25 mg once daily
Neuroeffector blocker		
Guanethidine (Ismelin)	0.2 mg/kg/day	10, 25 mg once daily
Guanadrel (Hylorel)	10 mg b.i.d. in adult; ? in child	10, 25 mg b.i.d.
Calcium channel blocker		
Verapamil (Calan)	80 mg/dose, 240 mg/day in adult, ? in child	80, 120 mg q6h
Nifedipine (Adalat, Procardia)	10–20 mg/dose, 30–60 mg/day in adult, ? in child	10 mg q6–8h
Diltiazem (Cardizem)	60–90 mg/dose; 60 to 180 mg/day in adult, ? in child	30, 60, 90, 120 mg q8h

Thiazide treatment for 2 to 3 weeks should lower the blood pressure in such individuals, assuming they take the medication. Diuretics should certainly be avoided in a child who has any propensity to lose salt, although a patient with a salt-wasting nephrologic abnormality or an adrenal disorder would certainly not be categorized as having childhood primary hypertension. One should avoid prescribing diuretics for athletes during warm weather. Furthermore, diuretic therapy should be avoided in the highly compulsive compliant child or teenager who may develop electrolyte abnormalities on a no-added-salt diet in combination with diuretic treatment.

Beta Blockers

Beta blockers may be especially helpful in the anxious child or teenager with hypertension, provided he or she has no asthmatic history. Because many runners, soccer players, and sprinters report a loss of athletic prowess while taking these agents, beta blockers should be avoided in such individuals. Furthermore, in the very young child, propranolol and other beta blockers are frequently associated with vivid dreams and night terrors. If these phenomena occur, drug treatment should be discontinued. Although sustained-release propranolol (Inderal-LA) has been very successful in the treatment of many adolescents in whom once daily dosing is important, malabsorption of the beads also may occur so that the patient may be compliant without the

agent being absorbed. In children with migraine, as in adults with migraine, beta blockers, especially propranolol, may be effective. While labetalol, with its combined alpha and beta blocking ability, appears to avoid some of the side effects seen after the use of beta blockers, its oral use in children and adolescents is still limited.

Vasodilators (Direct-Acting)

The direct-acting vasodilators such as hydralazine should not be used as first-line drug therapy for the child with primary hypertension. Frequently, their use is associated with flushing and perceptible tachycardia. With more potent and selective agents available (i.e., the angiotensin-converting enzyme inhibitors and calcium channel blockers), these vasodilators have been rendered archaic. Minoxidil, which had been frequently used for severe hypertension, is rarely necessary in this era of converting enzyme inhibitors and calcium entry antagonists.

Centrally Acting Agents

Children often become somnolent while receiving methyldopa, clonidine, guanabenz, and similar agents. For this reason limited use of these agents is recommended. Furthermore, clonidine use in children has been associated more frequently with rebound hypertension than in adults. For example, a young child with gastroenteritis may vomit several doses and then become severely hypertensive. On the other hand, my experience has indicated that adolescents who do not like to take pills will often take to the idea of clonidine patch therapy. The dose in such adolescents is the same as that used in adults and appears to be well tolerated.

Converting Enzyme Inhibitors

The converting enzyme inhibitors, captopril, enalapril, and lisinopril interfere with the production of angiotensin II. Data on these agents are scarce in children and adolescents, however, and even more limited in infants. Although the formal dosage recommendations are not available, the use of these agents by pediatric hypertension specialists, nephrologists, and cardiologists is increasing. Table 2 lists doses of these agents that have been used in the treatment of children. Given cautiously, converting enzyme inhibitors appear to be especially efficacious and well tolerated in the active school-age and adolescent child.

Calcium Channel Blockers

Whereas calcium channel blockers are especially effective in childhood hypertensive crisis, they have not gained much favor for the long-term pharmacotherapy for primary hypertension in children, mainly because of the side effects of tachycardia and fluid retention. These are such distressing side effects that other agents ought to be used as first-line therapy.

Step-Down Therapy

The concept of step-down pharmacotherapy in childhood hypertension is even more important than in adults. Because the long-term implications of pharmacotherapy are completely unknown, the control of blood pressure for 6 months to 1 year should support a trial of decreasing medication. My approach is to explain the concept of step-down therapy prior to the initiation of pharmacotherapy. At that time the patient and family are told that medication will be given for a specified time and that I would then supervise a step-wise decrease in medication. It may still be necessary to continue drug therapy if the blood pressure level increases after the attempted lowering of the dosage, or to restart medication if the blood pressure later increases. However, my

experience has shown it to be possible to stop drug therapy completely.

COMPLIANCE ISSUES

The statistics on compliance with suggested medical care in general are not encouraging. For a health problem such as primary hypertension in childhood where there are few, if any, symptoms, the accomplishment of compliance with medical recommendations can be very difficult indeed. Most studies concerning compliance issues reveal that adolescence (most children with primary hypertension present for evaluation and care in adolescence) is a particularly difficult time for getting patients to follow medical recommendations. Various adjuncts may be helpful in ensuring adherence to suggestions for hypertension evaluation and therapy in those children and adolescents who require it. Education in the form of interactive teaching sessions and written material are especially useful in promoting understanding. Home blood pressure monitoring is recommended because instrumentation is currently adequate, and because home monitoring will provide ongoing empiric data about blood pressure levels. The child and family may then be able to have a measure against which to monitor ongoing therapeutic maneuvers. Additional aids to patient compliance should include making necessary office visits as convenient as possible, enlisting the patient as a partner and colleague in therapy, and encouraging ongoing interchange about concerns about diet or medications.

SUGGESTED READING

Burke GL, Voors AW, Shear CL, et al. Blood pressure. Pediatrics 1987; 80(suppl):784–788.
Ingelfinger JR. Nutritional aspects of pediatric hypertension. Ann NY Acad Sci 1989; 65:1109–1120.
Lauer RM, Clarke WR. Childhood risk factors for high adult blood pressure: the Muscatine study. Pediatrics 1989; 84:633–641.
National Heart, Lung, and Blood Institute Report of the Second Task Force on Blood Pressure Control in Children. Pediatrics 1987; 79:1–25.
Sinaiko AR, Gomez-Marin O, Prineas RJ. Prevalence of "significant" hypertension in junior high school-aged children: the children and adolescent BP program. J Pediatr 1989; 114:664–669.

HYPERTENSION IN SELECTED POPULATIONS

JAMES R. SOWERS, M.D.,
MICHAEL B. ZEMEL, Ph.D.
PAULA C. ZEMEL, Ph.D.
DILEK K. SOWERS, M.D., F.A.C.E.P.

This chapter discusses several subgroups of the hypertensive population with respect to the pathogenesis of high blood pressure, hypertension-related morbidity and mortality, and general therapeutic approaches. The prevalence of hypertension is especially high in the black, diabetic, and elderly populations. The prevalence of pregnancy-induced hypertension is also very high in nulliparous, black, inner-city women. Hypertension in these populations is characterized by increased peripheral vascular resistance and abnormalities in cellular cation transport and insulin resistance. Dietary factors probably contribute significantly to the development of hypertension in these subgroups. Accordingly, dietary modifications are an important component of the nonpharmacologic approach to therapy for these patients. Certain classes of pharmacologic agents appear to be more efficacious, and their use in the treatment of hypertension in these subgroups is discussed in this chapter.

HYPERTENSION IN BLACKS

Hypertension in African-American individuals occurs more frequently and is associated with greater morbidity and mortality than in the rest of the U.S. population. Indeed, the prevalence of hypertension among blacks in the United States is 38.2 percent compared with 28.8 percent among nonblacks. Approximately 25 percent of blacks have uncontrolled hypertension compared with 16 percent of nonblacks. This higher prevalence, combined with greater severity, increases the risk of strokes, end-stage renal disease, congestive heart failure, and left ventricular hypertrophy (LVH). Blacks are two to four times more likely to incur strokes. In the southeastern United States they have a higher death rate from strokes than do blacks from other regions, perhaps because of the lower rates of hypertension control in that region. Hypertension was noted to be the main cause of end-stage renal disease in 27.7 percent of black patients and in 11.9 percent of white patients in maintenance dialysis. An increased prevalence of LVH in blacks may contribute to increased ventricular ectopy, impaired coronary reserve, and increased sudden death in this population.

A number of hypotheses have been set forth to explain the higher prevalence and severity of hypertension in blacks on a genetic basis. However, most studies have not demonstrated a genetic factor or marker to explain these pathophysiologic differences. Further, the prevalence of hypertension among blacks is considerably different in various parts of the world. For example, the prevalence of high blood pressure in rural Africans is considerably less than that in blacks in the United States and the Caribbean. These observations suggest that environmental factors play a large role in determining the prevalence of hypertension.

Factors such as decreased access to preventive health care, lower educational and income levels, greater environmental stress, and poorer nutritional status are probably contributory. In this regard, current efforts appear to be promising in lowering the "black-white gap" in hypertension-related morbidity and mortality. For example, the Hypertension Detection and Follow-up Program showed that blacks and whites responded equally well to an aggressive systematic treatment of hypertension. Black patients appeared to benefit from free medication, free transportation, baby sitting services, and convenient clinic hours, suggesting that overcoming the barriers to good health care eliminated differences in blood pressure control.

Pathophysiology

High blood pressure in blacks is characterized by a low plasma renin, expanded intravascular volume, and salt sensitivity. Regardless of the methods used to classify renin status, black hypertensives have been found to have low-renin status twice as frequently as white hypertensives. The tendency to a low renin state in blacks is observed in childhood. A suppressed plasma renin level is usually associated with expanded plasma volume; however, even with normal or contracted plasma volumes, blacks often manifest a suppressed renin state. Expanded plasma volume in black hypertensives does not result from increased dietary intake of salt, although several studies have demonstrated decreased dietary potassium and calcium consumption in the black population. In this regard, it has been demonstrated that an increase in dietary consumption of potassium produces natriuresis, a negative sodium balance, and increased plasma renin in black but not white children. Other studies have shown that increased calcium intake by blacks is also associated with natriuresis, elevations in plasma renin, and a more negative sodium balance. These observations suggest that deficient dietary intake of potassium and calcium play an important role in mediating salt sensitivity in blacks.

Investigations of salt sensitivity have shown that blacks (both normotensive and hypertensive) have greater changes in blood pressure associated with varying salt content of the diet. The mechanism underlying this heightened salt sensitivity is only partially understood. Decreased ability to generate endogenous renal natriuretic factors such as dopamine, prostaglandins and kinins may be contributory. For example, urinary dopamine excretion is decreased in blacks with salt-sensitive hypertension. Also, dietary salt-induced increases in urinary dopamine excretion are considerably less in salt-sensitive blacks than in whites. These observations are important in view of the considerable evidence suggesting a relationship between renal production of dopamine and the ability of the kidney to excrete a salt load. Reduced urinary excretion of kallikrein, the enzyme-mediating synthesis of the dilating and diuretic kinins, has been observed in blacks. This reduction in kallikrein excretion has been observed in normotensive black adolescents, making it less likely to be secondary to hypertensive damage to the kidney. Levels of other natriuretic factors have been observed to be decreased in the black population.

Racial differences in cellular cation metabolism may also contribute to the increased prevalence of salt-sensitive hypertension in blacks. For example, elevated erythrocyte sodium concentrations, particularly after increased dietary salt intake, have been observed in blacks as opposed to nonblacks. Increased platelet ionized calcium levels have also been reported. Racial differences have likewise been noted in membrane cation transport mechanisms, which may account for the observed increased intracellular sodium and calcium concentrations. Decreased active (ouabain-sensitive adenosine triphosphatase [ATPase]) and passive (ouabain-insensitive) sodium-potassium transport activity of erythrocyte membranes has been observed in both normotensive and hypertensive blacks. In hypertensive blacks, and also in young blacks with a family history of hypertension, there is distinctly lower erythrocyte sodium-potassium-chloride cotransport. Furthermore, the latter correlates with both salt sensitivity and insulin resistance in young blacks with borderline hypertension.

Recent reports have demonstrated a linkage of insulin resistance/hyperinsulinemia to the clustering of essential hypertension, non–insulin-dependent diabetes mellitus (NIDDM), and obesity. Insulin resistance in blacks has been addressed by studying insulin-stimulated glucose uptake in healthy lean young adult males, employing the euglycemic hyperinsulinemic clamp technique. Compared with normotensive individuals, borderline hypertensives exhibited a reduction in insulin-stimulated glucose uptake, consistent with insulin resistance. The borderline hypertensive individuals also were noted to have higher fasting plasma insulin concentrations than the normotensive subjects despite lack of difference in adiposity. Nevertheless, upper body fat (central obesity) is closely linked to hypertension, insulin resistance/hyperinsulinemia, type II diabetes mellitus, and cardiovascular disease. Insulin resistance/hyperinsulinemia associated with central obesity in blacks may contribute to the higher prevalence of both hypertension and type II diabetes in this population.

We have observed that hyperinsulinemia and insulin resistance occurring in the first trimester is a predictor of pregnancy-induced hypertension in urban black nulliparous women. It is unclear whether insulin resistance is inherited or acquired in conjunction with hypertension secondary to environmental influences. Various patho-

physiologic characteristics of the black hypertensive are listed in Table 1.

Therapy

As might be predicted from the hemodynamic and hormonal profiles, hypertension in black patients characteristically responds less well to drugs that inhibit the renin-angiotensin systems or that decrease cardiac output, than do nonblack hypertensive patients. Studies have generally shown that monotherapy with converting enzyme inhibitors or beta-blockers is less efficacious than in white hypertensives. However, racial differences in responses to converting enzyme inhibitors disappear when these agents are combined with thiazide diuretics. Calcium channel blockers and thiazide diuretics have been shown to be as effective as in nonblack hypertensives.

HYPERTENSION IN DIABETICS

Both diabetes mellitus and hypertension are common medical disorders in Westernized industrialized cultures. In individuals with NIDDM the prevalence of hypertension is elevated twofold over the nondiabetic population. Hypertension in diabetic patients is associated with accelerated atherosclerosis as well as microvascular disease. An estimated 2.5 million Americans have both diabetes mellitus and hypertension. The prevalence of hypertension in the diabetic population increases with age, and the prevalence of these coexist-

Table 1 Pathophysiologic Characteristics of Black Hypertensive Patients

Demographics
  Lesser education
  Lower socioeconomic status
  Less accessibility to health care
  More environmental stress
Cardiovascular Hemodynamics
  Increased peripheral vascular resistance
  Expanded intravascular volume
  Normal or reduced cardiac output
  Normal or reduced renal blood flow
Hormonal Factors
  Low plasma renin activity
  Normal or elevated plasma aldosterone levels
  Hyperinsulinemia and insulin resistance
Cellular Cation Alterations
  Increased intracellular sodium and calcium levels
  Altered membrane cation transport
Renal Factors
  Increased salt retention
  Decreased dopamine production
  Decreased kallikrein production
  Decreased renin production
  Increased renal vascular resistance
Dietary Factors
  Central obesity
  Low dietary calcium intake
  Low dietary potassium intake

ent conditions is almost twice as great in blacks. Important determinants of elevated blood pressures, particularly systolic blood pressure, in the diabetic population are age, race, greater body mass, duration of diabetes, and the presence of persistent proteinuria.

Hypertension doubles the risk of cardiovascular mortality in diabetics. Diabetic patients with hypertension have a strikingly higher frequency of strokes and myocardial infarction than normotensive diabetics. Hypertension accelerates the progression of both diabetic retinopathy and nephropathy; progression of retinopathy is slowed with effective antihypertensive treatment. Renal disease associated with diabetes mellitus is the single most common cause of new end-stage renal disease in the United States. The 5-year survival of diabetics with end-stage renal disease receiving dialysis is less than half that of patients without diabetes.

Pathophysiology

Several lines of evidence suggest that many of the disturbances in blood pressure regulation in patients with diabetes are very similar to those observed in elderly patients with hypertension (Table 2). Like elderly hypertensives, diabetics with hypertension manifest greatly enhanced peripheral vascular reactivity, a tendency to a low-renin state, decreased cardiopulmonary and sinoaortic baroreceptor sensitivity, and apparent salt sensitivity. Premature atherosclerosis and senescent changes in resistance vessels may explain, in part, the exaggerated vascular reactivity.

Alterations in vascular smooth muscle cation metabolism may also underlie the increased vascular reactivity. We and others have observed decreased activity of erythrocyte membrane Ca^{2+}-ATPase in hypertensive NIDDM patients. This decrease was associated with an increase in erythrocyte Ca^{2+} concentration. In animal models of insulin resistance, we have found

Table 2 Pathophysiologic Characteristics of Diabetic Hypertensive Patients

Cardiovascular Hemodynamics
  Increased peripheral vascular resistance
  Increased pressor responses to angiotensin II and norepinephrine
  Intravascular volume often expanded
  Decreased cardiopulmonary and sinoaortic baroreceptor
    sensitivity
Renal Factors
  Reduced renal production of kallikrein and prostaglandins and
    possibly other natriuretic factors
  Glomerular hyperfiltration and proteinuria
  Increased renal vascular resistance
  Decreased renin (particularly active renin) secretion
Cellular Cation Abnormalities
  Increased cell calcium and sodium
  Decreased Ca^{2+}-ATPase activity
  Altered sodium-lithium countertransport
Other Metabolic Factors
  Decreased cell insulin activity (insulinopenia or insulin resistance)
  Obesity
  Dyslipidemia

widespread reductions in Ca^{2+}-ATPase activity; in addition, the regulatory effects of insulin on calcium transport are markedly diminished in this model. These observations support the notion that regulation of intracellular calcium by insulin is impaired in states of insulin resistance and hypertension. This may lead to increased intracellular calcium and increased calcium in the vascular smooth muscle cells, which would enhance vasoconstriction, and thereby increase systemic vascular resistance.

Decreased activity of the ouabain-sensitive (Na^+, K^+)-ATPase cell membrane pump has also been observed in rat models of diabetes. Reduced pump activity will increase intracellular sodium, decrease Na^+-Ca^{2+} exchange, and increase intracellular calcium. Thus, abnormalities in vascular smooth muscle cation metabolism may contribute to the increased peripheral vascular resistance in patients with subtle and overt abnormalities of glucose metabolism.

There is also evidence that hyperinsulinemia, per se, may play a role in the pathogenesis of hypertension. Investigators have reported that hyperinsulinemia is associated with elevated erythrocyte sodium levels, obesity, and hypertension. Altered membrane cation transport is a characteristic shared in states of obesity, glucose intolerance, and hypertension associated with hyperinsulinemia. Hyperinsulinemia could theoretically increase renal tubular sodium reabsorption and thus account for increases in exchangeable sodium and volume expansion. Thus, hyperinsulinemia could be a common factor in the hypertension associated with NIDDM and obesity. Studies have also suggested that hyperinsulinemia accelerates the development of atherosclerosis. In animal models, insulin promotes diet-induced lesion development and overrides lesion regression and estrogen protection against atherosclerosis. Insulin has been shown to stimulate subintimal smooth muscle and fibroblast cells in culture, and to increase the uptake and esterification of lipoprotein-cholesterol by these cells. Thus, hyperinsulinemia may directly accelerate the rate of atherogenesis, as well as indirectly influence this process by elevating blood pressure.

Dyslipidemia is common in the diabetic state. The most common alteration of lipoproteins in NIDDM is an elevation in very-low-density lipoproteins (VLDL), as reflected by either increased total triglyceride levels or VLDL-triglyceride concentrations. Abnormalities in both the production and clearance of VLDL have been observed in NIDDM. Overproduction of VLDL may be induced by hyperglycemia or the attendant hyperinsulinemia, since production normalizes when glycemia is improved. Increased production and decreased clearance of VLDL apo B have also been reported in NIDDM patients. Decreases have been observed in adipose tissue lipoprotein lipase activity in NIDDM patients that have paralleled and may partially explain the decrease in clearance of VLDL triglyceride in NIDDM. Decreased rate of high-density lipoprotein (HDL) synthesis and perhaps increased clearance may explain the low HDL cholesterol levels often seen in NIDDM. A negative relationship between insulin resistance and HDL cholesterol have been observed, suggesting that insulin resistance may dictate low HDL levels. Increased levels of LDL cholesterol have been reported in some NIDDM patients related to increased production and/or decreased clearance of LDL cholesterol. Thus, elevations of VLDL and reductions in HDL cholesterol are very common in NIDDM patients, elevations in LDL cholesterol being less common in these individuals.

Therapy

Because hypertension is an especially powerful risk factor in diabetics, and because diabetics often have other concomitant risk factors for cardiovascular disease, it is important to treat hypertension in the diabetic patient aggressively. However, diabetics are more prone to the side effects of antihypertensive medications, including orthostatic hypertension, cerebral and renal hypoperfusion, sexual dysfunction, reduced cardiac reserve, and metabolic disturbances (hypertriglyceridemia, hypercholesterolemia, hypokalemia, hypomagnesemia).

A number of nonpharmacologic approaches serve the dual purpose of improving glycemic control and lowering blood pressure. For example, weight reduction in the obese NIDDM patient is often accompanied by a decrease in blood pressure as well as improvement in glucose tolerance. Glycemic control is important in treating hypertension, because good control lessens problems with fluid retention as well as with potassium and magnesium loss from osmotic diuresis. Glycemic control may also be important in protecting the kidney from increased intraglomerular pressure and hyperfiltration. These problems are engendered by increased osmotic load and increased secretion of atrial natriuretic peptide in association with hyperglycemia. One study in diabetic hypertensive individuals showed that systolic blood pressure was higher in diabetic patients whose glucose levels were poorly controlled than in those whose levels were well controlled. Salt restriction appears to be generally effective in lowering blood pressure in diabetic patients, as these individuals appear to have a propensity for salt sensitivity.

In choosing drug therapy for the diabetic hypertensive patient, it is important to remember that some antihypertensive agents (diuretics and beta-blockers) can worsen insulin resistance and diabetic control as well as worsen the lipoprotein profile in these patients. In this regard, calcium channel blockers, alpha-adrenergic blockers, and angiotensin converting enzyme (ACE) inhibitors appear to be the most appropriate antihypertensive agents available for treating these patients.

THE ELDERLY HYPERTENSIVE PATIENT

Hypertension is an important risk factor for cardiovascular disease in the elderly. In the Framingham study, borderline hypertension (levels of 140/90 to 160/95) was associated with an increase in mortality from stroke and coronary artery disease, and the increased mortality rate was more evident with advancing age. Isolated systolic hypertension, which occurs in up to one-third of individuals over 65, is a greater cardiovascular risk factor than is diastolic hypertension. In one study of a geriatric population, the cardiovascular mortality rate was seven times greater in individuals with elevated systolic hypertension than in a matched control group with blood pressures below 140/90 mm Hg. Myocardial infarction occurred twice as often in those with elevated systolic blood pressures, and strokes were almost three times as frequent.

Pathophysiology

Age-associated increases in the prevalence of hypertension are especially notable in Westernized and industrialized societies. In the United States, approximately 40 percent of whites and 50 percent of blacks 65 to 74 years of age have systolic-diastolic hypertension or isolated systolic hypertension; diastolic blood pressures begin to rise in early adulthood, peak in the 45- to 55-year range, and then fall slightly with advancing age. Systolic pressures continue to rise with advancing age. The differences in high blood pressure prevalences between blacks and whites and between individuals from industrialized areas and those from agrarian cultures become increasingly pronounced with advancing age. These observations suggest that environmental factors such as diet, physical activity, and perhaps stress may account for these age-dependent differences in hypertension prevalence.

In Westernized industrialized societies, advancing age is associated with body composition changes. There is a loss of lean body mass and an increase in adipose tissue. Increased adiposity, particularly central or "android" adiposity, is associated with an increased prevalence of hypertension, insulin resistance and NIDDM, and cardiovascular disease. Obesity probably contributes to the high prevalence of hypertension through associated insulin resistance/hyperinsulinemia (the mechanism is discussed above) and via enhanced sympathetic nervous system activation (seen in both obesity and aging).

Elderly hypertensive people in our society tend to be salt sensitive, but this does not appear to be associated with age-related increases in either sodium or salt intake. Although it has been suggested that the reduced taste acuity for salt that occurs with aging causes the elderly to consume more salt than do young adults, no association was found between salt consumption and hypertension in the elderly in the NHANES I population. This suggests that if salt sensitivity in the elderly is related to and possibly modified by diet, nutrients other than salt must be considered. Indeed, evidence has accumulated to suggest that suboptimal intakes of calcium, and possibly potassium, may be predisposing factors to hypertension in general, and to salt sensitivity in particular.

A high prevalence of salt sensitivity in the elderly may also be related to senescent changes in the kidney and the consequent reduced ability to excrete a salt load. This age-related decline in renal function is more striking in blacks, and this may explain, in part, the higher rate of salt-sensitive hypertension in the aging black population. In addition, an age-related decrease in the natriuretic response to increased dietary salt may result from a reduced ability to generate natriuretic substances such as dopamine and prostaglandin E_2 (PGE_2). The renal excretion of PGE_2, a vasodilator with natriuretic properties, declines with age. Salt sensitivity in the elderly may also be accentuated by alterations in cellular cation metabolism. For example, reductions in both erythrocyte and myocardial membrane NA^+/K-ATPase activity has been observed in aged animal models. It has been suggested that the resultant increase in intracellular sodium may account for the increase in vascular resistance (by virtue of reduced Na^+/Ca^{2+} exchange). Increased vascular smooth muscle intracellular calcium may in turn help mediate a state of insulin resistance and accompanying hyperinsulinemia that are also characteristic of aging in industrialized societies. Hyperinsulinemia may further contribute to age-related reductions in renal excretion of a salt load by increasing renal tubular sodium reabsorption.

Structural changes in the vasculature with senescence are important in the pathogenesis of hypertension, especially isolated systolic hypertension, in the elderly. With aging, vascular rigidity increases and elasticity of the aorta and other large vessels decreases. These senescent alterations are caused, in part, by the fracturing and uncoiling of elastic fibers and the deposition of calcium and collagenous matrix within the vessel walls. Because of the decreased elasticity and compliance, the pulse generated during systole is transmitted to the aorta and its large tributaries, resulting in a steeper rise in pressure per unit volume of blood pumped into these large vessels and a disproportionate rise in systolic pressure. With aging, arterioles also undergo hyaline degeneration of the media, which decreases the lumen-to-wall ratio and overall cross-sectional area of the lumen. These alterations in precapillary arterioles may increase vascular resistance in response to ambient circulating vasoactive factors such as norepinephrine and angiotensin II. Other age-related changes in the cardiovascular systems of the elderly include a decline in cardiac output, stroke volume, heart rate, and systemic and renal blood flow. Cardiac hypertrophy is characteristic of the latter stages of hypertension in the elderly and reflects elevated left ventricular stroke work against elevated peripheral vascular resistance, with a decrease in intravascular volume.

Abnormalities in baroreceptor function may play a role in the pathogenesis of hypertension in the elderly. Decreased baroreceptor sensitivity probably contributes to increased sympathetic nervous system activity and elevated plasma norepinephrine levels.

Plasma renin activity declines with advancing age and is more pronounced in the hypertensive state. This reduction is probably unrelated to salt retention and extracellular fluid volume expansion. In fact, several studies have demonstrated that blood volume is actually reduced in older hypertensive individuals with low renin activity. Also, renin activity is low in the elderly even when a fixed sodium diet is given after diuretic-induced volume contraction (Table 3).

Evaluation and Management

Variability in blood pressure, particularly systolic pressure, increases with advancing age. Therefore, multiple blood pressure measurements should be obtained before initiating or altering antihypertensive therapy in the elderly. Blood pressure should be measured during each of three separate office visits over a period of several weeks before therapy is initiated. Another condition that may increase the difficulty of accurately determining blood pressure by the usual methods is "pseudohypertension," which in the elderly is a phenomenon associated with rigid sclerotic brachial arteries that cannot be occluded by the sphygmomanometer cuff.

Coexisting diseases often complicate the treatment of many elderly hypertensive patients. Geriatric hypertensive patients are more likely to have concomitant LVH and congestive heart failure. Hypertension in geriatric patients with chronic obstructive pulmonary disease is also a challenging problem. Beta-blockers must, of course, be used with considerable caution, as they may induce bronchospasm. Many of the sympathomimetic agents used in the treatment of obstructive pulmonary disease lead to increases in blood pressure.

Diabetes mellitus often coexists in elderly hyperten-

Table 3 Pathophysiologic Characteristics of Elderly Patients with Hypertension

Cardiovascular Hemodynamics
   Increased peripheral vascular resistance
   Normal or decreased cardiac output
   Normal or reduced intravascular volume
   Decreased baroreceptor sensitivity
   Increased blood pressure variability
   Normal or reduced renal blood flow
Renal Factors
   Tendency to salt retention
   Decreased renal production of prostaglandins and other
      natriuretic factors
   Decreased renin production
   Increased renal vascular resistance
Metabolic Factors
   Tendency to increased adiposity
   Enhanced sympathetic nervous system activity
   Hyperinsulinemia and insulin resistance
Cellular Cation Abnormalities
   Increased intracellular sodium and calcium
   Decreased sodium pump activity
   Decreased Ca^{2+}-ATPase with insulin resistance
Dietary Factors
   Relatively high salt intake
   Low dietary potassium, calcium, and magnesium
   Relatively high-fat diets
   Relatively low-fiber intake

sive patients. These patients frequently have some degree of cardiac and renal decompensation. Diuretics and beta-blockers often worsen glucose intolerance in these patients, and beta-blockers may mask as well as prolong hypoglycemia. These considerations, along with the decrease in drug metabolism seen in the elderly, make the older hypertensive population more subject to adverse drug effects.

A nonpharmacologic approach should be the initial therapy for most patients with mild to moderate hypertension. This is particularly true for elderly patients, who are perhaps more likely to experience complications from antihypertensive drugs. Even if such agents are necessary, nonpharmacologic therapy should be continued in conjunction with drug therapy.

Weight reduction is clearly beneficial in reducing blood pressure. Obese hypertensive patients may be more motivated to lose weight if told that a significant reduction in blood pressure occurs with only a modest weight loss (5 to 10 percent). Walking for 15 to 20 minutes each day is usually well tolerated by older individuals. Sodium restriction is also an effective form of therapy, particularly in low-renin forms of hypertension, typically seen in the elderly. Potassium and, perhaps, calcium and magnesium supplementation may also be indicated in elderly hypertensive patients who are deficient in these nutrients.

The choice of pharmacologic agent to initiate therapy in elderly hypertensive patients depends on a number of factors. Cost, frequency of dosing, and side effects must be considered. Diuretics are frequently employed to treat hypertension in the elderly. Diuretics of intermediate duration, such as hydrochlorothiazide and chlorthalidone, should be used in smaller dosages in elderly patients, in the range of 12.5 to 25 mg per day. Larger dosages may lead to hypokalemia and hypomagnesemia, which can cause serious cardiac arrhythmias. This is especially true for elderly patients who may have underlying heart disease and who are also taking digitalis. In larger dosages, diuretics may also promote magnesium deficiency through excess renal excretion of this cation. Magnesium deficiency may in turn make it more difficult to correct potassium deficiencies. Hypokalemia is also partially responsible for the glucose intolerance associated with diuretic use. Furthermore, hyperosmolar-nonketotic diabetic coma is more likely to occur with thiazide therapy in elderly patients with renal impairment. Other side effects such as increased uric acid, altered lipoprotein metabolism, and impotence can also result from diuretic therapy. These derangements, and their possible role in increasing cardiovascular morbidity and mortality, make diuretics somewhat less than ideal therapy. Newer agents such as calcium channel blockers, alpha-adrenergic blockers, and ACE inhibitors are being used increasingly as first-line antihypertensive therapy in the elderly. All of these drugs are discussed in the chapter *Hypertension in the Elderly*.

Compliance is a concern in treating elderly patients with antihypertensive drugs. Improved compliance can be accomplished by using a simple regimen with a minimum of side effects. Because of an age-related loss of homeostatic adaptability, the elderly are particularly prone to side effects from antihypertensive medications. Dizziness and orthostatic falls are more likely to occur in the elderly because of reduced baroreceptor sensitivity, decreased cerebral blood flow autoregulation, and limited compensatory cardiovascular responses to reductions in intravascular volume. Thus, one must use considerable caution when prescribing drugs that have a tendency to cause orthostatic hypotension. It is also important to avoid other classes of drugs that can aggravate hypertension in the elderly. For example, decongestants and bronchodilators, both of which can elevate blood pressure, are commonly used by the geriatric population. Nonsteroidal anti-inflammatory agents, commonly used in older patients, may cause salt and water retention and compromise renal productive mechanisms called forth to overcome renal ischemia (i.e., renal prostaglandin production). Compliance can also be improved in elderly patients by carefully instructing them and their families in the mechanics of taking the medication, and by emphasizing the importance of compliance in preventing cardiovascular events.

PREGNANCY-INDUCED HYPERTENSION (PIH)

High blood pressure development, de novo, during pregnancy is referred to as pregnancy-induced hypertension (PIH). When this condition is accompanied by proteinuria, it is often referred to as preeclampsia, although proteinuria is just one of the many clinical manifestations of the severity of this disorder. PIH and preeclampsia affect at least 5 to 6 percent of all nulliparous pregnant women and up to 10 percent of nulliparous, indigent, inner-city pregnant women, causing striking increases in both maternal and fetal/neonatal morbidity and mortality.

Pathophysiology

The pathophysiology of PIH is poorly understood but may include alterations in systemic hemodynamics, renal hemodynamics, cellular cation metabolism, prostaglandin metabolism, endocrine function, and uteroplacental function. Enhanced maternal vascular reactivity is generally considered to be an important factor in the pathogenesis of PIH. Increased vascular pressor sensitivity to angiotensin II has been observed even in the normotensive phase of pregnancies that progress to PIH. This enhanced vascular responsivity is in sharp contrast to normal pregnancy, which is characterized by reduced peripheral vascular resistance, as well as blunted vascular responsiveness to the pressor effects of angiotensin II.

Increased intracellular calcium in the vascular smooth muscle is a major determinant of peripheral vascular resistance. Platelets have been used as surrogates for study of intracellular calcium in vascular smooth muscle because of their accessibility and because they have anatomic and functional similarities to vascular smooth muscle. In prospective studies we have found that platelets from women with PIH displayed substantially greater intracellular calcium in response to the vasoconstrictor vasopressin. This abnormality was manifested in the first trimester of pregnancy (preceding differences in vascular resistance) and it persisted through the second and third trimesters. In fact, discriminant analysis demonstrated that this abnormal response predicted the subsequent development of PIH (Table 4).

Dietary factors have been suggested to be important in the pathogenesis of PIH. For example, studies conducted in populations with a high incidence of PIH and a relatively low dietary calcium intake have shown that dietary calcium supplementation significantly reduces the incidence of PIH. Other animal and human studies have indicated the possibility that dietary deficiencies of essential fatty acids and magnesium may play a role in the pathogenesis of PIH. The roles of excessive caloric intake and obesity are poorly delineated for this disease.

Nonpharmacologic and Pharmacologic Approaches to Management

At present, insufficient clinical data are available to support the use of supplements of calcium, magnesium, and essential free fatty acids to prevent PIH. Good general maternal health care and well-rounded diets appear prudent. Several decades ago some experts recommended dietary salt restriction to prevent and treat PIH. Today, however, most authorities no longer advocate dietary salt restriction or the use of diuretics, because both interventions tend to aggravate the hypovolemic state already present in PIH, and potentially worsen renal and placental function. Further, there have been no well-controlled studies to determine the efficacy of volume expansion in PIH. Bed rest and hospitalization are generally considered appropriate interventions for PIH. Bed rest with lateral recumbency appear to be associated with the mobilization of interstitial fluid to the intravascular space, reductions in activity of the sympathetic nervous system, reductions in vascular resistance, and improved uterine and renal blood flow.

Preliminary data suggest that low-dose aspirin may reduce the incidence of PIH. More extensive controlled trials, currently in progress, must be completed before the safety and efficacy of low-dose aspirin can be determined. Further, the safety and effectiveness of theophylline and beta-adrenergic agents in decreasing peripheral vascular reactivity are still in the investigational stage and remain to be documented. Specific thromboxane receptor inhibitors are currently being tested for safety and efficacy in PIH.

Pharmacologic therapy for PIH has traditionally depended on the use of antihypertensive agents such as methyldopa (Aldomet) and hydralazine (Apresoline) over a number of years. Of the newer products currently on the market, the calcium channel blockers probably offer the most potential in treating PIH. Studies conducted in Europe have primarily evaluated nifedipine, which appeared to be both safe and effective in several clinical studies employing this agent for blood pressure reduction in hospitalized patients with PIH. Larger controlled trials need to be conducted to better determine the safety and efficacy of various calcium antagonists in the treatment of PIH.

Table 4 Pathophysiologic Characteristics of Pregnancy-Induced Hypertension

Cardiovascular Hemodynamics
  Increased peripheral vascular resistance
  Enhanced pressor responses to angiotensin II and other vasoactive agonists
  Normal to increased cardiac output
  Reduced intravascular volume
  Increased platelet aggregation
  Vascular endothelial dysfunction (?)
Demographic Factors
  More common in:
    Nulliparous women
    Indigent women
    Black inner-city women
    Populations with low dietary calcium
Cation Abnormalities
  Increased intracellular calcium
  Increased cell-free calcium responses to vasoactive agents such as vasopressin
  Decreased cell membrane Ca^{2+}-ATPase activity
Metabolic Factors
  Hyperinsulinism and insulin resistance
  Elevated levels of atrial natriuretic peptide
  Elevated levels of digitalis-like sodium pump inhibitor
  Imbalance between thromboxane (inappropriately high) and inappropriately low prostacyclin production
  Decreased progesterone production

SUGGESTED READING

Falkner B. Differences in blacks and whites with essential hypertension. Biochem Endocr Hypertens 1990; 15:681–686.

Lindheimer MD, Katz AI. Hypertension in pregnancy. N Engl J Med 1985; 313:675–680.

Otsfeld ASM. Epidemiologic overview. In: Horan MJ, Steinberg GM, Dunbar JB, Hadley EC, eds. Blood pressure regulation and aging. New York: Biomedical Information Corporation, 1987:3.

Sowers JR. Hypertension in the elderly. Am J Med 1987; 82(Suppl 1B):1–8.

Sowers JR, Levy J, Zemel MB. Hypertension in diabetes. Med Clin North Am 1988; 72:1399–1414.

Sowers JR, Zemel MB. Clinical implications of hypertension in the diabetic patient. Am J Hypertens 1990; 3:415–424.

Sowers JR, Zemel MB, Bronsteen RA, et al. Erythrocyte cation metabolism in preeclampsia. Am J Obstet Gynecol 1989; 161: 441–445.

Sowers JR, Zemel MB, Zemel P, et al. Salt sensitivity in blacks. Salt intake and natriuretic substances. Hypertension 1988; 12:485–490.

Zemel MB, Zemel PC, Berry S, et al. Altered platelet calcium metabolism as an early predictor of increased peripheral vascular resistance and preeclampsia in urban black women. N Engl J Med 1990; 323:434–438.

HYPERTENSIVE HEART DISEASE

EDWARD D. FROHLICH, M.D., F.A.C.C.

Cardiac disease in the patient with hypertension may be expressed in a myriad of clinical forms. Most frequently, it may be considered as an adaptive response of the left ventricle (LV) to the increasing afterload imposed on it by the continually rising total peripheral resistance (TPR) and arterial pressure produced by the progressive vascular disease of essential hypertension. Under these circumstances, the ventricle increases its mass by the structurally adaptive mechanism of concentric left ventricular hypertrophy (LVH) in order to minimize the net pathophysiologic consequences of this afterload and to increase its efficiency of contraction. When the heart can no longer adapt functionally or structurally to this progressing afterload, congestive heart failure (CHF) supervenes.

In part, the foregoing concept is correct. However, the myocardial response of hypertrophy does not necessarily follow the functional changes; these two adaptive processes occur simultaneously. Thus, coincident with the increased demands to which the LV is subjected by the increasing afterload, the biologic "transducers" of the cardiac myocyte respond by increasing its force of contraction and by initiating the structural process of adaptive hypertrophy.

Also, the heart does not seem to be subjected in each patient with hypertension to a pure pressure overload. In some patients, there may be an additional component of volume overload. Although the circulating intravascular volume contracts in proportion to the increasing systemic resistance in most patients with essential hypertension, in most patients with essential hypertension, in some patients (e.g., blacks and the elderly) volume contracts to a lesser degree. In still other patients, there is a direct correlation between the height of arterial pressure and an increase in the circulating blood volume, i.e., those with exogenous obesity, steroidal dependence, or parenchymal disease of the kidney. It is this volume component that serves as an increased LV preload, promoting a structural adaptation that may be reflected as an eccentric form of LVH. Thus, in these patients, there is a dual overload of the LV, thereby promoting a "dimorphic" hypertrophic structural response that facilitates the likelihood of CHF and that increases the cardiac risk in these patients.

One further concept should be considered. Hypertension is frequently associated with other diseases, the most common being atherosclerotic (i.e., ischemic coronary arterial) heart disease. Other diseases that often coexist with hypertension are diabetes mellitus, exogenous obesity, hyperlipidemia, and hyperuricemia; and each of these problems complicates the formulation of a meaningful therapeutic program for the individual patient. These concepts should be kept in mind as we consider the therapy for the specific patient with the general problem of "hypertensive heart disease."

BORDERLINE OR MILD ESSENTIAL HYPERTENSION

Any patient with an elevated arterial pressure, even if the problem is one of borderline or mild essential hypertension, has hypertensive heart disease. The heart is already subjected to an increased pressure overload for which it must adapt functionally and structurally. Borderline hypertension exists in an individual whose diastolic pressure is intermittently elevated (i.e., greater than 89 mm Hg). Recent studies (the Framingham and Tecumseh Heart Studies) have demonstrated that these patients are at increased risk of cardiovascular morbidity and mortality and their condition may already be associated with target organ involvement from hypertension (including LVH).

Pathophysiology

Frequently, patients with this early expression of hypertension demonstrate physiologic evidence of a hyperkinetic circulation. This may be manifested by a faster heart rate, enhanced myocardial contractility, elevated cardiac output, and a normal TPR. However, were normotensive individuals to have the same degree of cardiac output elevation, their TPR would be reduced; hence, their TPR is "inappropriately normal." Furthermore, the elevated cardiac output is in direct proportion to the increase in venous return and cardiopulmonary volume. Since the intravascular volume is not expanded, the increased cardiopulmonary volume reflects a redistributed circulating volume to the central circulation from the periphery as a result of peripheral venoconstriction (because the circulating volume is primarily contained in the veins and venules). Thus, patients with borderline and mild essential hypertension provide evidence of a hyperdynamic circulation associated with both arteriolar and venular constriction. Moreover, a number of studies have related these changes to increased circulating levels of norepinephrine.

Therapy

These changes suggest that the presence of increased participation of adrenergic mechanisms could be suppressed best by adrenergic inhibiting agents, and the beta-adrenoceptor blocking drugs have been used in some of these patients with safety and efficacy. These agents (e.g., propranolol, timolol, nadolol, atenolol, metoprolol) reduce arterial pressure, heart rate, and cardiac output, but tend to increase TPR. However, there are regional differences in the effect of beta-blockers on vascular resistance; renal vascular resistance frequently decreases, whereas coronary, skeletal muscle, and splanchnic vascular resistance increases. With the introduction of newer agents (e.g., labetalol) that also inhibit alpha-adrenergic receptor sites, a reduction in TPR is possible. More recently, a new generation of beta-adrenergic inhibiting drugs has been introduced that inhibit $beta_1$, and stimulate $beta_2$ receptor sites. The hemodynamic consequence is that these agents inhibit the cardiac beta-receptors (to reduce cardiac contractility and heart rate) but stimulate vascular beta-receptors (to reduce TPR), thereby reducing arterial pressure.

HYPERDYNAMIC BETA-ADRENERGIC CIRCULATORY STATE

For hundreds of years, practitioners of medicine have been aware of a population of patients having symptoms of cardiac awareness (e.g., palpitations, awareness of irregularity of cardiac action, chest discomfort), flushing, and feelings of anxiety or hysteria. These patients have been reported since the time of Avicenna (the first description I have found). The condition has been described variously as the soldier's heart syndrome, irritable heart syndrome, neurocirculatory asthenia, hyperkinetic heart syndrome, and, more recently, as the hyperdynamic beta-adrenergic circulatory state.

Pathophysiology

Some of these patients may have an elevated arterial pressure, although some may be normotensive; also, those patients who are normotensive may demonstrate an inordinate delay in the return of arterial pressure to normotensive levels after exercise. Not infrequently, these patients develop cardiovascular symptoms associated with normal (physiologic) adrenergic stimulation (e.g., when assuming upright posture, with exercise, or with emotional disturbances). When evaluated clinically, they may have flushed skin, inappropriate diaphoresis, dilated pupils, cardiac dysrhythmias, an inappropriately fast heart rate, a systolic apical click suggesting a mitral valve prolapse, a systolic ejection–type flow murmur, and perhaps an elevated arterial pressure (isolated systolic hypertension or diastolic hypertension). It is of interest that laboratory studies are usually unrevealing, including studies of thyroidal function; studies to exclude pheochromocytoma (although serum or urinary catecholamine levels may be slightly elevated, they are not in the range of levels compatible with that diagnosis); and studies of 5-hydroxy-indoleacetic acid (to exclude the possibility of carcinoid).

When studied physiologically, these patients demonstrate an elevated cardiac output and increased myocardial contractility associated with the faster heart rate. Upright tilting may provoke an excessive increase in heart rate, cardiac output, myocardial contractility, and arterial pressure. These hemodynamic findings are not provoked by intravenous administration of atropine. However, even in the supine position, if the beta-adrenotropic agonist isoproterenol is infused, it will provoke the abnormal hemodynamic findings associated with the same disturbing symptoms (including frank hysteria) that had precipitated the patient's need to seek medical advice. Indeed, beta-adrenergic receptor responsiveness in these patients is increased. Normally, a low dose of isoproterenol (0.01 µg per kilogram per minute) will induce an increase in heart rate of 4 to 8 beats per minute; with higher doses (0.02 to 0.04 µg per kilogram per minute), heart rate will increase to a maximum of 12 to 18 beats per minute. By contrast, in the patient with the hyperdynamic circulatory state, heart rate may increase by 32 to 40 beats per minute at the lowest dose of isoproterenol.

Therapy

Each of the above abnormal clinical and hemodynamic findings can be either prevented or corrected by slow intravenous injection of propranolol (10 mg). Moreover, with prolonged daily oral treatment with any of the usual beta-adrenergic receptor blocking drugs, (e.g., propranolol, 160 mg or atenolol, 100 mg), the symptoms and abnormal findings will be reversed and normalized.

IDIOPATHIC MITRAL VALVE PROLAPSE SYNDROME

As might be inferred from the discussion of the symptoms and findings in patients with the hyperdynamic beta-adrenergic circulatory syndrome, the condition of these patients often suggests the possible diagnosis of idiopathic mitral valve prolapse syndrome. Indeed, if the patient shows the findings of this condition (e.g., systolic click, echocardiographic demonstration of mitral valve prolapse), the diagnosis is likely. I have found that many patients with borderline or mild essential hypertension, or with the hyperdynamic beta-adrenergic circulatory state, also have idiopathic mitral valve prolapse syndrome. It may well be that each clinical problem is but a forme fruste of the same problem. Thus, the increased responsiveness of the myocardial beta-adrenergic receptors serves to pull the posterior leaflets of the mitral valve downward, so that a functional prolapse and insufficiency of the mitral valve result. This may occur in both normotensive and hypertensive patients; the findings may be provoked by isoproterenol infusion and may remit with beta-adrenergic blockade.

LEFT VENTRICULAR HYPERTROPHY

Mechanisms

As indicated earlier, as hypertensive vascular disease progresses, TPR increases, and so does the afterload imposed on the LV. Also as stated, the structural response of the myocardium is one of a concentric LVH. Occasionally there is an eccentric component to the LVH that may be due to genetic factors or to superimposed volume overload. The hemodynamic factors that overload the LV are of primary clinical concern, although in recent years it has been determined that other factors participate in the development of LVH. Among these nonhemodynamic factors are age, race, and gender; the stage and severity of the hypertensive disease; associated clinical diseases (e.g., coronary arterial disease, atherosclerosis, exogenous obesity, diabetes mellitus); humoral and tissue growth factors; and the antihypertensive agents employed.

Diagnosis

Clearly, the chest roentgenogram and electrocardiogram (ECG) have been useful for the clinical detection of LVH. Many ECG criteria have been employed to identify LVH, but there are a number of associated false-positive and false-negative diagnoses. Nevertheless, as shown by the Framingham Heart Study, when these LVH criteria are present, a very severe and ominous independent risk is imparted to the affected patient.

Some of the earliest ECG findings that precede the QRS voltage, ST-segment, and T-wave changes of LVH are the ECG findings of left atrial enlargement. This abnormality reflects early development of LVH and its associated reduced distensibility that impairs LV filling during diastasis. As a result, the atrium enlarges and hypertrophies in order to assist with diastolic filling of the LV. This, then, represents an ECG correlate of abnormal (i.e., impaired) diastolic filling.

A far more sensitive means for detecting LVH is by echocardiography. Thus, many patients with normal ECG findings may already demonstrate echocardiographic evidence of LVH, as indicated by an increased LV mass and its posterior and septal wall thicknesses. Furthermore, these patients all have left atrial enlargement and impaired LV filling indices, and may also demonstrate evidence of impaired LV systolic contractile function (e.g., reduced LV ejection fraction and fiber shortening rate).

With increasing arterial pressure, therefore, there is a greater likelihood that LVH will be detected by these diagnostic modalities. However, there are patients with elevated arterial pressures whom one might expect to have LVH, but who do not; conversely, there are patients whose arterial pressures are not severely elevated, yet LVH is evident.

Risk

LVH confers an independent risk of premature morbidity and mortality. However, we do not know at this time whether a decrease of LV mass will reverse the increased risk. Moreover, we are not certain which factor or factors promote the increased risk associated with LVH. Is it the LVH itself; cardiac dysrhythmias or sudden death associated with LVH; associated

absolute (or even relative) decrease in coronary blood flow or flow reserve; other factors alone; or a combination of the above changes that account for the risk? It is important that this problem be approached by effective control of arterial pressure and, it seems reasonable with reversal of the hypertrophy process (as long as no other abnormalities are induced by treatment).

Therapy

All patients with elevated arterial pressure, whether it is associated with LVH or not, should be treated. This treatment should provide the best control of arterial pressure that is feasible using the fewest antihypertensive drugs, at their lowest possible dosages, and, if possible, by administering this therapy once daily. Today, these therapeutic possibilities are not only feasible but readily available. Detailed discussion concerning the selection of initial pharmacologic therapy is presented in the chapter *Initial Pharmacologic Therapy,* and subsequent chapters outline appropriate therapy for specific patient groups.

A major goal of any reasonable antihypertensive treatment program is to prevent the development of LVH. However, once LVH has occurred, most antihypertensive drug regimens will attenuate or even reverse the hypertrophic process if used for a sufficient time.

In recent years, certain classes of antihypertensive therapeutic agents have been said to reverse LVH better than others. Among these have been centrally active adrenergic inhibiting compounds (the prototype of which is methyldopa), beta-adrenergic receptor blocking agents, angiotensin converting enzyme (ACE) inhibitors, and calcium antagonists. These agents predictably diminish LV mass, and they are highly effective antihypertensive drugs in controlling arterial pressure. The reason they have been said to be better is that they have been shown to diminish LV mass in a very short time (4 to 12 weeks).

Selection of Antihypertensive Therapy

How does one select an agent for a patient with LVH? I generally prescribe a beta-blocker for the patient with LVH associated with a hyperkinetic circulation, idiopathic mitral valve prolapse, or supraventricular ectopic beats. I may also use a beta-blocking agent if the patient has coronary arterial disease with angina pectoris. On the other hand, if the foregoing conditions are not present, if there are contraindications, or if the angina pectoris is not adequately controlled with the beta-blocking drug, I prescribe a calcium antagonist or an ACE inhibitor. However, if the patient has had a previous myocardial infarction, I may continue with the beta-blocker (perhaps at a higher dose) or add a calcium antagonist to a lower dose of the beta-blocker. However, if the patient has evidence of impaired systolic function or if there are findings that suggest CHF, an ACE inhibitor may be selected.

Hypokalemia

The patient with LVH is highly predisposed to ventricular irritability. For this reason, if the patient is already receiving a diuretic, particular care must be taken to prevent hypokalemia. Thus, if one wishes to maintain the diuretic together with other antihypertensive therapy, a potassium-retaining agent (e.g., triamterene, amiloride, or spironolactone) may be added to the treatment program in combination with the thiazide diuretic. This concern about hypokalemia should be kept in mind, especially if the patient is already receiving a digitalis preparation, whether or not diuretic-induced hypokalemia is encountered. Thus, if both agents (digitalis and a diuretic) are being used, it is important that particular care be taken to prevent hypokalemia and cardiac dysrhythmias.

HYPERTENSIVE AND ISCHEMIC HEART DISEASE

Pathophysiology

As already indicated, hypertensive heart disease, with or without associated LVH, facilitates the development of atherosclerosis, particularly of the coronary arteries. Thus, coexistent symptomatic or asymptomatic coronary arterial disease should always be considered as a possibility in a patient with hypertension. This possibility of ischemic heart disease is even more likely in the presence of LVH. Under these circumstances, the elevated arterial pressure and the increased cardiac size both serve to increase myocardial wall tension, and thus, myocardial oxygen demands. In this latter situation, occlusive coronary arterial disease may not even be present.

Therapy

In all patients with hypertension and LVH, when any situation occurs to suggest underlying coronary arterial insufficiency, it is important to assess the patient for possible ischemic heart disease. This may be suggested by the appearance of symptoms indicating early CHF, angina pectoris, or the development of cardiac dysrhythmias during everyday activities, on exercise treadmill, or by Holter monitoring studies. Under these circumstances, particularly if there is no evidence of coronary arterial disease (from other studies) or if there is no indication for surgical intervention, an agent that directly dilates the coronary arteries (e.g., a calcium antagonist) is particularly indicated. In these patients, a situation may exist that is not unlike silent ischemia for a nonhypertensive patient. The calcium antagonists are indicated for the treatment of hypertension in these patients, but particular care should be exercised in selecting these agents (e.g., verapamil, diltiazem) if there is any concern about negative inotropic effects or undue slowing of cardiac rate.

HYPERTENSION AND CARDIAC FAILURE

Left ventricular failure may supervene when the LV can no longer adapt to its increasing overload. Under this circumstance, when CHF exists, the use of an ACE inhibitor is particularly indicated. The agent may be administered cautiously as a single dose. If the patient is already receiving antihypertensive therapy, it is important to prescribe the ACE inhibitor initially in its lowest dosage. A rapidly acting agent, such as captopril, can be given in a dosage of 12.5 to 25 mg in the office setting where the patient can be observed for a few hours to make certain that undue hypotension is not produced. The same agent (or another ACE inhibitor) can then be prescribed. It is important to emphasize that the patient with hypertension receiving an ACE inhibitor will be very sensitive (inordinate hypotension) to an administered diuretic agent. Thus, when prescribing therapy for an untreated patient with mild CHF, it is important not to overprescribe or use multiple therapy unless this is necessary.

Another condition noted in the patient with cardiac failure is secondary hyperaldosteronism. Under these circumstances, hypokalemic alkalosis is present, and it is important not to prescribe a diuretic unless the patient is protected from the attendant dysrhythmic complications of hypokalemia (and possibly also hypomagnesemia).

The patient with hypertension who suddenly develops CHF should be suspected to have significant myocardial ischemia or infarction. Clearly, the usual diagnostic and therapeutic interventions should be pursued for such a patient. After a myocardial infarction, antihypertensive treatment with an ACE inhibitor may be particularly appropriate. The ACE inhibitor will control arterial pressure and any attendant CHF, and (as recent studies have suggested) may even remodel the myocardium and prevent the further progression of CHF.

DISCUSSION

The physician should consider any patient with hypertension as having hypertensive heart disease. The mere elevation of arterial pressure increases the myocardial demand for oxygen delivery. Superimposed on this state are the augmented needs of the hypertrophied LV for oxygen as myocardial wall tension increases further. When the heart can adapt no longer through the processes of hypertrophy, cardiac failure will supervene. The best way to treat LVH and CHF in hypertension is to control arterial pressure early so as to prevent the development of LVH. It is not known whether reversal of LVH by pharmacologic means will reduce the independent risk that is imparted by this abnormality. Nevertheless, most antihypertensive therapy that controls arterial pressure will attenuate or reverse the hypertrophic process if administered for sufficient time.

Certain agents reverse hypertrophy in a short period (4 to 12 weeks). In this case, selection of an ACE inhibitor is particularly suitable if there is additional suggestion of LV failure, and selection of a calcium antagonist is likewise suitable for a patient with coexisting coronary arterial insufficiency (with or without coexisting occlusive disease). In patients with angina pectoris or a previous myocardial infarction, a beta-adrenergic blocking agent is also merited. Moreover, beta-blockers are also useful for patients with a hyperdynamic circulation, whether it be related to borderline or mild essential hypertension, hyperkinetic heart syndrome, hyperdynamic beta-adrenergic circulatory state, associated idiopathic mitral valve prolapse, or ectopic or supraventricular extrasystoles. In the final analysis, the best therapy for hypertensive heart disease is vigorous treatment and control of arterial pressure before cardiac involvement is clinically manifested.

SUGGESTED READING

Bakris GL, Frohlich ED. The evolution of antihypertensive therapy: An overview of four decades of experience. J Am Coll Cardiol 1989; 14:1595–1608.

Frohlich ED. Left ventricular hypertrophy: An independent factor of risk. In: Frohlich ED, Brest AN, eds. Preventive aspects of coronary heart disease. Philadelphia: FA Davis, 1990:85.
Frohlich ED. Hypertension. In: Rakel RE, ed. Conn's current therapy 1989. Philadelphia: WB Saunders, 1989:225.
Frohlich ED. LVH, cardiac diseases and hypertension: Recent experiences. J Am Coll Cardiol 1989; 14:1587–1594.
Frohlich ED. Overview of hemodynamic and non-hemodynamic factors associated with LVH. J Mol Cell Cardiol 1989; 21:3–10.
Frohlich ED (state of the art). The first Irvine H. Page lecture: The mosaic of hypertension: past, present, and future. J Hypertens 1988; 6(Suppl 4):S2–S11.
Frohlich ED. Cardiac hypertrophy in hypertension. N Engl J Med 1987; 317:831–833.
Frohlich ED. Evaluation and management of the patient with essential hypertension. In: Parmley WM, Chatterjee K, eds. Cardiology. Vol 2. Cardiovascular disease. Philadelphia: JB Lippincott, 1987:1.
Frohlich ED. Hypertensive emergencies: A paradigm for tailoring antihypertensive therapy. J Intensive Care Med 1987; 2:123–125.
Frohlich ED, Tarazi RC, Dustan HP. Clinical-physiological correlations in the development of hypertensive heart disease. Circulation 1971; 44:446–455.
Frohlich ED, Tarazi RC, Dustan HP. Hyperdynamic beta-adrenergic circulatory state: Increased beta receptor responsiveness. Arch Intern Med 1969; 123:1–7.
The Joint National Committee on the Detection, Evaluation, and Treatment of High Blood Pressure (member). The 1988 report. Arch Intern Med 1988; 148:1023–1038.

HYPERTENSIVE EMERGENCIES

C. VENKATA S. RAM, M.D.
ALEXANDER S. KHOURY, M.D.

Hypertensive crises occur in many clinical syndromes in which rapid blood pressure reduction is indicated to prevent serious complications. Although less common in clinical practice, a hypertensive crisis should be promptly diagnosed and treated. Any form of hypertension may be associated with the development of hypertensive crisis, the chief determinant being the level of blood pressure rather than the cause of the hypertension. A crucial factor in the development of hypertensive crisis is the rapidity with which the blood pressure rises as this factor seems to affect the development more than does the absolute level of blood pressure in certain clinical situations—e.g., acute onset of hypertension in children with acute glomerulonephritis, eclampsia acquired during pregnancy, and drug-induced hypertension. In some clinical circumstances the immediate reduction of blood pressure is indicated not because of its absolute level but because the coexisting complications may make even moderate hypertension dangerous, as in aortic dissection or acute left ventricular failure.

Hypertensive crises are conveniently categorized into emergencies and urgencies in Table 1. Hypertensive emergencies carry poor prognoses unless the blood pressure declines rapidly, whereas hypertensive urgencies pose less immediate danger; they become emergencies, however, if the blood pressure is not vigorously controlled.

ACCELERATED AND MALIGNANT HYPERTENSION

The characteristic difference between uncomplicated and accelerated or malignant hypertension is the presence of acute vascular lesions in the kidney and in other target organs in accelerated or malignant hypertension. Accelerated hypertension is identified by the presence of severe retinal abnormalities (without papilledema) in the form of exudates, hemorrhages, arteriolar narrowing, and spasm. Malignant hypertension, an extension of the accelerated form, is distinguished by the presence of papilledema. Both the accelerated and malignant forms of hypertension are associated with clinical evidence of severe vascular injury to the kidney and other target organs. Studies have shown that when effective antihypertensive therapy is unavailable, malignant hypertension runs a short clinical course that culminates in renal failure and death. With the advent of effective antihypertensive therapy, how-

Table 1 Examples of Hypertensive Emergencies and Urgencies

Emergencies	Urgencies
Hypertensive encephalopathy	Hypertension associated with coronary artery disease
Acute aortic dissection	
Pulmonary edema	Accelerated and malignant hypertension*
Pheochromocytoma crisis	
MAO inhibitor + tyramine interaction	Severe hypertension in patient receiving kidney transplant
Intracranial hemorrhage	Postoperative hypertension
Eclampsia	Uncontrolled hypertension in the patient who requires emergency surgery

*This condition is categorized as either hypertensive emergency or urgency.

ever, the prognosis has improved, with more than 90 percent of the treated patients surviving more than 5 years; also, no significant difference has been found in the course of accelerated or malignant disease, which suggests that the two types of hypertension can be considered part of the same process.

Pathogenesis

What transforms a previously stable hypertension state to a "malignant" course? Usually, it is the level of blood pressure; a critical feature does not explain the onset of malignant hypertension, however, as considerable overlap has been found between blood pressure levels in patients with uncomplicated and malignant hypertension. The stimulation of various vasoactive mechanisms such as renin-angiotensin, catecholamines, vasopressin, the kallikrein-kinin system, and hemostasis have been implicated in the genesis of malignant hypertension. To date, however, no convincing evidence has been presented to relate the vascular abnormalities of malignant hypertension to any of these neurohumoral derangements. The arteriolar lesions responsible for the clinical manifestations and course of malignant hypertension are found in many organs including kidney, brain, heart, intestine, and pancreas.

The consequence of obstructive vascular lesions is a decrease in perfusion to the affected organs, with the kidney bearing the main damage. Two different renal lesions have been described in malignant hypertension: proliferative arteritis and fibrinoid necrosis. The combination of these lesions is also referred to as *hyperplastic arteritis, fibrinoid intimal hyperplasia,* and *musculomucoid intimal hyperplasia* (Fig. 1). Fibrinoid necrosis presumably results from the leakage of fibrin and other plasma elements into the arteriolar wall thereby resulting in obstruction and compromising the function of the organ involved, which is usually the kidney. The precise link between the blood pressure level and arteriolar lesions is not established. It has been suggested that vascular permeability increases as a result of alternating contracted and dilated segments in the arterial vessels and that, with the treatment of hypertension, these abnormalities are eliminated. The immediate treatment of

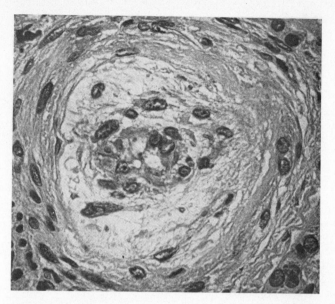

Figure 1 Characteristic changes of an interlobular artery in malignant hypertension. (From Kincaid-Smith P. Participation of intravascular coagulation in the pathogenesis of glomerular and vascular lesions. Kidney Int 1975; 7:242; with permission.)

hypertension arrests or even reverses the arteriolar damage, thus paving the way for functional restoration.

Plasma renin activity is markedly elevated in patients with malignant hypertension. One mechanism postulates an initial spontaneous sodium loss as the most likely cause. In experimental malignant hypertension, the lumen of the efferent renal arteriole remains unchanged, whereas the caliber of the afferent arteriole increases in size. Angiotensin sensitivity is augmented in the afferent arteriole, whereas the efferent arteriole shows hypersensitivity to both norepinephrine and angiotensin. This differential in sensitivity to circulating levels of angiotensin increases intraglomerular pressure and promotes natriuresis, which in turn stimulates the release of renin, vasopressin, and norepinephrine, thereby initiating a vicious cycle. Initial weight loss, a phenomenon observed in patients with malignant hypertension, may be caused by the loss of salt and water. The course of malignant hypertension has been curtailed in experimental and clinical studies by administering a saline load. The renin-angiotensin system may therefore play some role in the pathogenesis of malignant hypertension. This system is obviously also involved in hypertension caused by renovascular disease. In one series reported by Davis and co-workers, renal artery stenosis was detected in 35 percent of 123 patients with malignant hypertension. Cigarette smoking, immunologic changes, and oral contraceptive use have also been implicated in the development of malignant hypertension.

Clinical Manifestations

The blood pressure level in patients with malignant hypertension is usually very high, with diastolic levels often reaching to more than 130 to 140 mm Hg, but the degree of blood pressure elevation is not the sole diagnostic attribute. The elevation of blood pressure has to occur abruptly, and, most importantly, it is the extent of vascular damage that determines the clinical manifestations and course. Headache with or without coexisting encephalic disorder is the most common symptom that prompts the patient to seek medical attention. Typically, the headache is occipitally located and more intense in the morning hours. Weight loss, as discussed earlier, may occur in some patients with malignant hypertension as a result of salt and water loss. A majority of patients with malignant hypertension report visual symptoms. Drowsiness and altered mental status are commonly observed in patients with malignant hypertension. Any worsening of these symptoms may indicate progression to encephalic abnormalities or cerebral hemorrhage.

Congestive heart failure can occur in patients with malignant hypertension as a direct consequence of left ventricular dysfunction or as a result of volume retention from associated renal insufficiency. Azotemia, a common feature of malignant hypertension, may be associated with proteinuria. Without effective treatment, renal function deteriorates rapidly and even with appropriate treatment, the renal function may decline temporarily because of reduced renal perfusion. Although hypertension can result from chronic renal disease, renal failure in patients with malignant hypertension is a result rather than a cause of severe hypertension. Anemia is also a common finding in patients with malignant hypertension. The degree of anemia may give a clue as to the proximate cause; severe anemia suggests underlying chronic renal disease whereas mild-to-moderate anemia may reflect microangiopathic hemolysis.

The diagnosis of accelerated and malignant hypertension can be made at the bedside on the basis of the patient's history and clinical examination. Simple investigations such as chest radiography, electrocardiography (ECG), a complete blood count (CBC), blood urea nitrogen (BUN) analysis, creatinine and electrolyte measurements, and urinalysis are sufficient for the initial management of malignant hypertension.

Management

Patients with accelerated or malignant hypertension should be treated in the hospital, as the goal is not simply to lower the blood pressure level but to monitor, stabilize, and reverse the damage to target organs and to exclude reversible causes. Ideally, the patient should be treated in an intensive care unit. In the absence of significant target organ dysfunction, however, these patients can be managed safely on the medical wards.

Although sodium restriction was successfully used to treat malignant hypertension decades ago, as discussed earlier, sodium wasting may be a feature of this condition. Therefore, sodium restriction is not necessary during early treatment unless there is evidence of fluid overload. Similarly, the need for immediate diuretic therapy must be individualized. Diuretic therapy may be

needed to potentiate the hypotensive effects of certain vasodilators such as nitroprusside or hydralazine; therefore, this therapy is a common clinical practice used to co-administer intravenous furosemide when these drugs are used as well.

Sodium nitroprusside is the drug of choice for use in the immediate reduction of blood pressure levels. The details of its use are discussed later in this chapter. Thiocyanate, a product of nitroprusside metabolism, accumulates in patients with renal failure, and thiocyanate toxicity can occur in patients who receive high-dose or prolonged infusions of nitroprusside. This problem is rarely encountered unless the infusion is maintained beyond 48 to 72 hours. A prompt reduction in blood pressure levels can similarly be accomplished by bolus injections or by slow infusion of diazoxide or labetalol. Trimethapan offers some advantages in patients with acute aortic dissection by virtue of its ability to decrease the force and velocity of left ventricular contraction. Oral drug therapy should be started once the blood pressure has been stabilized at a desired level—only then should the patient be weaned off the intravenous drips.

Although parenteral therapy is often used in the initial treatment of malignant hypertension, various oral therapies can also be successfully used. Captopril, minoxidil, clonidine, prazosin, labetalol, and nifedipine have all been used in the initial treatment of malignant hypertension. The choice between oral and parenteral therapy depends on the monitoring facilities, condition of the patient, and coexisting complications. Once the blood pressure level stabilizes, long-term therapy must be initiated with the appropriate agent or agents based on the renal, cardiac, and neurologic status of the patient.

HYPERTENSIVE ENCEPHALOPATHY

Hypertensive encephalopathy is one of the most serious complications of severe hypertension. Although encephalopathy occurs in patients with malignant hypertension, it also complicates the rapid onset of hypertension of short duration. Despite its rarity, hypertensive encephalopathy should be quickly recognized and effectively treated because it carries a poor prognosis if left untreated but reverses rapidly if treated properly. The clinical manifestations of hypertensive encephalopathy are precipitated not only by the degree of blood pressure elevation but also by the abrupt onset of hypertension in a previously normotensive individual. Hypertensive encephalopathy usually occurs more frequently when the hypertension is complicated by renal insufficiency than when kidney function is normal.

The pathogenesis of hypertensive encephalopathy has been extensively studied and divergent opinions exist as to its mechanisms. Normally, cerebral blood flow remains relatively constant despite extensive fluctuations in systemic blood pressure levels (Fig. 2). This constancy is accomplished by autoregulation of the cerebral blood flow: When there is a severe elevation in

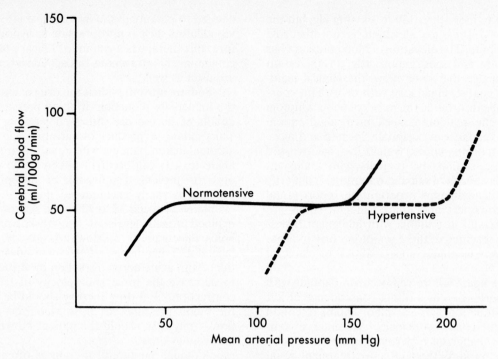

Figure 2 Cerebral blood flow autoregulation in normotensive and hypertensive individuals. (Modified from Strandgaard S, et al. Autoregulation of brain circulation in severe arterial hypertension. Br Med J 1973; 1:507; with permission.)

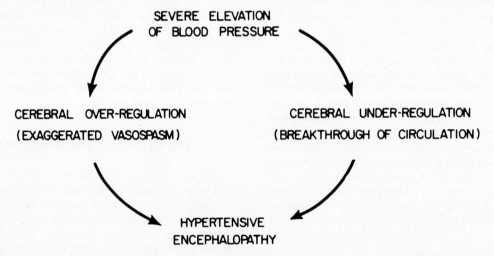

Figure 3 Pathogenetic mechanisms of hypertensive encephalopathy. (From RAM CVS. Hypertensive encephalopathy: recognition and management. Arch Intern Med 1978; 138:1851; with permission.)

the systemic blood pressure level, cerebral arterioles constrict; with a decline in blood pressure level, they dilate to maintain adequate cerebral blood flow. In patients with hypertensive encephalopathy, cerebral autoregulation is deranged to such a degree that cerebral blood flow becomes seriously affected. It was once thought that over-regulation (vasoconstriction) occurs in hypertensive encephalopathy, but a breakthrough of circulatory response with a consequent increase in cerebral blood flow has been found to result in cerebral

edema (Fig. 3). Which of these explanations is correct is immaterial in the management of hypertensive encephalopathy as the syndrome resolves after a prompt reduction in systemic arterial blood pressure.

Clinical Features

Major manifestations of hypertensive encephalopathy are depicted in Table 2. Severe and often generalized headache is the usual initial clinical manifestation.

Table 2 Clinical Features of Hypertensive Encephalopathy

Marked elevation of blood pressure
Headache
Nausea, vomiting
Papilledema
Visual complaints
Transient neurologic deficits (seizures)
Altered mental status; confusion

Altered neurologic function consisting of confusion, somnolence, and stupor may appear simultaneously with or following the onset of headache. Ultimately, if left untreated, progressive clouding of the sensorium occurs, which culminates in coma and death. The patients may be very restless during the initial stages of the syndrome. Other clinical features may include projectile vomiting, visual disturbances that range from blurring to frank blindness, and transient focal neurologic deficits. Sometimes (especially in children), generalized or focal seizures may dominate the clinical picture.

In a clinical examination, the blood pressure level is invariably found to be elevated but there is no arbitrary level of blood pressure above which encephalopathy is likely to occur. The fundi reveal generalized arteriolar spasm with exudates or hemorrhages. Although papilledema occurs in most patients with this complication, its absence does not exclude the presumptive diagnosis of hypertensive encephalopathy.

Diagnosis

A patient with poorly controlled hypertension who has severe headache, altered mental status, papilledema, and various neurologic deficits is likely to have hypertension encephalopathy, which must be distinguished from other acute neurologic complications of hypertension such as cerebral infarction or hemorrhage and uremic encephalopathy. Meticulous but rapid evaluation of the patient should be carried out to consider these differential diagnoses. Finally, the possibility of reflex elevation in systemic blood pressure as a response to cerebral ischemia should be considered in the differential diagnosis. The only definitive criterion that exists to confirm the diagnosis of hypertensive encephalopathy is a prompt favorable response of the patient's condition to antihypertensive therapy.

Management

Once the diagnosis of hypertensive encephalopathy is made, the blood pressure should be lowered rapidly to near normal levels; however, the diastolic blood pressure level should probably remain at or slightly above 100 mm Hg. A rapid reduction in the blood pressure produces prompt, dramatic, and significant relief in the symptoms of hypertensive encephalopathy. The patient preferably should be treated in an intensive care unit to monitor the response to therapy. The most important aspect of therapy is the prevention of permanent neurologic

damage. The most useful and dependable drug to use toward this end is sodium nitroprusside. Specific details concerning this and other antihypertensive agents are discussed later in this chapter. Although effective oral agents such as minoxidil, nifedipine, and captopril can control severe hypertension, parenteral drugs are preferred in treating a potentially lethal condition such as hypertensive encephalopathy.

SEVERE HYPERTENSION WITH "CEREBROVASCULAR ACCIDENTS"

A patient who has had an acute stroke and severe hypertension poses a challenging, complex therapeutic dilemma. When intracerebral pressure rises as a result of hemorrhage or thrombotic infarction, cerebral blood flow may no longer be controlled by normal autoregulation. Therefore, a reduction in the systemic blood pressure may conceivably further compromise cerebral blood flow. Conversely, persistent severe hypertension may worsen the stroke. In many patients with acute stroke, initial hypertension may resolve spontaneously within 48 hours. The need for a reduction in blood pressure in this setting should be individualized on the basis of the patient's clinical course. If antihypertensive therapy is warranted, agents with short and rapid onsets of action are preferred to reduce the risk of harmful effects of a lower blood pressure. Although there are no guidelines concerning the standard approach in managing these patients, a drastic reduction in blood pressure should be avoided. A safe therapeutic goal is to bring the diastolic level to no less than 100 mm Hg. Such a controlled reduction in blood pressure can only be accomplished with the use of nitroprusside. Drugs with central mechanisms of action such as reserpine, clonidine, and methyldopa should not be used as they may interfere with the neurologic evaluation of the patient.

ACUTE AORTIC DISSECTION

Hypertension is an important predisposing factor in the development of acute aortic dissection. Mortality from acute aortic dissection results not from the intimal tear itself but from the course taken by the dissecting hematoma, which may rupture anywhere along the aorta or which may obliterate blood supply to a major organ. Therefore, therapy should be implemented promptly after the appearance of the tear in order to arrest the complicating course. Aggressive and immediate treatment of hypertension is essential to the survival of the patient and to the enabling of surgical treatment if needed.

Severe and persistent chest or abdominal pain is the most common hallmark of acute aortic dissection. The precise location and radiation of the pain depends on the site and extent of the dissecting process. Hemoptysis, orthopnea, and dyspnea sometimes occur in patients with dissection of the thoracic aorta. Signs such as sudden loss of pulse in an extremity or sudden appearance of a new diastolic murmur should signal the possibility of acute dissection. Syncope, paralysis, and blindness may occur as a result of dissections that involve the carotid and innominate vessels. Dissection of the abdominal aorta may cause various gastrointestinal and genitourinary disturbances.

Diagnosis

The diagnosis of an acute aortic dissection should be suspected whenever a patient with hypertension has an abrupt onset of severe chest or abdominal pain, pulse deficits, and signs of circulatory compromise to a major organ. Obviously, one has to consider in the differential diagnosis entities such as myocardial infarction, pulmonary embolism, cerebrovascular accidents, and past surgery of the abdomen. The initial diagnosis is made by computed tomography, echocardiography, or magnetic resonance imaging and is later confirmed by digital or standard angiography.

Management

The initial management of both proximal and distal dissections should include measures to reduce the blood pressure and heart rate and to relieve the pain. Once the patient's condition is stabilized, definitive therapy is undertaken. For most patients with proximal dissection (type I and II, class A) and for some with distal dissection (type II, class B), surgical repair of the aortic dissection and associated complications, such as aortic regurgitation, is indicated.

If the patient has hypertension, the blood pressure should be reduced rapidly to the lowest level tolerable by the patient, keeping in mind that the force and velocity of ventricular contraction (dp/dt) and the pulsatile flow are crucial factors that determine the shearing force acting on the aortic wall. Therefore, blood pressure reduction should be accomplished with the administration of drugs that decrease, rather than increase the dp/dt. Trimethaphan, a ganglion-blocking agent, is a logical choice because it produces prompt and smooth reduction in blood pressure to a desired level while blunting the sharpness of the pulse wave generated by the heart. The same goal can be achieved with the use of labetalol or sodium nitroprusside in addition to beta-blocker therapy. Drugs that stimulate myocardial contraction, e.g., diazoxide and hydralazine, should be avoided because of their adverse hemodynamic actions. Stated simply, the medical management for acute aortic dissection should include the rational use of antihypertensive drugs that calm as opposed to stimulate the heart. Once the blood pressure and clinical status of the patient are stabilized, definitive therapy (surgical or medical) should be planned without undue delay. Although the presenting manifestations of acute aortic dissection are ominous, aggressive medical and surgical therapy provide considerable therapeutic benefits.

ACUTE LEFT VENTRICULAR FAILURE

Acute left ventricular failure (pulmonary edema) in a hypertensive patient is an indication for prompt blood pressure reduction. The higher the blood pressure, the harder the ventricle must work. Therefore, decreasing the workload of the failing myocardium improves the pump action of the heart. Features of a failing heart include an increased end-diastolic fiber length, increased ventricular volume, and a reduced ejection fraction, factors that increase myocardial oxygen requirements. This increase could be particularly deleterious in patients who have coexistent coronary artery disease. A prompt reduction in blood pressure induced through the use of a balanced vasodilating agent such as nitroprusside is indicated in this circumstance. Sodium nitroprusside decreases both preload and afterload with restoration of myocardial function and cardiac output. Although the angiotensin-converting enzyme (ACE) inhibitors may be useful in this situation because of their pharmacologic actions, there is a paucity of clinical experience concerning the therapeutic response to ACE inhibition in patients with acute left ventricular failure. Drugs that increase the cardiac work, such as hydralazine and diazoxide, should not be used. Along with the treatment of hypertension, other measures for managing pulmonary edema should be instituted.

SEVERE HYPERTENSION ASSOCIATED WITH OCCLUSIVE ISCHEMIC HEART DISEASE

Systemic hypertension increases myocardial oxygen consumption by increasing intraventricular pressure and left ventricular diameter. Patients with myocardial infarction and severe hypertension should therefore theoretically benefit from blood pressure reduction but there are no conclusive data to prove that treatment is beneficial. Reduction of systemic blood pressure reduces the cardiac work, wall tension, and oxygen demand and may thus limit myocardial necrosis in the early phase of infarction. However, there are conflicting data in the literature about the value of reducing blood pressure (to reduce infarct size) in the absence of pulmonary congestion. Although hypertension usually precedes the onset of chest pain, a marked rise in blood pressure may follow the onset of coronary insufficiency. Therefore, an acute elevation of blood pressure in the setting of acute myocardial infarction may be transient and not harmful, but some investigators have observed that the mortality rate and incidence of cardiac failure are significantly greater in patients with severe systolic hypertension and acute myocardial infarction.

A reduction in systemic arterial pressure early in the course of acute myocardial infarction has been shown to protect the myocardium, as reflected by the reduced release of creatinine phosphokinase enzyme activity. The cautious treatment of hypertension in patients with acute myocardial infarction is therefore likely to be beneficial. Parenteral agents such as sodium nitroprusside can be used. Diazoxide and hydralazine should not be used in the presence of myocardial infarction because of their adverse hemodynamic effects. It must be emphasized that the degree of blood pressure reduction should depend solely on the demonstration of a beneficial hemodynamic response obtained in a given patient and not on any predetermined level. Aortic diastolic pressure is a major determinant of coronary blood flow, and unnecessary reductions in the blood pressure could compromise an already critical situation.

MISCELLANEOUS CONDITIONS

Pheochromocytoma Crisis

Pheochromocytoma crisis has striking clinical features. Typically, the blood pressure is markedly elevated during the paroxysm and the patient may have profound sweating, marked tachycardia, pallor (especially of the face), numbness, tingling, and coldness of the feet and hands. A single attack will last from a few minutes to hours and may occur as often as several times a day to once a month or less.

If pheochromocytoma is suspected, the alpha-adrenergic blocking drug, phentolamine, should be given in a dose of 5 to 10 mg intravenously, to be repeated in a few minutes if needed. An alternative to phentolamine would be sodium nitroprusside, but phentolamine is more specific. A beta-blocking drug may be useful if the patient has a concomitant cardiac arrhythmia. The administration of beta-blocking agents should always be preceded by that of either phentolamine or phenoxybenzamine. If these latter drugs are not administered, the beta-blockade can aggravate the unopposed alpha-mediated peripheral vasoconstriction. Labetalol, a combined alpha- and beta-receptor blocking drug, has also been successfully used to treat this condition.

Clonidine Withdrawal Syndrome

A syndrome that mimics pheochromocytoma crisis has been reported following the abrupt discontinuation of therapy with the antihypertensive drug clonidine. Clonidine exerts its antihypertensive effect by stimulating the alpha receptors in the brain stem, thus reducing peripheral sympathetic activity. When clonidine therapy is abruptly discontinued, or even sometimes rapidly tapered, a specific syndrome has been noted that includes symptoms of nausea, palpitations, anxiety, sweating, nervousness, and headache in addition to a marked elevation in blood pressure. In some patients the blood pressure rises beyond the pretreatment level. The probable mechanism of the clonidine withdrawal syndrome is a sudden resurgence of sympathetic activity. The incidence of this peculiar syndrome is extremely low and in some cases blood pressure decreases rapidly toward the pretreatment level but never surpasses it.

Symptoms of clonidine withdrawal can be alleviated by the reinstitution of therapy with clonidine. If there is a marked elevation in blood pressure and the patient is experiencing severe and annoying symptoms such as palpitations, chest discomfort, or epigastric discomfort the intravenous administration of phentolamine or labetalol is recommended.

Hypertensive Crisis Associated with Drug and Food Interactions: Monoamine Oxidase Inhibitors

Patients receiving monoamine oxidase (MAO) inhibitors are at risk for developing hypertensive crisis if they also take drugs such as ephedrine or amphetamines, or ingest foods that contain high quantities of tyramine. In the presence of an MAO inhibitor, tyramine and indirectly acting sympathetic amines escape oxidative degradation, enter the systemic circulation, and potentiate the actions of catecholamines. Sympathomimetic amines such as those contained in nonprescription cold remedies can also provoke this response.

The hypertensive attack occurs with an abrupt onset from 1 to 2 hours after intake of the offending agent and sometimes lasts up to several hours. The patient characteristically feels acutely ill with headache, sweating, and palpitations, and the blood pressure is often elevated to alarming levels. The manifestations of food and drug interactions with MAO inhibitors closely resemble those of pheochromocytoma. Guidelines for immediate treatment are similar in both conditions.

Hypertensive Crisis in the Postoperative Period

Open heart surgery and surgical manipulation of the carotid artery are sometimes followed by severe hypertension in the immediate postoperative period. Hypertension, even of moderate degree, may jeopardize the integrity of the vascular suture lines; it should therefore be managed promptly with the use of parenteral agents. Sodium nitroprusside is usually the agent of choice, although nerve blockers and other drugs may be effective.

Hypertensive Crisis in Quadriplegic Patients

Hypertensive crises have been reported in patients with transverse lesions of the spinal cord that usually occur above the origins of the thoracolumbar sympathetic neurons. The stimulation of dermatomes and muscles supplied by nerves below the injury may evoke severe hypertension, profound headache, and bradycardia. The blood pressure crisis is the result of excessive stimulation of sympathetic neurons, and the associated bradycardia is probably caused by excitation of the baroreceptor reflexes. Given the pathophysiologic basis for such hypertensive reactions, these critical blood pressure elevations can be prevented by avoiding excessive stimulation of the susceptible portion of dermatomes. Treatment is dictated by the severity of hypertension and the status of target organ function.

Hypertension Associated with Head Injury

Patients with head injury may have marked elevations in blood pressure. The mechanism for these elevations is likely complex and may involve the medullary vasomotor centers which, when rendered ischemic, may elevate the blood pressure by reflex action. Increased intracranial pressure in itself may induce certain cardiovascular changes that result in hypertension. The dilemma for treatment is whether to induce a blood pressure reduction under such circumstances. The same principles apply as were discussed under the section that dealt with cerebrovascular accidents.

Hypertensive Crisis as a Result of Systemic Vasculitis

An abrupt onset of severe hypertension has been known to occur as a complication of necrotizing vasculitis. The mechanism of action in this complication has not been clearly delineated. Possible mechanisms include a direct increase in peripheral vascular resistance as a result of the vasculitic process itself or as a result of activation of the renin-angiotensin system. Acute necrotizing vasculitis should be considered in the differential diagnosis when a young patient develops a hypertensive crisis.

Hypertensive Crisis Induced by Metoclopramide

Hypertensive crises induced by the administration of metoclopramide have been reported in previously normotensive patients and in patients with pheochromocytoma. The exact mechanism by which metoclopramide, a dopamine agonist, causes a hypertensive response is not known. The drug could act by sensitizing the vascular endothelium to the pressor effects of catecholamines or by causing a release of catecholamines from the adrenal medulla or adrenergic neurons.

MANAGEMENT OF HYPERTENSIVE CRISES

Patients with hypertensive crises should be hospitalized. Whether they should be treated in the intensive care unit depends on the level of blood pressure and the extent of associated complications. The acute treatment of hypertension should be implemented with careful monitoring of blood pressure as well as cardiac, renal, and neurologic functions. Drugs that can be administered parenterally to reduce blood pressure are listed in Tables 3 and 4. A major consideration in treating patients with hypertensive emergencies is the rapidity of onset and duration of action of the drug given. The

Table 3 Parenteral Drugs Useful in the Immediate Control of Severe Hypertension

Drug	Route and Dosage	Onset	Offset	Comments
Nitroprusside	IV infusion, 0.25 μg/kg/min to 8 μg/kg/min	Seconds	3–5 min	Thiocyanate toxicity may occur with prolonged (> 48 hrs) or high-dose infusion (> 15 μg/kg/min), particularly in renal insufficiency
Diazoxide	IV, 50–150 mg q 5 min or as infusion of 7.5–30 mg/min	1–5 min	4–24 hrs	Should not be used for patients with angina pectoris, myocardial infarction, dissecting aneurysm
Trimethaphan	IV infusion pump, 0.5–5 mg/min	1–5 min	10 min	Drug of choice for treatment of aortic dissection
Labetalol	IV, 20 mg q 10 min (can increase to 80 mg doses)	5 min or less	3–6 hrs	Prompt response; can be followed with same drug taken orally
Hydralazine	IM/IV, 10–20 min	10–30 min	2–4 hrs	May precipitate angina, myocardial infarction
Nicardipine	IV, 5–15 mg/hr	5–15 min	30–40 min	May cause reflex tachycardia

Table 4 Indications for Use of Parenteral Drugs in the Treatment of Severe Hypertension

	Nitroprusside	Labetalol	Nicardipine
Severe hypertension	Yes	Yes	Yes
Chronic heart failure	Yes	No	Yes
AV block	Yes	No	Yes
Asthma and COPD*	Yes	No	Yes
Renal insufficiency	No	?	Yes
Vascular disease	?	?	Yes
Cerebrovascular accident	?	Yes	Yes
Aortic dissection	?	Yes	–
Switch to same drug orally	No	Yes	Yes

*COPD = chronic obstructive pulmonary disease.

physician must be aware of the pharmacologic and hemodynamic actions of the drug to be used, as the aim is not just to lower the blood pressure but to do so with minimal adverse effects.

Parenteral Agents

Nitroprusside

Extensive clinical use over time has shown that sodium nitroprusside is the most potent and effective drug for the treatment of hypertensive crisis. The drug solution must be made at the moment of use and it must be shielded from light during the infusion because the substance is photosensitive. The drug's hypotensive response occurs within seconds after the infusion is started and disappears almost as rapidly when the infusion is discontinued (Fig. 4). Nitroprusside acts by relaxing both the arteries and the veins, thereby reducing systemic arterial and venous pressures along with systemic and pulmonary vascular resistances. The exact mechanism by which nitroprusside dilates the vessels has not been firmly established.

Because of its rapid onset of action and potency, the infusion of nitroprusside must be closely monitored by means of an infusion pump or a microdrip regulator, as well as by intra-arterial blood pressure recording. A safe initial dose is 0.3 μg per kilogram per minute, which can be increased every 5 minutes until the desired blood pressure is obtained.

Once the desired effect from therapy with nitroprusside is achieved, the infusion usually can be maintained with minimal adjustment, but blood pressure should be continuously monitored. Parenteral treatment of hypertensive crisis generally is needed only for 12 to 48 hours and drug therapy should be discontinued as soon as alternate modes of therapy have been proved effective. Because of a short duration of action, the effects of stopping nitroprusside therapy will be seen within a few minutes. If indicated, treatment can be resumed promptly. Hypotension is the most common side effect of nitroprusside therapy, a consequence of inadequate regulation of the infusion rate.

The immediate metabolic product of nitroprusside is cyanide, which is liberated by the direct combination of nitroprusside with the sulfhydryl groups in red blood cells and tissues. The circulating cyanide rapidly converts to thiocyanate in the liver through the action of the enzyme rhodanate or by transsulfarase; thiocyanate in turn is removed almost exclusively by the kidneys and has a half-life of approximately 1 week.

Cyanide toxicity from nitroprusside use, although extremely rare, has occurred. The prophylactic infusion of hydroxocobalamin (Vitamin B_{12a}) at 25 mg per hour has been shown to decrease the cyanide concentration and tissue hypoxia that results from nitroprusside infusion during surgery. Hydroxocobalamin has one cyanide radical less than does cyanocobalamin and, therefore, allows cyanide to combine and form cyanocobalamin, which is then excreted in the urine.

Thiocyanate toxicity secondary to nitroprusside therapy is uncommon and occurs only with high doses and in the presence of renal failure. Symptoms of thiocyanate toxicity include fatigue, nausea, anorexia, skin rashes, headaches, disorientation, and psychotic behavior. These symptoms tend to occur at plasma levels of 5 to 10 mg per deciliter; levels greater than 20 mg per

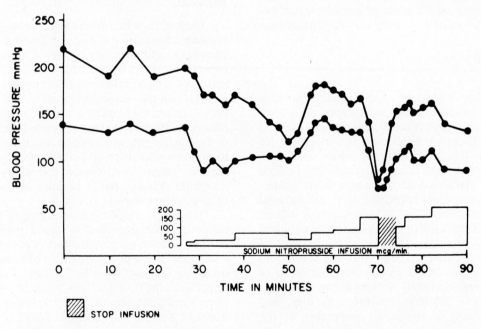

STOP INFUSION

Figure 4 Blood pressure regulation with nitroprusside. Note that excessive hypotension was readily reversed when the infusion was stopped for a few minutes. (From Gifford RW. Management and treatment of malignant hypertensive emergencies. In: Genest J, et al, eds: Hypertension. New York: McGraw-Hill Book Co., 1977:1024; with permission.)

deciliter are dangerous. Therefore, during high-dose infusions of nitroprusside, and especially when renal function is impaired, plasma thiocyanate levels should be determined periodically; treatment should be interrupted when the thiocyanate level reaches close to 10 mg per deciliter. Plasma thiocyanate levels need not be monitored as long as the patient's clinical status is monitored closely. The treatment of thiocyanate toxicity demands discontinuation of the drug therapy and institution of dialysis.

Nicardipine Infusion

Recent clinical studies have indicated that intravenous administration of the calcium antagonist, nicardipine, produces a prompt decline in blood pressure in patients with severe hypertension. Nicardipine is a dihydropyridine agent like nifedipine but, unlike the latter, it is a water-soluble compound, which makes it suitable for intravenous use. The intravenous administration of nicardipine exerts a prompt hypotensive effect (Fig. 5) and the desired blood pressure level can be maintained with appropriate adjustments to the infusion rate. Thus, nicardipine pharmacodynamics resemble those of nitroprusside in terms of onset, duration, and offset of action. Because of its mechanism of action, nicardipine may be useful in preserving tissue perfusion. This property may be particularly beneficial in patients with ischemic disorders such as coronary, cerebrovascular, or peripheral vascular disease. Our clinical experience with the use of nicardipine suggests that this agent may turn out to be a useful therapeutic option in the management of severe hypertension with or without target organ damage. This mode of therapy is particularly attractive because the route of administration can easily be switched to oral by using the oral formulation of the drug.

Trimethaphan

Trimethaphan camsylate is a ganglion-blocking agent. The hypotensive effect of trimethaphan is accompanied by a reduction in left ventricular ejection rate and cardiac output. These attributes make it a drug of choice for the medical treatment of acute aortic dissection. When administered, a rise in cardiac output may be seen in hypertensive patients with congestive heart failure, which reflects a reduction in the venous return induced by this drug, a property it has in common with sodium nitroprusside. Trimethaphan has a rapid onset of action and its effects dissipate within a few minutes of discontinuation of therapy. The head of the bed should be elevated to augment the antihypertensive effect of this agent. Like nitroprusside, trimethaphan should be administered as a continuous intravenous drip, and constant monitoring is necessary, preferably in the intensive care unit. The usual starting dose of the drug should be 1 mg per minute titrated to obtain the desired blood pressure level. After prolonged infusion, tachyphylaxis may result from intravascular volume expan-

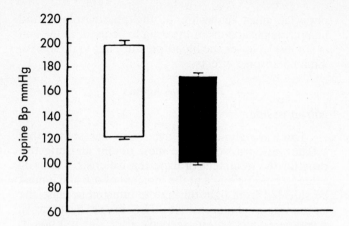

Figure 5 Decline in blood pressure levels during the infusion of nicardipine in patients with uncontrolled hypertension. (Adapted from Ram CVS. Current concepts in the diagnosis and management of hypertensive urgencies and emergencies. Keio J Med 1990; 39:225; with permission.)

sion, which can be partially overcome by the initiation of effective diuretic therapy.

The major disadvantage to the use of trimethaphan is that it causes parasympathetic inhibition, which results in paralytic ileus, urinary retention, and mydrasis. These effects are particularly likely to occur when the drug is administered for more than 1 to 2 days. The patient's respiratory status should be monitored closely— particularly if large doses of trimethaphan are used— because of the remote possibility of respiratory depression caused by the use of this drug.

Diazoxide

Diazoxide, when given intravenously, has a direct relaxant effect on the vascular smooth muscle, which prompts a rapid decrease in arterial blood pressure. The hypotensive effect of diazoxide is associated with striking increases in heart rate and cardiac output. Diazoxide has no effect on the capacitance vessels and, therefore, the venous return to the heart is not impeded. Diazoxide has no direct effect on the myocardium, but reflex increases in the cardiac output and heart rate may pose a problem to patients with intrinsic cardiac disease. Expansion of plasma volume and edema formation occur during diazoxide therapy, partly because of the drug's direct tubular antinatriuretic action.

The intravenous administration of diazoxide produces a rapid decrease in blood pressure within 1 minute, and the maximum effect is achieved within 2 to 5 minutes. The hypotensive effect of a single injection of diazoxide may last for 3 to 15 hours, but if there is no effect from the first injection, an additional dose can be given within 30 minutes. The previously recommended dose of diazoxide was 300 mg or 5 mg per kilogram given as a rapid intravenous injection. To be maximally effective, the dose should be injected rapidly—in 10 to 30 seconds—to overcome protein binding of the drug. The sudden depressor effect that follows intravenous bolus injection may be deleterious to cerebral blood flow.

Rapid injection of this relatively large single dose may cause hypotension with resultant myocardial and cerebral ischemia. Smallar bolus injections (Fig. 6) and slow intravenous infusions of diazoxide for the treatment of severe hypertension have been used in an attempt to reduce the dangers of a drastic and precipitous reduction in blood pressure. Based on results from these studies, mini-bolus injections of diazoxide (i.e., 50 mg given every 5 minutes) or 20- to 30-minute infusions at a rate of 15 to 30 mg per minute may be effective in rapidly controlling severe hypertension while providing the advantage of ease of administration and relative freedom from side effects.

The most common side effects reported with diazoxide use include nausea, vomiting, abdominal discomfort, sodium and water retention, and a sensation of warmth along the vein. The excessive hypotensive effect of diazoxide is particularly likely to occur in patients who have had prior antihypertensive therapy.

To counteract fluid retention, 40 or 80 mg of furosemide must be given intravenously. The hyperglycemic effect of diazoxide rarely necessitates therapy but blood glucose levels should be monitored, particularly in patients with impaired carbohydrate metabolism and with repeated injections of diazoxide. The need to use diazoxide has been nearly eliminated by the availability of safe alternative drugs.

Hydralazine

The hypotensive action of hydralazine results from a direct relaxation of the vascular smooth muscle and is accompanied by reflex increases in stroke volume and heart rate, which can precipitate myocardial ischemia. An intramuscular or intravenous administration of hydralazine results in an unpredictable but definite decrease in blood pressure. In the treatment of hypertensive emergencies, the initial dose should be 10 to 20 mg. The onset of the hypotensive effect occurs within 10 to 30 minutes and its duration of action ranges from 3 to 9 hours. The dose and frequency of administration necessary to control blood pressure vary substantially. The delayed onset and unpredictable degree of hypotensive effect present difficulties in titration. Nevertheless, hydralazine continues to be successfully used in the treatment of severe hypertension and is especially effective in the treatment of eclampsia secondary to hypertension.

Labetalol

Labetalol is a combined alpha- and beta-blocking drug that can be given parenterally or orally for the treatment of hypertensive crises. Labetalol administered intravenously in bolus injections or as a slow infusion produces a prompt decrease in blood pressure by decreasing peripheral vascular resistance without inducing tachycardia. Patients treated with parenteral labetalol can be subsequently given the oral form for the

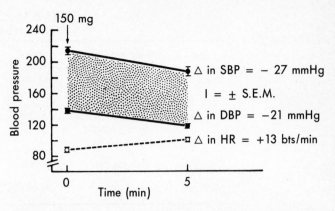

Figure 6 Response to injection of diazoxide, 150 mg. (From Ram CVS, Kaplan NM. Individual titration of diazoxide dosage in the treatment of severe hypertension. Am J Cardiol 1979; 43:627; with permission.)

long-term management of hypertension. Because of its dual adrenergic blocking properties, labetalol is particularly indicated for the acute treatment of hypertension associated with increased circulating catecholamines, such as in pheochromocytoma and drug withdrawal hypertension. Administration should be avoided in situations in which a beta-blockade is contraindicated; otherwise, the use of labetalol is an excellent option in the immediate management of severe hypertension.

Phentolamine

Phentolamine, an alpha-receptor blocking agent, is specifically indicated for the treatment of hypertensive crises associated with increased circulating catecholamines—e.g., pheochromocytoma crisis, certain cases of clonidine withdrawal syndrome, and crises resulting from the interaction of MAO inhibitors with drugs or food. The hypotensive effect of a single intravenous bolus injection is short-lived and lasts less than 15 minutes.

Nitroglycerin

Nitroglycerin dilates the venous capacitance vessels as well as the resistance arterioles. As a result, it reduces both left ventricular preload and afterload. Although no comparative data exist, nitroglycerin infusion may be particularly helpful in the treatment of patients with severe hypertension with concomitant coronary artery disease.

Orally Effective Drugs

Certain orally effective antihypertensive drugs decrease the blood pressure promptly and are useful in the management of hypertensive urgencies (Table 5). Clinical experience suggests that these orally effective drugs can be conveniently used to lower the blood pressure for conditions in which parenteral drugs have been used in the past.

Table 5 Acute Oral Therapy for the Immediate Control
of Severe Hypertension

Drug	Route and Dosage	Onset	Offset	Comment
Nifedipine	10–20 mg PO or sublingual	5–15 min	3–5 hrs	Generally good response; short duration of action for optimal dosage not standard
Clonidine	0.2 mg PO initially, then 0.1 mg/hr, up to 0.8 mg total	0.5–2 hrs	6–8 hrs	Prominent sedation
Captopril	6.5–25 mg PO	15 min	4–6 hrs	Generally good, sometimes excessive response
Minoxidil	5–10 mg PO	30–60 min	12–16 hrs	Tachycardia, fluid retention

Minoxidil

Minoxidil is a powerful direct vasodilator and has been successfully used in the treatment of refractory or severe hypertension. Because of its relatively rapid onset of action and sustained duration, this drug has been used for the treatment of hypertension crises. Minoxidil in doses ranging from 2.5 to 10 mg can be given every 4 to 6 hours initially in the treatment of severe hypertension. The drug works best when given along with a diuretic agent, and an adrenergic blocker is necessary to counteract reflex tachycardia.

Clonidine

Clonidine, when given in incremental doses, has been shown to cause a significant reduction in blood pressure levels in patients with severe hypertension. Although this form of therapy may be convenient, the sedative effects of clonidine may alter the neurologic function of patients who have severe hypertension.

Nifedipine

Nifedipine, a calcium antagonist, reduces arterial pressure rapidly and is useful in the management of hypertensive urgencies as well as crises. Its major advantages are a rapid onset of action and a lack of central nervous system depression. In its capsular formulation, it may produce reflex tachycardia, and heart rate and cardiac output increase in response to the rapid reduction in total peripheral arterial pressure. Because the duration of action of nifedipine is short, patients receiving this drug should be monitored to make certain that re-administration is appropriate. If the patient can take oral medications, nifedipine can be given orally with an equally satisfactory response.

In contrast with clonidine therapy, nifedipine therapy preserves or increases cerebral blood flow. It should be kept in mind that many vasoactive drugs that do penetrate the blood-brain barrier and dilate cerebral vessels may lead to uneven cerebral perfusion as a result of an intracranial steal effect. This possibility is especially relevant in elderly patients with atheromatous disease of intracranial or extracranial vessels.

Many patients with severe hypertension may have coronary artery disease. In addition, potent peripheral arterial dilators such as nifedipine can induce a sudden marked decrease in blood pressure. These drugs, therefore, have the potential to lower coronary artery perfusion pressure, which could result in a coronary artery steal phenomenon. In fact, nifedipine-associated myocardial ischemia or infarction has been reported in patients being treated for hypertensive urgencies.

Angiotensin-Converting Enzyme Inhibitors

Captopril, a converting enzyme inhibitor, has been found to be effective in the treatment of hypertensive crises. Captopril acts to decrease the blood pressure promptly without causing tachycardia, and thus offers a distinct hemodynamic advantage over direct arteriolar dilators. However, the maximal effect from orally administered captopril may not be attained for as long as 2 hours. On the other hand, some reports have documented the effectiveness of sublingual captopril in the treatment of hypertensive crisis. Because the experience with sublingual captopril is limited, further data have to be generated to define the role of this drug in the acute management of hypertensive crisis. High renin states such as malignant hypertension associated with scleroderma renal crisis are particularly responsive to captopril. Enalaprilat, an intravenous converting enzyme inhibitor, has also been found to be effective in the treatment of hypertensive crises. Patients with volume depletion merit closer surveillance as converting enzyme inhibition in this setting may cause profound hypotension and azotemia.

COMPLICATIONS OF THERAPY

Renal Function

Accelerated or malignant hypertension and hypertensive encephalopathy are more commonly seen in patients with underlying renal insufficiency. The effective control of hypertension in such circumstances may result in transient deterioration of renal function, and temporary dialysis may sometimes be necessary. The long-term treatment of severe hypertension, however, is likely to stabilize or even improve renal function.

Cerebral Function

Normally, cerebral blood flow (CBF) is maintained with a safe margin despite great fluctuations in systemic blood pressure levels. However, CBF may be disrupted in certain hypertensive crises—e.g., hypertensive encephalopathy and antihypertensive therapy may adversely influence cerebral circulation. Experimental data obtained from hypertensive rats suggest that different antihypertensive drugs may have different effects on cerebral blood flow. For example, diazoxide maintains the CBF at a fairly constant level until the systemic blood pressure decreases to a very low level; hydralazine causes disruption of CBF independent of changes in systemic blood pressure; and converting enzyme inhibitors and calcium antagonists appear to have a favorable impact on CBF. The relevance of these observations in humans remains to be determined.

Other Complications

The treatment of extremely elevated blood pressure has its risks as well as its benefits. The complications of antihypertensive therapy usually result from hypotension and sometimes from the nature of therapy, such as with diazoxide causing cardiac ischemia and nitroprusside causing thiocyanate toxicity. Sometimes, worsening of neurologic status follows an acute reduction in blood pressure. These complications can be avoided by careful evaluation of the patient and by choosing an appropriate antihypertensive agent. In this respect, drugs with a short duration of action offer an advantage because unwanted hypotension can be quickly reversed by adjusting the dose or stopping the therapy.

In patients recovering from acute cerebrovascular accident or hypertensive encephalopathy, centrally acting agents such as methyldopa or clonidine should not be used because of their sedative effects. One common error in managing hypertensive crises is to introduce drugs by oral route of administration prematurely. Another error is the failure to monitor the standing blood pressure in a patient who has been receiving potent antihypertensive agents in the supine position.

RECOMMENDATIONS

The most important immediate decision made in the management of hypertensive emergencies is to assess the patient's clinical state and to ascertain whether the patient's condition truly needs emergency management. A patient with true hypertensive crisis should be ideally treated in an intensive care unit. The choice of oral versus parenteral administration depends on the urgency of the situation as well as the patient's general condition. The level to which the blood pressure should be lowered varies with the type of hypertensive crisis and

should be determined on an individual basis. There is no predestined level for the goal of therapy. Complications of therapy, mainly hypotension and ischemic brain damage, can occur in patients who are given multiple potent antihypertensive drugs in large doses without adequate monitoring. Such complications can be minimized by gentle decreasing of blood pressure, careful surveillance, and individualization of therapy. Relatively asymptomatic patients who have severe hypertension, i.e., a diastolic blood pressure ranging from 130 to 140 mm Hg, need not be treated with parenterally administered drugs. Patients who fit this category should be managed on an individual basis and the usual course would be to intensify or alter the previous antihypertensive therapy.

Once hypertensive crisis has resolved and the patient's condition is stable, one should investigate possible factors that might have contributed to the precipitous elevation of the blood pressure, such as nonadherence to prescribed therapy or the presence or progression of a secondary form of hypertension such as renal artery stenosis.

SUGGESTED READING

Abe M, Orita Y, Nakashima Y, Nakamura M. Hypertensive crisis induced by metoclopramide in patients with pheochromocytoma. Angiology 1984; 35:122–128.

Adelman RD, Russo J. Malignant hypertension: recovery of renal function after treatment with antihypertensive medications and hemodialysis. J Pediatr 1981; 98:766–768.

Anderson RJ, Hart GR, Crumpler CP, et al. Oral clonidine loading in hypertensive urgencies. JAMA 1981; 246:848–850.

Barcenas CG, Eigenbrodt E, Long DL, Hull AR. Recovery from malignant hypertension with anuria after prolonged hemodialysis. South Med J 1976; 69:1230–1233.

Barry DI, Jarden JO, Paulson OB, et al. Cerebrovascular aspects of converting-enzyme inhibition I: effect of intravenous captopril in spontaneously hypertensive and normotensive rats. J Hypertens 1984; 2:589–597.

Barry DI, Strandgaard S, Graham DI, et al. Effect of diazoxide-induced hypotension on cerebral blood flow in hypertensive rats. Eur J Clin Invest 1983; 13:201–208.

Bauer JH, Alpert MA. Rapid reduction of severe hypertension with minoxidil. J Cardiovasc Pharmacol 1989; 2(suppl):S189–S199.

Beer N, Gallego I, Cohen A, et al. Efficacy of sublingual nifedipine in the acute treatment of systemic hypertension. Chest 1981; 79:571–574.

Bertel O, Conen D, Radu E, et al. Nifedipine in hypertensive emergencies. Br Med J 1983; 286:19–21.

Biollaz J, Waeber B, Brunner HR. Hypertensive crisis treated with orally administered captopril. Eur J Clin Pharmacol 1983; 25:145–149.

Cottrell JE, Casthely P, Brodie JD, et al. Prevention of nitroprusside induced cyanide toxicity with hydroxocobalamin. N Engl J Med 1978; 298:808–811.

Davis VA, Crook JE, Vestel LE. Prevalence of renovascular hypertension in patients with Grade III or IV hypertensive retinopathy. N Engl J Med 1979; 301:1273–1279.

DiPette DJ, Ferraro JC, Evans RR, Martin M. Enalaprilat, an intravenous angiotensin-converting enzyme inhibitor, in hypertensive crises. Clin Pharmacol Ther 1985; 38:199–204.

Dunn FG, Jones JV, Fife R. Malignant hypertension associated with use of oral contraceptives. Br Heart J 1975; 37:336–338.

Flaherty JT, Magee PA, Gardner TL, et al. Comparison of intravenous nitroglycerin and sodium nitroprusside for treatment of acute hypertension developing after coronary artery bypass surgery. Circulation 1982; 65:1072–1077.

IV Nicardipine Study Group. Efficacy and safety of intravenous nicardipine in the control of postoperative hypertension. Chest 1991; 99:393–398.

Fox KM, Tomlinson JW, Portal RW, Aber CP. Prognostic significance of acute systolic hypertension after acute myocardial infarction. Br Med J 1975; 3:128–130.

Garrett BN, Kaplan NM. Efficacy of slow infusion of diazoxide in the treatment of severe hypertension without organ hypoperfusion. Am Heart J 1982; 103:390–394.

Garrett BN, Ram CVS. Acute aortic dissection. Cardiol Clin 1984; 2:227–238.

Ghose RR, Mathur YB, Upadhyay M, et al. Treatment of hypertensive emergencies with oral labetalol. Br Med J 1978; 2:96.

Gibson TC. Blood pressure levels in acute myocardial infarction. Am Heart J 1978; 96:475–480.

Graham DI. Ischaemic brain damage of cerebral perfusion failure type after treatment of severe hypertension. Br Med J 1975; 4:739.

Gudbrandsson T, Hansson L, Herlitz H, et al. Immunological changes in patients with previous malignant essential hypertension. Lancet 1981; 1:406–408.

Haft JI, Litterer WE III. Chewing nifedipine to rapidly treat hypertension. Arch Intern Med 1984; 144:2357–2359.

Hansson L, Hunyor SN, Julius S, Hoober SW. Blood pressure crisis following withdrawal of clonidine. Am Heart J 1973; 85:605–610.

Isles C, Brown JJ, Cumming AMM, et al. Excess smoking in malignant-phase hypertension. Br Med J 1979; 1:579–589.

Kaneda H, Yamauchi T, Murata T, et al. Treatment of malignant hypertension with infusion of sodium chloride: a case report and a review. Tohoku J Exp Med 1980; 132:179–186.

Karachalious GN, Georgiopoulos AN. Treatment of hypertensive crisis with sublingual captopril. Clin Pharmacol 1989; 8:90–91.

Kincaid-Smith P. Malignant hypertension. Cardiovasc Rev Rep 1980; 1:42–50.

Kincaid-Smith P. Malignant hypertension: mechanisms and management. Pharmacol Ther 1980; 9:245–269.

Mitchell HC, Graham RM, Pettinger WA. Renal function during long-term treatment of hypertension with minoxidil. Ann Intern Med 1980; 93:676–681.

Mohring J, Mohring B, Peter M, et al. Studies on the pathogenesis of malignant course of hypertension in rats. Kidney Int 1975; 8:S174–S180.

Mohring J, Petri M, Szokol M, et al. Effects of saline drinking on malignant course of renal hypertension rats. Am J Physiol 1976; 230:849–857.

Naftchi NE, Tuckman J. Hypertensive crisis in spinal man. Am Heart J 1979; 97:536–538.

O'Connell MT, Kubrusly DB, Fournier AM. Systemic necrotizing vasculitis seen initially as hypertensive crisis. Arch Intern Med 1985; 145:265–267.

O'Mailia JJ, Sanders GE, Giles TD. Nifedipine-associated myocardial ischemia or infarction in the treatment of hypertensive urgencies. Ann Intern Med 1987; 107:185–186.

Ram CVS, Boldrick RW, Heller J, Kaplan NM: Rapid control of severe hypertension with intravenous infusion of nicardipine: a new therapeutic approach. J Clin Pharmacol 1989; 29:835.

Ram CVS. Current concepts in the diagnosis and management of hypertensive urgencies and emergencies. Keio J Med 1990; 39: 225–236.

Ram CVS, Engelman K. Abrupt discontinuation of clonidine therapy. JAMA 1979; 242:2104–2105.

Ram CVS. Hypertensive emergencies: recognition and management. Curr Probl Cardiol 1982; VII(1):1–70.

Ram CVS, Kaplan NM. Individual titration of diazoxide dosage in the treatment of severe hypertension. Am J Cardiol 1979; 43:627–630.

Ramos O. Malignant hypertension: the Brazilian experience. Kidney Int 1984; 25:209–217.

Shell WE, Sobel BE. Protection of jeopardized ischemic myocardium by reduction of ventricular afterload. N Engl J Med 1974; 291:481–486.

Sheridan C, Chandra P, Jacinto M, et al. Transient hypertension after high doses of metoclopramide. N Engl J Med 1982; 307:1346.

Singh A, Bedi VP. Transient paraplegia following sudden lowering of blood pressure. J Indian Med Assoc 1984; 82:214–228.

Still JM, Cottom D. Severe hypertension in childhood. Arch Dis Child 1967; 42:34–39.

Strandgaard S, MacKenzie ET, Jones JV, Harper AM. Studies on the cerebral circulation of the baboon in acutely induced hypertension. Stroke 1976; 7:287–290.

Taylor D, Ramsay J, Day S, Dillon M. Infarction of the optic nerve head in children with accelerated hypertension. Br J Ophthalmol 1981; 65:153–160.

Wallace JD, Levy LL. Blood pressure after stroke. JAMA 1981; 246:2177–2180.

Wheat MW. Treatment of dissecting aneurysms of the aorta: current status. Prog Cardiovasc Dis 1973; 16:87–101.

Wilson DJ, Wallin JD, Vlachakis ND, et al. Intravenous labetalol in the treatment of severe hypertension and hypertensive emergencies. Am J Med 1983; 75:95–102.

HYPERLIPIDEMIA IN PATIENTS WITH VASCULAR DISEASE

DAVID H. BLANKENHORN, M.D.
HOWARD N. HODIS, M.D.

Patients with lipid disorders and definite clinical evidence of myocardial, cerebrovascular, or peripheral ischemia are at very high risk for continued disease progression. They require special attention in the form of aggressive lipid-lowering therapy. The list of high-risk patients includes those with bypass grafts, angioplasty, myocardial infarction, and stroke. Treatment of patients with symptomatic vascular disease should begin as soon as possible. We believe it prudent to begin lipid-lowering therapy before the placement of grafts or angioplasty; if this is precluded by management of acute problems, it should begin as soon as practical thereafter.

Patients with hypertension and coexistent hyperlipidemia are also at increased risk for the development of atherosclerosis. The special need in this group is for coordinated treatment to provide adequate control of blood pressure with antihypertensive agents that do not adversely affect blood lipid levels.

EVALUATION OF PATIENTS

A first step in evaluation is to determine blood lipid levels. All patients with definite vascular disease or hypertension require a low-density lipoprotein cholesterol (LDL-C) determination, since therapeutic decisions and interventions are based on LDL-C. The standard battery of tests for this purpose includes total cholesterol (TC), triglyceride (TG), and high-density lipoprotein cholesterol (HDL-C). A minimal 8-hour fast is advised. The usual clinical laboratory procedure to determine LDL-C is to measure TC, HDL-C, and TG directly and then to apply the formula LDL-C = TC − HDL-C − (TG/5). This formula cannot be used if the TG is greater than 400 mg per deciliter (4.52 mmol per liter). Confirm LDL-C levels greater than 130 mg per deciliter (3.36 mmol per liter). This can be done as early as 1 week after the first determination, and the average of two values can be used unless they vary by more than 30 mg per deciliter (0.78 mmol per liter), in which case a third determination is obtained and an average of the three values is used. LDL-C may be temporarily lowered for 6 weeks to 3 months after a myocardial infarction and should be rechecked at later intervals. It is desirable to use a laboratory participating in the Lipid Standardization Program of the Center for Disease Control, where daily analytical variation should be less than 5 percent.

Secondary causes of lipid disorders (Table 1) should be considered. A medication history and family history of diabetes mellitus should be taken from all patients. Measurement of free unbound thyroxine (FT_4) (or thyroid-stimulating hormone [TSH]), alkaline phosphatase, serum creatinine, and a fasting blood glucose level, plus urinalysis for albumin, will identify most secondary hyperlipidemias. The most common secondary cause of hyperlipidemia is type II diabetes mellitus. A 2-hour glucose tolerance test with 100 g of oral glucose should be performed in patients who have a family history of diabetes if they are more than 30 pounds over ideal body weight or have elevated TG levels. If the 2-hour blood glucose level exceeds 165 mg per deciliter at age 40, 180 mg per deciliter at age 50, or 190 mg per deciliter at age 60 and above, consider the blood lipid problem secondary to diabetes and initiate a program to reduce fasting blood sugar levels. These diagnostic criteria are designed to identify individuals with hyperlipidemia at an early stage of type II diabetes mellitus.

Antihypertensive agents that increase blood lipid levels (Table 2) are another common cause of secondary

Table 1 Secondary Causes of Lipid Disorders

Endocrine
  Diabetes mellitus
  Hypothyroidism
  Hypopituitarism
  Acromegaly
  Anorexia nervosa
Renal
  Nephrotic syndrome or nephrotic range proteinuria
  Uremia
Hepatic
  Primary biliary cirrhosis
  Extrahepatic biliary obstruction
  Acute hepatitis
Immunologic
  Dysglobulinemia
  Lymphoma
  Systemic lupus erythematosus
Drugs
  Alcohol
  Antihypertensives (see Table 2)
  Oral contraceptives
  Glucocorticoids

Table 2 Lipoprotein Effects of Commonly Used Antihypertensive Agents

	LDL-C	TG	HDL-C
Diuretics			
Thiazides	↑	↑	↓ ↔
Loop	↑		↓ ↔
Potassium-sparing	↑ ↔	↑ ↔	↓ ↔
Indapamide	↔	↔	↔
β-Blockers			
Nonselective	↑ ↔	↑	↓
B_1-Selective	↔	↑	↓
α/β Blocker	↔	↔	↔
With ISA	↔	↔	↔
α-Blockers			
Nonselective	↓ ↔	↓ ↔	↑ ↔
$α_1$-Selective	↓ ↔	↓ ↔	↑ ↔
CNS α-agonists			
Clonidine	↓	↓	↑
Guanabenz		↔	
Methyldopa	↓ ↔	↑ ↔	↓ ↔
Calcium channel blockers	↔	↔	↔
ACE inhibitors	↔	↔	↔
Physiologic vasodilators	↔	↔	↔

For abbreviations, see text.

hyperlipidemia, particularly in moderate to heavy social drinkers who are overweight. Hypothyroidism is a poor third among the common causes of secondary hyperlipidemia, but should always be given consideration when LDL-C levels fail to respond to bile acid–binding resin therapy. Patients with hypothyroidism usually require increased oral thyroid replacement when treated with bile acid–binding resins because of reduced intestinal absorption. The presence of renal disease can influence treatment of hyperlipidemia in two ways: (1) the nephrotic syndrome can cause secondary elevations of both LDL-C and TG levels and (2) reduced dosage of fibrate drugs may be required if renal insufficiency from any cause is present. If a correctable secondary cause of hyperlipidemia is identified, treat it before instituting lipid-altering medication.

Blood lipid evaluation should be coupled with assessment of nonlipid coronary risk factors for atherosclerosis (Table 3). If nonlipid factors that cannot be altered are present, the need for blood lipid lowering is increased. A program to reduce those factors that can be modified, particularly smoking, should be coordinated with antilipid therapy.

TREATMENT GOALS

The treatment goal for patients with definite vascular disease is normalization of all lipoprotein levels. The LDL-C level should be lowered below 130 mg per deciliter (3.36 mmol per liter) and ideally to under 100 mg per deciliter (2.59 mmol per liter), since current evidence indicates that levels under 100 mg per deciliter (2.59 mmol per liter) are associated with atherosclerotic lesion regression. Total TG should be lowered below 150 mg per deciliter (1.69 mmol per liter) and HDL-C levels ideally increased to 52 mg per deciliter (1.34 mmol per liter) or greater in males and 66 mg per deciliter (1.71 mmol per liter) or greater in females.

An additional treatment goal is to have patients adopt dietary and life style patterns that produce a long-term reduction in all risk factors and maintain body weight as close as possible to the ideal. These life style changes should include as much exercise as the cardiovascular status allows, and should give high priority to abstinence from smoking.

DIETARY THERAPY

Reduction in dietary fat and cholesterol intake are a prerequisite for optimal lipid alteration and must play a substantial role in treatment of all patients (Table 4). The key elements are (1) reduction of dietary cholesterol, (2) reduction of all fats with emphasis on reduction of saturated fats, and (3) weight control. This strategy potentiates the action of hypolipidemic therapy and frequently allows use of lower doses, reducing the risk of side effects. At times, dietary modification can obviate the need for drug therapy. Medications should be used only in the setting of appropriate dietary changes. Drugs

Table 3 Risk Factors for Atherosclerosis

Family history of myocardial infarction or sudden death in a parent or sibling before age 55
Cigarette smoking
Male gender
Diabetes mellitus
Hypertension
Obesity ($\geq 30\%$ overweight)
HDL–C <35 mg/dl
(Postmenopausal state)

Table 4 Dietary Guidelines for Lipid Disorders (Percentage of Calories)

Nutrient	Step 1	Step 2
Saturated fat	<10%	<7%
Polyunsaturated fat	<10%	<10%
Monounsaturated fat	10–15%	10–15%
Total fat	<30%	<30%
Protein	10–20%	10–20%
Carbohydrates	50–60%	50–60%
Cholesterol	<300 mg/day	<200 mg/day

should not be considered a substitute for dietary therapy; the efficacy of medication is significantly reduced by diets high in saturated fat and cholesterol. When an urgent need to achieve substantial lipid reduction leads to early initiation of drug therapy, the importance of dietary modification should be emphasized to the patient.

Drug and dietary therapy should be initiated simultaneously in high-risk patients. The additional dietary change most frequently needed is greater reduction of dietary fat, because cholesterol intake has declined in recent years, particularly among educated, older, upper-income individuals in whom daily cholesterol intake of 200 mg is not uncommon, but whose usual fat intake is 35 percent of calories. It is wise to start dietary therapy with knowledge of an individual's current dietary habits. A one-page questionnaire that covers foods accounting for approximately 75 percent of the fat in American diets is shown in Figure 1. The form is designed for analysis by IBM compatible desk top computers and provides a written report within minutes.

Dietary therapy is greatly facilitated by a team approach, which includes a registered dietitian and/or nurse educator to offer intensive patient education, counseling, and reinforcement. Other family members, especially the food preparer and shopper, should be involved. Guidelines for food preparation and selection are given in Tables 5 and 6. The American Heart Association Cookbook is an excellent source of recipes. Counseling by a registered dietitian with experience in outpatient therapy is particularly recommended to meet Step-Two dietary guidelines. The physician and team should provide feedback on dietary and drug progress in

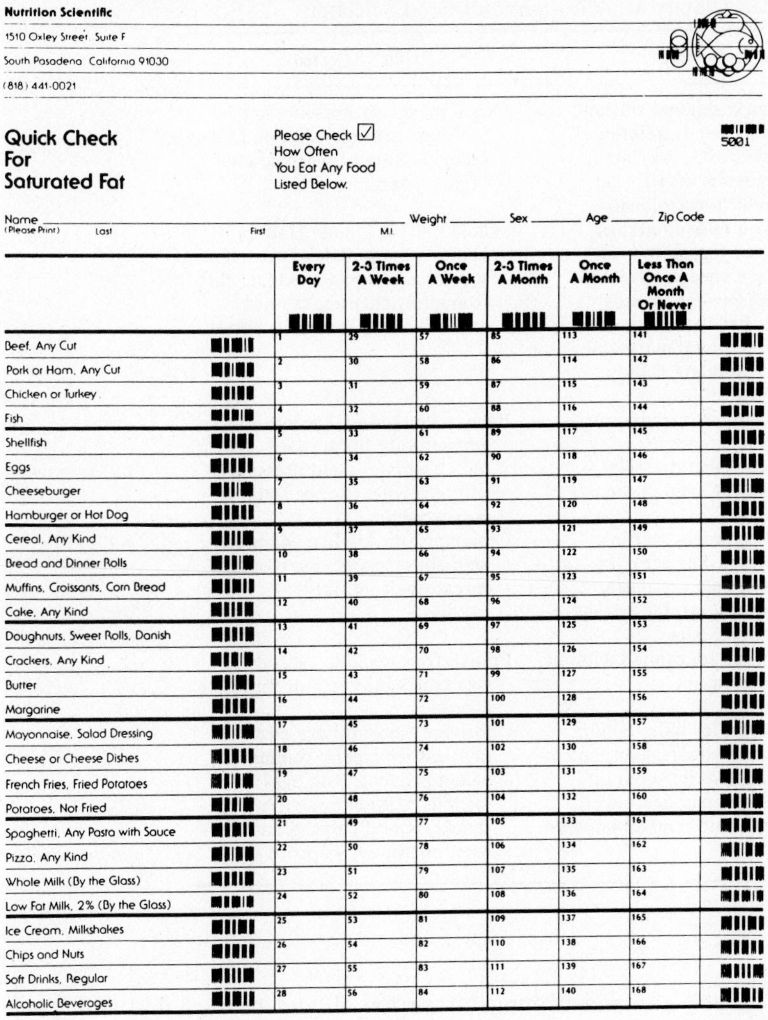

Nutrition Scientific

1510 Oxley Street, Suite F

South Pasadena, California 91030

(818) 441-0021

Quick Check For Saturated Fat

Please Check ☑ How Often You Eat Any Food Listed Below

5001

Name (Please Print) Last First M.I. — Weight ____ Sex ____ Age ____ Zip Code ____

Food	Every Day	2-3 Times A Week	Once A Week	2-3 Times A Month	Once A Month	Less Than Once A Month Or Never	
Beef, Any Cut	1	29	57	85	113	141	
Pork or Ham, Any Cut	2	30	58	86	114	142	
Chicken or Turkey	3	31	59	87	115	143	
Fish	4	32	60	88	116	144	
Shellfish	5	33	61	89	117	145	
Eggs	6	34	62	90	118	146	
Cheeseburger	7	35	63	91	119	147	
Hamburger or Hot Dog	8	36	64	92	120	148	
Cereal, Any Kind	9	37	65	93	121	149	
Bread and Dinner Rolls	10	38	66	94	122	150	
Muffins, Croissants, Corn Bread	11	39	67	95	123	151	
Cake, Any Kind	12	40	68	96	124	152	
Doughnuts, Sweet Rolls, Danish	13	41	69	97	125	153	
Crackers, Any Kind	14	42	70	98	126	154	
Butter	15	43	71	99	127	155	
Margarine	16	44	72	100	128	156	
Mayonnaise, Salad Dressing	17	45	73	101	129	157	
Cheese or Cheese Dishes	18	46	74	102	130	158	
French Fries, Fried Potatoes	19	47	75	103	131	159	
Potatoes, Not Fried	20	48	76	104	132	160	
Spaghetti, Any Pasta with Sauce	21	49	77	105	133	161	
Pizza, Any Kind	22	50	78	106	134	162	
Whole Milk (By the Glass)	23	51	79	107	135	163	
Low Fat Milk, 2% (By the Glass)	24	52	80	108	136	164	
Ice Cream, Milkshakes	25	53	81	109	137	165	
Chips and Nuts	26	54	82	110	138	166	
Soft Drinks, Regular	27	55	83	111	139	167	
Alcoholic Beverages	28	56	84	112	140	168	

Figure 1 The bar-coded questionnaire is used to record the patient's name, weight, sex, age, zip code, and frequency of intake of 28 foods. Data are entered by bar code wand into an IBM compatible personal computer, and results are immediately obtained. (With permission from Nutrition Scientific, South Pasadena, CA.)

Table 5 Guidelines for Food Preparation

Recommend
  Trim all visible fat before cooking
  Allow fat to drain before eating
  Remove skin and underlying fat from poultry before cooking
  Steam, bake, broil, grill, stir fry with limited quantities of nonsaturated fats
  Avoid cooking oils by preparing food in microwave or nonstick pans
  Chill soups and remove top fat layer before eating
  Replace whole eggs with 1 or 2 egg whites in recipes or use egg substitutes
Avoid
  Cooking or frying in saturated fats
  Cooking or covering foods in fat–rich sauces or butter
  High–cholesterol, high–fat salad dressings

a series of scheduled appointments. During the early stages of treatment, food records and blood cholesterol levels should be analyzed and discussed at each visit. Later visits are used to continue the educational process, introduce further improvements in dietary habits, and guard against relapse. The goal is a permanent alteration in eating habits.

Eating away from home should take place in restaurants that follow the American Heart Association dietary guidelines, and foods prepared according to these guidelines should be chosen (Table 5). Patients should be taught to recognize 3-oz portions and to take the rest home when larger portions of meats, poultry, and fish are served. Patients should also be taught to read food labels and to monitor the cholesterol and saturated fat content of food purchases. They should know that some "low-cholesterol" and "cholesterol-free" foods contain substantial amounts of fat. The major ingredients of prepared foods must appear in rank

Table 6 Recommended Dietary Modifications and Food Selection

Food	Recommended	Avoid or Decrease
Meats 3 oz/meal; 6 oz total per day	Fish 3 times/wk; skinless chicken, turkey (white meat preferable); leanest cuts beef, pork, lamb, veal; lunchmeats with 1 g fat per oz; shellfish occasionally	Organ meats; processed meat— hot dogs, sausages, bacon, salami, bologna; fatty or marbled cuts of meat; sardines
Dairy products	Nonfat or skim milk; nonfat or low–fat (1%) yogurt; low–fat (2%) cottage cheese; vegetable oil cheeses; low–fat cheeses (≤4 g oz); low–fat mayonnaise (≤1 g sat. fat/tbls); margarine (≤2 g sat. fat/tbls); <3 egg yolks/wk; egg whites	Whole milk; 2% milk; Half and Half; cream; nondairy creamers; sour cream; swiss, cheddar, blue, Roquefort cheeses; coconut milk; whole milk yogurt; butter
Fats, oils ≤ 6 tsp/day	Corn, olive, safflower, sunflower, sesame, canola, cottonseed, soybean oils; salad dressings with 0 g sat. fat; baking cocoa	Palm, palm kernel, coconut, hydrogenated oils; butter, lard, beef fat; chocolate; salad dressings with egg yolk, cheese, sour cream, cream
Bread Cereal	Nonegg bagels; bread, muffins, rolls (0–1 g sat. fat/slice); low–fat crackers; rice; nonegg pasta; cereals with 0 g sat. fat; barley; buckwheat; rye; oats	Croissants; doughnuts; egg breads; high–fat crackers; egg pasta; cereals with sat. fats
Vegetables Fruits	Fresh, frozen, dried, canned without sauces or butter	French fries made in sat. oils; vegetables in sauces or butter; avocados
Desserts Snacks Limit foods high in sugar in persons with high TG or excess weight	Sherbert; sorbet; ice milk; nonfat, low–fat frozen yogurt; light ice cream (≤1 g sat. fat/serving); nonfat cookies, pastries; cakes, pies; pretzels; air–popped popcorn	Chocolate; coconut; egg custard; high–fat ice cream; commercial baked products with eggs and sat. fats; corn chips, cheese snacks, potato chips, granola bars, microwave popcorn

order, and one safe rule is to avoid products that list any of the following among the first three: fat, animal fat, and hydrogenated fat or oil.

If a gradual change in dietary habits appears likely to increase compliance, therapy can proceed according to the National Cholesterol Education Program Step-One and Step-Two dietary guidelines (see Table 4). This strategy is for a progressive reduction in the intake of saturated fat and cholesterol, plus a reduction of excess calories for overweight patients. In general, patients with moderately severe lipid elevations who are on high-fat, high-cholesterol diets will show the greatest responses to dietary change.

Regular exercise augments the effects of dietary modification by assisting weight loss and raising HDL-C levels. It can also assist in smoking cessation, which itself results in an increase in HDL-C levels. Sustained regular aerobic exercise lasting for 20 to 30 minutes at least three to four times a week is recommended if the patient's cardiovascular status permits it. It is a valuable component for the treatment of most lipid disorders. Aerobics, walking, jogging, swimming, cycling, and rowing are all acceptable forms of exercise for patients with minimal cardiac damage who can be encouraged to work up to 80 percent of maximal heart rate (220 − patient's age × 0.80) for the entire exercise period. A warm-up

and cooling off period should be included with each exercise session. Lower-level exercise can also improve blood lipid control in patients who cannot or will not attempt more strenuous activity.

DRUG THERAPY

General Guidelines

Begin with one drug directed specifically at the predominant lipoprotein abnormality (Table 7). Add other drugs, one at a time, to treat remaining abnormalities. The drugs of choice for an elevated LDL-C without hypertriglyceridemia are the bile acid sequestrants colestipol and cholestyramine. Bile acid resin treatment has been shown to reduce ischemic heart disease rates, and a bile acid resin has been used in every drug trial to date to provide angiographic evidence of atherosclerosis regression. Lovastatin is a drug of second choice until it has been shown to produce atherosclerosis regression when used as a sole agent. It is attractive because of ease of administration. Lovastatin is useful in combination with the bile acid sequestrants for severely elevated LDL-C levels, and this combination has been shown to produce angiographic evidence of regression. If a low

Table 7 Lipid–Altering Drug Therapy Based on Primary
Lipid Abnormality

Lipid Level	Lipid–Lowering Drugs
Category 1 LDL–C >130 mg/dl TG <250 mg/dl	Cholestyramine Colestipol Lovastatin Nicotinic acid Cholestyramine or colestipol can be used in combination with lovastatin if LDL–C reduction is insufficient; nicotinic acid or gemfibrozil may be added as a second drug if HDL–C is concurrently low
Category 2 TG >250 mg/dl LDL–C >130 mg/dl	Nicotinic acid Gemfibrozil Add cholestyramine, colestipol, or niacin if LDL–C is not reduced sufficiently
Category 3 TG >250 mg/dl LDL–C <130 mg/dl	Nicotinic acid Gemfibrozil
Category 4 HDL–C <35 mg/dl LDL–C >130 mg/dl and/or TG >250 mg/dl	Nicotinic acid Gemfibrozil LDL–C and TG should be normalized primarily with appropriate agents, then low HDL–C can be treated
Category 5 HDL–C <35 mg/dl LDL–C <130 mg/dL and/or TG <250 mg/dl	Nicotinic acid Gemfibrozil

HDL-C occurs with an elevated LDL-C, gemfibrozil or nicotinic acid are appropriate second drugs to add to bile acid resins for further reduction of LDL-C and elevation of HDL-C levels. Nicotinic acid and gemfibrozil are the drugs of choice for isolated hypertriglyceridemia and when elevations of both TG and LDL-C are present. Angiographic evidence of regression has not been demonstrated with sole use of either nicotinic acid or gemfibrozil, but both drugs used alone have been shown to reduce ischemic heart disease mortality rates. If LDL-C remains elevated after TG levels are normalized, either a bile acid sequestrant or lovastatin can be added for combination therapy. The combination of nicotinic acid and a bile acid resin has been shown to produce angiographic evidence of regression in two controlled clinical trials. The combination of gemfibrozil and lovastatin should be used with caution in all patients, and not used at all in patients with renal disease or on immunosuppressive therapy.

Specific Drugs

Colestipol and Cholestyramine

Bile acid sequestrants are nonabsorbable anion exchange resins that bind bile acids within the gastrointestinal tract, decreasing their enterohepatic circulation. A decrease in the hepatic pool of bile acids stimulates compensatory synthesis and depletes hepatic cholesterol stores, which in turn results in increased hepatic LDL-C receptor activity. Reduction of the blood LDL-C level follows because of LDL-C removal and catabolism. Bile acid resins are the drugs of first choice for treating isolated elevated LDL-C levels because of their long-term safety profile, proven effects in reducing coronary heart disease events, and association with atherosclerosis regression, as mentioned previously. They are the safest agents to use in children and pregnant women. Use of bile acid resins as single agents in the treatment of hypertriglyceridemia is contraindicated because they can increase hepatic very-low-density lipoprotein (VLDL) production and plasma TG levels.

Bile acid sequestrants are dispensed as a powder in cans or packets. Cholestyramine is also available in candy bar form with three flavors. Colestipol is unflavored and each packet or scoop contains 5 g. Cholestyramine is orange flavored and comes in two powder forms: a regular formulation in which each packet or scoop contains 4 g of resin and 5 g of excipients for flavoring, and as cholestyramine light in which each packet contains 5 g of powder of which 4 g is resin. Cholybars contain 4 g of resin.

Treatment is initiated with the equivalent half-maximal dosages, 4 g of cholestyramine three times a day or of colestipol 5 g three times a day. Twice-daily dosing is acceptable if it increases compliance, but three times a day is the preferred regimen. If the bar form of cholestyramine enhances compliance at lunchtime or at times away from home, it can be substituted for the powder form of either colestipol or cholestyramine.

If the LDL-C level is not sufficiently reduced by half dosage, increase to maximal dosage, 8 g of cholestyramine three times a day or 10 g of colestipol three times a day. The maximal effect to be expected from bile acid–binding therapy is a 30 percent reduction in LDL-C. If progression from half dosage to maximal dosage does not produce a further reduction in LDL-C, return to the lower dose and add a second drug. Bile acid resins should be taken at mealtime even if a meal is not eaten. However, observe for gastritis if this occurs consistently. Bile acid resins can help curb appetite and assist in weight reduction if taken immediately before meals. Digitalis preparations, thyroxine, warfarin, beta-blockers, and thiazide diuretics must be taken 1 hour before or 4 hours after bile acid resins, because the resins can interfere with their absorption.

Patients should be told in advance that these agents have a gritty consistency that can be partially masked by chilling or mixing with pulpy fluids. They also produce constipation, which is most marked during the first weeks of use. Less frequent gastrointestinal side effects include bloating, nausea, abdominal pain, bulky stools, and aggravation of hemorrhoids. Most of these side effects, except bulky stools, are transient and can be reduced by having patients experiment with dosage schedules and methods of preparing the powders. Some patients unable to take colestipol are able to take cholestyramine, and vice versa. Either powder should be slurried into a minimal 8 oz of a liquid and allowed to stand for at least 5 minutes. A wide variety of drinks are acceptable and patients should be encouraged to experiment.

Constipation can be reduced by taking a stool softener and mixing 3.4 g of psyllium hydrophilic mucilloid (1 teaspoon of Metamucil or the equivalent) with each resin dose and drinking plenty of fluids throughout the day. A bonus from this dose of psyllium is an additive effect in reducing cholesterol levels. Although bile acids are not systemically absorbed, they can cause mild transient elevations in hepatic transaminase and alkaline phosphatase levels. Because bile acid–binding resins reduce the absorption of warfarin and fat-soluble vitamins, prothrombin times and vitamin A or carotenoid levels should be checked at yearly intervals when large doses are used. Routine vitamin supplementation in adults is not recommended. Bile acid sequestrants do not lower lipid levels in the presence of complete biliary obstruction, but do improve pruritus from biliary cirrhosis. In patients with pre-existing constipation, pretreat with a stool softener for 1 week before beginning resin therapy.

Nicotinic Acid

Nicotinic acid is one of the most effective and least expensive agents available. This water-soluble vitamin B has multiple effects on lipid metabolism. Nicotinic acid decreases hepatic synthesis of VLDL, which in turn reduces LDL-C because LDL-C is derived directly from VLDL. Reduced hepatic VLDL synthesis results from inhibition of adipose tissue lipolysis, with a consequent decrease in plasma fatty acid levels, as well as decreased esterification of hepatic triglycerides. Nicotinic acid can be used as a first-line agent in the treatment of isolated LDL-C elevations, but more common uses are for treatment of isolated hypertriglyceridemia, concurrent TG and LDL-C elevations, and low HDL-C levels. The effects of nicotinic acid are dose dependent. This agent is capable of lowering LDL-C 10 to 20 percent and TG 20 to 80 percent, and raising HDL-C 35 to 60 percent.

Nicotinic acid is started at 100 mg three times a day with meals and increased as tolerated by the patient, usually 100 mg three times a day each week. Some patients are able to double the dosage on a weekly basis. Compliance may be increased by twice-daily dosing, but administration three times a day reduces the incidence of flushing. Sustained-release nicotinic acid may decrease flushing symptoms, but we avoid these preparations because of a greater risk of serious liver toxicity.

Flushing, dry skin, and gastric irritation limit the acceptance of nicotinic acid. Flushing is reduced by increasing the dose slowly and taking the medication on a very regular schedule. Taking nicotinic acid with meals reduces flushing and helps to avoid gastric irritation. Patients should be told that flushing can also be reduced by small daily doses of aspirin. Flushing is a prostaglandin-mediated process that can be reduced by taking one-half or one adult aspirin every morning during the early stages of treatment. Larger doses of aspirin are not more effective and increase the incidence of gastric irritation. As a rule, patients flush only once a day, and the flush lasts 4 to 5 minutes. Once a flush has started, the taking of aspirin will not shorten the duration. Tolerance to the flushing usually develops by the sixth week of therapy at a constant dose, but may reappear when the dosage is increased.

Nicotinic acid uniformly causes reversible increases in hepatic transaminase levels, but significant liver toxicity is extremely rare. Glucose intolerance and hyperuricemia are common. The hyperuricemia can lead to symptomatic gout, but is easily controlled with small doses of allopurinol. Fasting plasma glucose, uric acid, and liver enzymes should be determined before initiating therapy and every 4 to 6 weeks while increasing the dosage. Once the optimal dosage has been determined, routine monitoring should take place every 3 months. Nicotinic acid can be given in doses as high as 12 g per day, but most patients are limited by gastric irritation to 3 to 6 g per day. Supraventricular tachyarrhythmias can occur with nicotinic acid, which should be used with caution in patients with a history of arrhythmias. Nicotinic acid is contraindicated in patients with complete left bundle branch block, active peptic ulcer, and severe liver dysfunction. It should be used with caution in patients with a history of peptic ulcer. Retinal edema with loss of visual acuity is a rare but reversible side effect.

Lovastatin

Lovastatin is one of a new class of agents that are competitive inhibitors of the rate-limiting enzyme in cholesterogenesis, 3-hydroxy-3-methylglutaryl coenzyme A reductase (HMG-CoA reductase). Pravastatin and simvastatin are other agents in this class. These agents are very effective in decreasing LDL-C levels by direct inhibition of hepatic cholesterol synthesis. This decreases the hepatic cholesterol pool and increases hepatic LDL receptor activity, which in turn increases the removal and catabolism of plasma LDL-C. Lovastatin produces very few short-term side effects except elevation of liver enzymes, although information about its long-term safety is limited. Lovastatin can lower LDL-C 20 to 45 percent and TG 10 to 30 percent, and raise HDL-C 5 to 15 percent. Its main indication is for the treatment of elevated LDL-C levels, and it should be reserved for patients who cannot tolerate the bile acid sequestrants or who have not had a sufficient LDL-C response to those agents.

Lovastatin is started at 20 mg per day with the evening meal, because cholesterogenesis occurs mainly during the late night to early morning hours. The dosage is increased as indicated by the LDL-C level every 4 to 6 weeks; the maximal dose is 80 mg per day, which should be divided between morning and evening doses.

Lovastatin causes reversible elevations of liver transaminase in 2 to 5 percent of patients. Nausea, headaches, and rash are less frequent. Liver enzymes should be determined before starting lovastatin, every 4 to 6 weeks while increasing the dosage, and then at 3-month intervals. If the liver enzymes persistently exceed three times normal, dosage should be reduced or lovastatin discontinued. Lovastatin has no effect on steroidogenesis. An eye examination for cataracts should be performed before using lovastatin and then on a yearly basis. A possible increase in cortical lenticular opacities has been a concern but has not been demonstrated.

Caution must be exercised when using lovastatin in combination with nicotinic acid or gemfibrozil. Both lovastatin and gemfibrozil as single agents can cause myopathy, which begins with myalgia and elevated creatine kinase (CK) levels and may progress to rhabdomyolysis, renal insufficiency, or severe ventricular arrhythmia. When both agents are used together, patients should be monitored closely for symptoms of muscle pain, weakness, or tenderness. In addition, CK levels should be determined before instituting this drug combination, after 4 to 6 weeks, and periodically thereafter. Lovastatin is contraindicated in patients treated with cyclosporine; the incidence of severe myopathy is approximately 30 percent. Lovastatin should also be stopped temporarily if erythromycin is administered, otherwise rhabdomyolysis may occur. Lovastatin is contraindicated in severe hepatic disease and never used in pregnancy or during lactation. It causes fetal damage, and women in the childbearing years must be warned that it may be advisable to terminate a pregnancy that occurs during lovastatin treatment.

Gemfibrozil

A fibric acid derivative, gemfibrozil is structurally related to clofibrate and has largely supplanted this earlier agent. Like other fibric acid derivatives, gemfibrozil exerts its main lipid-lowering effects on TG levels by potentiating the activity of lipoprotein lipase, an enzyme responsible for catabolism of VLDL. To a lesser extent, these agents indirectly reduce hepatic VLDL secretion by inhibiting peripheral lipolysis and decreasing hepatic extraction of free fatty acids, thereby decreasing hepatic TG production. The reduction in plasma TG levels is accompanied by a variable effect on LDL-C levels. Decreased VLDL production tends to reduce LDL-C levels, but increased VLDL catabolism can lead to an increase in hepatic LDL-C production. If LDL-C levels are elevated by gemfibrozil, the addition of either a bile acid–binding resin or nicotinic acid usually is corrective.

Although gemfibrozil as a sole agent can reduce LDL-C levels, it is not recommended primarily for this purpose. The main use for gemfibrozil is in isolated TG elevations and in the common problem of concurrent elevations in TG and LDL-C levels, where it will reduce LDL-C 10 to 20 percent and TG 35 to 50 percent, and raise HDL-C 10 to 20 percent. It is also useful in correcting low HDL-C levels, but is not as effective as nicotinic acid for this purpose. Gemfibrozil used alone in asymptomatic men has reduced the risk of coronary heart disease. Fenofibrate and bezafibrate are more potent fibric acid agents used in Europe and are currently under consideration for use in the United States.

The maximal dose of gemfibrozil is 1,200 mg per day, divided between a morning and an evening dose. It is available in 300-mg and 600-mg capsules and can be given or started at 600 mg per day if side effects occur or if the lipid disorder is not too severe.

There are two serious side effects from fibrates; both can be avoided with proper precautions. These agents potentiate the effects of warfarin, and so when beginning or changing the dose prothrombin time must be measured frequently until it stabilizes. The second serious side effect of fibrates is a rare myopathy, observed first with clofibrate, which begins in the first week of therapy; it can cause malaise, fever, and muscle pain and can progress to multifocal ventricular arrhythmias unless the agents are stopped. Fibrate excretion is 70 percent through the urine, and reduced doses are required in patients with renal insufficiency. The manner in which fibrates reduce triglyceride levels is inherently lithogenic, and published data for clofibrate, the most extensively studied agent of the class, indicate that clinical event rates are low but higher than with placebo treatment. Gemfibrozil is contraindicated in primary biliary cirrhosis and severe liver disease.

A variety of minor gastrointestinal side effects have been reported, including dyspepsia, abdominal pain, and nausea. Other reported but uncommon side effects include atrial fibrillation, hyperesthesia, paresthesia, and fluid retention. Elevation of liver enzymes as well as

LDH and alkaline phosphatase levels is not uncommon, and requires observation but not discontinuance of the medication unless levels rise progressively or exceed three times normal. Liver enzyme levels should be monitored 4 to 6 weeks after starting the medication and then at 3-month intervals.

Probucol

Probucol is a lipophilic antioxidant which is transported by LDL and stored in depot fat. The mechanism of action of probucol is incompletely defined, but it appears to increase the fractional catabolic rate of LDL partly through a non–receptor-mediated pathway. It produces relatively small reductions of LDL-C (10 to 15 percent) and lowers HDL-C (5 to 20 percent). Probucol is well tolerated; the most common side effects are loose stool, abdominal pain, flatulence, and nausea occurring in less than 5 percent of patients. This agent is contraindicated because of the risk of serious cardiac arrhythmia in patients with a prolonged QT interval on the electrocardiogram (ECG), and should be used with caution when hypokalemia is possible. Probucol can induce the regression of xanthomas, and evidence from animal studies indicates that its antioxidant properties impart an antiatherogenic effect independent of changes in the blood lipid level. However, probucol is a second-line drug for the treatment of elevated LDL-C levels because of its adverse lowering effect on HDL-C. Its use is limited to patients who are unable to take the drugs of choice for lowering LDL-C, and it is occasionally used with the first-line drugs when other medications used in combination are not tolerated. Probucol is never used to treat hypertriglyceridemia. Because probucol is stored in adipose tissue, blood levels decline slowly after therapy is discontinued; it therefore should be used with caution in women of childbearing age. The starting dose of probucol is 250 mg twice a day, and this may be increased to 500 mg twice a day.

SPECIAL SITUATIONS

Isolated or Predominant Hypertriglyceridemia

Patients with an isolated or predominant elevation of TG and definite vascular disease should have TG reduced below 150 mg per deciliter insofar as possible. Type II diabetes mellitus is a common unrecognized underlying cause, and so the family history should be reviewed with special care for diabetes. If fasting blood sugar shows even borderline elevation, perform formal glucose tolerance testing. Be sure to learn about alcohol intake and have a dietitian obtain a quantitative estimate of the percentage of total calories that alcohol provides. If alcohol furnishes more than 7 to 10 percent of total calories, treatment of hypertriglyceridemia will be difficult until intake is reduced. Alcohol intake as high as 20 percent of calories can be encountered in social drinkers who limit other calories for weight control. Secondary causes of hypertriglyceridemia, including oral contraceptives, corticosteroid therapy, and antihypertensive therapy, need to be corrected if present (see Table 2). If patients are more than 20 percent over the ideal body weight, the primary dietary change should be restriction of calories. Dietary patterns meeting Step-One guidelines are appropriate if the calories are adequately restricted (Table 8). If TG levels exceed 1,000 mg per deciliter (11.29 mmol per liter), nicotinic acid, a fibric acid derivative, or a combination of both drugs will probably be required. However, drug therapy may not be effective until after 2 to 3 weeks of rigid dietary fat restriction where no more than 10 percent of total calories derived from fat is used to reduce chylomicronemia.

Drug treatment should be initiated simultaneously with dietary therapy and exercise. Exercise is an extremely important adjuvant to drug therapy in overweight hypertriglyceridemic patients, especially since lipid-lowering medications may have minimal effects until the patient begins to exercise and lose weight. Gemfibrozil and nicotinic acid are both effective single agents and are also effective when used together. Treatment of elevated TG levels often results in elevations of HDL-C levels. Currently, fish oil supplements are not recommended for treatment of hypertriglyceridemia.

Isolated Low HDL-C

A predominant lipid abnormality in a subgroup of patients with definite vascular disease is a low HDL-C (< 35 mg per deciliter, 0.91 mmol per liter). LDL-C levels (typically < 130 mg per deciliter, 3.36 mmol per liter) are normal, as are TG levels (< 150 mg per deciliter, 1.69 mmol per liter). Although there is no direct evidence indicating that raising HDL-C levels will reverse atherosclerotic disease, there is substantial evidence that low levels increase the risk of clinical cardiac disease. Therefore, patients with definite vascular disease should be aggressively treated. Nonpharmacologic therapy should include as vigorous physical exercise as cardiac status allows, maintenance of ideal body weight, and cessation of smoking. Medications that lower HDL (Table 9) should be reduced or replaced with alternatives. Nicotinic acid is by far the most effective medication capable of raising HDL-C, especially in conjunction with exercise; gemfibrozil is a poor second (see Table 7). Alcohol in moderate amounts also raises HDL-C in patients with low or normal TG levels, but because of the multitude of other adverse health consequences, it is not recommended as a drug for this purpose. The amount of HDL-C increase that can be obtained by any means is inversely proportional to the degree of the abnormality. HDL-C levels between 30 mg per deciliter (0.78 mmol per liter) and 35 mg per deciliter (0.91 mmol per liter) are significantly more responsive than lower levels.

Table 8 Nonpharmacologic Therapy
for Hypertriglyceridemia

Exercise
Cessation of cigarette smoking
Maintenance of ideal body weight
Discontinuation of medications that elevate triglycerides (see
　Tables 1 and 2)
Step–One dietary guidelines in addition to:
　Restriction of simple sugars
　Restriction of alcohol intake (abstinence)
　Increase in fish intake
　Increase in soluble fiber intake

Table 9 Causes of Low HDL–C Levels

Nonpharmacologic	Pharmacologic
Cigarette smoking	Antihypertensives
Male gender (after puberty)	(see Table 2)
Postmenopausal state	Androgens
Obesity	Progestins (unopposed)
Diabetes mellitus	Probucol
Hypertriglyceridemia	Anabolic steroids
Lack of exercise	
Familial hypoalphalipoproteinemia	

Concurrent Hypertension and Hyperlipidemia

Antihypertensive medications that can cause elevations in LDL-C and TG levels, as well as lower HDL-C levels, should be changed to lipid-neutral agents (see Table 2). Before a decision to institute lipid-altering medications is made, allow an 8-week "wash-out" period for antihypertensive agents that adversely affect lipid levels, during which time the lipid levels will equilibrate. Most diuretics, including the thiazide and loop diuretics, as well as beta-blockers without alpha-blockade or intrinsic sympathomimetic activity, should be avoided. Medications with neutral lipid effects, such as the calcium channel blockers verapamil, nifedipine, and diltiazem, and the angiotensin converting enzyme (ACE) inhibitors enalapril, captopril, and lisinopril, are excellent alternatives as first-step agents. The indole diuretic indapamide, which is free of adverse lipid effects, can also be used as a sole first-step agent or in conjunction with other nondiuretic antihypertensive agents if monotherapy is inadequate for hypertension control. If thiazide agents are considered essential for therapy, they should be used in low dosages of 12.5 to 25 mg per day. However, thiazide agents alone or in combination with other antihypertensives should be avoided if possible.

If monotherapy fails to control hypertension, drugs with different modes of action are combined. Medications with lipid-neutral or lipid-positive effects for consideration include the alpha$_1$-selective antagonists prazosin and terazosin, centrally acting alpha-agonists clonidine and guanabenz, and the physiologic vasodilators hydralazine and minoxidil. Minoxidil is usually reserved for patients with severe hypertension unresponsive to other agents and in whom the medication regimen can be simplified with the addition of this agent. Hydralazine is generally used in patients with hypertension and congestive heart failure.

Drug interactions occur between lipid-altering and antihypertensive agents. Bile acid–binding resins can interfere with the absorption of beta-blockers and thiazide diuretics. Antihypertensive agents should be taken 1 hour before, or 4 hours after, bile acid–binding resins. Nicotinic acid also can potentiate the effects of vasodilating agents.

Lowering body weight to as close to the ideal as possible with exercise and caloric restriction is a vital component in the treatment of patients with coexistent hyperlipidemia and hypertension, because both lipoprotein levels and blood pressure levels are reduced. Alcohol and tobacco avoidance is of prime importance, because these risk factors independently cause blood pressure elevation and have adverse effects on lipid levels. Restriction of salt intake to 4 to 6 g per day is a mandatory adjunct in the treatment of hypertension, since this can obviate the need for antihypertensive agents in some patients with mild to moderate hypertension and allow reduced dosages in others.

SUGGESTED READING

Ames RP. The effects of antihypertensive drugs on serum lipids and lipoproteins. I. Diuretics. Drugs 1986; 32:260–278.

Ames RP. The effects of antihypertensive drugs on serum lipids and lipoproteins. II. Non-diuretic drugs. Drugs 1986; 32:335–357.

Blankenhorn DH. Preventive treatment of atherosclerosis. Menlo Park, CA: Addison-Wesley, 1984.

Blankenhorn DH, Nessim SA, Johnson RL, et al. Beneficial effects of combined colestipol-niacin therapy on coronary atherosclerosis and coronary venous bypass grafts. JAMA 1987; 257:3233–3240.

Canner PL, Berge KG, Wenger NK, et al. Fifteen year mortality in Coronary Drug Project patients: Long-term benefit with niacin. J Am Coll Cardiol 1986; 8:1245–1255.

Consensus Conference. Treatment of hypertriglyceridemia. JAMA 1984; 257:1196–1200.

Frick MH, Elo O, Haapa K, et al. Helsinki Heart Study: Primary-prevention trial with gemfibrozil in middle-aged men with dyslipidemia. Safety of treatment, changes in risk factors, and incidence of coronary heart disease. N Engl J Med 1987; 317:1237–1245.

The Lipid Research Clinics Coronary Primary Prevention Trial. Results: I. Reduction in incidence of coronary heart disease. JAMA 1984; 257:351–364.

Report of the National Cholesterol Education Program Expert Panel on Detection, Evaluation, and Treatment of High Blood Cholesterol in Adults. Arch Intern Med 1988; 148:36–39.

SECONDARY HYPERTENSION

RENOVASCULAR HYPERTENSION

RICHARD N. RE, M.D.

Hemodynamically significant stenosis of one or both renal arteries can produce significant, indeed often severe, hypertension and at the same time impart a predisposition for the subsequent loss of renal function. Thus, renovascular hypertension challenges clinicians not only to improve patients' blood pressure, and thereby reduce a major cardiovascular risk factor, but also to prevent the deterioration of renal function. At the same time, clinicians are confronted with the problem of determining which of their many patients with hypertension are at risk for renovascular hypertension and should therefore receive extensive evaluation and therapy.

Although renovascular hypertension is the most common form of secondary hypertension, its prevalence is estimated to range only from about 1 to 6 percent of all hypertensive individuals. Therefore, cost-benefit considerations argue strongly against evaluating all patients with hypertension for possible renal artery stenosis and renovascular hypertension, if diagnosis depends on costly or potentially dangerous studies. For this reason, routine intravenous urography has been abandoned in the evaluation of hypertensive patients in favor of a more selective diagnostic strategy. However, it must be kept in mind that, as screening tests are developed that are more specific and sensitive while at the same time less expensive and associated with less risk than current screening tests, this strategy may have to be re-evaluated.

PATHOPHYSIOLOGY

For the purposes of clinical management, renovascular stenosis may be considered a disorder in which diminished renal blood flow to one or both kidneys stimulates enhanced secretion of the enzyme renin.

Renin, either in the circulation or following uptake into the vascular wall, generates angiotensin I from the hepatically synthesized alpha$_2$-globulin angiotensinogen. Angiotensin I is a decapeptide that is converted by angiotensin converting enzyme (ACE) to the octapeptide angiotensin II. Angiotensin II is a potent vasoconstricting agent and a secretagogue for aldosterone. Thus, a diminished blood flow to the kidney results in an elevation of the angiotensin II concentration in blood, which in turn produces vasoconstriction and a rise in blood pressure. At the same time, the diminution of glomerular filtration rate (GFR) caused by renal artery stenosis and the enhanced secretion of aldosterone produced by hyperreninemia result in sodium retention and subsequent volume expansion. This secondary volume expansion has the effect of suppressing plasma renin activity. Thus, in established renovascular hypertension, circulating plasma renin activity need not be frankly elevated. Although it is unusual in renovascular hypertension for circulating plasma renin activity to be extremely low (in the absence of renin-suppressing drugs), it cannot be assumed that the presence of a normal, or even low-normal, plasma renin activity excludes the diagnosis of renovascular hypertension. Thus, plasma renin activity obtained under standardized circumstances is only one piece in a clinical mosaic that may lead a clinician to evaluate a patient aggressively for renovascular hypertension. For this and other reasons, it is generally assumed that the obtaining of blood for plasma renin activity is not a cost-effective screening measure in the general hypertensive population. While there is debate on this point, it should be noted that in patients suspected on other grounds of suffering from renovascular hypertension, the renin level, both stimulated and unstimulated, becomes an important component in the overall clinical mosaic that influences the decision to proceed with more aggressive evaluation.

In patients under 40 years of age, arterial fibrodysplasia is the most common cause of renovascular hypertension. This group of disorders is commonly referred to as fibromuscular hyperplasia, and each of its forms has a characteristic natural history. According to the Mayo and Cleveland Clinic classification, three forms of arterial fibrodysplasia may be distinguished: intimal fibroplasia, medial fibromuscular dysplasia, and perimedial fibrodysplasia. These dysplastic arterial processes can involve arteries other than the renal arteries. Although these disorders are more frequent among young patients suffering from renovascular hypertension, they can be found in all age groups. A full discussion of these disorders is beyond the scope of this chapter, but as in other forms of renovascular, the physician must be concerned with the progression of the vascular disease to the point of renal compromise as well as the correction of hypertension. The choice of therapeutic strategy and the degree of vigor with which such strategies are pursued in patients suffering from arterial fibrodysplasia depends not only on their clinical state, but also on the known natural histories of each disorder. In general, however, when intervention is chosen in these patients, angioplasty has proved generally effective, particularly for medial fibroplasia.

In the older patient population, atherosclerotic renal artery stenosis clearly is more common than fibromuscular hyperplasia or other causes of renal artery stenosis. Atherosclerotic vascular disease may be limited to the renal artery but more commonly involves multiple arteries, including the carotids and the coronary arteries. The abdominal aorta and the iliac and femoral vessels may also be involved. Physicians should approach patients with atherosclerotic renovascular hypertension as they would patients harboring a systemic vascular disease. This has important implications for both diagnosis and therapy (see below). Atherosclerotic lesions usually occur at the orifice of the renal arteries or in the proximal 2 cm of the artery and may be associated with post-stenotic dilatation. Thrombosis or dissection may entirely obliterate the renal artery.

A potential complication of atherosclerotic arterial disease is cholesterol embolization, which may lead to renal insufficiency. Thus, the progressive loss of renal function in older hypertensive patients should suggest to the clinician the possibility of either progressive renal artery stenosis or renal artery stenosis and atherosclerotic vascular disease complicated by cholesterol embolization. Unfortunately, atherosclerotic renal artery stenosis tends to progress in about 50 percent of cases. Progression to total occlusion is noted in about 16 percent of involved renal arteries. Thus, intervention to preserve renal function is often warranted and aggressive follow-up of medically treated patients is required. Indeed, because restenosis after angioplasty and other interventions is common, aggressive long-term follow-up of all patients is necessary.

Finally, physicians must recall that a variety of other disorders can be associated with renovascular hypertension, albeit uncommonly. Included in this group are entities such as renal artery dissection, vasculitis, neurofibromatosis, congenital bands, pheochromocytoma hydronephrosis, and others. It also should be noted that primary renin-secreting tumors of the juxtaglomerular cells (reninomas), as well as renin-producing hypernephromas and Wilms' tumors, can be associated with all the clinical and laboratory manifestations of renovascular hypertension.

DIAGNOSIS

Although improved screening tests may well be on the horizon, the development of which may greatly simplify the diagnosis of remediable renovascular hypertension in the near future, current practice requires that the diagnosis and evaluation of patients suspected of having renovascular hypertension proceed in a stepwise fashion. Because of the relatively low prevalence of the disease, it is impractical, cost ineffective, and possibly dangerous to subject all hypertensive patients to radiographic screening procedures. Although a few selected centers are exploring the use of outpatient angiography and outpatient renal vein renin sampling early in the diagnostic evaluation of patients, most centers proceed in a stepwise fashion.

Clinical Suspicion

In general, the patient who should be aggressively evaluated is one who develops hypertension for the first time not in middle age but at a young or old age; whose stable or controlled hypertension suddenly worsens or becomes uncontrollable; who is, or becomes, refractory to therapy; who displays an extremely elevated blood pressure; who has hypertension and a unilateral small kidney; who has progressive unilateral or bilateral reductions in renal mass; or who presents on physical examination with clinical evidence suggestive of renovascular hypertension, such as a systolic-diastolic abdominal bruit. Similarly, hypertension in the presence of renal insufficiency after ACE inhibition therapy is suggestive of renovascular hypertension. The presence of diffuse atherosclerotic vascular disease in a hypertensive patient also raises the possibility of atherosclerotic renovascular hypertension. In general, any patient who meets these criteria should be subjected to further work-up.

Plasma Renin Activity

As a first step, it is not inappropriate to determine plasma renin activity normalized for sodium intake. This test is imprecise, but an extremely high level suggests renovascular hypertension, while an extremely low level argues against the diagnosis. Ideally, the patient should not be taking any medication at the time of this test, but if medication is required to control blood pressure, the results of the test must be interpreted with an understanding of the renin-stimulating or renin-suppressing effects of the medication employed. Recently, it has been suggested that both the blood pressure response and the degree of renin stimulation observed after the administration of captopril can serve as a useful diagnostic screening test for renovascular hypertension. This captopril-stimulated renin test ("captopril fling") is deemed to be suspicious for renovascular hypertension if the plasma renin activity at baseline is greater than 5 ng per milliliter per hour and rises above 10 per milliliter per hour 1 hour after ingestion of 25 mg of captopril, but these normative values depend on the methods used to assay renin activity and the testing protocol employed. Although this test may be useful, its specificity and sensitivity are debated currently and it cannot yet be recommended as an established procedure. The test appears to be less reliable in patients with renal insufficiency and those recently treated with ACE inhibitors or diuretics than in others. Also, if the clinicians choose to use this test, they must understand that administration of a fast-acting ACE inhibitor to patients who actually suffer from significant renovascular hypertension can produce a profound and rapid fall in blood pressure. Physicians must be aware of this possible complication and must be assured of patients' ability to withstand any such fall in blood pressure before subjecting them to the test. In general, the rapid infusion of saline and the assumption of a supine posture rapidly restore blood pressure in these patients.

Imaging

Typically, screening procedures for the detection of remediable renovascular hypertension involve imaging the kidneys. In use today are hypertensive intravenous urography, renography, captopril renography, and angiography. In general, intravenous digital subtraction angiography has not proved sufficiently sensitive and specific for this purpose. With the possible exception of the captopril renogram, however, the remaining procedures have sensitivities of approximately 80 percent and specificities of 70 to 80 percent. The captopril renogram involves a determination of GFR using Tc-DPTA or some comparable tracer followed by the ingestion of captopril and a repeat study approximately 1 hour later. A wide variety of protocols are currently employed. The test hinges on the fact that in renovascular hypertension GFR is maintained by angiotensin II–induced efferent vasoconstriction. The elimination or reduction of circulating angiotensin II concentrations results in the release of efferent vasoconstriction and diminution in GFR. This can be detected on the postcaptopril renogram. Some authors report that ^{131}I-hippuran renography is more sensitive than [99m]TC-DTPA scintigraphy in detecting renal cortical hold-up of tracer following captopril. Although the sensitivity and specificity of these procedures have not been well established, partly because a variety of protocols are being employed, the captopril renogram does appear to be useful and is rapidly gaining support for the purpose of diagnosing renovascular hypertension. Indeed, a recent study reports a specificity of 95 percent and a sensitivity of 96 percent, albeit in one preselected study population. Nonetheless, the captopril renogram must be further studied and standardized before its true specificity and sensitivity for remediable renovascular hypertension can be ascertained and its proper role in the diagnostic work-up determined. Currently, it provides the physician with an important piece of diagnostic informa-tion that, taken with others, leads to the diagnosis of renovascular hypertension.

Arteriography

Once the initial screening tests have been completed and found to be consistent with the diagnosis of renovascular hypertension, selective arteriography is generally performed either before, after, or in conjunction with renal vein renin sampling. When physicians' index of suspicion is high, they may proceed directly to invasive diagnostic procedures without using screening procedures, and similarly may do so in the presence of a negative screening test. Although it has been argued that renal vein renin sampling does not offer sufficient predictive information to warrant the use in all patients, numerous studies have confirmed its usefulness of this procedure. Not all stenotic lesions demonstrated on arteriography are associated with hemodynamically significant reductions in blood flow or with remediable renovascular hypertension, and therefore a variety of predictors of physiologically relevant stenosis have been studied. During renal vein sampling, blood should be sampled from each renal vein and from the inferior vena cava either simultaneously or as close to simultaneously as possible. Plasma renin activity is measured in each sample. Vaughn and colleagues developed criteria for renin gradients across normal and stenotic kidneys in patients not on antihypertensive therapy. They further demonstrated that the renin concentration in the inferior vena cava below the renal arteries is approximately equal to that in the renal artery. Thus, gradients of renin across the kidney can be determined without actually sampling arterial blood. These gradients are of considerable use in determining the inappropriate secretion of renin from one or both kidneys.

Other groups have used a variety of secretagogues in order to enhance renin secretion and improve the sensitivity and specificity of renal vein renin sampling. Hydralazine, furosemide, and upright tilting have all been studied as well as other interventions. Early on, my group demonstrated that ACE inhibition using the peptide converting enzyme inhibitor teprotide is an effective renin secretagogue that enhances the diagnostic discrimination of renal vein renin sampling. The administration of ACE inhibitors results in a dramatic increase in the renal vein renin ratio between the two kidneys in favor of the post-stenotic kidney. Subsequently, Lyons and Thibonnier and their colleagues obtained similar data regarding the use of captopril. It is now common to administer captopril 25 mg by mouth 20 to 60 minutes before renal vein sampling. Blood is drawn from each renal vein and from the inferior vena cava above and below the renal arteries. Again, it should be emphasized that the acute administration of captopril, be it during a captopril renin stimulation test, a captopril renogram, or captopril-stimulated renal vein renin sampling, may be associated with significant and rapid falls in blood pressure in patients suffering from renovascular hypertension. Physicians and radiologic teams must be prepared for this possibility. Indeed, it is not unreasonable for physicians to obtain a plasma renin activity before admitting patients to the hospital for renal vein renin sampling. Generally, if the peripheral renin activity is extremely high, no secretagogue need be used and the risk of hypotension can be avoided. If, on the other hand, the peripheral renin level is extraordinarily low as the result of antihypertensive therapy, even captopril may not adequately stimulate the system. Patients therefore should be placed on drugs that provide good blood pressure control and yet a detectable plasma renin activity before they undergo renal vein renin sampling.

In my institution, renal arteriography is generally performed at the same time as renal vein renin sampling. This provides direct visualization of the renal arteries, and the information obtained complements that derived from renal vein sampling so that one can estimate the probability of future loss of renal mass, as well as the probability that correctable hypertension exists. Often, at the time of angiography, I ask my radiologic colleagues to be prepared to perform angioplasty if a significant lesion is found. This is done in patients who have been evaluated to exclude the possibility that relatively abrupt falls in blood pressure will induce myocardial infarction, cerebrovascular insult, or other ischemic events. I also require vascular surgery standby during angioplasty so that, should vascular rupture or some other vascular catastrophe occur, surgical intervention can immediately be undertaken. In general, therefore, if a patient is to have angiography with angioplasty standby, not only is the vascular surgery team alerted, but a bed is reserved in the intensive care unit. When a pre-emptive angioplasty is performed, based on the degree of narrowing produced by a lesion, it can nonetheless be helpful to obtain renal vein renin samples before the procedure. This helps confirm the initial diagnosis if the patient's blood pressure does not improve after an apparently successful angioplasty. When possible, renal vein renin levels are determined after the procedure as well.

One final point regarding angiography, angioplasty, and surgery in patients with renovascular disease centers on the possibility of angiography- or surgery-induced cholesterol embolization. Extreme care must be employed during all interventional procedures in patients suffering from widespread atherosclerotic disease to reduce the likelihood of cholesterol embolization with subsequent ischemia of vital organs. Similarly, during surgery care must be taken to avoid severe hypotension that might lead to infarction of vital organs, such as bowel, whose blood supply might be compromised by atherosclerotic disease. Thus, it is often worthwhile before planning a therapeutic intervention to evaluate carefully the intra-abdominal aorta, and in particular the mesenteric arteries, so as to have some estimate of risk before undertaking interventional therapy.

THERAPY

The goals of therapy for renovascular hypertension are the improvement or cure of hypertension and the preservation of renal mass. In some patients, renal ischemia may have been of sufficient degree and severity essentially to preclude the possibility that revascularization of the ischemic kidney will lead to a functioning organ or substantially reduce hypertension secondary to hypersecretion of renin. In these patients, either nephrectomy or medical therapy is clearly indicated. No absolute guidelines can be provided to indicate when a kidney is salvageable and when it is not, but certain findings can help physicians make this determination. Assessment of GFR by renography or intravenous pyelography provides a quantitative estimate of remaining renal function. Evidence of function in these studies suggests that a viable, functioning renal mass will be present after corrective surgical procedures. Renal size likewise is an indication of salvageable renal mass. In general, kidneys whose length exceeds 9 or 10 cm can be considered candidates for revascularization. The presence of abundant collateral blood supply and back-bleeding from the kidney at the time of surgery are also guides to the existence of salvageable renal mass. Intraoperative renal biopsies that demonstrate viable glomeruli also can be helpful.

Surgery

Because of the often systemic nature of the vascular disease seen in patients with renovascular hypertension, many authors recommend that after the decision to intervene surgically is made, a full evaluation for potentially life-threatening vascular stenosis should be undertaken before surgery or angioplasty, because of the theoretical possibility of acute blood pressure lowering after this procedure. It has been argued that screening for both carotid arterial disease and coronary arterial disease should be undertaken with such measures as ultrasonography, and possibly even carotid angiography in the case of carotid evaluation, and thallium stress tests, SPECT stress tests, dipyridamole stress tests, or even coronary arteriography where appropriate in screening for coronary artery disease. Again, before invasive correction of renal artery stenosis, physicians must familiarize themselves, to the extent clinically prudent, with any associated aortic vascular disease that might complicate the procedure.

Once the decision to intervene invasively to correct renal artery stenosis has been made, the physician must choose from an assortment of procedures. Surgical intervention is the standard mode of invasive therapy and a variety of procedures have been developed for use in specific clinical circumstances.

Angioplasty

This procedure has proved effective in many younger patients suffering from fibrodysplasia. In general, these patients achieve greater long-term remissions in blood pressure and sustain fewer complications than patients suffering from atherosclerotic renal artery stenosis. Long-term improvement in hypertension is hard to obtain with angioplasty in patients with atherosclerotic disease, and many of these lesions are ostial and therefore not amenable to angioplasty. Nonetheless, percutaneous transluminal renal angioplasty is an attractive alternative for some patients with atherosclerotic disease and can be repeated if necessary. Similarly, surgery is generally more effective and associated with fewer complications in younger patients with unilateral fibrodysplasia, close to 90 percent of whom benefit from surgical treatment, as contrasted with older patients suffering from atherosclerotic disease.

Thrombolysis

Finally, patients occasionally present with acute thrombotic or embolic occlusion of the renal artery, often associated with flank pain. These can sometimes be benefited by thrombolytic therapy, angioplasty, or surgery.

Pharmacotherapy

A variety of medications can be used to treat patients with renovascular hypertension in lieu of performing surgery or angioplasty, but if this course is chosen, the status of the involved kidney must be carefully monitored. In general, once the diagnosis of remediable renovascular hypertension is made, invasive therapy is recommended unless the patient's condition precludes this because of the risk involved. Irrespective of the indication for choosing medical as opposed to surgical therapy, it is important that the status of the involved kidney be carefully monitored. Progressive renal loss can occur even in the absence of acceleration of hypertension. Therefore, ongoing evaluation of renal function and morphology (e.g., using renography and determinations of endogenous creatine clearance) should be undertaken. Indeed, even when surgical or angioplasty intervention is chosen, renal function and mass properly should be monitored on a regular and ongoing basis to be certain that no recurrence of the disorder takes place. The patient who has not received the benefit of an invasive procedure is presumably at greater risk than one who has, and therefore should be followed even more closely. In general, the medical treatment of renovascular hypertension employs renin-suppressing agents, diuretics, calcium channel blockers, and often ACE inhibitors. One should remember that the use of ACE inhibitors in patients with renal artery stenosis relieves efferent arterial tone and reduces GFR. Although this diminution in renal function is often reversible, it need not always be, and therefore extreme caution should be used when ACE inhibitors are administered to patients with known renovascular hypertension. Renal function must be diligently followed in this circumstance.

SUGGESTED READING

Bergentz SE, Bergqvist D, Weibull H. Optimal reconstruction of the renal arteries. Acta Chir Scand Suppl 1990; 555:227–235.

Burnier M, Waeber B, Nussberger J, Brunner HR. Effect of angiotensin converting enzyme inhibition in renovascular hypertension. J Hypertens 1989; 7:S27–S31.

Case DB, Atlas SA, Lorogh JH. Reactive hyper-reninaemia to angiotensin blockade identifies renovascular hypertension. Clin Sci 1979; 57:3135–3165.

Frederickson ED, Wilcox CS, Bucci CM, et al. A prospective evaluation of a simplified captopril test for the detection of renovascular hypertension. Arch Intern Med 1990; 150:569–572.

Gifford RW. Evaluation of the hypertensive patient with emphasis on detecting curable causes. Milbank Mem Fund Q 1969; 47:170.

Grim CE, Freidrich CL, Yune HY, et al. Percutaneous transluminal dilation in the treatment of renal vascular hypertension. Ann Intern Med 1981; 95:439.

Harrison EG Jr, McCormack LJ. Pathologic classification of renal arterial disease in renovascular hypertension. Mayo Clin Proc 1971; 46:161–167.

Hillman B. Imaging advances in the diagnosis of renovascular hypertension. Am J Radiol 1989; 153:5–14.

Hunt JC, Strong CG. Renovascular hypertension mechanisms, natural history and treatment. Am J Cardiol 1973; 32:563.

Lyons DF, Kem DC, Brown RD, et al. Captopril stimulation of differential renins in renovascular hypertension. Hypertension 1983; 5:615.

Muller FB, Sealey JE, Case DB, et al. The captopril test for identifying renovascular disease in hypertensive patients. Am J Med 1986; 80: 633.

Novick AC, Straffon RA, Stewart BH, et al. Diminished operative morbidity and mortality following revascularization for atherosclerotic renovascular disease. JAMA 1981; 246:747–753.

Olin JW, Vidt DG, Gifford RW, et al. Renovascular disease in the elderly: an analysis of 50 patients. J Am Coll Cardiol 1985; 5:1232–1238.

Re R, Novelline R, Escourrou MT, et al. Inhibition of angiotensin-converting enzyme for diagnosis of renal artery stenosis. N Engl J Med 1978; 298:582.

Sheps SG, Kincaid OW, Hunt JC. Serial renal function and angiographic observations in idiopathic fibrous and fibromuscular stenoses of the renal arteries. Am J Cardiol 1972;30:55.

Sos TA, Pickering TG, Phil MB, et al. Percutaneous transluminal renal angioplasty in renovascular hypertension due to atheroma or fibromuscular dysplasia. N Engl J Med 1983; 309:274.

Thibonnier M, Joseph A, Sassano P, et al. The improved diagnosis of unilateral renal artery lesions after captopril administration. JAMA 1984; 251:56.

Vaughn ED Jr, Buhler FR, Laragh JH, et al. Renalvascular hypertension: renin measurements to indicate hypertension and contralateral suppression, estimate renal plasma flow, and score for surgical curability. Am J Med 1973; 55:402.

Vidt DG. Advances in the medical management of renovascular hypertension. Urol Clin North Am 1984; 11:417–424.

Vidt DG, Eisele G, Gephardt GN, et al. Atheroembolic renal disease: association with renal arterial stenosis. Cleve Clin J Med 1989; 407–413.

ENDOCRINE HYPERTENSIONS

CAREN G. SOLOMON, M.D.
ROBERT G. DLUHY, M.D.

Endocrine causes for hypertension can often be suspected after a careful review has been done of the patient's clinical and family history in combination with a directed physical examination. For example, a history of steroid ingestion or use of oral contraceptive is clear-cut, and complaints of proximal muscle weakness and easy bruising in an individual with a buffalo hump and purple striae should immediately raise suspicion for Cushing's syndrome. In other instances, the routine chemistry profile may suggest an underlying endocrine abnormality in a hypertensive patient who has no obvious symptoms—e.g., hypokalemia in hyperaldosteronism, and hypercalcemia in hyperparathyroidism. When suspicion is raised by such clues, the clinician should order additional laboratory tests to confirm hormonal overproduction and then radiologic testing to localize the source of overproduction. Severe or refractory hypertension is another indication for seeking a secondary cause, which would include a suspicion of pheochromocytoma even where other suggestive history may be absent.

Although screening for endocrine causes of hypertension is critical where indicated, the routine screening of unselected hypertensive patients is not recommended; fewer than 5 percent of cases of hypertension are caused by an associated endocrine abnormality. This chapter describes the endocrine disorders that can underlie hypertension (Table 1), the recommended evaluation when they are suspected, and options for therapy when they are diagnosed.

MINERALOCORTICOID EXCESS

Primary Hyperaldosteronism

Primary hyperaldosteronism accounts for approximately 1 percent of cases of hypertension. Elevated blood pressure in this condition has been attributed to volume expansion associated with sodium retention, but more recently has been linked to peripheral vasoconstriction in the setting of increased amounts of intracellular sodium.

Symptoms and Signs

The symptoms found in hyperaldosteronism are basically similar to those found in hypokalemia—muscle cramps, weakness, and polyuria. Notably, edema is not a feature of this syndrome, due to "escape" from the sodium-retaining effects of aldosterone. As symptoms of hyperaldosteronism are nonspecific, suspicion of the

Table 1 Endocrine Causes of Hypertension

Adrenal
  Cortex
    Primary hyperaldosteronism
      Aldosterone-secreting adenoma or carcinoma
      Bilateral adrenal hyperplasia
      Glucocorticoid-suppressible hyperaldosteronism
    Congenital adrenal hyperplasia
      11β-hydroxylase deficiency
      17α-hydroxylase deficiency
    Deoxycorticosterone (DOC)-secreting tumor
    Cushing's syndrome
      Cortisol-secreting adenoma or carcinoma
      Cushing's disease (pituitary)
      Ectopic ACTH syndrome
  Medulla
    Pheochromocytoma

Extra-adrenal
  Renovascular (see the chapter *Renovascular Disease*)
  Hypothyroidism
  Hyperthyroidism
  Acromegaly
  Exogenous
    Mineralocorticoids (licorice, chewing tobacco, fluorinef)
    Glucocorticoids
    Oral contraceptives

diagnosis rests mainly on the recognition of spontaneous hypokalemia ($K^+ < 3.5$ mEq per liter) or severe hypokalemia ($K^+ < 3.0$ mEq per liter) with diuretic therapy. However, serum potassium levels may occasionally be normal in individuals with this condition, which is probably attributable to a low-sodium diet with less distal sodium delivery and thus, less K^+ wasting. Another laboratory finding consistent with the diagnosis is mild metabolic alkalosis; mild hypernatremia and hyperglycemia may result from the decreased release of antidiuretic hormone (ADH) and insulin, respectively.

Screening

A low serum potassium level, exacerbated by diuretic therapy, is so commonly related to primary hyperaldosteronism that it serves as an effective screen for the disorder. To rule out the diagnosis, as well as to safeguard against dangerous hypokalemia in any patient given potassium-wasting diuretic agents, potassium levels should be checked in all hypertensive patients prior to the initiation of diuretic therapy and at regular intervals while the drug is being used. Hypokalemia prior to the use of diuretics is an indication for further evaluation for hyperaldosteronism. If significant hypokalemia (e.g., $K^+ < 3.4$ mEq per liter) develops with diuretic therapy, the medication should be temporarily discontinued and potassium should be repleted; a diet high in sodium (150 to 200 mEq daily), which results in increased distal sodium delivery and hence Na^+/K^+ exchange, should then be instituted for 1 week, and potassium levels should be rechecked. A normal potassium level under these conditions essentially rules out the diagnosis.

After confirmation of spontaneous hypokalemia, plasma renin activity (PRA) and plasma aldosterone (PA) levels should be measured, and a 24-hour urine test for sodium to evaluate sodium balance should be done (Fig. 1). A normal or high PRA virtually excludes the diagnosis of primary hyperaldosteronism, as a chronically suppressed renin-angiotensin system is anticipated. However, a low PRA (< 2.5 ng per milliliter per hour), consistent with primary hyperaldosteronism, is also seen in up to 30% of patients with essential hypertension. A ratio of PA to PRA of greater than 20 is another marker suggestive of primary hyperaldosteronism. However, many antihypertensive agents have independent effects on potassium, PRA, and PA levels that can confound the use of these measurements as screening tests. The potassium-wasting diuretics tend to decrease PA and raise PRA, whereas the potassium-sparing diuretics spironolactone and amiloride often reverse the suppressed PRA levels expected with hyperaldosteronism. Beta blockers, moreover, induce lower PRA, and calcium-channel blockers (at least nifedipine) may lower PA levels. Thus, most antihypertensive therapy should be discontinued for 1 to 2 weeks, and spironolactone therapy, for at least 6 weeks before definitive diagnostic testing for primary hyperaldosteronism is pursued. Where medication is clearly needed, the alpha-receptor antagonist, prazosin, is a good choice, as it does not seem to affect these values.

Another screening test involves the measurement of PRA and PA levels after administration of a 50 mg dose of captopril. The normal response, a decrease in PA levels and an increase in PRA, is not seen in patients who have primary hyperaldosteronism as a result of chronic suppression of the renin-angiotensin system. However, a lack of sensitivity and specificity limit the usefulness of this test.

Diagnosis

To establish the diagnosis of hyperaldosteronism, a diet low in sodium (< 2 g) and high in potassium (100 to 200 mEq per day) is instituted on an outpatient basis for 3 days prior to hospital admission. After admission and achievement of a low salt balance while ingesting a diet containing only 10 mEq of sodium daily, the patient should undergo an upright posture study. PRA, PA, and K^+ levels are measured with the patient in the recumbent position at the beginning of the study and then again after the patient has been ambulating for 2 hours. Sodium restriction coupled with the further stimulatory effect of upright posture normally results in a PRA of more than 2.5 ng per milliliter per hour. The failure of PRA to rise as expected in this setting is consistent with primary hyperaldosteronism, but also occurs with low-renin essential hypertension. Extremely low PRA levels near the detection limits of the assay, however, are more suggestive of primary hyperaldosteronism, which reflects the profound suppression of the renin-angiotensin system in this condition. Normalization of a previously low potassium level while maintaining the low salt diet is likewise supportive of the diagnosis.

Following the posture study, the patient undergoes salt loading with 3 L of normal saline infused intravenously at 500 ml per hour over 6 hours. Because hypokalemia with its attendant risk for cardiac arrhythmia may be potentiated by salt loading in a patient with nonsuppressible aldosterone secretion, potassium should be repleted prior to saline infusion. Hypomagnesemia, which often occurs with primary hyperaldosteronism, also should be treated to facilitate potassium replacement and to avoid cardiac risks associated with this electrolyte disturbance. Prior sodium depletion minimizes the risks for severe hypokalemia or volume overload associated with the saline infusion. Nonetheless, we do not perform this test in patients who have had a recent myocardial infarction, congestive heart failure, or stroke within the past 6 months.

Serum potassium, aldosterone, and cortisol levels are measured at hourly intervals throughout the study. The potassium level is measured again prior to hospital discharge, because the appearance of hypokalemia may be delayed. As noted, the development of significant hypokalemia with salt infusion suggests primary hyperaldosteronism. More importantly, the failure of aldosterone to suppress to less than 5 ng per deciliter by the end of 6 hours is virtually diagnostic of this condition. The simultaneous measurement of cortisol rules out the possibility that nonsuppressed aldosterone levels are secondary to stress, with high adrenocorticotropic hormone (ACTH) levels stimulating the adrenal glands.

While awaiting results of diagnostic testing, we begin the administration of spironolactone, an aldosterone antagonist. Dosages and potential adverse effects of this agent are discussed in the section that describes therapy for hyperaldosteronism.

Differential Diagnosis

Once a patient is found to have primary hyperaldosteronism, appropriate therapy depends on the cause. The differential diagnosis includes aldosterone-producing adenoma, bilateral adrenal hyperplasia, glucocorticoid-suppressible hyperaldosteronism, and, very rarely, adrenal carcinoma. Aldosterone-producing adenomas were initially believed to underlie the disorder in almost two-thirds of cases, but this estimate may be skewed by the more severe hypertension and hypokalemia that is associated with solitary adenomas versus bilateral hyperplasia, the other common cause.

Radiologic evaluation is the first step in distinguishing between these possibilities. We initially do an abdominal computed tomographic (CT) scan, which is 90 percent sensitive in identifying adenomas and will localize virtually all that are larger than 1 cm in diameter. When CT fails to demonstrate a unilateral adrenal mass, bilateral adrenal hyperplasia becomes the more likely cause of hyperaldosteronism, but definitive exclusion of a small solitary adenoma requires adrenal vein sampling,

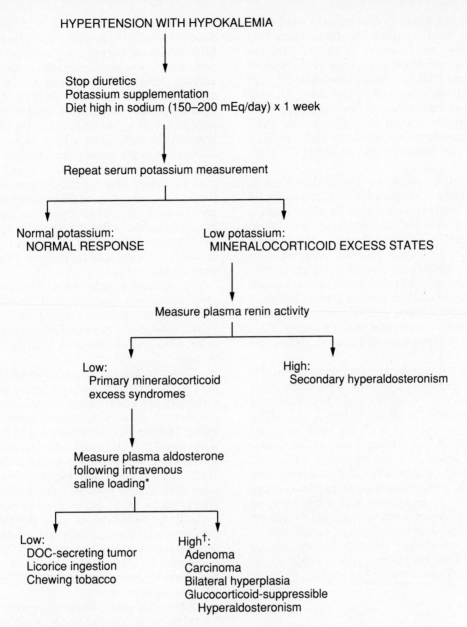

Figure 1 Algorithm for evaluting patients with suspected primary hyperaldosteronism.
*See text for contraindications
†To distinguish diagnostic possibilities, CT scan ± adrenal venous sampling are necessary. When there is a family history of early onset hypertension associated with hypokalemia, a 4-week trial of glucocorticoids is indicated. See text for details. (Adapted from Williams GH, Dluhy RG. Diseases of the adrenal cortex. In: Wilson JD, et al., eds. Harrison's principles of internal medicine, 12th ed. New York: McGraw-Hill, 1991:1726; with permission.)

which is a more sensitive procedure. Adrenal vein sampling notably carries a not insignificant risk for adrenal vein thrombosis or rupture, adrenal infarction, and failure to sample adequately; it should only be performed by a radiologist practiced in the procedure. Outflow from both adrenal glands is sampled simultaneously and compared with respect to aldosterone and cortisol levels. Equal levels indicate bilateral adrenal hyperplasia, while lateralization is consistent with an adenoma.

Alternative approaches have been suggested to distinguish between adenoma and bilateral hyperplasia. Iodocholesterol scanning relies on the uptake of a radionuclide by steroid-synthesizing cells; however, this test is costly and not widely available, lacks sensitivity, and involves radiation exposure that far exceeds that of a CT scan. The measurement of 18-OH corticosterone and aldosterone levels at the time of the posture study may also be helpful. Aldosteronomas are frequently associated with elevated 18-OH corticosterone levels (> 100 ng per deciliter) and in some cases with unexpected posturally related decreases in the aldosterone levels. These tests lack sensitivity and specificity as well and do not eliminate the need for CT confirmation.

Another possible cause of hyperaldosteronism, aldosterone-secreting adrenal carcinoma, can easily be identified by CT scan. The sensitivity for carcinomas is even higher than that for adenomas, as carcinomas are typically larger (generally >6 cm) at the time of presentation. The distinction between adenoma and carcinoma in the absence of demonstrable metastatic disease depends on surgically discovered abnormalities, although biochemical markers such as urinary ketosteroid levels are often elevated with carcinoma. Notably, aldosterone-secreting carcinomas are extremely rare, with an incidence of approximately 1 case per 100 million individuals.

Glucocorticoid-suppressible hyperaldosteronism is inherited as an autosomal dominant trait. Individuals with a family history of hypertension of early onset or of hypertension associated with hypokalemia should be given a trial of prednisone at 5 mg twice daily or dexamethasone at 0.5 mg twice daily for 6 weeks. Normalization of blood pressure, potassium, PRA, and aldosterone levels at the end of this period is consistent with the diagnosis. Temporary improvement may occur at the start of therapy in patients with other forms of hyperaldosteronism, but will not be sustained. Definitive diagnosis in affected individuals may be established by detection of the abnormal "hybrid" steroids 18-OH cortisol and 18-OH cortisone in affected family members, but these tests are not widely available.

Therapy

Therapy for an aldosterone-secreting tumor involves surgery in the absence of contraindications to this approach, such as severe cardiovascular disease or metastatic disease. Surgery results in resolution of hypokalemia and hypertension in more than 95 percent of individuals with an adenoma within 3 to 6 months. Hypertension may recur in up to 25 percent of these patients within the next 2 to 3 years, but is typically easily controlled and not accompanied by recurrent hypokalemia.

Perioperatively, patients receive high-dose steroids, a precaution in case the contralateral "normal" adrenal gland is unable to produce cortisol appropriately. A continuous intravenous infusion of hydrocortisone is given at a rate of 10 mg per hour beginning just prior to surgery and continuing for 24 hours, and is then decreased in rate by 50 percent daily for the subsequent 24 to 48 hours. Once the patient is eating, steroid

administration is changed to oral hydrocortisone at a dose of 40 mg in the morning and 20 mg in the afternoon. Hydrocortisone therapy is gradually tapered over the next 4 to 6 weeks, during which time the uninvolved adrenal gland should return to normal function. Recovery is assessed toward the end of the taper by changing to alternate-day administration of steroids given as one dose in the morning and measuring a morning cortisol level on the "off" day; a level higher than 10 μg per deciliter suggests normal endogenous cortisol production. Hypoaldosteronism may be seen for up to 6 months postoperatively due to the long-term suppression of PRA. Adequate salt and fluid intake should be encouraged during this time and the patient should be monitored closely for dehydration and hyperkalemia, but the use of the mineralocorticoid, fluorinef, is best avoided, as its use may perpetuate adrenal glomerulosa suppression.

In contrast to adenomas, bilateral adrenal hyperplasia does not respond well to surgery. Although bilateral adrenalectomy corrects hypokalemia and high aldosterone levels, hypertension persists in 85 percent of cases. Thus, the treatment for this disorder involves drug therapy.

Drug therapy for patients with bilateral hyperplasia, as well as for those with adenoma who are awaiting surgery or for whom surgery is not elected, involves the aldosterone antagonist spironolactone as a first-line agent. This medication is started at 50 mg twice daily and is increased at 1- to 2-week intervals until blood pressure is controlled; the maximum dosage is 200 mg twice daily. While hypertension and hypokalemia are adequately controlled in most patients treated with this agent, side effects occur in as many as 20 percent of patients. Particularly disturbing in male patients are problems attributable to the androgen-antagonizing effect of the medication, including gynecomastia, loss of libido, and impotence. Gastrointestinal distress, including cramping and diarrhea, and complaints of lethargy and fatigue are also not uncommon.

When the side effects of spironolactone are intolerable, an alternative agent is amiloride. This medication acts through an aldosterone-independent mechanism to block distal tubule sodium channels and thus decrease the sodium-potassium exchange and potassium wasting. The starting dose is 10 mg daily, which can be increased at 1- to 2-week intervals to a maximum dose of 40 mg daily until blood pressure is controlled. This medication is often better tolerated than spironolactone, although it too can cause gastrointestinal distress and fatigue. Although potentially less toxic than spironolactone, amiloride frequently is less effective, particularly in the setting of bilateral adrenal hyperplasia. During treatment with either amiloride or spironolactone, serum potassium levels must be checked on a regular basis. When used prior to the surgical resection of adenoma, therapy with these medications should be discontinued at the time of admission for surgery.

Patients with glucocorticoid-suppressible hyperaldosteronism are usually treated with prednisone, 5 mg twice daily. Some patients require higher doses, however. In cases in which the doses of prednisone required to control hyperaldosteronism are associated with significant steroid side effects, therapy with spironolactone or amiloride is preferable.

Congenital Adrenal Hyperplasia

Symptoms and Signs

Two forms of congenital adrenal hyperplasia, 11β-hydroxylase deficiency and 17α-hydroxylase deficiency are associated with hypertension (Fig. 2). Occurring in either a classic (early-onset) or attenuated (late-onset) form, 11β-hydroxylase deficiency is associated with overproduction of androgens, which leads to virilization or less severe manifestations of androgen excess such as hirsutism, acne, or oligomenorrhea. In contrast, 17α-hydroxylase deficiency is associated with an absence of development of secondary sexual characteristics at the time of puberty in both sexes, due to an inability to produce androgens and estrogens. Elevated blood pressure and hypokalemia in both syndromes result from high ACTH levels in the setting of inadequate cortisol production causing overproduction of deoxycorticosterone (DOC), which acts as a potent mineralocorticoid. Volume overload and hypertension lead to suppression of plasma renin activity, with resultant low aldosterone levels.

Diagnosis

Suspicion of these syndromes depends on recognition of the disorders of androgen excess in females and abnormal secondary sexual development in association with the elevated blood pressure. The measurement of plasma 17-OH progesterone and urinary 17-ketosteroids confirms the diagnoses; these levels are elevated in patients with 11β-hydroxylase deficiency and essentially absent in 17α-hydroxylase deficiency. The 11-deoxycortisol level is also typically elevated with 11β-hydroxylase deficiency and increases markedly with ACTH stimulation testing.

Therapy

Therapy for both disorders involves suppression of adrenal function with administration of glucocorticoids. Because patients are typically very sensitive to this type of drug, one should find the smallest dose of glucocorticoid possible that will control overproduction of ACTH and thus, steroid intermediates. Therapy may be complicated by the development of Cushing-like features or other problems associated with cortisol excess (discussed in section on Cushing's syndrome).

Exogeneous Mineralocorticoid Excess

Hypertension and hypokalemia may also occur with the ingestion of substances that result in increased mineralocorticoid activity. Licorice (which must be eaten in abundance) is perhaps the best known of the offenders, but others include chewing tobacco and carbenoloxone, an ulcer medication. The former two contain glycyrrhizic acid, and carbenoloxone is a derivative of this substance. Glycyrrhizic acid has been found to inhibit the enzyme 11β-hydroxysteroid dehydrogenase in the kidney. As a result, excessive levels of cortisol accumulate and bind to mineralocorticoid receptors, where they exert mineralocorticoid activity. Fluorinef, used occasionally in the treatment of orthostatic hypotension, is a potent mineralocorticoid with hypertensive effects.

These rare causes of hypertension are recognized by careful history taking. Supportive laboratory values are low serum potassium levels in the setting of low aldosterone levels, low plasma renin activity, and lack of elevation of steroid precursors. Treatment involves discontinuation of ingestion of the offending substance.

Deoxycorticosterone-Secreting Tumors

An extremely rare cause of hypertension associated with hypokalemia is the production of deoxycorticosterone by an adrenal tumor. In such cases, PRA and, as a result, PA levels become suppressed. CT scanning should detect essentially all cases, as such tumors are large at the time of presentation. Treatment involves surgical excision unless contraindicated by the presence of metastatic disease.

GLUCOCORTICOID EXCESS

Cushing's Syndrome

Cushing's syndrome, the hypersecretion of cortisol, is associated with elevations in blood pressure in more than 80% of patients. Postulated mechanisms include increases in PRA and angiotensin-converting enzyme, inhibitory effects on vasodilatory prostaglandins, and, in small part, mineralocorticoid effects. Cushing's syndrome may be caused by adrenal adenoma or, rarely, carcinoma, pituitary ACTH hypersecretion with resultant bilateral adrenal hyperplasia, or ectopic ACTH production. Exogeneous glucocorticoids given in supraphysiologic doses may also cause this syndrome.

Symptoms and Signs

Cushing's syndrome should be suspected when hypertension occurs in combination with other evidence of cortisol excess, including central adiposity (e.g., with moon facies, buffalo hump, supraclavicular fat pad), easy bruising, wide purple striae, proximal myopathy, and osteopenia. Concomitant androgen excess frequently results in menstrual irregularities, hirsutism, and acne in females. Although none of these findings is universal, each occurs in a majority of patients with the disorder.

Laboratory results occasionally seen with Cushing's syndrome include mild leukocytosis (typically with a left

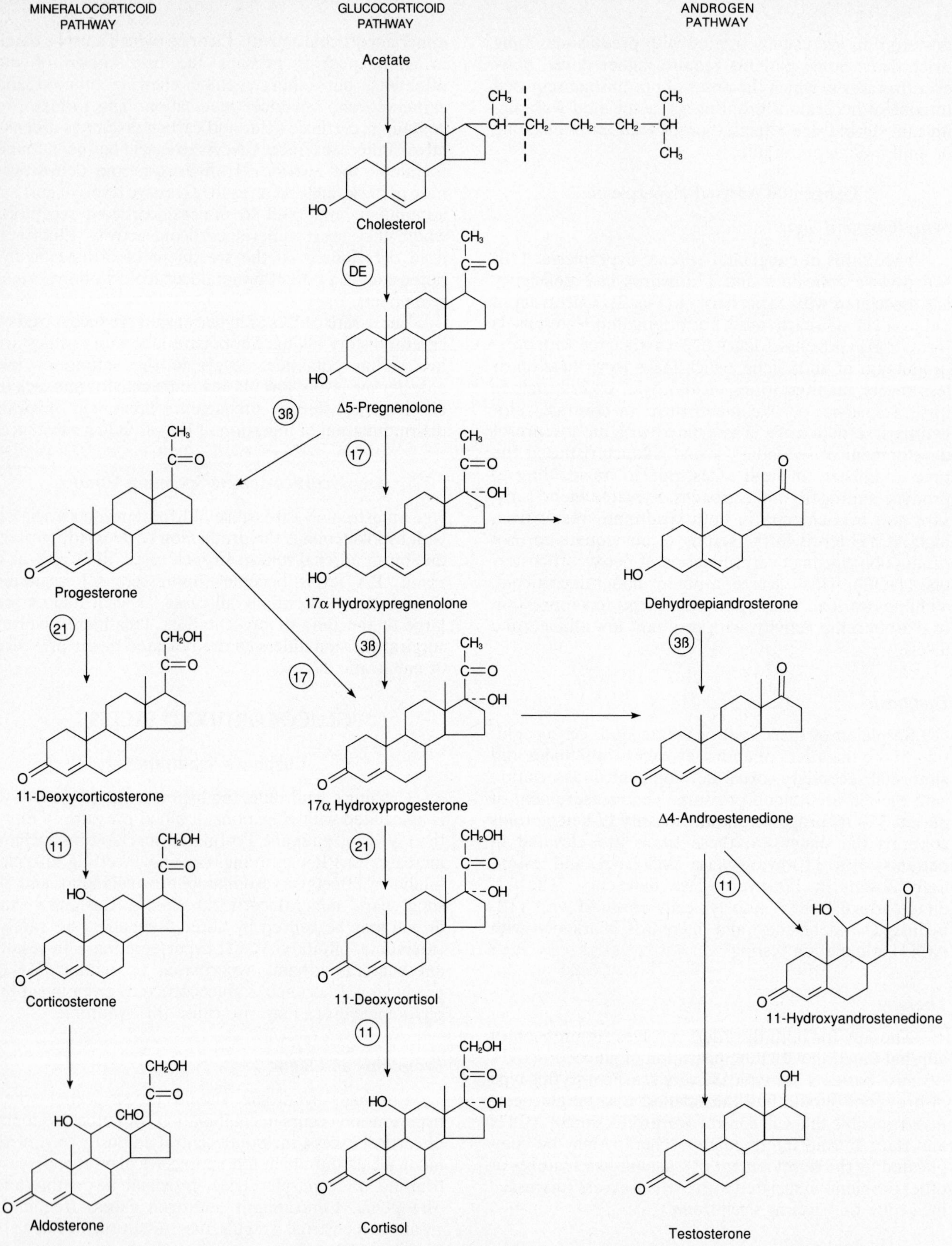

Figure 2 Biosynthetic pathways for adrenal steroid production; major pathways to mineralocorticoids, glucocorticoids, and androgens. Circled letters and numbers denote specific enzymes: DE = cholesterol side chain cleavage enzyme; 3β = 3β-ol-dehydrogenase with $\triangle^{4.5}$ isomerase; 11 = C-11 hydroxylase; 17 = C-17 hydroxylase; 21 = C-21 hydroxylase. (From Williams GH, Dluhy RG. Diseases of the adrenal cortex. In Wilson JD, et al., eds. Harrison's principles of internal medicine, 12th ed. New York: McGraw-Hill, 1991:1714; with permission.)

shift), and, occasionally, hyperglycemia and hypercholesterolemia. Hypokalemic alkalosis is observed commonly when excess cortisol secretion occurs secondary to adrenal carcinoma or ectopic ACTH production, but it is rarely found in conjunction with other sources.

Screening

The best screen for Cushing's syndrome is a 24-hour urine-free cortisol measurement (Fig. 3). A value of more than 100 μg per 24 hours raises suspicion for the diagnosis. An alternative screening test is an overnight dexamethasone suppression test, in which morning cortisol levels are measured following a 1 mg dose of dexamethasone the preceding evening. The failure of cortisol to suppress to less than 5 μg per deciliter is also suggestive of Cushing's syndrome. However, a lack of suppression may occur with simple obesity, as well as with the anticonvulsants dilantin, phenobarbital, and primidone, which accelerate the metabolism of dexamethasone; none of these agents affect urine free cortisol measurements. False-positive results obtained with either screening test may be seen in patients with alcoholism (so-called pseudo Cushing's syndrome) or depression.

When screening tests raise concern, the next step is to perform a low-dose dexamethasone suppression test. Dexamethasone, 0.5 mg, is given every 6 hours for 48 hours and is followed by a measurement of plasma cortisol levels the following morning or of 24-hour urine-free cortisol levels on the second day of dexamethasone administration. The failure to suppress with this regimen (to less than 5 μg per deciliter or less than 20 μg per 24 hours, respectively) confirms excessive cortisol secretion.

Additional biochemical tests help to distinguish possible causes of cortisol excess. ACTH, measured by a sensitive immunoreactive assay (normal range 20 to 100 pg per milliliter) can not be detected in hypercortisolemia of adrenal origin, is usually moderately elevated (40 to 100 pg per milliliter) with a pituitary tumor, and is often very high (usually greater than 200 pg per milliliter) with ectopic sources of ACTH. High-dose dexamethasone testing, involving 2 mg doses of dexamethasone every 6 hours for 48 hours, also may be useful. Cortisol excess from an ACTH-secreting pituitary tumor is generally suppressed to less than or equal to 50 percent of baseline levels by this regimen, whereas other causes fail to show suppression (see Fig. 3).

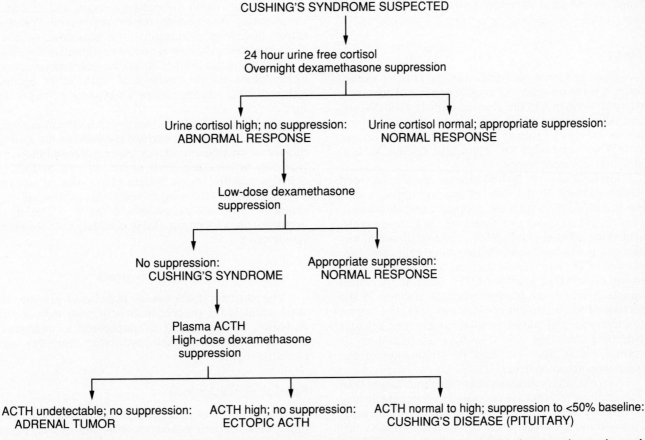

Figure 3 Algorithm for evaluating patients with suspected Cushing's syndrome. See text for details of suppression testing and causes of false-positive and false-negative findings. (Adapted from Baxter JD, Tyrrell JB, The adrenal cortex. In: Felig P, et al, eds. Endocrinology and metabolism, 2nd ed. New York: McGraw-Hill, 1987:609; with permission.)

Radiologic Diagnosis

The focus of radiologic imaging depends on results of the testing described previously. When an adrenal source is suspected (i.e., undetectable ACTH levels), an adrenal CT scan should be the initial approach. As is the case with aldosteronoma, sensitivity for a cortisol-secreting adrenal tumor is higher than 90% because most tumors measure more than 1 cm. Magnetic resonance imaging (MRI) may help to distinguish adrenal adenoma from carcinoma, as carcinomas typically appear somewhat brighter on T2-weighted images; however, there is significant overlap, and the much larger size of most carcinomas (usually >6 cm) is of greater value in distinguishing the two possibilities radiologically. When a pituitary tumor seems the likely diagnosis, MR imaging of the pituitary gland is pursued first. If the findings are equivocal or normal, and suspicion is high, petrosal sinus sampling for ACTH levels is indicated. In the setting of a pituitary source of excess ACTH, petrosal vein levels of this hormone are typically at least two times greater than those of peripheral blood sampled simultaneously.

Where suspicion of an ectopic source is high (e.g., with hypokalemic alkalosis, very elevated ACTH levels, failure of cortisol to suppress with high-dose dexamethasone testing, absence of classic Cushing-like features), imaging should be directed elsewhere. The pancreas and lungs are the most common sources of ectopic ACTH secretion.

Therapy

Therapy varies with the cause of cortisol excess. Surgery is the treatment of choice for adrenal adenoma, adrenal carcinoma in the absence of metastatic disease, and ACTH-secreting pituitary tumor. It is also appropriate for the treatment of those sources of ectopic ACTH not associated with metastatic disease, such as localized carcinoid tumors.

Stress doses of hydrocortisone should be used perioperatively. In the case of adrenal tumor, excess cortisol production from the neoplasm suppresses pituitary ACTH secretion and, therefore, the function of the remaining adrenal gland. With pituitary adenoma, any remaining "normal" ACTH-secreting cells are suppressed by the elevated cortisol levels, as are these cells in the presence of ectopic ACTH secretion. A typical approach to steroid administration is outlined in the section on the treatment of aldosteronoma. In contrast to surgery for hypoaldosteronism, surgery for Cushing's syndrome does not result in hypoaldosteronism, as cortisol excess does not lead to suppression of the renin-angiotensin system.

Large pituitary tumors (macroadenomas larger than 1 cm in diameter) that are not completely resectable may be treated with radiation as an adjunctive therapy. Hypopituitarism is the major complication of both this therapy and surgical resection; its development following radiation therapy may take years. Following surgery or radiation therapy, all patients require at least an annual evaluation of levels of hormones that are regulated by the pituitary gland so that development of partial or complete pituitary insufficiency can be recognized and treated.

In cases in which treatment directed at the pituitary gland is not successful, an alternative surgical treatment is bilateral adrenalectomy. Although this approach definitively eliminates excessive cortisol production, ACTH levels may become even higher in the absence of any feedback suppression from the adrenal gland. One result is development of hyperpigmentation caused by the melanocyte-stimulating effects of the ACTH precursor, pro-opiomelanocortin. A greater concern is enlargement of a pre-existing pituitary tumor or the appearance of one not previously discovered (Nelson's syndrome).

In cases in which surgical resection is not an option because of concomitant medical problems, invasive pituitary tumor, or metastatic disease, medical therapy may provide much needed palliation. Ketoconazole, developed as an antifungal medication, decreases cortisol production in dosages of up to 1200 mg per day. However, the drug often causes gastrointestinal distress and hepatotoxicity. Metyrapone, which blocks the 11β-hydroxylase enzyme in the adrenal cortex, also causes gastrointestinal problems as well as headache and occasionally, leukopenia.

In the case of metastatic adrenal cortical carcinoma, mitotane can inhibit steroid production and in some cases result in objective tumor regression. Adverse effects include gastrointestinal and neurologic toxicity. Cytotoxic chemotherapy is another alternative for therapy. Cis-platin has been of limited benefit in many cases, either alone or in combination with other agents, although renal toxicity, nausea, and vomiting complicate its use.

The efficacy of medical therapy should be monitored by measuring urine-free cortisol levels or, in the setting of adrenal cortical carcinoma, other hormonal markers that may be elevated, such as the adrenal androgen, dehydroepiandrosterone sulfate (DHEAS), or urinary 17-ketosteroids. Radiologic tests that delineate the extent of malignant disease should also be repeated, as hormonal markers do not always correlate with objective tumor mass.

Pheochromocytoma

Pheochromocytoma causes high blood pressure in approximately 0.1 percent of hypertensive individuals. Although uncommon, it is important to recognize because of its considerable associated morbidity and potential mortality.

Familial Versus Sporadic

The majority of pheochromocytomas occur as sporadic cases, but their association with familial syndromes in approximately 10 percent of cases underscores the importance of taking a careful family history in patients in whom the diagnosis is suspected. Pheochromocytoma occurs with hyperparathyroidism and medullary carcinoma of the thyroid gland in the MEN (multiple endocrine neoplasia) 2a syndrome, and with the medullary carcinoma of the thyroid gland along with mucosal neuromas and a marfanoid habitus in the MEN 2b syndrome. In these syndromes, pheochromocytomas may be of early onset and are frequently bilateral, although involvement of the two sides is often not simultaneous. Adrenal medullary hyperplasia has been noted to precede the development of pheochromocytoma in familial studies. Other syndromes associated with pheochromocytoma are neurofibromatosis and von Hippel-Lindau syndrome, which involves hemangiomoblastomas of the retina and cerebellum.

Symptoms and Signs

Symptoms most suggestive of pheochromocytoma include palpitations, sweats, and headache. Whereas all three occur in only a fraction of patients, the absence of any of these symptoms makes the diagnosis extremely unlikely, with a frequency of probably less than 0.01 percent. Anxiety, fatigue, nausea, and chest and abdominal discomfort are among other manifestations. Symptoms are paroxysmal in approximately 50 percent of cases, occuring as often as several times daily and usually lasting less than 1 hour.

The "hallmark" of pheochromocytoma is considered to be paroxysmal hypertension, but paroxysms occur in only about 50 percent of patients; sustained hypertension occurs in the other 50 percent. Even in the absence of clear paroxysms, lability of blood pressure is common. Orthostatic hypotension is frequent due to the peripheral vasoconstriction and hypovolemia associated with catecholamine excess. Hypertension provoked by palpation of the abdomen, anesthesia, or administration of certain medications (e.g., opiates, tricyclic antidepressants) raises a suspicion of pheochromocytoma.

Symptoms and signs may differ if a pheochromocytoma secretes primarily epinephrine. In these infrequent cases, paroxysmal hypotension as well as cardiac arrhythmias and pulmonary edema may be seen. Often, secretion of norepinephrine accompanies that of epinephrine.

Laboratory tests may reveal mild-to-moderate elevation in hematocrit values that is at least in part secondary to hemoconcentration (contracted plasma volume). Mild hyperglycemia may result from the suppression of insulin release by high levels of catecholamines. Hypercalcemia may also be seen as a result of hemoconcentration, release of parathyroid hormone (PTH)-related peptide from the tumor, or concomitant hyperparathyroidism, which is seen when pheochromocytoma occurs as part of the MEN 2a syndrome.

Screening

When pheochromocytoma is suspected, biochemical screening is indicated. A 24-hour urine specimen should be analyzed for levels of the catecholamine metabolites metanephrine and vanillylmandelic acid (VMA), as well as for unmetabolized or "free" catecholamines, which may be fractionated to epinephrine and norepinephrine. Creatinine is are also measured to assess the adequacy of the urine collection. Although generally all of these levels are elevated, tumors may occasionally be associated with abnormalities in only one. The measurement of metanephrines is considered to be the most sensitive of these tests, and that of VMA, the most specific. The occurrence of a paroxysm during the period of sample collection heightens the sensitivity of the tests, so that a normal finding in the setting of a paroxysm during the period of sample collection essentially excludes the diagnosis. Nonetheless, elevated levels are typically seen with pheochromocytomas even in the absence of paroxysms. Elevations in any of these levels to values above the normal range should be viewed as suspicious. Certain medications, however, may cause false-positive or false-negative results. Methyldopa and sympathomimetic agents, for example, may elevate levels of free catecholamines; MAO inhibitors, which alter catecholamine metabolism, lead to increased metanephrine levels and decreased levels of VMA.

The measurement of plasma catecholamine levels has been suggested to be a more sensitive screening test. Levels higher than 1,000 pg per milliliter are highly suggestive of pheochromocytoma. However, the accurate measurement of plasma levels necessitates that the patient lie in a quiet room with an intravenous line in place for at least 20 minutes before a blood sample is drawn. Even with these precautions, both false-negative and false-positive findings have been documented. Urine testing as described previously thus seems preferable, providing an integrated measure of catecholamine secretion and accurately diagnosing pheochromocytoma in 95 percent of patients.

In equivocal cases, particularly those in which plasma catecholamine levels measure between 500 and 2000 pg per milliliter, a clonidine suppression test can help to distinguish between pheochromocytoma and essential hypertension. Three hours following administration of a 0.3 mg dose of clonidine, norepinephrine levels should decrease to less than 500 pg per milliliter in normal patients, but fail to decrease with pheochromocytoma. Notably, blood pressure decreases in both cases, and hypotension is one of the potential adverse effects of the test. The measurement of plasma catecholamine levels after provocative testing with glucagon, a test previously promoted by some investigators, is not recommended given the dangers associated with inducing a hypertensive crisis.

Radiologic Diagnosis

Once biochemical screening has proved abnormal, CT or MRI of the abdomen is the best initial approach to localizing pheochromocytoma. Ninety percent of pheochromocytomas are intra-adrenal, and most of the remainder are para-aortic, along the sympathetic chain; almost all measure well over 1 cm at the time of presentation and thus are easily visualized by either modality. MRI may be of additional value in that pheochromocytomas classically appear extremely bright on T2-weighted images with a signal intensity greater than three times that of liver, a characteristic that distinguishes them from "incidentalomas," which are discussed later.

If adrenal imaging procedures fail to identify a mass when catecholamine levels are elevated, radionuclide scanning with meta-iodobenzylguanine (MIBG) is indicated, if available, to localize an extra-adrenal lesion. MIBG is taken up fairly selectively by chromaffin cells; abnormal tests in the absence of pheochromocytoma rarely occur with some uncommon neuroendocrine tumors. Where MIBG is not available, CT or MRI of the pelvis and chest may identify pheochromocytomas at unusual sites (e.g., bladder or posterior mediastinum). A bone scan may identify bony metastases.

Therapy

The treatment for pheochromocytoma is surgical unless metastatic disease contraindicates this approach. Critical to successful surgery is preoperative preparation to prevent hypertensive crises with anesthesia and intraoperative tumor manipulation. Patients should begin receiving phenoxybenzamine, an alpha-receptor antagonist, at least 1 week prior to surgery. The initial dose is 10 mg twice daily, which is increased by 10 mg twice daily increments until the blood pressure is well controlled and there is mild orthostatic hypotension. As volume contraction is typical with pheochromocytoma, a pressure reduction will restore plasma volume. If this is not adequate, an increased sodium diet (150 to 200 mEq sodium daily) for the week before surgery will assist in restoring euvolemia. Secondary effects of phenoxybenzamine also help to correct volume status. Patients who are or become tachycardic with alpha-blockade, or who experience significant ectopy, are also given beta-receptor blockers such as propranolol (Inderal). Alpha blockade is always initiated prior to a beta blockade to avoid unopposed alpha-receptor stimulation. An alternative to phenoxybenzamine used at some centers is nifedipine, which both vasodilates and may decrease catecholamine secretion from pheochromocytomas. Therapy with these medications is continued up to surgery, which is carried out with careful hemodynamic monitoring and intraoperative infusion of nitroprusside or labetolol as needed.

Adrenalectomy results in the cure of hypertension in over 80 percent of patients. Those with sustained rather than paroxysmal hypertension prior to surgery tend to have a somewhat lower cure rate (67 percent). Pre-existing essential hypertension or renal vascular damage secondary to longstanding hypertension may explain the persistence of elevated blood pressure. Inadequate resection or tumor recurrence may explain other cases. It is particularly important in pheochromocytoma associated with MEN syndromes to exclude bilateral disease preoperatively. Some investigators advocate bilateral adrenalectomy for all pheochromocytomas associated with these syndromes in view of the frequency of bilateral involvement, but the very long intervals before appearance of many contralateral tumors and the morbidity of bilateral adrenalectomy provide a sound argument for a more conservative approach.

Following surgery, catecholamine levels must be monitored to ensure complete resection and the absence of recurrence. It is not useful to check these levels within the first 1 or 2 weeks postoperatively, as false-positive test results may occur as a result of postsurgical stress or a still expanded catecholamine pool. Urinary catecholamine, metanephrine, and VMA levels are measured 1 month after surgery, at 6-month intervals for 2 years, then yearly. Another marker, chromogranin A, a peptide synthesized and secreted by chromaffin cells, is often elevated in patients with pheochromocytoma. This test is currently not as studied as the measurement of catecholamine levels in the monitoring for recurrence of pheochromocytoma.

The importance of continued surveillance cannot be overemphasized, as a surprising amount of pheochromocytomas may prove malignant during a prolonged follow-up. Although the incidence of malignant pheochromocytomas has been quoted at 10 percent or less, longer periods of follow-up have revealed an incidence of between 20 and 40 percent. Malignant potential may be difficult to recognize at surgery, as there are no specific pathologic markers for this, and the diagnosis rests on the appearance of metastases. Large size and extra-adrenal location, however, are associated with an increased likelihood of malignant behavior. In this regard, surveillance of the entire family of patients with MEN 2a syndrome is also exceedingly important.

Patients who are not candidates for surgery because of other medical problems and those who have metastatic disease are treated medically. Phenoxybenzamine is used in this setting as well, with or without a beta blocker. Patients refractory to maximal doses of phenoxybenzamine may be treated with metyrosine, an agent that blocks catecholamine synthesis. Calcium channel blockers, mentioned previously, may be a useful alternative therapy. Malignant pheochromocytomas have been treated with external radiation, chemotherapy, and therapeutic doses of MIBG, but reports of successful results are largely anecdotal, and the overall impact of these approaches is questionable.

Incidentally Discovered Adrenal Masses

With the increasing use of abdominal CT scanning for many varied indications, unsuspected or incidentally discovered adrenal masses have become a well-described finding, occurring in 0.6 percent of scans. Evaluation and follow-up of these "incidentalomas" in series of patients have indicated that only a few are of clinical significance.

In general, masses of importance are those that are hormonally functioning or those measuring larger than 6 cm. Although the relative rarity of adrenal cortical carcinoma (incidence, approximately 1 in 1 million) makes this diagnosis unlikely, all adrenal masses larger than 6 cm should be surgically resected whether functional or not, as masses of this size are much more likely than smaller masses to be malignant. Biochemical assessment, outlined below, is indicated preoperatively to guide management (e.g., alpha blockade for pheochromocytoma) and identify baseline markers for postoperative comparison.

When an adrenal neoplasm smaller than 6 cm is found incidentally on a CT scan, a directed personal and family history taking and physical examination should be done to screen for those states of hormonal excess described in the preceding sections, as well as for possible androgen or estrogen overproduction. Where indicated, appropriate biochemical evaluation as previously outlined should follow; where inappropriate virilization or feminization is suggested, testosterone and DHEAS levels, or estradiol levels, should be measured, respectively.

Hormonal excess may be clinically inapparent, and thus a limited biochemical evaluation is indicated even in the absence of characteristic symptoms and signs. As cortisol-secreting tumors may rarely be associated with normal levels of urine-free cortisol, low-dose dexamethasone testing (0.5 mg PO every 6 hours for 48 hours) should be done to assess suppressibility. The most cost-effective approach to evaluation, which requires only one 24-hour urine collection, is to assess free cortisol, 17-ketosteroid, and catecholamine levels on the second day of low-dose dexamethasone testing; cortisol levels of more than 20 μg per 24 hours, 17-ketosteroid levels of more than 10 mg per 24 hours, or elevated catecholamine levels indicate the presence of a functioning tumor.

Functioning tumors should be surgically resected in the absence of contraindications, as described in the preceding sections. A mass that measures less than 6 cm and is nonfunctional should be followed with repeat CT scanning at 3 and 12 months. If the tumor remains unchanged over time, it can presumably be safely followed; growth over time indicates an increased risk for malignancy and the need for repeat biochemical assessment and surgical resection.

OTHER ENDOCRINE DISORDERS ASSOCIATED WITH HYPERTENSION

Hypothyroidism

Hypothyroidism may account for 1 to 2 percent of cases of diastolic hypertension in the general population. Postulated mechanisms include extracellular volume expansion and elevation in systemic vascular resistance.

Symptoms and Signs

The diagnosis of hypothyroidism is suggested by a history of weight gain, lethargy, hair loss, cold intoler-

ance, and, in females, menstrual irregularities. A family history of thyroid or other autoimmune disease is suggestive of chronic thyroiditis (Hashimoto's disease), the most common cause of hypothyroidism. A history of treatment with radioactive iodine or external radiation involving the neck area, as in Hodgkin's disease, is also important, as these procedures often result in destruction of the thyroid gland. A physical examination may reveal periorbital edema, a hoarse voice, and delayed deep tendon reflexes; in severe cases, myxedema is seen. Laboratory tests may reveal low sodium levels, elevated creatine kinase levels (secondary to reduced renal clearance), and hyperlipidemia.

Diagnosis

The diagnosis rests on thyroid function tests, specifically those for thyroid-stimulating hormone (TSH), thyroxine (T4), and thyroid hormone binding resin (THBR). A measurement of TSH concentration alone is a very reasonable screen for hypothyroidism in otherwise healthy patients, as over 90 percent of hypothyroidism is primary, due to thyroid gland destruction, and therefore is associated with an elevated TSH level (>5 μU per milliliter; normal, 0.5 to 5 μU per milliliter). Antimicrosomal antibodies are often useful in establishing the cause of hypothyroidism, as they are found in the serum of approximately 90 percent of patients with Hashimoto's disease.

In some patients, TSH levels may be elevated while the T4 level remains well within the normal range, a condition referred to as "subclinical hypothyroidism." While some individuals with this condition appear to benefit symptomatically or with respect to lipid levels from thyroid hormone replacement, there are currently no data to our knowledge to suggest that hypothyroidism of this mild degree induces diastolic hypertension or that treatment will cause a blood pressure reduction in such patients.

Therapy

The treatment for hypothyroidism involves thyroxine replacement. Most individuals require a dose of approximately 0.8 μg per lb of body weight, although requirements do not always correlate with weight. In the presence of advanced age, documented or suspected coronary disease, or severe hypothyroidism, the treatment should start at a low dose, such as 0.025 mg daily. Thyroid function test results should be checked every 3 to 4 weeks, and thyroxine should be increased in 0.025 mg increments until TSH levels fall to within the normal range, unless this protocol is contraindicated by development or worsening of symptoms of ischemic heart disease. When treating primary hypothyroidism, suppression of TSH to undetectable levels should be avoided, as this amount of suppression has been shown to accelerate bone loss.

Thyroxine replacement therapy will lower blood pressure in most patients and result in normal blood pressure in approximately one-third. Those in whom it is not effective presumably have concomitant essential hypertension.

Hyperthyroidism

In contrast to the diastolic hypertension associated with hypothyroidism, hyperthyroidism usually causes elevated systolic blood pressure.

Symptoms and Signs

Symptoms of hyperthyroidism include anxiety, sweating, increased appetite, weight loss, heat intolerance, and palpitations. A history of recent iodine exposure, such as to intravenous radiographic contrast agents or medications such as amiodarone, raises a suspicion of iodine-induced hyperthyroidism, which is characteristically seen in the setting of a multinodular goiter. A family history of thyroid or other autoimmune disease suggests the possibility of Graves' disease, the most common cause. A recent pregnancy raises the question of postpartum thyroiditis, while subacute painful thyroiditis may follow an upper respiratory infection.

Characteristic physical findings in hyperthyroidism regardless of cause include expanded pulse pressure, tachycardia, fine tremor, hyperreflexia, lid lag, and stare. Other infiltrative eye findings such as exophthalmos, extraocular muscle entrapment, and chemosis, as well as a diffusely enlarged thyroid gland, are typical of hyperthyroidism due to Graves' disease. The thyroid gland may be tender if hyperthyroidism is due to subacute thyroiditis, or nodular if a hyperfunctioning nodule is present (either solitary or as part of a multinodular goiter). There are no routine laboratory abnormalities characteristic of hyperthyroidism, although mild hypercalcemia may be noted; the erythrocyte sedimentation rate is generally elevated when subacute thyroditis is present.

Diagnosis

As with hypothyroidism, the diagnosis is based on thyroid function tests. Using the currently available supersensitive TSH assay, a suppressed TSH level (< 0.5 µU per milliliter) is the best indicator of hyperthyroidism. Elevated T4 and THBR levels are confirmatory. In some cases referred to as T3 toxicosis, the T4 level is not above the normal range, but T3 is elevated; it is therefore useful to check this value if the TSH level is suppressed without concomitant T4 elevation. Rarely, TSH levels are suppressed in the absence of hyperthyroidism due to side effects from medications (e.g., from steroids) or the presence of an autonomous thyroid nodule. Causes may be distinguished by iodine uptake, which is high in Graves' disease and multinodular goiter and low in thyroiditis or with exogenous thyroxine ingestion.

Therapy

Treatment generally first involves the use of the antithyroid medications, propylthiouracil (PTU) or methimazole, which block thyroidal iodine organification. PTU has the advantage of also inhibiting peripheral conversion of T4 to T3 at higher doses. However, the shorter half-life of PTU often necessitates dosing three times a day, in contrast to the twice-daily dosing regimen used with methimazole. Because both agents can rarely cause agranulocytosis, or, more commonly, granulocytopenia, patients must be instructed to be alert to fever or other evidence of infection such as a persistent sore throat, which would then indicate a need for the white blood cell count to be checked.

Definitive treatment of hyperthyroidism involves the use of radioactive iodine or surgery. Both commonly result in permanent hypothyroidism (often delayed for years following radioiodine therapy), which then necessitates thyroxine replacement.

Hyperparathyroidism

Hyperparathyroidism has been identified in slightly less than 1 percent of hypertensive patients, in contrast to its overall incidence of 0.1 percent in the general population. Conversely, approximately 40 percent of individuals with hyperparathyroidism are hypertensive. Renal dysfunction secondary to this condition may account for some cases of high blood pressure, but a more important factor seems to be hypercalcemia itself, which can cause elevated systemic vascular resistance.

Familial Versus Sporadic

Hyperparathyroidism may occur as part of the familial syndromes MEN 2a (see section on pheochromocytomas) or MEN 1 (which also involves pituitary and pancreatic tumors, most commonly, gastrinoma). In such cases, hyperparathyroidism is most commonly caused by four-gland hyperplasia. Much more often, hyperparathyroidism occurs sporadically, usually as a result of a solitary parathyroid adenoma. Sporadic cases may also be caused by hyperplasia or, very rarely, by parathyroid carcinoma.

Symptoms and Signs

Hyperparathyroidism may be associated with renal stones, bony pains or fractures, gastrointestinal distress including peptic ulcer disease and constipation, and neuropsychiatric disturbances. However, more often symptoms are subtle if present, and hyperparathyroidism is considered when routine chemistry profiles reveal an elevated calcium level. Other frequent serum abnormalities are low phosphorus, elevated chloride, and elevated creatinine levels; urine tests typically reveal a high or normal calcium level in the absence of dehydration or significant renal insufficiency, and a high phosphorus level.

Diagnosis

In the setting of elevated serum calcium (corrected for albumin level), an elevated or high normal level of parathyroid hormone confirms the diagnosis. Parathyroid hormone is best evaluated with an immunoreactive assay for intact hormone.

Therapy

In the presence of any complications of hyperparathyroidism as described above, and the absence of contraindications to surgery, the preferred treatment is parathyroidectomy. Some clinicians recommend this approach even for mild uncomplicated disease (e.g., serum calcium levels < 11.5 mg per deciliter), but some evidence indicates that surgery is not necessary in this setting as long as patients are monitored for the development of renal dysfunction and bone loss. Medical therapy to decrease serum calcium levels where surgery is not elected may involve phosphate supplementation or estrogens in female patients. Phosphate administration, best limited to hypophosphatemic patients, is complicated by the development of diarrhea in many patients, as well as a risk for calcium-phosphate precipitation if the calcium-phosphate product increases above approximately 60.

Importantly, there is debate over the efficacy of parathyroidectomy in reversing the hypertension associated with hyperparathyroidism. An optimistic estimate is that up to 54 percent of individuals may have a significant decrease in blood pressure following successful parathyroidectomy. It is theorized that many of the remainder may in fact have essential hypertension co-existing with hyperparathyroidism, as both are common disorders. In others, irreversible renal dysfunction secondary to longstanding hypercalcemia may perpetuate hypertension, although it is clear that blood pressure does sometimes improve despite persistently elevated serum creatinine levels.

Acromegaly

Acromegaly, caused by excessive secretion of human growth hormone (hGH), may also cause high blood pressure. Sodium retention with resultant extracellular volume expansion appears to underlie the hypertension in this disorder, but the mechanism(s) remain unclear.

Symptoms and Signs

Acromegaly is suspected when enlargement of the hands and feet occurs after normal growth is completed. A change in ring or shoe size is characteristic. Enlargement of the tongue may result in sleep apnea secondary to intermittent airway obstruction. Other suggestive manifestations are profuse sweating (which appears to correlate with disease activity), arthritis, and, in females, menstrual irregularities. Galactorrhea or loss of libido may result from associated hyperprolactinemia.

In addition to acral enlargement and macroglossia, the physical examination may reveal prognathism, frontal bossing, salivary gland enlargement, and multiple skin tags. Distal sensory or motor impairment, resulting from nerve entrapment or axonal demyelination, may also be seen; carpal tunnel syndrome is the most common neurologic manifestation of this disorder. Routine chemistry profiles reveal fasting hyperglycemia in approximately 25 percent of cases, as a result of insulin resistance induced by excessive hGH secretion.

Diagnosis

The diagnosis of acromegaly is based on a nonsuppressible elevation in hGH levels. Following a 3-hour oral glucose tolerance test, hGH levels fall in normal patients to less than 2 ng per milliliter. Failure to suppress is diagnostic of acromegaly. Random hGH measurements should not be used in diagnosis because of the normal sporadic nature of hGH secretion. An alternative approach to diagnosing acromegaly is a measurement of insulin-like growth factor (IGF) 1, also known as somatomedin C, a peptide made in the liver through which GH exerts its effects. Because of its long half-life, this peptide serves as an integrated measure of GH secretion.

Once the diagnosis is confirmed biochemically, MR imaging of the pituitary gland is done to look for an hGH-secreting adenoma, by far the most likely cause of acromegaly. If this test is normal, chest or abdominal CT may reveal an ectopic source of GH-releasing hormone (GHRH), but these sources account for less than 1 percent of cases. In the presence of a normal pituitary MRI scan, the measurement of plasma GHRH levels is an option to consider prior to pursuing extrapituitary evaluation.

Therapy

Pituitary adenomas and ectopic sources of GHRH should be surgically resected when possible. Radiation may be used as an adjunctive therapy for incompletely resected pituitary tumors. Where surgery is contraindicated or fails to eliminate hGH hypersecretion, medical therapy may be tried. Bromocriptine, an ergot derivative that acts as a dopamine agonist, may decrease GH secretion in up to 50 percent of cases. However, its use is frequently associated with nausea and transient hypotension; these side effects can be minimized by starting with a very small dose, such as 1.25 to 2.5 mg, given at night with food, and increasing the dose in small increments until hGH secretion is controlled. Usually, large doses of bromocriptine (more than 20 mg per day) are required to diminish hGH secretion in responsive patients. Approximately 25 percent of patients with a biochemical response to this medication will show objective shrinkage in tumor size. A newer alternative agent is octreotide, a somatostatin analogue that is a potent inhibitor of hGH secretion. Octreotide is associated with an increased risk for gallstones and must be administered by subcutaneous injection twice daily.

SUGGESTED READING

Bravo EL, Gifford RW. Pheochromocytoma: diagnosis, localization and management. N Engl J Med 1984; 311:1298–1303.

Copeland PM. The incidentally discovered adrenal mass. Ann Intern Med 1983; 98:940–945.

Diamond TW, Botha JR, Wing J, et al. Parathyroid hypertension: a reversible disorder. Arch Intern Med 1986; 146:1709–1712.

Kaye TB, Crapo L. The Cushing syndrome: an update on diagnostic tests. Ann Intern Med 1990; 112:434–444.

Streeten DHP, Anderson GH, Howland T, et al. Effects of thyroid function on blood pressure: recognition of hypothyroid hypertension. Hypertension 1988; 11:78–83.

White PC, New MI, Dupont B. Congenital adrenal hyperplasia (second of two parts). N Engl J Med 1987; 316:1580–1586.

Young WF, Hogan MJ, Klee GG, et al. Primary aldosteronism: diagnosis and treatment. Mayo Clin Proc 1990; 65:96–110.

RENAL PARENCHYMAL DISEASE AND HYPERTENSION

MOHAMED H. SAYEGH, M.D.
J. MICHAEL LAZARUS, M.D.

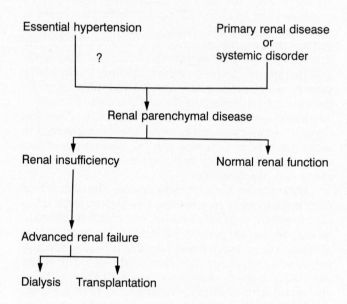

Figure 1 Approach to the management of elevated blood pressure in patients with renal parenchymal disease.

Essential hypertension accounts for approximately 90 to 95 percent of hypertension in patients with elevated blood pressure. Of the remaining, so-called secondary hypertension, renal parenchymal disease is the most common cause. Whether benign essential hypertension progresses to nephrosclerosis and subsequently to renal insufficiency is unclear. It is apparent, however, that poorly controlled hypertension hastens the decline in glomerular filtration rate (GFR) in the presence of underlying renal parenchymal disease. This effect is thought to be mediated by increased intraglomerular hydraulic pressure due to loss of renal autoregulation. Patients with diabetic nephropathy and underlying abnormalities of the renal circulation induced by the diabetic milieu are especially vulnerable to the added renal injury from hypertension. Therefore, therapy for hypertension in patients with renal parenchymal disease not only prevents the nonrenal complications of hypertension, but also may slow the progression of renal dysfunction. The approach to the management of elevated blood pressure in patients with renal parenchymal disease depends on whether they have renal insufficiency, and if so the degree of this insufficiency (Fig. 1). In that regard, and for the purpose of this chapter, we define mild renal insufficiency as a serum creatinine level of less than 3 mg per deciliter and a creatinine clearance of more than 30 ml per minute; moderate renal insufficiency as a serum creatinine of 3 to 6 mg per deciliter and a creatinine clearance of 10 to 30 ml per minute; and advanced renal insufficiency (end-stage renal disease) as a serum creatinine of more than 6 mg per deciliter and a creatinine clearance of less than 10 ml per minute.

The prevalence of hypertension in patients with mild to moderate renal insufficiency varies, depending on the etiology of the underlying renal parenchymal disease. Elevated blood pressure is more frequent in patients with glomerulonephritis and diabetic glomerulosclerosis than in those with polycystic kidney disease or chronic interstitial nephritis. Moreover, among patients with chronic glomerulonephritis, the prevalence of hypertension varies with the histologic lesion. Irrespective of the etiology, by the time advanced chronic renal insufficiency is reached, hypertension occurs in 80 to 90 percent of this patient population (Table 1).

An understanding of the pathophysiologic mechanisms involved in the initiation and maintenance of elevated blood pressure in patients with renal parenchymal disease is important when considering different therapies. In brief, when the GFR decreases, an increase in total exchangeable sodium or extracellular fluid (ECF) volume leads to increased cardiac output and a subsequent increase in total peripheral resistance. In patients with mild to moderate renal insufficiency, hypertension is primarily mediated by an increase in total systemic peripheral resistance mediated by renin

Table 1 Prevalence of Hypertension in Renal Parenchymal Disease

Disease	Percentage of Patients With Hypertension
Nephrosclerosis	100
Primary glomerular disease	
Focal glomerulosclerosis	75–80
Membranoproliferative glomerulonephritis	65–70
Membranous nephropathy	40–50
Mesangioproliferative glomerulonephritis	35–40
IgA nephropathy	30
Minimal change disease	15–20
Diabetic glomerulosclerosis	65–75
Polycystic kidney disease	50–60
Scleroderma	52
Vasculitis	40–60
Chronic interstitial nephropathy	30
Advanced renal insufficiency (? etiology)	80–90

and angiotensin. In patients with advanced renal insufficiency, elevated blood pressure is usually sustained by the added factor of expanded extracellular volume.

There are ample epidemiologic data suggesting that a relative deficiency of dietary potassium increases the risk of hypertension, and several clinical studies have shown that supplemental potassium has a modest antihypertensive effect. Whether potassium deficiency contributes to elevated blood pressure in patients with renal insufficiency is unknown. Most of these patients, however, have problems handling a potassium load, and supplemental potassium may lead to dangerous clinical hyperkalemia. Similarly, there is some evidence that calcium supplements lower the blood pressure in different patient populations. Further study of this observation in patients with renal insufficiency will be important, because most of these patients are on both vitamin D supplements and calcium carbonate.

MANAGEMENT OF HYPERTENSION IN PATIENTS WITH RENAL PARENCHYMAL DISEASE

The treatment of hypertension in patients with renal disease without renal insufficiency is not very different from that of essential hypertension. Experimental evidence suggests that angiotensin converting enzyme (ACE) inhibitors or calcium entry blockers may slow the progression of renal disease, particularly when used early. This remains to be proved, but in the absence of known contraindications, these agents may be considered as first-line therapy for patients with renal parenchymal disease.

Effective treatment depends on dietary factors as well as pharmacologic therapy. Sodium restriction is useful in patients with abnormal renal function. However, it is important to realize the limitations of dietary interventions in patients with renal insufficiency. Most of these patients are on one or more special diets involving low protein, low potassium, low phosphate, and sometimes low cholesterol. When these individuals are asked to restrict sodium, there is difficulty with compliance. Thus, in this group diuretics play a special role in reducing total body sodium.

In patients with malignant hypertension or severe nephrosclerosis with long-term hypertension, regardless of the pharmacologic or dietary therapies, an initial transient reduction in renal function may be observed. This is presumably due to a decrease in perfusion pressure in a system in which GFR has become adapted to the higher pressure. Over a period of weeks to months of treatment, renal function may stabilize or improve.

Diuretics

Recent studies have advocated the use of drugs other than diuretics as first-line therapy for patients with essential hypertension. This approach is also appropriate in patients with renal parenchymal disease and minimally reduced renal function. Conversely, in patients with significant renal insufficiency, sodium and ECF volume are increased, and thus dietary sodium restriction and diuretics are very important as first-line therapy. In patients who have other complicating conditions (Table 2), it may be advisable to start with other antihypertensive medications.

Thiazide diuretics are effective when the creatinine clearance is above 30 ml per minute. However, because of a reduced ability to concentrate urine, patients with mild renal insufficiency on thiazide diuretics are susceptible to volume depletion and hyponatremia. In diabetic patients, thiazide diuretics can worsen glucose control. Because of the increased incidence of hyperlipidemia and the possible associated risk of increased cardiovascular mortality, lipid profile should be carefully monitored while patients are on thiazide diuretics.

When the creatinine clearance drops below 30 ml per minute, loop diuretics and/or metolazone are more efficacious. Occasionally, very high dosages (200 to 400 mg of furosemide or 5 to 10 mg of bumetanide every 8 to 12 hours) of loop diuretics alone or in combination with metolazone (2.5 to 20 mg per day) are required to achieve diuresis and adequate blood pressure control in patients with advanced renal insufficiency prior to initiation of dialysis. In such situations, it is rare to use diuretics alone; their role is adjunctive with that of other antihypertensive agents. In hypertensive patients with massive edema who are resistant to oral therapy, intravenous furosemide, with or without concomitant administration of albumin, can help mobilize the edema and produce a significant diuresis. Patients with salt-losing nephropathy, although rarely hypertensive, and patients on nonsteroidal anti-inflammatory drugs (NSAIDs), are particularly susceptible to the development of volume depletion and prerenal azotemia. Ototoxicity is a potentially disabling and irreversible complication of ethacrynic acid. Interstitial nephritis has been reported in nephrotic patients receiving high doses of loop diuretics.

Table 2 Antihypertensive Therapy for Patients With Associated Complicating Conditions

Condition	Agents to Avoid	Preferred Agents
Congestive heart failure	Beta-blockers	Diuretics, ACE inhibitors
Coronary artery disease	Vasodilators	Beta-blockers, calcium entry blockers, ACE inhibitors, diuretics
Diabetes	Beta-blockers, thiazides	Calcium entry blocker, vasodilators, ACE inhibitors
Sexual dysfunction	Beta-blockers, diuretics, sympatholytic agents	Calcium entry blockers, vasodilators, ACE inhibitors
Dementia, depression	Beta-blockers, sympatholytic agents	Calcium entry blockers, diuretics, ACE inhibitors
Obstructive pulmonary disease	Beta-blockers	Calcium entry blockers, vasodilators, ACE inhibitors, diuretics
Peripheral vascular disease	Beta-blockers (?)	Calcium entry blockers, vasodilators, ACE inhibitors, diuretics

Potassium-sparing diuretics (spironolactone, amiloride, and triamterene) are potentially dangerous in patients with renal insufficiency and should be avoided except in rare patients with tubulointerstitial disease and hypokalemia. Mannitol, a diuretic agent used in the past, is rarely used to treat hypertension. Diuretics have no role in the treatment of the dialysis patient.

Beta-Adrenergic Blocking Agents

If attention to dietary sodium and judicious use of an appropriate diuretic regimen do not result in optimal control of blood pressure, a second antihypertensive medication should be added to control the blood pressure. The choice of agent depends on the patient's clinical condition. Table 2 summarizes recommendations for the use of different antihypertensive medications in patients with renal insufficiency and other complicating conditions.

Beta-blockers can be effective in controlling blood pressure, but several considerations in patients with renal insufficiency warrant mentioning. It is necessary to know the route of metabolism and excretion of the drug selected to avoid those agents dependent on renal excretion, or to adjust the dosage and interval of administration (Table 3). Moreover, because of the high incidence of cardiac disease in patients with renal failure, and the fact that beta-blockers may precipitate cardiac decompensation in patients with congestive heart failure, caution should be taken in starting patients on these agents. Agents with intrinsic sympathomimetic activity (e.g., pindolol) may be of more value in this regard. In patients with coronary artery disease, when there is no ventricular systolic dysfunction, beta-blockers can be beneficial.

These agents may mask symptoms of hypoglycemia in diabetics, and may precipitate overt diabetes in patients with impaired carbohydrate tolerance. They may also cause hyperkalemia, which can be clinically

Table 3 Beta-blockers in Patients with Renal Insufficiency

Agent	Excretion	Dose Adjustments
Propranolol	Hepatic	None
Metoprolol	Hepatic	None
Pindolol	Hepatic	None
Timolol	Hepatic	None
Labetalol	Hepatic	None
Atenolol	Renal	Half dose at clearance 10–50 ml/min
		Quarter dose at clearance < 10 ml/min
Nadolol	Renal	Half dose at clearance 10–50 ml/min
		Quarter dose at clearance < 10 ml/min

significant in patients with underlying renal insufficiency. Sexual dysfunction, which is already prevalent in this patient population, may be induced or worsened and can result in decreased patient compliance with beta-blocker medication. Symptoms of lethargy and fatigue caused by this class of antihypertensives may be difficult to distinguish from the symptoms of progressive anemia and renal insufficiency. In addition, labetalol can cause liver dysfunction. The potential complications described above should be carefully evaluated in individual patients to avoid serious side effects, improve compliance, and increase blood pressure control.

Calcium Entry Blocking Agents

Calcium entry blockers have proved effective in controlling blood pressure in patients with essential hypertension. Some investigators recommend them as first-line agents in patients with renal disease and hypertension. Fewer data are available on their efficacy in patients with hypertension and renal insufficiency, but in our experience they are very useful. Recent studies suggest that they may have a beneficial effect secondary to decreased intraglomerular pressure, although they do not have the postglomerular dilatory effect seen with ACE inhibitors. No dosage adjustments are required for the three most commonly used agents (nifedipine, diltiazem, and verapamil) in this patient population. Sublingual or chewable nifedipine has been successfully used to decrease the blood pressure in severe or urgent hypertension. In chronic hypertension, the combination of nifedipine and beta-blockers can be useful, minimizing the negative vasodilator consequences of nifedipine such as headaches, flushing, and palpitations. Dependent edema, not an uncommon side effect of nifedipine, may not respond to diuretics but usually regresses with time. These side effects are also seen with diltiazem and verapamil, but to a lesser extent. Verapamil, on the other hand, can cause troublesome constipation, especially in elderly patients. Both agents should be used cautiously with beta-blockers because of additive adverse effects on atrioventricular conduction and ventricular function. Calcium entry blockers are particularly useful in patients with decreased ventricular compliance and diastolic dysfunction related to long-standing hypertension, a combination frequently observed in renal failure patients. The recent introduction of extended-release tablets may promote better compliance, especially in patients with renal insufficiency, but one should start with a low dose because the duration of action in renal insufficiency may be prolonged.

Angiotensin Converting Enzyme (ACE) Inhibitors

Because of their preferential vasodilation of the glomerular efferent arterioles, ACE inhibitors (captopril, enalapril, and lisinopril) may be particularly useful in patients with hypertension and renal disease. These agents not only decrease systemic blood pressure, but also decrease glomerular hydraulic pressure, an effect that may reduce the progression of renal dysfunction. This has been extensively studied in animal models and there are several ongoing clinical trials examining this issue in humans. These agents have been very useful in patients with renal parenchymal disease and normal function, and clinicians are beginning to use them as the initial drugs of choice. As renal insufficiency advances, these agents may be less useful. The incidence of some side effects of ACE inhibitors, including rash, hyperkalemia, proteinuria, and leukopenia, increases with the degree of renal impairment. Hyperkalemia is a particularly serious complication. More important, acute worsening of renal function has been seen in patients who are started on ACE inhibitors, especially patients with bilateral renovascular disease, unilateral renovascular disease in one functioning kidney, severe congestive heart failure, and vasculitis. This phenomenon usually occurs within a few days from the time the medications are started and is most commonly seen when patients are also on a diuretic agent. It is usually reversible with discontinuation of the medication. Because the available ACE inhibitors are excreted by the kidney, the usual initial starting dose should be reduced by 50 percent in patients with moderate renal insufficiency and by 75 percent in patients with advanced renal failure.

Vasodilators and Miscellaneous Agents (Hydralazine, Minoxidil, Prazosin, Clonidine, Alpha-Methyldopa, and Reserpine)

Hydralazine has received extensive use in the past in these patients. When ACE inhibitors or calcium entry blockers are contraindicated, hydralazine alone or in combination with beta-blockers is effective. It seems to produce a low incidence of side effects in this patient population. Minoxidil, a related but more potent vasodilator, is very effective in controlling blood pressure in resistant hypertension with renal disease. Sodium retention and hirsutism are common and pericardial effusion is potentially a serious side effect, especially in end-stage renal disease patients on dialysis. Thus, minoxidil should be used as a last resort in renal disease patients and only in those with resistant hypertension. We have found prazosin to be ineffective as monotherapy in renal failure patients. Rarely, it may cause severe hypotension with the first dose. Because of the availability of more effective antihypertensive medications with fewer side effects (especially fatigue, postural hypotension, and adverse effects on sexual function in males), the centrally acting sympatholytic agents clonidine and methyldopa have seen limited use in recent years. Reserpine causes sedation and depression and is of little use in this patient population.

Intravenous diazoxide is rarely used now to treat hypertensive emergencies; it can cause severe unpredictable hypotension and can precipitate angina in patients with coronary artery disease. Intravenous infusion of nitroprusside is the therapy of choice for the acute treatment of malignant hypertension. Signs of thiocyanate toxicity should be carefully sought, with frequent monitoring of blood levels in patients with renal insufficiency, and the drug should be used only temporarily until blood pressure is controlled and other agents are started. Intravenous labetalol, although this agent is not a direct vasodilator, is reported to be effective in patients with acute malignant hypertension.

HYPERTENSION IN DIALYSIS PATIENTS

By the time advanced renal insufficiency develops, close to 80 to 90 percent of patients will have significantly elevated blood pressure. It is estimated that two-thirds of hypertensive patients with end-stage renal disease can be managed by dialysis alone, provided that an adequate regimen of ultrafiltration is employed. The remaining one-third of dialysis patients will require drug therapy for blood pressure control. The aim of therapy in this patient population is to prevent the cardiovascular complications, the most common cause of morbidity and death in dialysis patients.

Diuretics are usually ineffective as renal function is lost; therefore, they have little to offer over ultrafiltration and should be withdrawn in these patients. Rarely, large doses of loop diuretics produce significant increments in urinary volume and thereby minimize intradialytic weight gains. The cost:benefit ratio is poor, however, and the risk of ototoxicity is increased with higher doses. The most important maneuver in the control of hypertension in dialysis patients is establishing a "dry weight," which is arbitrarily defined as the weight at which a normoalbuminemic patient experiences a drop in blood pressure to desired levels or to the level just before the onset of symptomatic hypotension (muscle cramping and nausea). Reducing patients' extracellular volume to this degree generally requires several dialysis sessions with gradual reduction in body weight. Determination of a true "dry weight" may be hampered by blood pressure medications, because they

lower blood pressure during dialysis, thus preventing optimal fluid removal. Antihypertensive medications should be withheld while this process is being carried out. In a small but significant number of patients, especially those who display hemodynamic instability during dialysis, it may be difficult to achieve "dry weight" unless special dialysis procedures are used. Such procedures are designed to minimize changes in osmolality that could induce vasodilation while fluid is removed.

As noted above, despite optimal fluid balance, one-third of hypertensive dialysis patients require additional antihypertensive medications to achieve blood pressure control. In patients who continue to need antihypertensive medications, it is advisable to avoid dosing them 4 to 6 hours before dialysis. Moreover, in order to limit intradialytic weight gains, dietary sodium should be restricted to 80 to 100 mEq per day. Most of these patients characteristically have elevated plasma renin activity and increased total peripheral resistance. In this regard, agents directed at lowering the activity of the renin-angiotensin system are logical choices. Indeed,

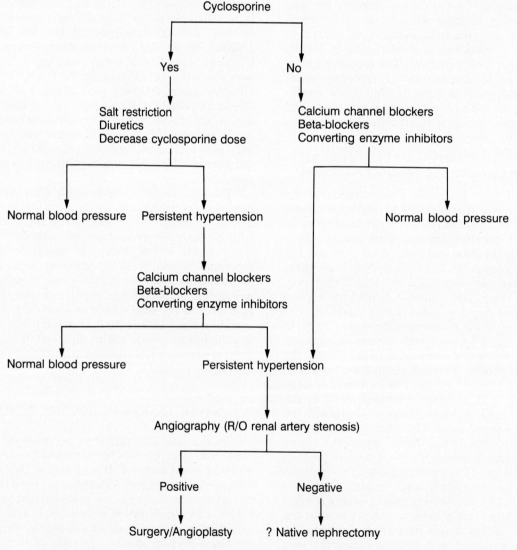

Figure 2 Approach to the management of hypertension after renal transplantation.

beta-blockers and ACE inhibitors have proved effective. Although calcium entry blockers have no apparent physiologic basis, they are being widely used in dialysis patients and are effective. If blood pressure is not controlled with these measures, patients' volume status should be reassessed to make sure that they are indeed at their "dry weight." A few patients with persistent hypertension, despite normal ECF volume and adequate doses of a first antihypertensive drug, require the addition of a second or even third drug (calcium entry blocker, ACE inhibitor, or beta-blocker). The centrally acting vasodilators are less useful in dialysis patients because of their tendency to induce postural hypotension.

It is important to note that more than 25 percent of patients treated with recombinant human erythropoietin, now used to correct anemia of chronic renal failure, require initiation of or increase in antihypertensive therapy. The exact mechanism of the changes in blood pressure is unclear, but hypertension in erythropoietin-treated patients is associated with the rate of rise in hematocrit. In a large multicenter study, more hypertension was noted in patients who had an increase in hematocrit of 4 or more in less than 2 weeks. Therefore, a decrease in erythropoietin dosage is recommended if the hematocrit increases by more than 4 in any 2-week period. Moreover, patients with uncontrolled hypertension should not receive erythropoietin until their blood pressure is brought under control.

Uncontrollable hypertension requiring nephrectomy is rare or nonexistent with current antihypertensive medications.

HYPERTENSION IN TRANSPLANT PATIENTS

Acute hypertension after transplant occurs during rejection or loss of function of the graft. Under these circumstances, elevated blood pressure usually responds to either dialysis therapy or the reversal of rejection with immunotherapy. Meanwhile, the patient may need one or more antihypertensive medications (Fig. 2).

The prevalence of chronic hypertension in kidney transplant patients averages 50 to 60 percent. The following factors have been associated with a higher likelihood of post-transplant hypertension: (1) renal allograft dysfunction manifested by an elevated serum creatinine level; (2) cadaveric allografts (which tend to have reduced function in comparison to living related allografts); (3) increased body weight; (4) the presence of native kidneys; (5) renal transplant artery stenosis; and (6) cyclosporine. Cyclosporine decreases the incidence of renal allograft rejection and permits a lower dosage of prednisone. Although steroid toxicity is minimized, cyclosporine itself can cause elevated blood pressure. Before cyclosporine, post-transplant chronic hypertension was thought to be due to increased total peripheral resistance due to activation of the renin-angiotensin system. Cyclosporine is a potent renal vasoconstrictor; hypertension in transplant patients on cyclosporine is less often associated with activation of the renin-angiotensin system and is more responsive to sodium restriction and diuretics. The addition of beta-blockers or ACE inhibitors may be necessary if patients do not respond to extracellular volume control. Calcium entry blockers are effective and may have the added benefit of minimizing cyclosporine nephrotoxicity.

It is difficult to determine how many hypertensive renal allograft recipients have angiographically and clinically significant renal artery stenosis, partly because angiography is not performed unless patients have resistant hypertension. The mean time for development of transplant artery anastomotic stenosis is approximately 2 years. In the absence of chronic rejection proved on biopsy, angiography should be performed in patients with persistent hypertension on an adequate medical regimen. If results are positive, correction of renal artery anastomotic stenosis, by either percutaneous transluminal angioplasty or vascular surgery, is recommended. Both procedures can be difficult and risky because of the intense scarring around the vessels of the transplant kidney. Thus, these procedures should be reserved for patients with poor blood pressure control despite adequate medical therapy. Figure 2 summarizes a practical approach to the management of patients with post-transplant hypertension.

One must be aware of possible interactions between cyclosporine and several antihypertensive medications commonly used in transplant patients (Table 4). Cyclosporine blood levels and renal function should be closely monitored when antihypertensive therapy is started or changed. Finally, in hypertensive renal allograft recipients in whom drug therapy has failed to control blood pressure and renal artery stenosis has been excluded, native kidney nephrectomy should be considered.

SUGGESTED READING

Bennett WM, McCarron DA. Pharmacotherapy of renal disease and hypertension. New York: Churchill Livingstone, 1987.

Table 4 Reported Interactions of Antihypertensive Medications With Cyclosporine

Agent	Cyclosporine Level	Effect
Diltiazem	Increased	Graft dysfunction, may prevent nephrotoxicity
Nifedipine	None	Increased gingival hyperplasia
Nicardipine	Increased	May cause graft dysfunction
Verapamil	Increased	May cause graft dysfunction, may prevent nephrotoxicity
		? Increased immunosuppression
Minoxidil	Unknown	Increased hirsutism
Metoprolol	Increased	Unknown
ACE inhibitors	Unknown	Synergistic effect to cause hyperkalemia

Laragh JH, Brenner BM. Hypertension: pathophysiology, diagnosis, and management. New York: Raven Press, 1990.

Milford E. Renal transplantation. New York: Churchill Livingstone, 1989.

Narins R, Stein J. Current trends in the treatment of hypertensive syndromes. Am J Kidney Dis 1989.

O'Rourke R. Hypertension and the heart. New York: Churchill Livingstone, 1984.

Rose BD. Pathophysiology of renal disease. 2nd ed. New York: McGraw-Hill, 1987.

IDIOPATHIC ORTHOSTATIC HYPOTENSION AND SUPINE HYPERTENSION

GARY L. SCHWARTZ, M.D.
ALEXANDER SCHIRGER, M.D.

Orthostatic hypotension (OH) is an abnormal decline in systolic and diastolic pressure that occurs with assumption of the upright position. OH becomes symptomatic when the reduction of blood pressure is severe enough and prolonged enough to result in symptoms of organ hypoperfusion.

The conditions associated with OH (see Table 1) are divided into primary and secondary disorders. OH arises from defects in the autonomic nervous system or is due to non-neurogenic factors. Non-neurogenic causes include disorders that result in low vascular volume or impair function of the heart or vasculature, reducing their ability to respond to the physiologic stresses that accompany standing. Transient mild orthostasis may occur as a benign condition in otherwise healthy people. More persistent and severe declines in standing blood pressure indicate a serious underlying disorder. Sufficient dysautonomia to result in OH may frequently accompany aging without other secondary etiologies.

This chapter concentrates on methods of managing patients with chronic OH. This is often due to conditions associated with degeneration of the autonomic nervous system.

HEMODYNAMIC PROFILE IN ORTHOSTATIC HYPOTENSION

The typical hemodynamic profile of arterial pressure and heart rate in patients with autonomic failure and chronic OH is shown in Figure 1. Standing, exercise, or the ingestion of food can cause the blood pressure to fall. Hypotension is often more frequent and severe in the mornings and less severe later in the day. Whatever the precipitating event, a corresponding rise in heart rate fails to occur. The expected decline in blood pressure that normally accompanies assumption of the supine position, as during sleep, fails to occur. In some persons, blood pressure may actually rise, occasionally to severe levels. It is helpful to keep this profile in mind when considering treatment strategies and discussing times of greatest risk for hypotension with the patient.

MANAGEMENT

General Principles

Before initiating specific therapy, a search should be made to identify reversible conditions that may aggravate or cause hypotension. These include drugs (Table 2), anemia, hypoxia, muscle deconditioning, electrolyte abnormalities, hypovolemia, hypothyroidism, and adrenal insufficiency.

Patients should be informed about both the cause of their symptoms (abnormally low blood pressure) and those factors likely to precipitate a fall in blood pressure. Because hypotension is usually worse in the mornings, in hot weather, and following the ingestion of food, prolonged standing or exertion in the upright position should be avoided or performed with caution at these times.

Autonomic failure frequently causes impaired sweating or absolute anhidrosis, making patients more susceptible to heat stroke. Prolonged heat exposure should be avoided and homes should be air conditioned if possible.

The Valsalva maneuver that accompanies straining with urination or defecation may cause syncope as the result of an acute decline in venous return to the heart and cardiac output. Patients with OH are particularly vulnerable to falls and serious injury when walking to the bathroom at night. Use of a bedside commode with a reclining back rest and an elevatable foot rest may reduce these risks. Constipation should be prevented with good hydration and stool softeners as needed.

Patients should avoid alcohol because it can cause sufficient vasodilatation to produce dramatic declines in blood pressure. This is particularly important during those times when the patient must stand for prolonged periods, such as at receptions.

Because there are a variety of medications that may aggravate hypotension, patients should be encouraged to use only medications (including over-the-counter medications) approved by the physician. When contemplating the use of any drug in such patients, the physician

Table 1 Disorders Causing Orthostatic Hypotension

Primary orthostatic hypotension
    Idiopathic orthostatic hypotension (primary autonomic failure)
    Idiopathic orthostatic hypotension with somatic neurologic deficit
       (primary autonomic failure with multiple system atrophy, Shy-
       Drager syndrome)
Secondary orthostatic hypotension
    Neurogenic
       Primary disorders of nervous system
          Tumors of the parasellar, hypothalamic, posterior fossa
          Multiple cerebral infarcts
          Wernicke's encephalopathy
          Tabes dorsalis
          Traumatic or inflammatory myelopathies
          Guillain-Barré syndrome
          Familial dysautonomia (Riley-Day syndrome)
          Holmes-Adie syndrome
          Acute pandysautonomia
          Dysautonomia of advanced age
          Hereditary system degenerations
          Parkinson's disease
          Syringomyelia
       Systemic diseases with autonomic neuropathy
          Diabetes mellitus
          Porphyria
          Primary systemic amyloidosis
          Carcinoma
          Uremia
          Alcohol neuropathy
          Vitamin B_{12} deficiency
          Botulism
          Tangier and Fabry's disease
       Iatrogenic causes
          Drugs (antihypertensive, psychotropic, antiparkinson)
          Extensive surgical sympathectomy
    Non-neurogenic
       Endocrine/metabolic disorders
          Adrenocortical insufficiency (Addison's)
          Pheochromocytoma
          Hypothyroidism
          Hypoaldosteronism
       Volume depletion
          Acute or chronic blood loss
          Fluid loss, vomiting, diarrhea
          Salt-losing nephropathy
          Altered capillary permeability syndromes
       Disorders impairing venous return
          Poor postural adjustment
          Varicose veins
          Venous obstruction (late pregnancy)
          Muscle wasting, prolonged recumbency
       Primary myocardial disease
          Myocardial infarction
          Arrhythmias
          Mitral valve prolapse
          Restrictive pericarditis
    Miscellaneous
       Hyperbradykininism
       Chronic renal hemodialysis
       Anorexia nervosa
       Mastocytosis
       Reduced aortic compliance (isolated systolic hypertension)
       Potassium depletion

must consider its potential impact on blood pressure, particularly in the upright posture. For example, angina pectoris may be precipitated in patients with autonomic failure by declines in blood pressure when upright. The use of sublingual nitroglycerin in this setting may cause profound hypotension, worsening the myocardial ischemia. More appropriate initial treatment of angina is to have patients assume the supine position, and then if angina persists, to have them use nitrates while supine.

Patients should rise slowly after prolonged periods of lying down. Dorsiflexion of the feet prior to sitting or standing may lessen the decline in blood pressure. Patients should routinely sit for several minutes before standing.

Heavy lifting, isometric or strenuous exercises, ingestion of large meals, taking of hot showers or baths, or working with the arms above the shoulder level for prolonged periods should be avoided, because all of these activities may aggravate hypotension.

Caveats of Treatment

Autoregulation of cerebral blood flow is shifted to lower levels of systemic blood pressure in patients with chronic OH. Therefore, patients often function well and are asymptomatic with low levels of blood pressure. Because interventions are associated with side effects and aggravate the tendency toward supine hypertension, treatment of low blood pressure should be reserved for patients who are symptomatic. The influence of any intervention on supine blood pressure, especially at night, must be assessed. Finally, in more severe cases of chronic neurogenic OH, limitations in life style are often necessary. This must be discussed honestly with the patient. The goal of therapy in severe autonomic failure may be limited to creating a window of time during the day in which the patient can carry out essential upright activities. Pressor therapy needs to be modified if patients become nonambulatory.

Nonpharmacologic Therapy

Nonpharmacologic therapy may be all that is required in mild cases and forms the foundation for treatment, even in patients with more severe disease (Table 3).

A daily sodium intake of at least 150 to 200 mEq (4 g of sodium) should be encouraged. This increases the vascular volume available for pooling and dampens the decline in venous return that occurs with standing. Caution should be used in patients with decreased cardiac or renal reserve in whom vascular overload could be precipitated.

Sleeping with the head of the bed elevated 10 to 12 inches (head-up tilt) can be accomplished by placing blocks beneath the headposts of the bed. This maneuver is associated with a lower blood pressure than that associated with the usual supine position, and this lower pressure may stimulate the renin-angiotensin-aldosterone axis, ultimately leading to a more expanded intravascular volume. This intervention is safe and rarely leads to volume overload.

Venous pooling in the upright posture may be inhibited by elasticized, graded pressure garments, which produce a gradient of counter-pressure with

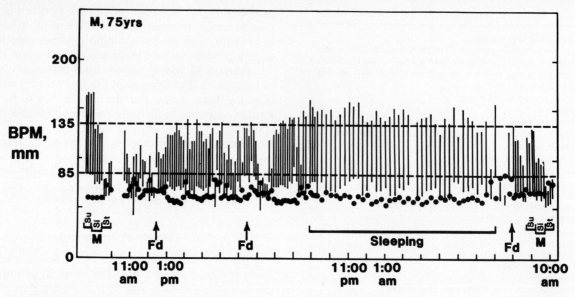

Figure 1 Ambulatory blood pressure profile of a 75-year-old man with autonomic failure. Each line represents a single determination of blood pressure. Su, supine; Si, sitting; St, standing; M, simultaneous manual and machine determinations of blood pressure; Fd, ingestion of food; •, heart rate; BPM, beats per minute; mm, millimeters of mercury.

Table 2 Drugs That May Cause Orthostatic Hypertension

Antihypertensives
  Diuretics
  Vasodilators (apresoline, minoxidil, calcium antagonists, nitrates, alpha-blockers [first dose effect])
  Adrenergic neuronal blockers (guanethidine, guanadrel)
  Alpha-adrenergic blocking drugs (Dibenzyline, labetalol)
  Central alpha-agonists (methyldopa, clonidine, guanabenz, guanfacine)
  ACE inhibitors
  Reserpine
Antipsychotics
  Phenothiazines, haloperidol
Antidepressants
  Tricyclics, MAO inhibitors
CNS depressants
  Narcotics, benzodiazepines, barbiturates, alcohol
Bronchodilators
  Beta-agonists
Anti-Parkinson medications
  Levodopa, bromocriptine
Appetite suppressants
  Amphetamine-like drugs

Table 3 Nonpharmacologic Therapy

High sodium intake (150–200 mEq sodium/day)
Head-up tilt at night
External pressure garments
Exercise as tolerated

support garments deconditions the myogenic response to stretch of the capacitance veins and may worsen standing hypotension when the garment is not worn.

Symptomatic orthostatic hypotension may be totally alleviated during immersion, and swimming may provide an excellent form of exercise and a respite for the patient whose daily activities are otherwise limited. Mild exercise may maintain the muscle pump function of the legs, which facilitates venous return. Vigorous exercise, however, may aggravate orthostasis, perhaps by depleting the available catecholamine reserve. However, under these circumstances, exercise-induced skeletal muscle vasodilatation may be associated with postexercise hypotension.

Pharmacologic Therapy

It should be made clear to patients at the outset that the treatment of OH due to autonomic nervous system dysfunction is often difficult and imperfect. The number of effective therapies is small. Many drugs cause unpleasant side effects and often fail to completely normalize blood pressure. Frequently, drugs must be given in combination, as in the treatment of essential hypertension. Pharmacologic therapies may be directed at several mechanisms to increase blood pressure. Some increase the fluid volume available for pooling, thus

maximal pressure in the lower legs. Chest-high garments impair splanchnic venous pooling as well as venous pooling in the legs and are preferred in severe cases. Waist-high garments may be sufficient in patients with milder disease. Use of these pressure garments can pose a problem because they are difficult to put on and take off and can be uncomfortable in hot climates. They can be fitted with zippers that make them easier to use and can be made with an open crotch to facilitate urination. Pressure garments should be put on in the morning while the patient is still recumbent and removed prior to recumbency in the evening. Chronic use of external minimizing the decline in venous return that occurs when upright. Others cause venous constriction in an attempt to decrease the size of the vascular space available for pooling. Several drugs exert their pressor effects by increasing either heart rate and contractility or peripheral vascular resistance. While each drug is associated with its own unique side effects, supine hypertension is a common problem with all of them.

Most Commonly Used Drugs

9α-Fludrohydrocortisone (Florinef) is the first drug to consider. Low doses may increase blood pressure through a variety of mechanisms, including sensitizing vascular adrenergic receptors to pressor stimuli; stimulating increases in the number of vascular alpha-receptors; increasing the release of norepinephrine and impairing its re-uptake; and increasing the fluid content of blood vessel walls, making them more resistant to stretch. Larger doses induce renal sodium retention and increase extracellular and vascular volume. The major potential complications of fludrocortisone are vascular congestion, hypokalemia, and aggravation of supine hypertension. Hypokalemia must be identified early and vigorously corrected, as it can aggravate hypotension and provoke cardiac dysrhythmias. This drug should be used cautiously in patients with reduced cardiac or renal reserve. The usual starting dose of 9α-fludrohydrocortisone is 0.1 mg given once or twice daily. While total daily doses of up to 2 mg may be used, it is rarely necessary to use more than 0.6 mg. Higher doses are associated with an increased incidence of side effects, including significant hypokalemia and vascular congestion.

Nonsteroidal anti-inflammatory drugs (NSAIDs) that block the formation of renal natriuretic and vasodilating prostaglandins may have a pressor effect in some patients. Indomethacin has been the most commonly used member of this class. It is most effective in doses of 25 to 50 mg given three times daily in combination with 9α-fludrohydrocortisone. The usual precautions regarding the use of NSAIDs must be observed. Because of the potential for gastric irritation and hemorrhage, NSAIDs should be given with meals and avoided in patients with known gastroparesis. One should keep in mind that gastroparesis frequently accompanies chronic OH due to autonomic failure. NSAIDs may induce acute renal dysfunction, and therefore serum creatinine levels must be monitored. If no benefit is noted after a 4- to 6-week trial, these agents should be discontinued.

A number of vasoconstrictor therapies are available. These include both direct-acting sympathomimetics (ephedrine, phenylephrine, phenylpropanolamine) and drugs that act indirectly to increase circulating catecholamines (methylphenidate, amphetamines, tyramine, and monoamine oxidase inhibitors). Because of their erratic effects on blood pressure, side effects (tachycardia, cardiac dysrhythmias, palpitations, insomnia, tremor, anxiety, piloerection), and tendency to cause severe supine hypertension, the use of many of these agents is not encouraged. Of this large group, ephedrine may be effective in doses of 25 to 50 mg given three times daily in mild cases. Phenylephrine is very short-acting and available as a nasal spray. This can be used prior to planned prolonged upright activity. Methylphenidate in doses of 5 to 20 mg given twice daily is probably the safest and most effective of these compounds. Drugs acting indirectly to increase circulating catecholamines are ineffective in advanced autonomic failure.

Caffeine may lessen postprandial hypotension by blocking adenosine-mediated splanchnic vasodilatation. The usual dose employed is 200 to 250 mg given once daily. This dose is found in two or three cups of coffee or can be given orally (No Doz). Tolerance tends to develop quickly, but this is a relatively benign intervention worth trying.

Drugs to Consider When Plasma Norepinephrine is Low

In the setting of low circulating catecholamines, there is often an increase in the number of vascular adrenal receptors (denervation hypersensitivity). In this setting, weak vascular adrenal receptor agonists may exert significant pressor effects. Plasma catecholamine levels can be measured and used as a guide for administration of these agents. Success with these drugs is seen in only a minority of cases, but a cautious trial is reasonable in selected patients.

Clonidine is an alpha$_2$-agonist. It acts in the central nervous system to inhibit sympathetic outflow, which accounts for its efficacy as an antihypertensive agent. Its peripheral action, however, is to increase venous and arteriolar tone. In the setting of autonomic neuronal damage, its peripheral action may dominate. Clonidine is usually given twice daily in a dose of 0.2 to 0.4 mg. Complications include hypotension, supine hypertension, dry mouth, and sedation. It has the best opportunity of exerting a pressor effect in complete postganglionic lesions.

If clonidine causes a depressor response, yohimbine may be tried. This alpha$_2$-antagonist acts centrally to enhance sympathetic outflow and also facilitates norepinephrine release from nerve terminals by blocking presynaptic alpha$_2$-receptors. Complications include tremulousness, nervousness, palpitations, and supine hypertension. The dose ranges from 2.5 to 5 mg given four times daily for a total daily dose of 10 to 20 mg.

Pindolol is a beta-adrenergic blocking drug with partial beta-agonist activity. In the setting of severe postganglionic autonomic disease, it may act as a pure beta-agonist. Blood pressure may rise as the result of beta-agonist–induced increases in heart rate and contractility. Complications include hypotension, bradycardia, and congestive heart failure. The drug should not be given to patients with a history of bronchospasm. The usual dose is 5 to 15 mg given once or twice daily.

Miscellaneous Drugs

Dopamine may exert vasodilator and natriuretic effects at physiologic concentrations. Metoclopramide is a dopamine receptor antagonist that may have pressor effects, especially when dopamine levels are excessive. Metoclopramide may be appropriate for use in patients with autonomic failure complicated by gastroparesis, because it facilitates gastric emptying. Side effects include the development of extrapyramidal symptoms. The usual dose of metoclopramide is 10 mg given one-half hour before meals and at bedtime.

Propranolol may increase blood pressure by blocking vasodilating beta-receptors and increasing exercise-induced adrenal catecholamine release. Major potential complications are hypotension, bradycardia, and congestive heart failure. Like pindolol, it should not be given to patients with bronchospastic lung disease. The usual dose employed is 40 to 240 mg given in divided doses.

Desmopressin acts on renal tubule receptors to inhibit water diuresis and thereby increases vascular volume. The drug can be given at bedtime, when it lessens the tendency for nocturnal polyuria often seen in chronic OH. The usual dose is 5 to 40 mg intranasally. The major potential complication is hyponatremia. Serum sodium must be monitored closely during the initiation of therapy.

The somatostatin analog Sandostatin prevents the release of gut vasodilatory peptides that follows the ingestion of food. It may prevent postprandial hypotension. Sandostatin is expensive and must be given subcutaneously two to three times per day. Potential complications include constipation, hepatitis, cholelithiasis, anxiety, galactorrhea, and hypothyroidism.

Investigational Drugs

We have had several years of experience with an investigational alpha-agonist, midodrine (Gutron). Midodrine increases blood pressure by inducing constriction of both arterioles and veins, thereby increasing both peripheral vascular resistance and venous return. It has few direct cardiostimulatory effects. The pressor effect is rather short-lived. Effective doses range from 2.5 to 15 mg given three or four times daily. Major potential complications include supine hypertension, piloerection, and nausea. This drug is currently widely available in Europe and Mexico and may be approved for use in the United States in the near future.

Dihydroergotamine exerts its pressor effects by constriction of venous capacitance vessels, thus facilitating venous return. A major problem with this drug is its poor oral bioavailability. It can be given once daily by intramuscular or subcutaneous injection. Major complications include supine hypertension and peripheral vasoconstriction.

Machines

Atrial tachypacing may be of benefit if severe bradycardia is present. Cardiac output, however, is often

Table 4 Treatment of Supine Hypertension

Avoid pressor therapies prior to periods of recumbency
Use a recliner for rest during the day
Bedtime snack
Small doses of ethanol at bedtime
Vasodilators at bedtime (calcium entry blockers, hydralazine)

only minimally increased unless venous return is simultaneously augmented. Initial enthusiasm for this procedure has waned. Often, bradycardia can now be treated with beta-blockers that contain partial beta-agonist activity (e.g., pindolol). This approach has largely replaced the use of pacemakers.

SUPINE HYPERTENSION

Characteristic of disorders associated with autonomic failure is loss of the usual decline in blood pressure with assumption of the supine position (see Fig. 1). In some cases, blood pressure actually rises into the hypertensive range, occasionally to severe levels. Patients may present with symptoms of headache associated with retinal hemorrhages on physical examination. All therapies for hypotension may cause further elevations in supine blood pressure. Therefore, supine blood pressure needs to be monitored, especially at bedtime.

Several therapies are available to treat supine hypertension (Table 4). Pressor therapies should not be taken prior to anticipated periods of prolonged rest. Patients should avoid the supine position during the day by resting in a recliner in a semiupright position. Upright tilt at night not only is potentially useful therapy to prevent daytime hypotension, but also decreases blood pressure when the patient is supine at night. The ingestion of food results in splanchnic vascular pooling and the release of vasodilatory peptides. Although these events cause bothersome hypotension during the day, they may act as effective antihypertensive therapy at bedtime. Alcohol given at bedtime will also exert a hypotensive effect owing to vasodilatation. Finally, small doses of several vasodilatory antihypertensive agents with relatively short durations of action may be given at bedtime. These include calcium channel blocking drugs (nifedipine, 10 to 20 mg; diltiazem, 30 to 60 mg; verapamil, 80 mg) or hydralazine (10 to 25 mg).

SUGGESTED READING

Bannister Sir R. Autonomic failure. 2nd ed. Oxford: Oxford University Press, 1988.

Lipsitz LA. Orthostatic hypotension in the elderly. N Engl J Med 1989; 321:952.

Onrot J, Goldberg MR, Hollister AS, et al. Management of chronic orthostatic hypotension. Am J Med 1986; 80:454–464.

Fealey RD, Schirger A, Thomas JE. Orthostatic hypotension. In: Spittell JA Jr., ed. Clinical medicine. Vol. 7. New York: Harper & Row, 1985:1.

CORONARY ARTERY DISEASE

CHRONIC ISCHEMIC HEART DISEASE: MEDICAL MANAGEMENT

JULES Y. T. LAM, M.D.
DAVID D. WATERS, M.D.

Angina pectoris is the clinical syndrome that results from an imbalance of myocardial oxygen demand and supply. The most common cause of this syndrome is a reduction in oxygen supply that results from large vessel epicardial coronary atherosclerotic disease. The atherosclerotic process may be limited to a single-vessel disease, or, more often, to multivessel coronary disease, and it may be focal or extensive in nature. The severity of symptoms may not necessarily correlate with the severity of coronary atherosclerosis, as severe angina may be associated with single-vessel disease, and conversely, the absence of symptoms does not exclude the presence of severe coronary disease. However, it is usually the symptoms of angina that will cause the patient to seek the care of a physician.

In this chapter we discuss the pharmacologic management of patients with chronic stable angina. The goal of drug therapy is primarily to minimize the frequency and severity of angina, thereby improving not only the patient's functional capacity but also his or her long-term prognosis. This treatment option must be individually tailored to take into consideration the patient's compliance, as well as side effects and costs of treatment. The benefits of drug therapy depend on an accurate diagnosis. Thrombolytic therapy can be disastrous in a patient whose chest pain is not caused by acute myocardial ischemia, and the incorrect diagnosis of angina can lead to years of fruitless medical therapy.

Once the diagnosis is certain and relevant coexistent medical problems are excluded, the introduction of medical therapy can be considered. If the anginal episodes occur infrequently (once or twice per month) with no limitation of normal physical activities, chronic antianginal therapy may not be necessary and sublingual nitroglycerin or nitroglycerin spray administered on an as-needed basis may be all that is needed for symptomatic control. If more frequent episodes of angina occur, a specific drug with a specific pharmacologic profile may be chosen, and its dose can be optimized according to the patient's clinical response. The rationale for using antianginal drug therapy is to decrease myocardial oxygen demand, increase coronary blood flow to ischemic myocardium, or both, so as to normalize the relationship between oxygen demand and supply. Three major classes of antianginal drugs are currently available: beta-adrenergic blocking drugs, slow-channel calcium entry blockers, and nitrates. These drugs can be used alone as the sole therapy or in combination. Although these drugs have been proved effective in the management of chronic stable angina, their limitations must be recognized and physicians must know when to turn to other treatment options such as coronary angioplasty or bypass surgery.

NITROGLYCERIN AND LONGER-ACTING NITRATES

Nitroglycerin has been used to treat angina for over a century. After sublingual administration it is absorbed within seconds and relieves attacks within 2 to 5 minutes. Several mechanisms that account for its beneficial effect have been described and the relative contribution of each of these to the clinical setting remains controversial. In comparison with its effect in reducing afterload, nitroglycerin decreases preload to a greater extent because of venous pooling. This agent dilates both epicardial coronary arteries and collateral vessels and prevents or relieves coronary spasm. Nitroglycerin is also capable of abolishing exercise-induced coronary vasoconstriction at sites of stenosis. This latter action may be the most relevant to the treatment of most cases of angina.

All patients with angina are routinely supplied with nitroglycerin and should be instructed in its proper use because misconceptions abound. The drug can cause headache, palpitations, dizziness, and syncope. It should not be used for symptoms other than those related to myocardial ischemia and patients should probably not take it while standing. The prophylactic use of nitroglycerin to prevent anginal attacks can greatly enhance the exercise capacity of many patients with stable, predictable angina.

Intravenously administered nitroglycerin is commonly used to treat patients with unstable angina, usually in association with beta-adrenergic and/or calcium channel blockers. This route of administration permits rapid titration of dosage in response to symptoms or to adverse events. In a randomized comparison between intravenously administered nitroglycerin and the combination of orally administered isosorbide dinitrate and topically applied nitroglycerin ointment in 40 patients with unstable angina, both regimens were found to be effective in reducing angina attacks; the difference between the two methods did not attain statistical significance (Curfman and co-workers, 1983). Recent evidence suggests that the antiplatelet activity of intravenously administered nitroglycerin may contribute to its beneficial effect in the treatment of unstable angina.

Few drugs can be administered in as many different ways as can nitroglycerin. In addition to the sublingual tablet and intravenous form, a lingual spray is available. This formulation does not lose potency with time and is probably more rapidly absorbed than the sublingual tablet, particularly if the mouth is dry. Sustained-release buccal formulations of nitroglycerin have also been shown to be effective antianginal agents. Isosorbide dinitrate is the most commonly used oral nitrate preparation in North America. Transdermal nitroglycerin patches have proved to be a very popular method of administration since their release in the United States in 1982.

The major problem with the long-term administration of nitrates by any route is the development of tolerance. Tolerance to the hemodynamic effects of nitroglycerin appears within 24 to 48 hours of chronic therapy and antianginal efficacy is completely attenuated after 7 to 10 days of continuous treatment. Intermittent therapy with nitrate-free intervals of 8 to 12 hours per day has been used with some success to circumvent the problem of tolerance. Isosorbide dinitrate should be prescribed in doses of two to three times per day with a drug-free overnight interval of at least 12 hours. Nitroglycerin patches should likewise be removed for at least 8 to 12 hours at night.

Unfortunately, even with intermittent dosing regimens, treatment with long-acting nitrates is associated with significant problems and limitations. Nitrate-related headache occurs in most patients treated with doses high enough to ensure antianginal efficacy and thus therapy is often discontinued. Nocturnal angina may occur more frequently with intermittent nitrate therapy than with placebo and patients receiving placebo have been shown to have better early morning exercise tolerance.

The mechanism of nitrate tolerance is unclear. It has been postulated that tolerance develops because of a reduced ability of the administered nitrate to undergo conversion to nitric oxide, the active metabolite of nitroglycerin. The depletion of intracellular thiol groups limits the conversion of nitrates to nitric oxide in the tolerant state. One strategy to prevent tolerance that is currently under investigation involves the administration of thiol donors such as captopril or N-acetylcysteine.

In light of these considerations, long-acting nitrate preparations are not recommended as the best choice in the prophylactic therapy for stable angina. However, in patients who do not tolerate or have contraindications to beta-adrenergic or calcium channel blockers, as in those with heart failure, long-acting nitrates are a reasonable therapeutic option to use. To minimize side effects, treatment should begin with low doses that are gradually increased. Intermittent therapy is essential and drug therapy should be discontinued if side effects or a lack of efficacy develops. Long-acting nitrates can also be used in patients with angina whose symptoms persist at an unacceptable level despite the use of other antianginal drugs. The combination of a long-acting nitrate and a beta-adrenergic blocker tends to act synergistically because the beta-blocker prevents any nitrate-induced acceleration in heart rate. The use of long-acting nitrates reduces the frequency of silent myocardial ischemia; however, the usefulness of these drugs in this condition has not been adequately investigated.

Intravenously administered nitroglycerin has been used in the acute phase of myocardial infarction to limit infarct size. A meta-analysis of controlled clinical trials suggests that such treatment reduces mortality by one-third, from 18 percent to 12 percent (95 percent confidence intervals: -18 percent to -49 percent). The benefit appears to be greatest in large, anterior, Q wave infarcts and may be due to the drug's salutary influence on ventricular remodeling. Subsequent treatment with an angiotensin-converting enzyme inhibitor is indicated to preserve left ventricular function by preventing left ventricular aneurysm formation.

BETA-ADRENERGIC BLOCKERS

The first beta-adrenergic blocker released in the United States was propranolol, in 1967. This drug is a competitive antagonist of both β_1 and β_2 stimulation and therefore results in negative chronotropic and inotropic effects in the heart, bronchoconstriction, and vasoconstriction. After oral administration, propranolol prolongs treadmill walking time to the onset of angina; total exercise time lasts from 1 to 12 hours.

Myocardial ischemia, with or without angina, occurs when coronary blood flow decreases or when myocardial oxygen consumption increases. The three major determinants of myocardial oxygen consumption are systolic wall tension, heart rate, and inotropic state of the myocardium. Propranolol and other beta-blockers reduce systemic arterial pressure, heart rate, and myocardial contractility both at rest and during exercise, which reduces myocardial oxygen consumption. In an early uncontrolled study of 63 patients with severe, stable angina (Warren and co-workers, 1976), the use of propranolol eliminated all episodes in 32 percent of patients and reduced episodes by at least half in 84 percent. During a follow-up period of 5 to 8 years, patients whose attacks were not reduced by at least half experienced a fourfold greater mortality compared with the others.

Propranolol is also effective in the therapy for hypertension, atrial and ventricular arrhythmias, thyrotoxicosis, essential tremor, hypertrophic cardiomyopathy, migraine, and glaucoma. Its antihypertensive action results in part from a lowering of plasma renin activity. Common side effects include fatigue, impotence, nightmares, and cold extremities. The drug can precipitate or worsen heart failure, conduction disturbances, and bronchoconstriction in susceptible individuals. In diabetic patients with labile blood glucose levels, propranolol can induce hypoglycemia; the drug also masks the premonitory symptoms of hypoglycemia. Abrupt withdrawal of therapy with propranolol can induce rebound with worsening angina or myocardial infarction. The use of propranolol increases serum triglyceride levels and slightly lowers high density lipoprotein (HDL) cholesterol concentrations; during long-term therapy these unfavorable metabolic effects could accelerate the progression of atherosclerosis.

The second beta-blocker to be released for clinical use in the United States was metoprolol, in 1978. This drug preferentially antagonizes the action of sympathomimetic amines on β_1-receptors and is therefore described as cardioselective. This cardioselectivity is only relative, however; at higher doses metoprolol also blocks β_2-receptors. Atenolol is also cardioselective and has a longer half-life so that it can be administered once per day.

Nadolol and timolol are nonselective beta-blockers with longer half-lives than propranolol. They do not have the membrane-stabilizing properties seen with propranolol; however, this quinidine-like effect on the cardiac action potential occurs only at very high doses and is unlikely to have any clinical relevance. Pindolol and acetabulol are beta-blockers with intrinsic sympathomimetic activity; that is, they not only block the β-receptor from catecholamine stimulation but also produce low-level beta stimulation themselves. Therefore, they reduce heart rate and myocardial contractility less than do other beta-blockers, potentially resulting in either fewer adverse effects or compromised efficacy, depending on one's viewpoint.

Are cardioselectivity and intrinsic sympathomimetic activity relevant to the treatment of angina? In a study that compared five different beta-blockers, including those with and without cardioselectivity and intrinsic sympathomimetic activity, no differences were seen in the degree of improvement in angina threshold (Thadani and co-workers, 1979). In patients with peripheral vascular disease or Raynaud's phenomenon, beta-blockers are often avoided entirely or cardioselective agents are used despite evidence from controlled studies that symptoms in these conditions do not worsen with the use of either type of beta-blocker.

Some features of the currently available beta-blockers are summarized in Table 1. Labetalol is a beta-blocker with alpha-blocking and direct vasodilating properties, making it useful for the treatment of hypertension. Esmolol is an ultra-short-acting beta-blocker with β_1 selectivity that is available only in an intravenous formulation. Its features make it ideal for the treatment of supraventricular arrhythmias or for use in patients at risk for serious adverse reactions to β-blockade. Sotalol, a beta-blocker that prolongs the action potential duration and increases refractoriness of cardiac tissue, appears to be effective for the treatment of many atrial and ventricular arrhythmias. However, higher drug concentrations appear to be necessary for its antiarrhythmic efficacy than for β-blockade. Sotalol has not yet been released in the United States.

A major positive feature of beta-blockers is their proven ability to reduce mortality in survivors of myocardial infarction. At least 25 randomized trials including over 23,000 patients have evaluated the

Table 1   Characteristics of Beta-Adrenergic Blocking Drugs

Drug	Potency vs that of Propranolol	Cardioselectivity	Intrinsic Sympathomimetic Activity	Membrane stabilizing	Elimination half-life
Acetabulol	0.3×	+	+	+	3–4 hrs
Atenolol	1.0×	+ +	0	0	6–9 hrs
Betaxolol	1.0×	+ +	0	+	15 hrs
Carteolol	10.0×	0	+	0	5–6 hrs
Esmolol*	0.02×	+ +	0	0	9 mins
Labetalol†	0.3×	0	+	0	3–4 hrs
Metoprolol	1.0×	+ +	0	0	3–4 hrs
Nadolol	1.0×	0	0	0	14–24 hrs
Oxprenolol	1.0×	0	+	+	2–3 hrs
Penbutalol	1.0×	0	+	0	27 hrs
Pindolol	6.0×	0	+ +	+	3–4 hrs
Propranolol	1.0×	0	0	+ +	3–4 hrs
Timolol	6.0×	0	0	0	4–5 hrs

*Available only in intravenous formulation.
†Also has alpha-blocking activity.
0 = none, + = mild, + + = moderate.

long-term use of these drugs after infarction. Overall, patients allocated to receive beta-blocker therapy enjoyed a 22 percent reduction in mortality and a 27 percent reduction in the rate of recurrent infarction (Yusuf and co-workers, 1988). The most impressive of the long-term trials is the Norwegian Multicenter Study with timolol, the beta-blocker Heart Attack Trial with propranolol, and the Göteborg metoprolol study. By contrast, three small trials using beta-blockers with intrinsic sympathomimetic activity did not reveal a reduction in postinfarction mortality in treated patients, although a recently completed French study showed benefit.

Controversy exists as to whether beta-blockers are necessary in low-risk survivors of myocardial infarction. In the beta-blocker Heart Attack Trial, the survival benefit was almost entirely restricted to patients with electrical or mechanical complications. Noninvasive testing can identify a large subset of patients postinfarction who have a 1-year mortality risk of less than 2 percent.

The administration of intravenous beta-blockers in the acute phase of myocardial infarction has also been shown to reduce mortality. In the ISIS-1 (International Studies on Infant Survival) trial, more than 16,000 patients were randomized to receive placebo or intravenously followed by orally administered atenolol; vascular mortality during the first week was reduced by 15 percent. Meta-analysis of early intravenous beta-blocker trials in the treatment of acute infarction suggests that about 200 patients would have to be treated to prevent one death, one reinfarction, and one cardiac arrest during the first week. In the United States this form of therapy is not widely practiced, probably because the risk for adverse events is perceived as being greater than the potential benefit and because thrombolytic therapy is more fashionable.

Most episodes of transient myocardial ischemia that occur in patients with coronary disease are unaccompanied by symptoms. The presence of silent ischemia has been reported to be an adverse prognostic factor in patients with stable and unstable angina and after myocardial infarction. Whether the treatment of silent myocardial ischemia with antianginal drugs improves prognosis is a hotly debated question that has not yet been definitely answered. Propranolol, atenolol, and metoprolol all reduce the frequency and duration of silent ischemia, and one study (Stone and co-workers, 1989) demonstrated a superiority of propranolol over nifedipine and diltiazem. However, antianginal drugs usually do not eliminate all spontaneous ischemic episodes and whether complete suppression of ischemia should be the goal of antianginal therapy is unknown.

The treatment of angina with beta-blockers requires dose titration because a favorable response may occur at any point over a wide range. Changes in heart rate are helpful in evaluating the effect of treatment. For example, if heart rate at rest remains at 70 beats per minute after the institution of chronic propranolol therapy at 160 mg per day, it is reasonable to increase the dose in an attempt to increase efficacy. However, if the heart rate at the same dose is 48 beats per minute with sinus rhythm, higher doses are not advisable because the risk for an adverse response outweighs any potential benefit.

In the absence of contraindications, beta-blockers are the antianginal drugs of choice in patients with previous infarction, and are also very useful in the treatment of patients with associated hypertension. In many patients beta-blockers are more effective than dihydropyridine calcium channel blockers or long-acting nitrates. Their effectiveness for a wide range of other cardiac and noncardiac conditions has been well documented over the past two decades.

CALCIUM CHANNEL BLOCKERS

Compounds that bind to specific receptor sites associated with the voltage-dependent calcium channel and inhibit cellular uptake of calcium come from diverse chemical groups. Of the four calcium channel blockers now available in the United States, two are dihydropyridines (nifedipine and nicardipine), one is a benzodiazepine (diltiazem) and one is a phenylalkylamine (verapamil). In contrast with beta-blockers, drugs that all have approximately similar hemodynamic effects, calcium channel blockers exhibit important differences that affect their clinical use. Some of the features of these drugs are listed in Table 2.

Each of these four drugs has been approved for the treatment of angina. Because the dihydropyridines

Table 2   Characteristics of Calcium Channel Blockers

	Nifedipine, Nicardipine	Diltiazem	Verapamil
Hemodynamic effects			
Heart rate	↑	↓	↓
Arterial pressure	↓	↓	↓
Myocardial contractility	↓	↓	↓ ↓
Electrophysiologic effects	no	yes	yes
Oral dose range*	10–30 mg t.i.d. or q.i.d.	30–120 mg t.i.d.	80–160 mg b.i.d. or t.i.d.

*Long-acting formulations of nifedipine, diltiazem, and verapamil are available.

increase heart rate and occasionally worsen angina, they are not the treatment of choice for stable angina. Diltiazem and verapamil do not cause reflex tachycardia and cause fewer side effects; they are thus preferable as the sole therapy for stable angina.

Variant angina, an uncommon syndrome in which myocardial ischemia is caused by coronary spasm, is not improved after therapy with beta-blockers. Calcium channel blockers are extremely effective in preventing angina in this condition and may also reduce the risk for myocardial infarction or sudden death. In unstable angina without evidence of coronary spasm, diltiazem and propranolol are equally effective in preventing angina but rarely eliminate all attacks and probably do not reduce the risk for infarction. The combination of nifedipine and propranolol for unstable angina have been shown to prevent episodes better than either of these two drugs used alone. Indeed, most patients with unstable angina are treated with two or three antianginal drugs, often including intravenously administered nitroglycerin, during the acute phase.

In an attempt to duplicate the positive results obtained with beta-adrenergic blocking drugs, at least nine controlled clinical trials were conducted to assess the effect on mortality of calcium channel blockers after myocardial infarction. Results from these studies are summarized in Table 3. In two of the five trials that evaluated nifedipine use, mortality was significantly higher in the group that received active drug compared with the group that received placebo (Muller and co-workers, 1984; SPRINT Study Group, 1988). The excess mortality caused by nifedipine appears to occur early, and while the exact mechanism is unknown, it may

be related to drug-induced hypotension or tachycardia in which the tenuous balance between myocardial oxygen demand and supply is upset in a susceptible minority of patients. These findings have generated the recommendation that nifedipine should be avoided in the acute phase of myocardial infarction unless a very compelling indication exists for its use.

Although diltiazem had no effect on overall mortality in the one large trial in which it was used (Multicenter Diltiazem Postinfarction Trial Research Group, 1988), the investigators noted an important two-directional effect related to left ventricular function. In patients with radiologic signs of pulmonary congestion during the acute phase of infarction, or an ejection fraction of less than 40 percent, mortality was higher in patients receiving diltiazem compared with that in those taking placebo. On the other hand, patients without pulmonary congestion benefited from therapy with diltiazem, with a risk reduction of 23 percent.

In another randomized, controlled trial in which diltiazem therapy was begun from 1 to 3 days after a non–Q-wave myocardial infarction and continued for up to 2 weeks, use of the drug significantly reduced the reinfarction rate, which was the primary endpoint of the study (Gibson and co-workers, 1986). The subset of patients with non–Q-wave infarction in the Multicenter Diltiazem Postinfarction Trial (MDPIT) study showed a significant survival advantage with diltiazem use. For these reasons, diltiazem is commonly used instead of a beta-adrenergic blocking drug to improve the outcome after an infarction of the non-Q type.

The purpose of the Danish Verapamil Infarction Trial II was to determine whether the administration of

Table 3 Mortality Found in Placebo-Controlled Trials of Calcium Channel Blockers After Myocardial Infarction

Drug	Number of patients	Duration of follow-up	Mortality (%)	
			Drug	Placebo
Nifedipine				
Muller et al	171	6 mos	10.1	8.5*
Norwegian Trial	227	6 wks	8.9	8.7
SPRINT	2,276	10 mos	5.8	5.7
TRENT	4,491	1 mo	6.7	6.3
SPRINT II	1,373	6 mos	15.8	12.6†
Verapamil				
DAVIT-I	1,436	6 mos	12.8	13.9
DAVIT-II	1,775	16 mos	11.1	13.8
Diltiazem				
MDPIT	2,466	25 mos	13.5	13.5
Lidoflazine				
MI Study Group	1,792	1–6 yrs	19.7	18.8

*At 2 weeks, mortality was 7.9 versus 0 percent (P = 0.018) in favor of placebo.
†Statistically significant difference in favor of placebo due to higher early mortality in nifedipine group.
SPRINT = Secondary prevention re-infarction Israeli nifedipine trial
TRENT = Trial of early nifedipine in acute myocardial infarction
DAVIT = The Danish verapamil infarctial trial
MDPIT = The multicenter diltiazem postinfarction trial

verapamil beginning 2 weeks after myocardial infarction and continuing for 12 to 18 months might reduce total mortality or the combined endpoint of death and reinfarction, when compared with placebo. Although the mortality difference did not attain statistical significance, the combined endpoint was significantly less in patients receiving verapamil. No benefit or adverse effect was seen in the subset of patients with heart failure. The degree of risk reduction in patients in this trial and in the patients without pulmonary congestion in the MDPIT study is equivalent to that seen in the beta-blocker trials. However, a beta-adrenergic blocker should be the drug of choice after myocardial infarction, particularly when left ventricular function is more compromised, based on the greater number of positive studies done with this class of drugs. Diltiazem or verapamil could be used if left ventricular function is well preserved and if there is a contraindication to the use of beta-blockers.

On theoretical grounds, calcium channel blockers are appealing as therapy for silent myocardial ischemia that occurs during daily life. Because most of these episodes occur at heart rates much below those seen with ischemia induced during exercise testing, it has been assumed that reductions in coronary flow are important in their pathogenesis. Although calcium channel blockers induce coronary vasodilatation and prevent coronary spasm, they do not seem to be superior to beta-adrenergic blockers in the treatment of silent ischemia.

In one uncontrolled study nifedipine reduced the number of ischemic episodes when added to baseline antianginal therapy; however, in a subsequent controlled study by Stone and co-workers the drug did not significantly decrease ischemic episodes. Diltiazem reduced ischemic episodes by 50 percent compared with placebo in a recently completed study that examined 60 patients with stable angina; the number of episodes was reduced by at least half in 70 percent of the cases. Whether medical treatment for silent ischemia improves the prognosis has not yet been established and, therefore, routine treatment for this condition can not be strongly recommended.

Calcium channel blockers are effective vasodilators, and acute and chronic vasodilator therapy has become an established approach to the management of heart failure. By reducing afterload, calcium channel blockers can increase cardiac output and produce short-term amelioration of symptoms. The dihydropyridines have an advantage over diltiazem and verapamil in these circumstances because their negative inotropic effects on the cardiac myocyte are more easily overcome by their salutary effect on afterload. However, even when these drugs induce persistent favorable hemodynamic effects, the renal and neurohumoral consequences usually induce clinical deterioration. Other vasodilators are preferable for the treatment of heart failure, and calcium channel blockers are not recommended for this condition.

Calcium channel blockers have been shown to inhibit the development of atherosclerosis in experimental models such as the cholesterol-fed rabbit. The mechanism for this beneficial effect is unknown but could include the preservation of endothelial integrity, modulation of low-density-lipoprotein (LDL) receptors to increase LDL binding, internalization and degradation by smooth muscle cells, reduction in smooth muscle cell proliferation and migration, or a reduction in the synthesis of matrix components.

Two controlled clinical trials have examined the potential of calcium channel blockers to influence coronary atherosclerosis. In the INTACT (International Nifedipine Trial on Antiatherosclerotic Therapy) study, no differences in the rates of progression or regression of coronary lesions were seen in an analysis by serial arteriography between patients given placebo and those treated with nifedipine. However, new lesions appeared at a reduced rate in the nifedipine-treated group. In a study by Waters and co-workers, nicardipine also had no effect on the incidence of progression and regression of established coronary lesions. Minimal stenoses, however—those 20 percent or lower in severity on the first arteriogram—were almost twice as likely to progress in patients given placebo as in those given nicardipine. Further studies are underway to clarify and confirm the antiatherogenic activity of this class of drugs.

The side effects associated with calcium channel blockers are usually mild and are sometimes consequences of their therapeutic effects. The dihydropyridines can cause dizziness, palpitations, headache, and peripheral edema. These problems are probably more common with the use of the original formulation of nifedipine due to rapid absorption and high peak serum levels than they are with the use of the longer-acting formulations or other dihydropyridines. The most common side effects of diltiazem are gastrointestinal upset, edema, and rash. Diltiazem is more likely to be tolerated than the dihydropyridines, but like verapamil, has the potential to induce or worsen conduction disturbances, particularly atrioventricular block. Verapamil and diltiazem are more likely to worsen heart failure than are the dihydropyridines and are contraindicated in patients with very low ejection fractions. Verapamil's most common adverse effects are headache and constipation.

The number of calcium channel blockers available for clinical use will increase over the next decade. Nisoldipine, nitrendipine, nimodipine, amlodipine, isradipine, and felodipine are all dihydropyridines that are nearing release or are already available in some countries. These agents differ in their duration of activity and their ability to cross the blood-brain barrier, but their similarities far outweigh their differences.

SUGGESTED READING

Curfman GD, Heinsimer JA, Lozner EC, Fung HL. Intravenous nitroglycerin in the treatment of spontaneous angina pectoris: a prospective, randomized trial. Circulation 1983; 67:276–282.

The Danish Study Group on Verapamil in Myocardial Infarction. Effect of verapamil on mortality and major events after acute myocardial infarction (The Danish Verapamil Infarction Trial II–DAVIT II). Am J Cardiol 1990; 66:779–785.

Diodati J, Théroux P, Latour JG, et al. Effects of nitroglycerin at therapeutic doses on platelet aggregation in unstable angina pectoris and acute myocardial infarction. Am J Cardiol 1990; 66:683–688.

Gibson RS, Boden WE, Théroux P, et al. Diltiazem and reinfarction in patients with non-Q-wave myocardial infarction. N Engl J Med 1986; 315:423–429.

ISIS-1 (First International Study of Infarct Survival) Collaborative Group: randomised trial of intravenous atenolol among 16,027 cases of suspected acute myocardial infarction: ISIS-1. Lancet 1986; 2:57–65.

Lichtlen PR, Hugenholtz PG, Rafflenbeul W, et al. Retardation of angiographic progression of coronary artery disease by nifedipine. Lancet 1990; 335:1109–1113.

Muller JE, Morrison J, Stone PH, et al. Nifedipine therapy for patients with threatened and acute myocardial infarction: a randomized, double-blind, placebo-controlled comparison. Circulation 1984; 69:740–747.

The Multicenter Diltiazem Postinfarction Trial Research Group. The effect of diltiazem on mortality and reinfarction after myocardial infarction. N Engl J Med 1988; 319:385–392.

Parker JO. Nitrate therapy in stable angina pectoris. N Engl J Med 1987; 316:1635–1642.

Rocco MB, Nabel EG, Campbell S, et al. Prognostic importance of myocardial ischemia detected by ambulatory monitoring in patients with stable coronary artery disease. Circulation 1988; 78:877–884.

Sirnes PA, Overskeid K, Pedersen TR, et al. Evolution of infarct size during the early use of nifedipine in patients with acute myocardial infarction: The Norwegian Nifedipine Multicenter Trial. Circulation 1984; 70:638–644.

The SPRINT Study Group. The secondary prevention re-infarction Israeli nifedipine trial (SPRINT): II. Results (abstr). Eur Heart J 1988; 9(suppl 1):350.

Stone PH, Gibson RS, Glasser SP, et al. Comparison of diltiazem, nifedipine, and propranolol in the therapy of silent ischemia. Circulation 1989; 80(suppl 2):II-267.

Subramanian VB, Bowles MJ, Khurmi NS, et al. Rationale for the choice of calcium antagonists in chronic stable angina. Am J Cardiol 1982; 50:1173–1179.

Thadani U, Davidson C, Singleton W, Taylor SH. Comparison of the immediate effects of five β-adrenoreceptor-blocking drugs with different ancillary properties in angina pectoris. N Engl J Med 1979; 300:750–755.

Warren SG, Brewer DL, Orgain ES. Long-term propranolol therapy for angina. Am J Cardiol 1976; 37:420–427.

Waters DD, Juneau M, Gossard D, et al. Limited usefulness of intermittent nitroglycerin patches in stable angina. J Am Coll Cardiol 1989; 13:421–425.

Waters D, Lespérance J, Francetich M, et al. A controlled clinical trial to assess the effect of a calcium channel blocker upon the progression of coronary atherosclerosis. Circulation 1990; 82:1940–1953.

Waters DD, Miller DD, Szlachcic J, et al. Factors influencing the long-term prognosis of treated patients with variant angina. Circulation 1983; 68:258–264.

Yusuf S, Wittes J, Friedman L. Overview of results of randomized clinical trials in heart disease. JAMA 1988; 260:2088–2093.

CHRONIC ISCHEMIC HEART DISEASE: ANGIOPLASTY AND OTHER CATHETER-BASED REVASCULARIZATION TECHNIQUES

TIM A. FISCHELL, M.D.

In September 1977 Andreas Gruentzig successfully performed the first percutaneous transluminal coronary angioplasty (PTCA) in man. Although the thought of inflating a balloon in an atherosclerotic coronary artery was initially met with great skepticism, the efficacy and relative safety of this therapeutic technique has led to the rapid and widespread acceptance of PTCA in the treatment of obstructive coronary artery disease. The explosive growth of this technique has been driven by a number of factors, including dramatic improvements in angioplasty equipment, greater operator experience, increases in the number of physicians performing PTCA, and patient preference for a nonsurgical approach. It is anticipated that approximately 300,000 PTCA procedures will be performed in the United States in 1991 (Fig. 1).

Along with the rapid proliferation in the number of procedures performed, there has been a significant expansion of the list of acceptable clinical indications for PTCA. It is now widely used for the treatment of patients with multivessel disease, unstable angina pectoris, acute myocardial infarction, diseased saphenous vein bypass grafts, and recent total coronary occlusions. Despite the impressive growth of PTCA as an accepted therapeutic modality, there remain a number of important limitations, including abrupt coronary artery closure with the need for emergency bypass surgery, the inability to effectively treat large subsets of patients with coronary artery disease (e.g., chronic total occlusions and diffuse disease), and, most important, restenosis. Nonetheless, the clinical efficacy of this procedure is now well established and has paved the way for new and innovative methods to treat obstructive coronary artery disease using other catheter-based revascularization techniques. This chapter discusses the pathophysiology and mechanism of PTCA, the clinical indications, the technical considerations and acute outcome with this procedure, and the complications and long-term results. There is also a limited discussion of the newer technologies, including atherectomy, intracoronary stents, and lasers.

HISTORICAL PERSPECTIVE

The therapeutic application of balloon dilatation is not new. Arnott described the modern application of such a technique in the early 1800s, when he used a catgut balloon dilating catheter to relieve urethral stenosis. In 1964 Dotter and Judkins were the first to

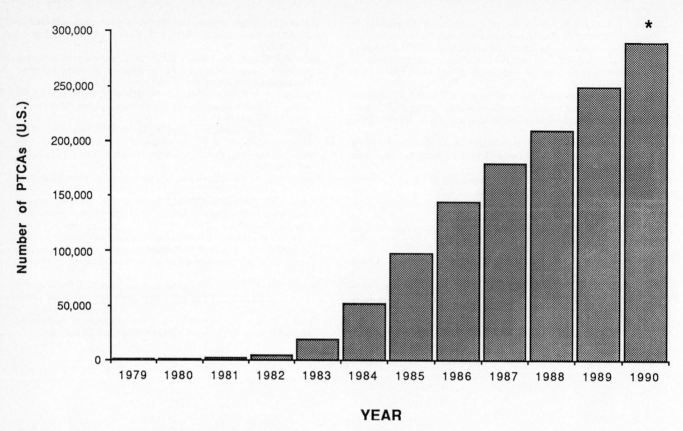

Figure 1 Bar graph showing the dramatic increase in the number of percutaneous transluminal coronary angioplasty (PTCA) procedures in the United States during the last 10 years. * represents the projected number of procedures for 1990.

describe the use of a percutaneous transluminal dilatation of an atherosclerotic obstruction in man. Using a series of sequentially larger, Teflon-coated catheters, they successfully dilated a lesion in a superficial femoral artery. This technique of increasing luminal area by mechanically dilating an atherosclerotic lesion was further refined for use in the peripheral circulation by Staple and Van Andel using a gradually tapered catheter. In 1974 Gruentzig and Hopff developed a double-lumen balloon dilating catheter that was successfully used in the treatment of obstructive iliac and femoral artery disease. After trials with a miniaturized balloon catheter in dogs and cadavers, Gruentzig performed the first PTCA in man in 1977. The initial angioplasty equipment allowed the treatment of primarily focal proximal disease with an overall success rate of only 60 to 70 percent, but the improvements in balloon catheter, guide wire, and guiding catheter technology now provide the capability to treat much more complex coronary disease with clinical success rates exceeding 90 percent.

TECHNICAL ASPECTS AND MECHANISMS OF SUCCESSFUL PTCA

The objective of PTCA is to safely increase the luminal dimensions in a stenotic coronary artery segment, thereby improving coronary blood flow and increasing coronary blood flow reserve, and thus decreasing or eliminating angina pectoris. Ideally, this should be accomplished in such a manner as to minimize the deep injury to the arterial wall and to maximize long-term vessel patency.

The detailed technical aspects of the procedure will not be described here. In brief, the balloon catheter is passed through a guiding catheter and advanced over a guidewire until it straddles the stenotic coronary lesion. Once the balloon is properly positioned under fluoroscopic guidance, the balloon is inflated. The ability to crack and dilate heavily calcified or very old lesions has been improved with the advent of newer balloon materials that can withstand inflation pressures in the 12 to 15 atmosphere range. The balloon is typically inflated for 30 to 90 seconds per inflation. Multiple inflation-deflation sequences are often required to achieve an optimal result. Successful dilatation in the cardiac catheterization laboratory is identified by either a significant drop in the trans-stenotic pressure gradient (e.g., to less than 20 mm Hg) as measured simultaneously from the proximally placed guiding catheter and the distal tip of the balloon catheter, or by angiographic assessment. Various definitions have been used to describe primary angiographic success. In general the procedure is considered successful when there is a 20 percent or greater reduction in the stenosis diameter, with a residual diameter stenosis of less than 50 percent.

Table 1 Indications for PTCA (Indications for Which There is General Agreement that PTCA is Appropriate*)

Single- or two-vessel coronary artery disease, with >50% diameter stenoses and objective evidence of ischemia
  Symptomatic patients on medical therapy (functional classes II to IV, unstable angina; lesion(s) subtend ≥ moderate area of viable
    myocardium) with:
    Evidence of myocardial ischemia on medical therapy during laboratory testing *or*
    Angina that is disabling or limits life style, not adequately responsive to medical therapy *or*
    Intolerance of medical therapy owing to side effects
  Asymptomatic or mildly symptomatic (~low-risk lesion morphology, lesion(s) subtend large area of viable myocardium)
    Severe ischemia at low-level exercise during laboratory testing *or*
    Resuscitated from cardiac arrest or sustained VT without myocardial infarction *or*
    Must undergo high-risk noncardiac surgery (e.g., abdominal aneurysm repair)
  Acute myocardial infarction (angioplasty during initial hospitalization, patients with morphologically ~low-risk lesion(s), dilatation of
    "significant" lesion(s) in infarct-related artery only), in patients with:
    Recurrent episodes of ischemic chest pain, particularly with associated ECG changes *or*
    Evidence of severe myocardial ischemia on medical therapy during predischarge laboratory testing *or*
    Recurrent (?ischemic related) ventricular tachycardia or fibrillation, despite intensive antiarrhythmic therapy

Adapted from ACC/AHA Task Force Report recommendations.
*Patients who do not fit into this set of indications may fall into a category for which there are mixed opinions regarding the appropriateness of PTCA, or into a category for which there is general consensus that PTCA is not appropriate (see Table 2).

Since there may be tremendous inconsistency when visual estimates of the percentage of stenosis are used, it is preferable to use either quantitative measures of this percentage or actual measurement of luminal dimensions to describe the adequacy of the angiographic result. Ultimately, clinical success is judged by the improvement in the patient's symptoms and/or functional capacity.

The probable mechanisms of successful PTCA are worthy of mention. Initially it was believed that the atherosclerotic plaque was compressed or compacted by the balloon inflation. Others postulated that there was plaque extrusion and embolization that accounted for the improvement in luminal dimensions. Both of these theories were disproved by postmortem studies and by in vitro studies performed by Chin and colleagues and others. Later experiments in rabbit arteries and cadaver tissue suggested that irreversible stretching of the media of the artery with aneurysm formation occurred after balloon angioplasty. More recently it has become evident that this irreversible active "stretching" with permanent paralysis of the medial smooth muscle layer does not occur in most cases during successful PTCA in man. Rather, it appears that the balloon dilatation cracks the rigid intimal plaque down to or through the internal elastic lamina, releasing the deeper medial and adventitial layers from the anchoring effects of the plaque, and thereby improving the compliance of the arterial segment, which is then passively distended by arterial pressure.

There are some differences of opinion regarding the optimal medication regimen to be used at the time of PTCA. However, there is little debate about the necessity to premedicate all patients with aspirin. This antiplatelet agent decreases the risk of abrupt coronary artery closure after PTCA. Given that coronary artery vasoconstriction and/or frank spasm occurs frequently after angioplasty, it is generally accepted practice to also administer nitroglycerin, with or without calcium channel blockers, during and after the procedure. There is little evidence to suggest any short- or long-term benefit from sodium warfarin (Coumadin), dextran, or other agents.

PATIENT SELECTION

Clinical Indications

Owing in large part to the significant improvements in equipment, the indications for PTCA have expanded in the last 10 years (Table 1). The most clear-cut indication is the patient with relatively focal single- or two-vessel coronary artery disease who has disabling or life style–limiting angina despite "reasonable" medical therapy, and shows objective evidence of ischemia during functional testing (i.e., treadmill test with or without thallium). "Reasonable" medical therapy obviously differs from patient to patient. Many cardiologists offer PTCA as an alternative to medical therapy for patients with appropriate coronary artery anatomy who would like to reduce or eliminate the need for medications.

Beyond this group of patients with moderate to severe symptoms and focal single- or two-vessel coronary artery disease, the indications are less well established. It is generally agreed, however, that PTCA is indicated in patients with suitable anatomy and one- or two-vessel coronary artery disease who have mild or possibly no symptoms, but demonstrate severe ischemia at a low work load, and have lesions that subtend a large area of viable myocardium. Likewise, such patients should be considered for the procedure prior to high-risk noncardiac surgery. Many cardiologists recommend and perform PTCA in patients with less suitable coronary anatomy (see below and Table 2) and in patients with three or more coronary lesions and/or diffuse disease. As mentioned above, the appropriateness of angioplasty in these settings is controversial.

In terms of coronary anatomy, the best candidates for PTCA are patients with coronary lesions that are relatively severe, focal, proximal, concentric, and noncalcified and are not situated on a tortuous portion of the vessel or at a branch. The long-term results are generally better in coronary vessels that are 2.5 mm in diameter or greater. If one performs PTCA in patients with modest stenoses (e.g., 50 to 60 percent in diameter), one runs the risk that the balloon injury will cause restenosis, which may actually accelerate the progression of the disease. The cardiologist who recommends angioplasty for a patient with a modest (e.g., 50%) coronary stenosis and minimal or no symptoms on medical therapy, using the argument "this procedure will prevent you from having a myocardial infarction," is doing the patient a disservice. The procedure also is generally avoided in diffusely diseased vessels (e.g., lesion length greater than 20 to 30 mm). In patients with this form of disease, particularly when it involves two or more vessels, medical therapy or bypass surgery is usually preferred. Eccentricity of the lesion is not a major contraindication, although it should be recognized that both the short- and long-term results are less favorable in eccentric than in concentric stenoses. Similarly, lesions that are severely calcified are often difficult to dilate adequately, even with the use of tougher balloon materials allowing high-pressure balloon inflations. Lesions that occur on a bend of more than 45 degrees and those that have an intraluminal filling defect on diagnostic angiography (i.e., evidence of intraluminal thrombus) are more prone to abrupt vessel closure and/or dissection. A thoughtful physician will bear in mind these anatomic considerations when weighing the risks and benefits of the procedure.

In some cases the indications for PTCA may be liberalized in patients who ordinarily would be candidates for coronary bypass graft surgery, but who have other severe medical problems (e.g., COPD or renal insufficiency) that would significantly increase the risks associated with open-heart surgery. This also may be an appropriate therapy for some elderly patients and patients with poor long-term prognoses due to other comorbidity (e.g., malignancy).

Contraindications to PTCA

A joint Task Force of the American College of Cardiology and the American Heart Association has established guidelines for contraindications to PTCA. Table 2 presents a summary of the relative and absolute contraindications based on the Task Force report and my experience. The absolute contraindications include the obvious case of a patient without a significant coronary stenosis, and patients with severe multivessel disease who are unequivocally better candidates for bypass surgery. Except in extraordinary circumstances, angioplasty should never be performed in patients with significant ("unprotected") left main coronary artery disease. In addition, angioplasty should be performed only at medical centers with an experienced cardiovascular surgical team to provide emergency bypass surgery in the event of failure (see "Complications" section). The relative contraindications, as listed in Table 2, include primarily situations in which there is either a reduced likelihood of success or an increased risk of serious complications.

Comparison with Bypass Surgery

Although PTCA has been clearly shown to provide palliation of symptoms and ischemia in patients with multivessel coronary artery disease, it must be viewed in comparison with bypass surgery. The latter can now be performed at experienced centers with an overall mortality rate of less than 2 percent. Approximately 70 percent of patients enjoy sustained symptomatic improvement and 50 percent are asymptomatic 5 years after surgery. With the increasing use of the internal mammary artery as a conduit, which has a better long-term patency rate than vein grafts (about 90 percent at 10 years for internal mammary versus about 50 percent patency at 10 years for vein grafts), the long-term efficacy of surgery may be improved over that

Table 2 Contraindications to PTCA

Absolute Contraindications
   No significant obstructing lesion (i.e., <50% diameter stenosis by caliper or other quantitative measurement)
   Multivessel disease with diffuse atherosclerosis in which bypass surgery would be unequivocally more effective
   Significant (>50%) obstruction of left main coronary artery that is not "protected" by at least one patent bypass graft*
   Absence of formal cardiac surgical back-up program within the institution
Relative Contraindications
   A hypo- or hypercoagulable state
   No clinical evidence of spontaneous or inducible myocardial ischemia
   Extensive myocardial jeopardy (occlusion at site of PTCA would result in loss of ≥50% of remaining viable myocardium)
   Dilatation of coronary stenoses in "noninfarct" vessel(s) in setting of acute or recent myocardial infarction
   Noncritical stenosis (<60%), particularly without objective evidence of ischemia or without angina refractory to medical therapy
   Presence of moderate left main coronary stenosis when firm guiding catheter engagement is needed to dilate stenosis
   Chronic total occlusion >3 months old, or subtotal occlusions >20 mm long
   Old (e.g., 8- to 10-year-old) vein grafts, particularly with diffuse disease
   Ostial stenoses of right coronary artery
   Variant or vasospastic angina is present in patients with moderate (≤60%) stenoses
   Stenoses involving major side branches that cannot be adequately protected
   Stenoses with associated intraluminal thrombus, or within severely angulated segment
   Extensive lesion calcification

Adapted in part from ACC/AHA Task Force Report recommendations.
*Graft to left anterior descending or left circumflex coronary artery.

observed in the Coronary Artery Surgery Study (CASS), VA, and European Cooperative studies from the 1970s. Bypass surgery may also be more effective in achieving "complete" revascularization than PTCA, particularly in patients with chronic total occlusions or diffuse disease. It is likewise important to recognize that surgery has been shown to improve survival in patients with left main disease and subsets of patients with three-vessel coronary artery disease, but there is currently little evidence that PTCA prevents myocardial infarction or prolongs life in comparison with medical therapy. On the other hand, one of the major advantages of PTCA is that it is clearly less traumatic and probably less costly in the long run than bypass surgery. The relative advantages and disadvantages of PTCA versus bypass surgery are summarized in Table 3. Several large randomized trials

are now under way comparing angioplasty with bypass surgery, primarily in patients with multivessel disease. The results from these trials should allow clinicians to make more rational decisions regarding the role of PTCA in the management of chronic ischemic coronary artery disease.

SAFETY AND EFFICACY OF PTCA IN VARIOUS PATIENT SUBGROUPS

Single-Vessel Coronary Artery Disease

PTCA has become the treatment of choice for most patients with symptomatic single-vessel coronary artery disease. In patients with single-vessel disease and an "ideal" lesion, the acute procedural (angiographic) success rate is 90 to 95 percent. In this setting the acute closure rate with a need for emergency coronary artery bypass surgery is approximately 3 percent. The risk of nonfatal myocardial infarction is approximately 3 percent and the mortality rate less than 0.5 percent. An example of successful PTCA in single-vessel disease is shown in Figure 2. The acute success rate of the procedure is lower for less favorable anatomy and for multilesion PTCA in patients with single-vessel disease. The primary angiographic and clinical success rate in patients with a long eccentric lesion, for example, may be only 70 to 80 percent, with a modestly higher complication rate. In the extreme situation of a chronic total occlusion, the acute success rate may be as low as 10 to 20 percent. One of the most important responsibilities of the physician performing PTCA is to be completely knowledgeable about the relative risks and predicted success rates of the procedure based on clinical and angiographic features, and to use this information effectively to allow appropriate patient selection. The

Table 3 Comparison of PTCA with Coronary Artery Bypass Grafting

Advantages of Bypass Surgery Compared with PTCA
  Ability to completely revascularize patients in nearly all cases
  More predictable outcome in terms of symptom relief
  Reduced need for repeat revascularization procedures in first year postoperatively
  Proved survival benefit for selected patient subsets (e.g,. left main disease)
Advantages of PTCA Compared with Bypass Surgery
  Lower initial cost
  No requirement for general anesthesia
  Much less traumatic, with brief hospitalization and substantially shorter disability
  Greater patient acceptance
  Ability to treat certain anatomic lesions that are not readily bypassable
  ? Decreased procedural mortality in most patients

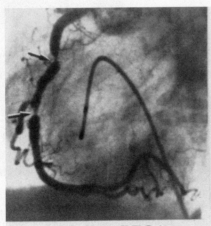 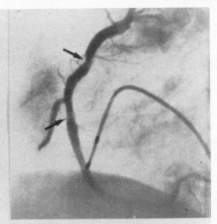

RCA Pre PTCA   RCA Post PTCA

Figure 2 Illustration of successful PTCA in a patient with single-vessel disease. In the left panel the right coronary artery is shown before PTCA with two discrete (focal) lesions in the proximal and middle right coronary artery respectively *(arrows)*. After the PTCA *(right panel)* there is only a minor residual stenosis at the two dilated sites.

significant improvements in primary success rates and reduction in complications in comparison to the original NHLBI PTCA Registry (see Table 4) are attributable to improved equipment and operator skills, and better case selection.

The large majority of patients with single-vessel disease (more than 80 percent) have relief of anginal symptoms after angiographically successful PTCA. Many patients will also note improvements in exercise-induced dyspnea. A variety of noninvasive measures to detect exercise-induced myocardial ischemia demonstrate unequivocal improvement in approximately 80 to 90 percent of patients after angiographically successful PTCA (Fig. 3). Interestingly, more direct invasive studies of coronary artery blood flow reserve have shown persistent reductions in coronary flow reserve immediately after angiographically successful PTCA that normalize within several weeks. The cause of this delayed improvement in coronary blood flow reserve is thought to be related to abnormalities in autoregulation after sudden reperfusion of a previously hypoperfused coronary artery bed.

Multivessel Coronary Artery Disease

PTCA is now frequently performed in patients with multivessel coronary artery disease. The evaluation of the risks and benefits of PTCA compared with bypass surgery or medical therapy is more complex in this group of patients. One of the major considerations is related to the issue of completeness of revascularization. Unlike bypass surgery, in which all lesions more than 50 percent in vessels of 1.5-mm diameter or greater are typically bypassed (i.e., the patient is "completely revascularized"), angioplasty operators often choose to treat only one or two "culprit" lesions in patients with multiple areas of coronary obstruction (i.e., "incompletely revascularized"). In this context a "culprit" lesion is defined as the lesion that is most clearly responsible for the patient's current symptoms of angina or threatened myocardial infarction, as determined by noninvasive

tests or angiographic assessment. As an example, in a patient with a 90 percent lesion in the left anterior descending (LAD) coronary artery and a 50 percent lesion in the right coronary artery who has T-wave inversions in precordial leads V1 to V4 during angina, one could reasonably consider the LAD lesion as the "culprit," particularly if other noninvasive testing fails to demonstrate signs of ischemia in the right coronary artery distribution. In such a patient, successful angioplasty of the LAD can be achieved with angiographic and clinical success rates similar to those for single-vessel disease (about 90 percent). Success rates are modestly lower in patients having dilatation of two or three lesions. The indications to perform the procedure in patients with four or more severe coronary lesions are controversial, and this cannot be routinely recommended. Complete revascularization using angioplasty is achieved in 80 to 90 percent of patients with single-vessel disease, 40 to 60 percent of those with two-vessel disease, and only 15 to 25 percent of those with three-vessel coronary artery disease. The inability to open chronic total coronary occlusions reliably is one of the primary reasons why PTCA fails to completely revascularize many patients with multivessel disease.

The risks associated with PTCA for multivessel disease are slightly higher than those associated with angioplasty of a single vessel. The risk of acute closure with the need for emergency bypass surgery is 2 to 6

Table 4 Comparison of Acute Results in Old (1977–1981) and New (1985) NHLBI PTCA Registry

	Old Registry (%)	New Registry (%)
Success of multivessel PTCA	25	53
Success by lesion (>20% improvement)	67	88
Clinical success*	61	78
Emergency bypass surgery	6.4	2.9
Nonfatal myocardial infarction	4.7	3.6
Death	1.0	0.7
Death, MI, or bypass surgery	11	5.9
Elective bypass surgery	18.5	2.2

From Detre K, Holubkov R, Kelsey S, et al. Percutaneous transluminal coronary angioplasty in 1985–1986 and 1977–1981. The National Heart, Lung, and Blood Institute Registry. N Engl J Med 1988; 318:265–270; with permission.

*All lesions improved by >20%, no MI, bypass surgery, or death.

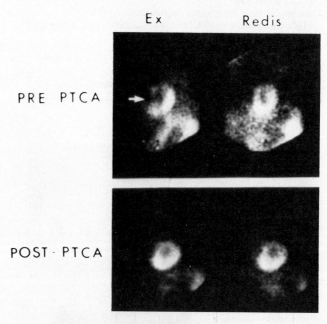

Figure 3 Improvement in exercise thallium test after successful single-vessel PTCA. Before PTCA (*upper panel*) the patient's thallium imaging shows a filling defect in the anteroseptal region during exercise (*arrow*) with redistribution to that segment during delayed imaging, consistent with a significant stenosis in the left anterior descending (LAD) coronary artery. After successful PTCA of a high-grade proximal LAD lesion, the exercise thallium study returns to normal without this redistribution defect (*bottom panel*).

percent, with a myocardial infarction rate of about 2 to 3 percent and an overall mortality risk of approximately 1.5 percent.

In appropriately selected patients PTCA is extremely effective in alleviating anginal symptoms in multivessel disease. Even when "incomplete revascularization" is performed with dilatation of only the "culprit" lesion or lesions, approximately 70 percent of patients are asymptomatic 1 year after the procedure. On the other hand, approximately 20 to 30 percent of patients with multivessel disease and an initially successful result need either repeat angioplasty or bypass surgery during this first year after PTCA, most often as the result of restenosis. Interestingly, the symptomatic status and the need for subsequent revascularization procedures 1 year after PTCA in patients with multivessel disease appears to be largely independent of the "completeness" of revascularization. This is consistent with recent unpublished data from the Coronary Artery Surgery Study (CASS) Registry, which suggests that even with bypass surgery the long-term benefits of complete revascularization are primarily limited to patients with severe angina and left ventricular dysfunction. As mentioned earlier, several large randomized trials are under way comparing PTCA with bypass surgery for patients with multivessel disease. The results from these trials will help to determine the appropriate role of PTCA in this subset of patients.

Unstable Angina

There is now much evidence demonstrating the relative safety and efficacy of PTCA in patients with unstable angina pectoris. In patients with unstable angina and a single high-grade stenosis, or with multivessel disease and an obvious "culprit" lesion, the primary angiographic and clinical success rate with PTCA is approximately 90 percent. In many of these patients there is angiographic evidence of an intraluminal filling defect, consistent with intracoronary thrombus, at the site of the "culprit" lesion. Since the presence of intraluminal thrombus significantly increases the risk of abrupt vessel closure during PTCA, it is often most reasonable in these patients to consider a 2- to 4-day course of intravenous heparin, in the hope that the thrombus burden will be decreased, before attempting PTCA. The role of intravenous or intracoronary thrombolytic agents in this setting is somewhat controversial, but they may be appropriate in selected patients. In patients with multivessel disease the successful dilatation of a "culprit" lesion is also effective for unstable angina.

There is a modestly greater acute complication rate associated with PTCA in the subgroup of patients with unstable angina. Whereas the acute closure occurs in approximately 3 to 4 percent of patients with stable angina, this complication occurs in about 8 to 10 percent of those with unstable angina. In patients with unstable angina and single-vessel or multivessel disease with a "culprit" lesion, successful PTCA is usually capable of achieving an event-free long-term result, although the restenosis rate may be slightly greater than that observed after PTCA in patients with chronic stable angina.

Diseased Saphenous Vein and Internal Mammary Artery Bypass Grafts

Saphenous vein coronary bypass grafts have limited longevity, and approximately 5 percent of grafts per year succumb to vein graft atherosclerosis.

Given the increased morbidity and mortality associated with repeat bypass surgery, PTCA is often an excellent option for treating symptomatic patients with focal disease in one or possibly two vein grafts. The primary angiographic and clinical success rate with angioplasty of vein grafts is similar to that of native vessels when the lesions are in the body of the graft or near the distal anastomosis (about an 80 to 90 percent success rate). In contrast, dilatation of lesions at the aortic anastomosis of a vein graft is much less effective, has a higher complication rate, and has a significantly higher restenosis rate (50 to 60 percent). PTCA of vein grafts is contraindicated in proximally occluded grafts and in grafts with diffuse disease. PTCA should also be avoided in vein grafts older than 8 to 10 years because of the increased embolic risks. Technically, the only significant difference between PTCA of native vessels and vein grafts is the appropriate use of somewhat oversized balloons in vein grafts. However, the restenosis rate after angioplasty of diseased vein grafts is higher. The restenosis rate is approximately 35 percent after dilatation at the distal anastomosis, 40 to 45 percent for lesions in the body of the graft, and 60 percent for lesions in the proximal graft. An example of successful PTCA in a diseased saphenous vein graft is shown in Figure 4.

PTCA is also effective in the treatment of diseased internal mammary artery bypass grafts. Although the internal mammary artery is relatively resistant to atherosclerosis, focal stenoses are often a problem at the distal (coronary) anastomosis of the graft. In many cases, these lesions are actually anatomically within the native coronary artery that has been grafted (e.g., LAD coronary artery). PTCA of these focal lesions has been very successful and often makes repeat bypass surgery unnecessary.

Total Occlusions

The most common indication for PTCA of an occluded vessel is the situation in which there is residual viable myocardium distal to the occlusion, and there are symptoms shown to be caused by ischemia in that territory as the result of inadequate collaterals. There is no demonstrated benefit in angioplasty of occluded vessels that supply only infarcted myocardium.

PTCA has been applied successfully for occluded vessels when the occlusion has been present for a short time. The most important determinant of the ability to pass a guidewire and balloon catheter through an occluded segment is the age of the occlusion. The

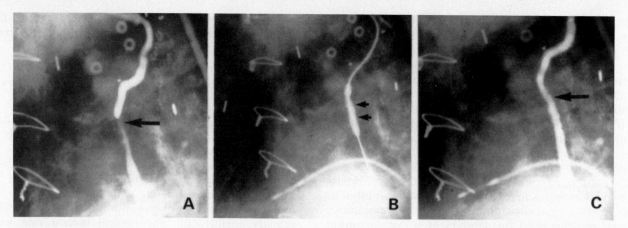

Figure 4 Example of successful PTCA in a focally diseased saphenous vein bypass graft. *A,* A high-grade stenosis *(arrow)* in a 5-year-old saphenous vein graft to the left circumflex coronary artery. The balloon catheter is advanced to the lesion and inflated. Arrows depict inflated balloon *(B).* After a total of three inflations, there is a significant improvement in vein graft patency *(C).*

Table 5 Strategies for Use of PTCA in Setting of Acute Myocardial Infarction

	Thrombolytic Therapy	Timing	Goals	Indications
Direct PTCA	No	Upon presentation As quickly as possible	Primary recanalization	Cardiogenic shock, or large MI and thrombolysis contraindicated
Immediate PTCA	Yes	As quickly as possible after thrombolytic therapy	Recanalization	? None
Rescue PTCA	Yes	60–90 min after thrombolytic therapy	Recanalization after failed thrombolysis	Very large MI, young or very-high-risk patient
Deferred PTCA	Yes	1–7 days after reperfusion	Prophylaxis for recurrent ischemic events	Probably not indicated
Delayed/"elective" PTCA	Yes	Within 1–2 wk after reperfusion	Prevent recurrent ischemia and/or infarction	Angina with ECG changes and/or positive exercise testing after reperfusion

primary angiographic success rates in PTCA of total occlusions is about 70 to 80 percent for occlusions less than 1 month old, about 40 to 50 percent for those 1 to 6 months old, and only about 10 to 15 percent for those over 6 months old. Although it is sometimes difficult to date the age of a total occlusion precisely, the angiographic appearance often provides clues. For example, if there is evidence of an intraluminal filling defect suggestive of thrombus, the occlusion is typically a recent event. If, on the other hand, there is a long segment of occlusion with bridging collateral vessels, this is indicative of a chronic occlusion. The other major determinant of success or failure in PTCA of total occlusions is the length of the occlusion: if this is more than 1.5 to 2.0 cm, the success rate is typically low (10 to 20 percent).

Angioplasty of occluded vessels carries less risk than PTCA of subtotal occlusions, because there is virtually no antegrade flow through these lesions, and abrupt closure after PTCA typically does not provoke ischemia or myocardial infarction. Rarely, there are complications related to distal embolization of thrombus at the site of occlusion, injury to side branches during guidewire manipulations or balloon inflations, or injury of the left main coronary artery related to vigorous guiding catheter engagement that is often required to cross these total occlusions. Overall, during PTCA of total occlusions, the risk of myocardial infarction is probably less than 2 percent and the mortality rate less than 0.5 percent.

Even when total occlusions can be successfully dilated, the restenosis rate is higher (40 to 50 percent) than that seen after routine single-vessel PTCA. Newer technologies such as lasers and slow rotational mechanical devices may significantly improve the short- and long-term results in this group of patients.

Acute Myocardial Infarction

Although PTCA has been applied successfully in the management of acute myocardial infarction, the appropriate timing and indications are controversial. A number of strategies have been proposed in the setting of acute myocardial infarction (Table 5).

Direct angioplasty refers to the emergent use of PTCA without the use of thrombolytic therapy. In large medical centers the acute angiographic success rate is approximately 90 percent. One caveat is that the reclosure rate in the first week ranges from 9 to 31 percent, which appears to be higher than that observed after successful thrombolytic therapy. Another difficulty with this approach is the need for a trained interventional team to be available on call 24 hours a day, with an associated high financial cost. This may not be practical in many areas in the United States. This approach also necessitates a rapid response time, since there is typically only a 2- to 4-hour window of opportunity after the onset of chest pain to achieve significant myocardial salvage by reperfusion. Direct angioplasty is the treatment of choice in most patients who present in the early hours of acute myocardial infarction with cardiogenic shock. The mortality rate of these patients is approximately 75 percent with medical therapy as opposed to 30 to 40 percent after successful emergency PTCA. This type of survival advantage in patients with cardiogenic shock has not been demonstrated with thrombolytic therapy. Direct PTCA is also a reasonable approach within the early hours of a large anterior infarction in patients with contraindications to thrombolytic therapy, or those who have resting electrocardiographic (ECG) abnormalities that make the accurate diagnosis of acute myocardial infarction difficult (e.g., left bundle branch block).

Immediate PTCA is the strategy whereby all patients given thrombolytic therapy undergo immediate PTCA to reduce any significant residual stenosis. This approach has been evaluated in several large randomized studies. Briefly, it appears that this costly approach offers no significant benefit with regard to left ventricular function or mortality. Indeed, it may add to morbidity and hospitalization costs compared with a strategy of thrombolytic therapy with PTCA performed only in patients with spontaneous or exercise-induced myocardial ischemia (i.e., delayed/elective PTCA). Similarly, there is little evidence to support the routine use of "deferred" PTCA in stable patients without evidence of ischemia after successful thrombolytic therapy. There are relatively few data regarding the value of "rescue" PTCA after intravenous thrombolytic therapy has failed to achieve reperfusion. Given the unreliability of intravenous thrombolytic therapy (only 50 to 80 percent of patients recanalize), it is reasonable to consider emergency cardiac catheterization with "rescue" PTCA in high-risk patients or young patients who present very early in the course of a large acute myocardial infarction. This approach is probably not appropriate for patients who present late after the onset of chest pain, and obviously can be offered as an option only at medical centers that can rapidly assemble an interventional team. This is a complex and rapidly evolving area of investigation. Readers interested in a more detailed discussion of these issues are referred to the recently published American College of Cardiology/American Heart Association guidelines.

Complications

A number of potentially serious acute complications may occur during angioplasty, including coronary occlu-

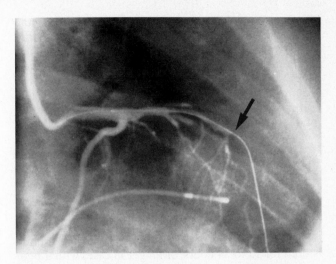

Figure 5 Acute coronary occlusion as a complication of PTCA. After two balloon inflations in the middle left anterior descending (LAD) coronary artery, there is evidence of a severe subintimal dissection with obliteration of the lumen (*arrow*) just beyond the dilated site. The guide wire can be seen traversing the occluded lumen. The patient experienced severe chest pain and underwent emergent coronary artery bypass grafting surgery.

sion, spasm, dissection, embolization, perforation, and rupture. Of these, abrupt coronary occlusion at the site of balloon dilatation is the most common serious complication, occurring in 3 to 5 percent of patients (Fig. 5). Occasionally, left main or right coronary artery dissection occurs secondary to guiding catheter trauma. Coronary occlusion is most often attributable to severe subintimal dissection, although coronary artery spasm and intraluminal thrombus formation may contribute to this process. The predictors of an increased risk of acute occlusion are the presence of an intraluminal thrombus; dilatation at an acute bend; eccentric, tubular, severe, or long lesions; and lack of antiplatelet therapy. The risk of coronary dissection is also increased when the balloon is oversized for the artery. Most abrupt occlusions occur in the cardiac catheterization laboratory, but subacute occlusion may occur within 24 to 48 hours of the PTCA, particularly when the final result after PTCA was poor, with evidence of an obvious dissection, thrombus, or slow distal blood flow.

Once an abrupt occlusion occurs, intracoronary nitroglycerin should be administered to try to reverse any spastic component of the occlusion. Intracoronary thrombolytic therapy may be helpful when there is evidence of intracoronary thrombus. Repeated inflations with the same or a slightly larger balloon will restore adequate blood flow in approximately 50 percent of cases. Recently, the availability of a perfusion balloon catheter with side holes has made it possible to perform long balloon inflations (for 20 to 30 minutes) while allowing continued perfusion and minimizing ischemia. This approach may be successful in recanalizing an occluded vessel in a minority of cases. The intracoronary stent, which is being used as an investigational device, has shown great promise as a means to "tack up" the intimal flap(s) obstructing blood flow so as to restore luminal patency. Should these measures fail, and if a substantial amount of myocardium is jeopardized, emergency surgery should be performed. In patients who require emergency bypass surgery for acute occlusion, there is a 30 to 40 percent incidence of myocardial infarction and about a 3 percent mortality rate.

POSTPROCEDURE CARE AND FOLLOW-UP

Immediately after a successful procedure, most patients return to the cardiac care unit or a specialized postangioplasty unit. The vascular access sheaths are typically left in place and intravenous heparin is administered for 12 to 24 hours, or longer in cases with a poor angiographic result (e.g., large intimal dissection). Patients should receive aspirin and a calcium channel blocker and/or long-acting nitrates to minimize coronary vasospasm. Most often, the sheaths are removed the morning after the procedure, and patients may be discharged the same evening if they are ambulating without complications. Local groin bleeding with hematoma formation may occur. Occasionally, significant local bleeding may be noted at the site of vascular access. This may at times precipitate a vasovagal reaction, leading to significant hypotension and the need for intravenous atropine and fluid resuscitation. The osmotic diuresis caused by contrast material given during PTCA, combined with limitation of oral intake on the day of the procedure, may cause hypotension due to volume depletion and require intravenous fluids. Patients who have recurrent anginal chest pain, particularly those with ischemic ECG changes, should immediately be brought back to the cardiac catheterization laboratory for repeat coronary arteriography. After an uncomplicated procedure, patients are discharged on a regimen that usually includes aspirin and a vasodilator (a calcium channel blocker and/or long-acting nitrates), although there is little clinical evidence that these medications affect the long-term results. Repeat outpatient exercise testing is usually recommended in the first 1 to 2 weeks after angioplasty, with a follow-up treadmill test at 4 to 5 months to screen for restenosis (see below).

LONG-TERM RESULTS AND RESTENOSIS

Approximately 30 percent of patients develop clinically evident restenosis within the first 6 months after successful single-vessel PTCA (Fig. 6). Several angiographic definitions of restenosis have been proposed; the most widely used is the loss of more than 50 percent of the initial luminal diameter improvement, and/or recurrence of a greater than 50 percent diameter stenosis. Restenosis usually occurs within the first 2 to 3 months after PTCA and is typically heralded by a return of symptoms or a clearly positive treadmill test. Ten to 15

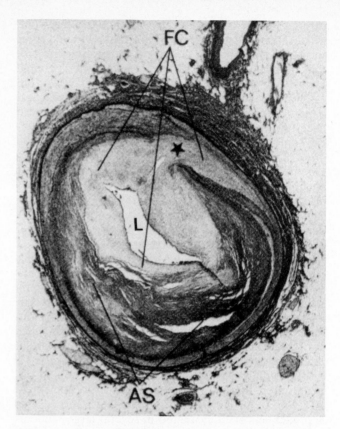

Figure 6 Photomicrograph showing the histologic appearance of restenosis after PTCA in a right coronary artery. The old atherosclerotic plaque (AS) can be seen with an intimal split still apparent from the initial balloon injury (star). The lighter staining material is the fibrocellular plaque (FC) that constitutes the restenotic lesion, narrowing the residual lumen (L) two months after the initially successful PTCA.

percent of patients have clinically silent restenosis (i.e., angiographic restenosis without return of symptoms). It is very unusual for restenosis to present as acute vessel closure with myocardial infarction without preceding warning symptoms.

Most patients (about 70 percent) who are symptom free with a normal exercise test at 6 months after single-vessel PTCA experience a low (5 to 10 percent) recurrence rate at the dilated site over the next 5 to 7 years. The cardiac mortality and myocardial infarction risk in the subgroup without restenosis is very low (about 1 percent per year). Higher rates of restenosis are observed after initially successful multivessel PTCA and in other higher-risk patient subgroups (Table 6).

Most cardiologists recommend repeat PTCA in patients who develop clinically evident restenosis. The restenosis risk after a second PTCA is approximately the same as that observed after the initial PTCA (about 30 percent). In patients who develop a second restenosis a third PTCA may be appropriate, particularly in those with single-vessel disease and relatively low-risk lesions. Some of these patients, however, are better served by

Table 6 Risk Factors for Restenosis After Successful PTCA

Clinical Variables
   Male sex
   Diabetes mellitus
   Recent angina
   Unstable angina
   Variant angina
   ? Smoking
Anatomic and Procedural Variables
   Stenosis in left anterior descending coronary artery
   Stenosis in saphenous vein graft (particularly proximal)
   PTCA of total occlusion
   PTCA of diffuse disease
   High initial degree of stenosis
   Poor final result (angiographic or hemodynamic)
   Absence of angiographic dissection

referral for bypass surgery. The restenosis rate becomes higher after a third PTCA, so after a third restenosis most patients should be referred for bypass surgery.

The pathophysiology of restenosis is complex. Pathologically, restenosis is caused by fibromuscular proliferation that occurs as a response to balloon-induced arterial injury. Medial smooth muscle cells migrate into the intima and proliferate in response to a variety of potent growth factors released at the site of injury by aggregating platelets, macrophages, endothelial cells, and possibly also smooth muscle cells themselves. After the cells proliferate, they elaborate an extracellular matrix that adds to the bulk of the lesion. It is not known why this process progresses in some patients but is limited in others.

A number of mechanical approaches to reduce or prevent restenosis have been proposed, including stenting, atherectomy, and lasers, but none of these have eliminated this vexing problem. Similarly, many conventional medical therapies such as calcium channel blockers, sodium warfarin, aspirin, and others have proved ineffective. High doses of fish oil begun before PTCA have been proposed as an effective regimen to prevent restenosis, but this remains controversial. New therapies are under development such as more potent antiplatelet agents and growth factor inhibitors.

NEW INTERVENTIONAL DEVICES

Many new interventional technologies are evolving to address the major problems associated with balloon angioplasty. Laser catheters, mechanical cutting devices ("atherectomy" catheters), and intravascular stents have been developed and are in various stages of clinical testing or approval.

Lasers

Ever since the early 1960s when the first lasers were developed, physicians and the lay public have been intrigued with the notion of harnessing this energy to treat a variety of medical conditions. However, the clinical application of laser technology to treat obstructive arterial disease did not evolve until the 1980s, when the success of balloon angioplasty, combined with the refinement of fiberoptics to transmit the energy along the length of a catheter, kindled intense interest in the promise of laser angioplasty. Early studies by Abela demonstrated the feasibility of continuous wave laser energy transmission (Nd:YAG and argon lasers) via flexible fiberoptics to ablate atheromatous plaque. The histopathology from these in vitro studies demonstrated a zone of ablation surrounded by areas of thermal injury, raising concerns regarding the focality of laser energy delivery. Severe thermal injury to the arterial wall associated with continuous wave laser application has been demonstrated to induce smooth muscle cell proliferation and collagen formation, leading to restenosis and limiting the long-term efficacy of continuous wave laser angioplasty. Subsequent studies have suggested that the use of pulsed delivery of laser energy at various wavelengths helps to minimize this thermal effect and has fueled interest in pulsed lasers for clinical application.

Despite the promise of laser angioplasty, this technology has had a number of limitations that have been difficult to overcome. The most important problem limiting the safe application of laser energy to atherosclerotic coronary artery disease has been the unacceptably high incidence of arterial perforation. Historically, this complication has resulted both from mechanical perforation due to the stiffness of bare fiberoptics, and from laser-induced perforation due to dispersion of laser energy to the more "normal" portion of the vessel wall. A variety of innovative approaches have been developed to try to overcome this problem, including encapsulation of the fiberoptic within an elliptical cap ("hot tip" laser), the use of pulsed laser delivery with multiple fibers delivered coaxially over a central guidewire (e.g., the AIS excimer laser, Fig. 7), the use of fluorescence (spectral feedback) guided laser delivery ("smart laser"), and the coaxial delivery of a divergent laser beam using a balloon catheter for centering the laser beam. The other current limitations of laser angioplasty include (1) the relatively small channel size created by laser catheters, often necessitating the use of adjunctive balloon angioplasty; (2) the potential for thermal injury (primarily with continuous wave lasers); (3) increased vessel wall thrombogenicity (e.g., excimer lasers); (4) arterial spasm (particularly with thermal injury); (5) the potential for embolic debris (as with pulsed laser); and (6) the substantial cost of purchasing and maintaining complex laser hardware. Despite these limitations, the newest generation of laser angioplasty catheters are beginning to show some clinical promise. It is possible that laser angioplasty will ultimately prove useful in the treatment of patients with diffuse disease and total occlusions. There are no convincing data at this time to suggest that laser angioplasty reduces the incidence of restenosis or acute complications.

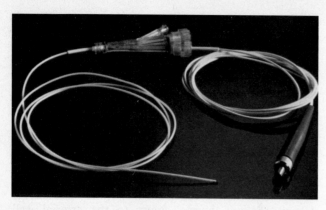

Figure 7 Multifiber excimer laser catheter (AIS) for coronary intervention.

Atherectomy

A number of mechanical systems have been developed during the last 4 to 5 years to treat obstructive peripheral and coronary artery disease. Three atherectomy devices are shown in Figure 8. Compared with laser angioplasty systems, mechanical devices have the potential advantages of greater predictability and decreased cost and complexity. Semantically, it is important to distinguish between *atherectomy* devices (e.g., Simpson AtheroCath and Pullback Atherectomy Catheter), which cut and remove obstructing atheromatous material, and *atheroablation* devices, such as the Rotablator, which grind the atheroma into small particles, allowing them to embolize distally. The relative advantages or disadvantages of these two approaches have not been compared in any controlled fashion. The idealized mechanical system should (1) efficiently debulk atheroma; (2) be flexible so as to allow device delivery to both proximal and distal coronary vessels; (3) be compatible with standard balloon angioplasty techniques and equipment; (4) minimize dissections, perforations, and closure; (5) be capable of treating eccentric stenoses; (6) minimize injury to the media and adventitial layers in order to decrease the incidence of restenosis; (7) create a smooth, cylindrical lumen to allow laminar blood flow, thus minimizing turbulence and shear-related platelet aggregation; (8) minimize embolic debris and remove tissue for study; (9) be capable of treating lesions that are anatomically unfavorable for PTCA; and (10) be capable of creating a luminal channel larger than the outer diameter of the atherectomy/atheroablation device. Some data suggest that atherectomy may reduce the incidence of restenosis compared with balloon angioplasty in certain subsets of patients, and that the incidence of abrupt vessel closure may be reduced with this approach. Atherectomy devices appear well suited to the treatment of lesions that are unfavorable for balloon angioplasty, such as ostial lesions, eccentric lesions, and lesions associated with intracoronary thrombus. However, like laser angioplasty, the mechanical approaches to atheroma removal are in an early stage of development.

Intracoronary Stents

An intravascular stent is a "scaffolding-like" device that is implanted within the vessel lumen in order to maintain a patent, roughly cylindrical luminal contour. The concept of intravascular stenting appeared in the earliest days of transluminal angioplasty when Charles Dotter first tested plastic tube and metallic coiled stents in canine iliofemoral arteries.

Some investigators have commented on the characteristics that are desirable for endovascular stents. In human coronary arteries, intravascular stents must meet a significant number of exacting specifications. The prosthetic device must be strong enough to oppose the "residual circumferential elasticity" of the arterial wall so that the structural integrity of the lumen is maintained. It must be flexible enough to allow its deployment in a tortuous vascular system. The device must have a favorable "expansion ratio" so that it can be tightly compressed on the delivery catheter; the higher the expansion ratio, the larger must be the diameter of the device after deployment. It should be either inert and durable or inert and readily degradable. Its deployment must result in very favorable flow dynamics through the "stented" arterial segment, and the device should result in little or no activation of thrombotic pathways. In general, the actual stent material should cover a small proportion of the intraluminal surface area (10 to 15 percent).

The practicalities of material science and current design capabilities have yielded a first generation of intracoronary stenting devices that fall short of the above "ideal" criteria. Nonetheless, a growing number of devices are becoming available for clinical use. Stents have been proposed for treatment of the following conditions: (1) threatened or actual acute closure of coronary artery segments after unsuccessful balloon angioplasty, (2) improvement and buttressing of the arterial segment after opening of chronic total occlusions, (3) improvement of the initial result after PTCA, and (4) prevention of restenosis by maintenance of vascular integrity through the buttressing of the vascular wall.

Intracoronary stents appear to be most promising as "bail-out" devices to restore luminal patency after acute closure following failed balloon angioplasty. It is uncertain at this time whether stenting will have a favorable effect on restenosis. The future development of stents that have antithrombogenic coating and are biodegradable may expand the applicability of this technology.

FUTURE DIRECTIONS

There has been rapid and widespread acceptance of PTCA and other catheter-based revascularization techniques in the last 10 years. More recently we have witnessed an explosion of new technologies, all intended to improve the short- or long-term efficacy of catheter-based revascularization. It is likely that the further evolution of this technology will ultimately improve the

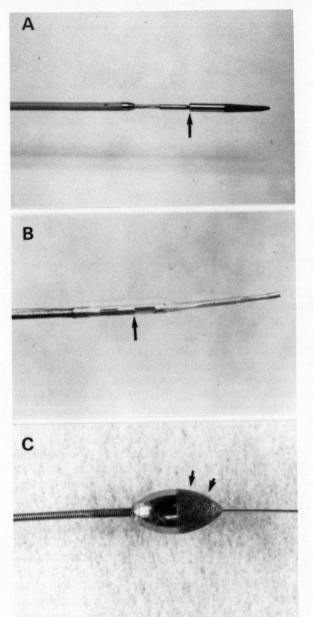

Figure 8 Three different mechanical systems for the treatment of coronary atherosclerosis. *A,* Distal tip of the pullback atherectomy catheter, shown here in its open configuration with the cylindric cutting blade exposed *(arrow).* Once the lesion has been crossed, the back portion of the device is pulled back; the blade tip is rotated at 2,000 rpm and pulled back through the lesion, collecting the cut plaque into the collection chamber. *B,* Distal aspect of the AtheroCath, another cut-and-collect atherectomy catheter. The capsule is advanced into the stenosis, and the balloon on the outer surface of the capsule is inflated, pushing plaque into the capsule window. The cylindric blade *(arrow)* is then advanced forward, cutting the plaque. This sequence is repeated as the device is rotated around the circumference of the lesion. *C,* Tip of the Rotoblator atheroabrasional device. The distal burr, which is coated with diamond particles *(arrows),* is spun at approximately 200,000 rpm to ablate the plaque into very small particles that embolize downstream.

safety and expand the applicability of catheter-based revascularization procedures. Many patients who now must undergo coronary artery bypass grafting may soon be reasonably treated by less invasive techniques that use more advanced balloon catheters or other devices. It is probable that several devices will eventually be shown to have utility in certain niches: lasers or an ultrasonic ablation catheter for total occlusions; retrograde atherectomy for treatment of ostial lesions; and stents, atherectomy, or laser thermal balloon for treatment of intimal dissection and abrupt coronary closure after PTCA. The ability of any of these devices to decrease restenosis compared with conventional balloon angioplasty remains uncertain. Ultimately, large randomized comparative clinical trials will be required to define the role of each of these new technologies in comparison with balloon angioplasty or coronary artery bypass graft surgery.

SUGGESTED READING

Bell MR, Bailey KR, Reeder GS, et al. Percutaneous transluminal angioplasty in patients with multivessel coronary diseases: How important is complete revascularization for cardiac event-free survival? J Am Coll Cardiol 1990; 16:553–562.

Detre K, Holubkov R, Kelsey S, et al. Percutaneous transluminal coronary angioplasty in 1985–1986 and 1977–1981. The National Heart, Lung, and Blood Institute Registry. N Engl J Med 1988; 318:265–270.

Dorros G, Lewin RF, Janke L. Multiple lesion transluminal coronary angioplasty in single and multivessel coronary artery disease: Acute outcome and long-term effect. J Am Coll Cardiol 1987; 10: 1007–1013.

Ellis SG, Roubin GS, King SB, et al. Angiographic and clinical predictors of acute closure after native vessel coronary angioplasty. Circulation 1988; 77:372–379.

Ellis SG, Roubin GS, King SB III, et al. In-hospital cardiac mortality after acute closure after coronary angioplasty: Analysis of risk factors from 8,207 procedures. J Am Coll Cardiol 1988; 11:211–216.

Fisch C, Beller GA, DeSanctis RW, et al. Guidelines for the early management of patients with acute myocardial infarction. J Am Coll Cardiol 1990; 16:249–292.

Fischell TA, Derby G, Tse TM, Stadius ML. Coronary artery vasoconstriction routinely occurs after percutaneous transluminal coronary angioplasty: A quantitative arteriographic analysis. Circulation 1988; 78:1323–1334.

Gruentzig AR, King SB, Schlumpf M, Siegenthaler W. Long-term follow-up after percutaneous transluminal coronary angioplasty: The early Zurich experience. N Engl J Med 1987; 316:1127–1132.

Leimgruber PP, Roubin GS, Hollman J, et al. Restenosis after successful coronary angioplasty in patients with single-vessel disease. Circulation 1986; 73:710–717.

Liu MW, Roubin GS, King SB. Restenosis after coronary angioplasty: potential biologic determinants and role of intimal hyperplasia. Circulation 1989; 79:1374–1384.

Topol EJ, Califf RM, George BS, et al. A randomized trial of immediate versus delayed elective angioplasty after intravenous tissue plasminogen activator in acute myocardial infarction. N Engl J Med 1987; 317:581–588.

CHRONIC ISCHEMIC HEART DISEASE: SURGICAL MANAGEMENT

GREGORY S. COUPER, M.D.

Most patients undergoing coronary revascularization today have chronic disabling exertional angina or rest angina unresponsive to medical therapy. Acute ischemic syndromes constitute a less frequent, albeit still significant indication for revascularization. This discussion focuses on surgical revascularization in chronic ischemic conditions.

The growth and development of catheter techniques (e.g., percutaneous transluminal coronary angioplasty [PTCA], laser angioplasty and atherectomy) have had a significant impact on the patient population referred for surgical revascularization. The general effect has been the channeling of symptomatic patients with single- or double-vessel disease who often have preserved left ventricular (LV) function toward angioplasty, and the referral of patients with multivessel disease for surgery. Consequently, the surgical population has changed greatly over the last decade. Numerous centers are reporting patients of more advanced age, a greater number of diseased vessels, worse LV function, and more concomitant comorbidities. These factors apply for patients presenting for both initial and repeat operations.

INDICATIONS

The usual indication for surgery in patients with stable or slowly progressive ischemic syndromes has been persistence of angina or anginal equivalents despite adequate medical treatment, generally consisting of multidrug therapy with beta-blockers, calcium channel blockers, and nitrates. The goals of surgery are complete relief of symptoms, restoration of a normal life style, and increased longevity.

The three widely quoted trials of the late 1970s comparing medical and surgical therapy were the Coronary Artery Surgery Study (CASS), the VA Cooperative Study (VA), and the European Coronary Surgery Study (ECSS). These prospective randomized studies were undertaken to elucidate the benefits, risks, and appropriate roles for these therapies. They continue to influence current philosophies regarding patient selection for coronary artery bypass grafting (CABG), despite the fact that they represent neither current surgical technique nor current medical management.

These three trials dealt in differing ways with patients with severe limiting exertional angina (class III) and angina occurring at rest or with any minimal physical activity (class IV). Believing that these indications for surgery were strong, the investigators of the CASS study excluded them from the randomized medical versus surgical trial. An observational study of these class III and IV patients demonstrated a survival benefit favoring surgery in patients with double- and triple-vessel disease, regardless of the presence or absence of LV dysfunction. The survival benefits were not seen in patients with single-vessel disease. However, significant relief of symptoms and improvement in exercise tolerance were demonstrated with surgery in the CASS trial. The VA study included class III and IV patients, and the ECSS, class III patients (excluding class IV), as significant minority components of their trials. Both also demonstrated long-term survival benefits in the surgically treated patients. Thus, in patients with severe stable angina (class III or IV), the indications for coronary artery bypass grafting include double- or triple-vessel disease with normal as well as diminished LV function.

Left main coronary stenosis, variably defined as greater than 50 or to 70 percent stenosis, has been the strongest indication for surgery. Reports from the VA and the ECSS trials clearly demonstrated better short- and long-term survival in surgically treated patients at 4 to 5 years (89 to 93 percent) compared with the medically managed cohort (65 to 67 percent). These data led the CASS investigators to specifically exclude patients with

70 percent or greater left main stenosis from the randomized trial.

Patients with mild to moderate anginal syndromes (classes I and II) constitute a large population from which selected subsets are referred for surgery. It is in these also that the greatest controversy surrounding coronary artery bypass grafting exists. Only the CASS randomized trial specifically segregated these patients for study; however, they constituted only 4.7 percent of patients in the overall CASS registry. Most patients were removed from consideration in the randomized trial because of class III or IV symptoms or left main stenosis. With respect to qualitative improvements, such as symptomatic relief, the CASS randomized trial in class I and II patients favored surgical management. Analysis of long-term survival benefits revealed improved longevity with coronary artery bypass grafting only in the selected subset with triple-vessel disease and an LV ejection fraction (EF) between 35 and 50 percent (patients with EF less than 35 percent were excluded from the CASS trial). Survival trends favored surgery with single- or double-vessel disease with LV dysfunction; however, low numbers precluded the achievement of statistical significance in these data.

One of the greatest deficiencies of these large prospective randomized trials of surgery versus medical therapy was the infrequent use (less than 10 percent) of internal mammary artery (IMA) grafting. This reflected the common practice of the time except at a few institutions. The significantly improved long-term patency of left internal mammary artery (LIMA) to left anterior descending (LAD) grafts (85 to 90 percent at 10 years and thereafter) relative to saphenous vein bypasses (approximately 60 to 70 percent at 8 to 10 years) has led to the routine use of IMA grafts in more than 90 percent of patients now. This improvement in graft patency has translated into a significant reduction in long-term mortality as evidenced by reports from the Cleveland Clinic, the CASS trial, and numerous other centers. The message we have learned is that the use of longer-lived conduits together with other methods of slowing both native artery and graft atherosclerosis (e.g., aspirin and dipyridamole [Persantine]) will result in even better longevity after surgery. This will probably widen the disparity in long-term survival between surgery and medical therapy, and possibly extend the indications to lesser degrees of symptoms with single- and double-vessel disease with or without LV dysfunction.

In general, I consider the following to be appropriate indications for revascularization surgery in patients with chronic ischemic heart disease:

1. Moderate to severe exertional angina, or rest angina (classes III and IV) despite an adequate medical regimen.
2. Left main stenosis greater than 50 percent.
3. Mild to moderate angina due to double- and triple-vessel disease associated with LV dysfunction (EF less than 50 percent).
4. Intolerance to medical therapy due to side effects or intolerable limitation of life style from the patient's perspective.
5. Significant coronary stenosis associated with other disorders requiring cardiac surgery; valvular disease represents the most common associated condition.

Less clear-cut indications include:

6. Significant silent ischemia detected by exercise tolerance test, ambulatory monitoring, or dipyridamole thallium ETT and associated with severe triple-vessel disease and LV dysfunction.
7. Severe double- or triple-vessel CAD, especially if associated with LV dysfunction, in a patient requiring a major vascular or other major surgical procedure.

An example of a high-risk application of bypass surgery is a procedure for the resolution of ischemic cardiomyopathy.

A steadily increasing proportion of bypass surgery consists of reoperations for progression of native coronary disease, or more likely, obliteration of bypass grafts by graft atherosclerosis. Currently, this may be as much as 15 to 20 percent of a center's volume. Considerations for reoperative bypass surgery need to take into account the higher morbidity and mortality rates and potentially greater technical difficulties encountered with reoperative surgery. Consequently, medical therapy is pursued further and more vigorously, and a greater degree of symptoms and limitation are generally required, before patients are accepted for repeat surgery.

RISK FACTORS

Once there are appropriate indications for surgery, a careful assessment of potential risk factors should be made before accepting a patient for surgery. A review of the coronary angiograms is generally an excellent predictor of the graftability of the coronary arteries. Extended endarterectomy can be applied successfully to either the left or right coronary vessels and can allow for grafting of diffusely diseased vessels previously considered ungraftable. It should be uncommon for poor distal vessels alone to be considered a contraindication for surgery, especially for an initial operation.

The major cardiac risk factor for poor postoperative outcome is extremely poor LV function (EF less than 20 percent). Most patients undergo some assessment of cardiac function, either right heart catheterization or left ventriculography, at the time of coronary angiography, or echocardiography/nuclear ventriculography. When severe LV dysfunction is consistently present on a variety of assessments on several occasions, serious concerns regarding operability arise. When significant angina exists and symptoms of congestive heart failure (CHF) are either transient or episodic or readily controlled medically, I presume there is ischemic but viable myocardium, so-called hibernating myocardium. Although the risks of low output state and mortality are somewhat increased in this situation, the vast majority recover satisfactorily.

When several evaluations demonstrate global LV ejection fractions below 10 to 15 percent, coronary artery bypass grafting should be restricted to patients with significant limiting angina, compensated CHF at worst, and of a relatively young physiologic age. In these patients, the use of ventricular assist devices (VADs) or subsequent cardiac transplantation would allow for recovery and long-term survival if severe low output syndrome or cardiogenic shock preclude weaning from cardiopulmonary bypass. Patients with ischemic cardiomyopathy whose symptoms are predominantly of fixed CHF and only minimal to mild angina are best approached as candidates for transplantation. When age or other factors render that option unsuitable, high-risk surgery can be considered; however, if the cardiomyopathy is irreversible because of diffusely nonviable myocardium, reasonable longevity is unlikely even if the patient survives surgery.

Comorbid conditions may impact on postoperative morbidity and mortality and eventually on long-term outcome. Potential deterioration in pre-existing pulmonary, cerebrovascular, or peripheral vascular disease can be anticipated and potentially prevented by careful routine assessment of these organ systems when signs or symptoms suggest dysfunction. Conventional pulmonary function testing with arterial blood gas sampling can only identify patients at greater risk for prolonged ventilatory support or pneumonia. It does not provide for any absolute contraindications to surgery, except in patients with severe limitations or end-stage pulmonary insufficiency secondary to intrinsic lung disease.

A detailed history and careful physical examination provide an adequate screen for peripheral or cerebrovascular disease. Significant diminution of femoral or more distal pulses, or the presence of bruits, is indicative of atherosclerotic peripheral vascular stenoses that might make insertion of an intra-aortic balloon pump (IABP) difficult, impossible, or threatening to limb viability. Symptomatic evidence of exercise or resting limb ischemia may dictate the choice, extent, and location of graft conduit to be harvested.

Perioperative stroke is a significant disabling, disheartening, and sometimes fatal complication of surgery. Considerable controversy still exists over the role of carotid endarterectomy in prevention of this complication, because carotid stenosis is only one of multiple causes of stroke in these patients. Patients with symptoms of recent stroke, transient ischemic attacks, or amaurosis fugax are screened with carotid ultrasonography and Doppler studies. If hemodynamically significant stenosis (more than 70 to 80 percent) is present, angiography is usually performed. Combined carotid endarterectomy and coronary artery bypass grafting is then performed, largely to eliminate the need for second admissions, repeat anesthesia, and subsequent carotid surgery. Asymptomatic patients with carotid bruits generally are not evaluated with noninvasive studies.

PREOPERATIVE PREPARATION

The medical preparation of the patient for upcoming surgery consists of optimizing cardiopulmonary function by appropriate treatment of CHF or chronic obstructive lung disease. Aggressive medical management of progressive or unstable anginal syndromes with beta-blockers, calcium channel blockers, and nitrates is indicated to keep patients stable. If an unstable clinical circumstance requires a more urgent or emergently needed surgery, the perioperative risks are significantly higher, largely because of the lesser margin of myocardial reserve.

Anticoagulants are stopped before admission to the hospital so as to minimize wasted hospital time while a satisfactory coagulation status is restored. Warfarin (Coumadin) is halted 2 days before admission. Generally the prothrombin time (PT) is only slightly elevated, therefore, at the time of admission. If surgery is unexpectedly deferred, intravenous heparin may be used to replace warfarin in inpatients. Unless aspirin is thought to be an essential component of an antianginal regimen, I discontinue it 7 to 10 days before elective surgery. Aspirin has generally been associated with increased postoperative mediastinal bleeding of a mild to moderate degree.

When the elective surgery is scheduled for 2 to 3 weeks after catheterization, patients with stable ischemic syndromes generally can donate at least two units of autologous blood. For patients undergoing an initial operation, this virtually ensures that they will not require any heterologous blood transfusions, with the attendant risks of transfusion-associated disease. For patients undergoing reoperation, autologous donation will significantly reduce but may not eliminate the need for heterologous transfusion.

A significant issue in assessment for upcoming coronary artery bypass grafting, especially for reoperations, is the presence of adequate conduits to perform bypass grafting. Patients with significant varicose veins, those who have had vein stripping or sclerotherapy, and those who have previously undergone coronary or lower leg revascularization that used saphenous veins, need to be evaluated carefully by cardiologists and cardiac surgeons. The adequacy or presence of the greater or lesser saphenous venous systems can be assessed noninvasively with vascular ultrasound mapping, or invasively by venography.

For reoperations in which remaining venous conduits may be poor or absent, an arteriographic assessment of the left and/or right internal mammary artery (LIMA and/or RIMA) is advised. If issues of potential conduit difficulties are considered before cardiac catheterization and coronary angiography, the additional angiograms can be readily performed simultaneously.

CHOICE OF PROCEDURE

The extent of coronary artery bypass grafting performed in individual patients has varied throughout the history of this procedure. The proportion of patients receiving only one or two grafts has decreased, largely because of fewer patients with only single- or double-vessel disease presenting for surgery. The vast majority of patients receive three, four, or possibly five grafts (a mean of about 3.5 grafts per patient). This is in keeping with the philosophy of global revascularization; i.e., revascularization of LAD, circumflex, and right coronary artery (RCA) territory in general. Use of more than five grafts generally is not indicated, because grafting of a myriad of small diseased coronary arteries does not improve the long-term results and certainly prolongs the procedure.

The extent of grafting is therefore based on angiographic demonstration of coronary stenoses in excess of 50 to 60 percent. This is modified, however, by the presence of akinetic or dyskinetic regions of myocardium detected by ventriculography or echocardiography. When a region is judged nonviable secondary to previous transmural infarction, the importance of grafting the responsible coronary artery is relatively diminished. This is especially so if the coronary artery is completely occluded or the distal vessel is diffusely diseased, rendering it less suitable for grafting.

Currently, the LIMA is the conduit of choice for LAD grafting because of the vastly greater longevity afforded. There are no absolute contraindications to its use except poor blood flow after harvesting, due either to traumatic injury or to small size or intrinsic disease. Circumstances in which a saphenous vein graft (SVG) is used in preference to an IMA should be unusual. These may include severely depressed LV function with extensive anteroseptal infarction, and severe pulmonary emphysema with hyperexpansion or severe bullous disease. Advanced age, even over 80 years, is not a contraindication to IMA grafting. Despite slightly higher overall risks in older patients, the LIMA graft has proved satisfactory.

The use of bilateral IMA grafting and/or other newer arterial grafts, such as gastroepiploic artery (GEA), inferior epigastric, or even radial artery autografts, is still controversial. Given the improved long-term results with the LIMA graft, it was natural to pursue increased use of arterial rather than venous conduits to further extend long-term results. To date, several studies point toward improved graft longevity but not necessarily improved patient survival. Currently, multiple arterial grafting is probably more important to younger patients (under 60 to 65 years of age) perceived at very high risk for recurrence of disease requiring reoperation. A relative contraindication to bilateral IMA grafting is significant diabetes mellitus, in which there is a greatly increased risk of sternal dehiscence or sternal wound infection. In these patients, alternative arterial conduits may be considered.

An additional circumstance in which multiple arterial grafts are helpful is the presence of significant atherosclerotic disease of the ascending aorta that may preclude the use of proximal vein graft anastomoses. Pedicled bilateral IMA or GEA grafts eliminate the need for proximal anastomoses. Free RIMA or RGEA can also be brought off the side of the LIMA pedicle, as can SVGs. This so-called no-touch technique has eliminated the atheroembolic complications seen with manipulation of the atherosclerotic ascending aorta.

CONDUIT PROBLEMS

The availability of adequate graft material is an increasing problem when patients present for second or third operations, or when the greater saphenous vein is varicose or sclerosed, or has been surgically removed because of intrinsic disease. Traditional alternatives to the greater saphenous vein, such as the lesser saphenous (posterior calf) or cephalic (arm) vein, do not approach its long-term patency rates. Consequently, alternative grafts such as RIMA, RGEA, and inferior epigastric artery grafts are increasingly used. Long-term studies may confirm the excellent short-term patency seen to date. Synthetic graft materials such as Gore-Tex have very poor long-term patency and are rarely considered. There is a resurgent interest in human saphenous vein allografts, in light of the dramatic advances in cryopreservation techniques.

MYOCARDIAL PROTECTION

Dramatic advances in myocardial protection techniques over the last 15 years are responsible for the steady improvements in operative risk. Better preservation has allowed more complicated procedures to be performed safely. Intermittent hypothermic ischemic arrest is rarely used today. Hypothermic fibrillation is still useful and the method of choice when aortic cross-clamping is contraindicated. Cold crystalloid and cold-blood cardioplegic arrest constitute the most widely and routinely used forms of myocardial protection. Benefits of blood cardioplegia are more evident when longer and more complex procedures are anticipated. Classically used by antegrade administration via the aortic root to the coronary arteries, it has been demonstrated that more uniform distribution, resulting in better protection, can be obtained with retrograde cardioplegia infusion via special coronary sinus catheters, especially when subtotal coronary occlusions or aortic insufficiency are present.

Special problems in operative technique are encountered during reoperative bypass grafting. Resternotomy, itself, rarely results in life-threatening injury to underlying structures such as the innominate vein or artery, the aorta, patent bypass grafts, or the right atrium or ventricle. Manipulation, however gentle, can result in atheroembolization from patent, atherosclerotic, or recently thrombosed vein grafts down the native coronary arteries, resulting in potentially lethal myocardial infarction. Various techniques have evolved to deal with these circumstances in order to minimize complications. Alternative methods of cardiopulmonary bypass, such as femoral vein–femoral artery perfusion, are used more commonly to reduce the risk to vascular, graft, or cardiac structures. Early detachment of patent diseased grafts and retrograde cardioplegia are used to minimize atheroembolism. Alternative surgical approaches for left coronary regrafting, such as left thoracotomy, avoid the risks of resternotomy.

POSTOPERATIVE CARE: COMPLICATIONS

Successful perioperative care depends on anticipating, preventing, and minimizing the usual significant complications. These are largely the result of three organ systems: cardiac, pulmonary, and neurologic.

Postoperative myocardial infarction is fortunately uncommon, with Q-wave infarction rates of approximately 3 percent overall. Ischemia is more often seen, but the vast majority of patients do not experience this complication. Routine use of intravenous nitroglycerin, nitroprusside, or sublingual nifedipine has reduced perioperative ischemia due to coronary spasm or graft spasm, especially with internal mammary or other arterial grafts. Incomplete revascularization, due to vessels that cannot be grafted to viable tissue, inability to find intramyocardial vessels, or excessive attempts at revascularization such as complex endarterectomies, account for many perioperative infarctions. Appropriate patient selection, reasonable grafting techniques, and use of adequate myocardial preservation techniques may reduce some of these problems. Aggressive means of hemodynamic support, such as intra-aortic balloon pumping or even VADs, can tide patients through the early difficult postoperative period and allow complete recovery. Unremitting evidence of ischemia despite these measures occasionally warrants recatheterization and reoperation for early graft complications.

Today, a common cause of cardiac mortality after surgery is the low output states associated with cardiogenic shock followed by multiorgan failure, often in the absence of perioperative ischemia or infarction. Restoration of satisfactory hemodynamics requires invasive monitoring, preferably with pulmonary artery catheters capable of enabling cardiac output to be estimated. Optimal volume loading and establishment of acceptable cardiac rate and rhythm are the initial steps. Atrial, ventricular, or atrioventricular sequential pacing are performed when necessary, using temporary epicardial wires placed at surgery. Pharmacologic aids in the form of inotropic or vasopressor agents are the next line of therapy. Dopamine, dobutamine, and epinephrine are the mainstays of treatment. Newer agents, such as the phosphodiesterase inhibitor amrinone, have frequently resulted in dramatic reversal of low-output states refrac-

tory to the usual agents. When pharmacologic means are unsuccessful, mechanical support such as an IABP is instituted. In some patients, considerable improvement may be seen with the recovery of stunned myocardium. VADs may temporarily provide sufficient circulation to allow restoration of organ function; if the myocardium recovers, the VAD can be discontinued.

Ventricular arrhythmias are responsible for a significant proportion of postoperative morbidity and mortality. Sustained ventricular tachycardia (VT) or ventricular fibrillation (VF) is commonly associated with electrolyte depletion (potassium or magnesium), perioperative ischemia or infarction, or pre-existing ischemic cardiomyopathy. Appropriate treatment includes prophylactic and therapeutic potassium and magnesium administration. Continuous electrocardiographic monitoring allows for detection and quantitation of ventricular ectopy. Lidocaine given intravenously is the first line of therapy for complex ectopy. If lidocaine fails to control or prevent further arrhythmia, progression to procainamide, bretylium, amiodarone, or combined therapy should be considered. Because of their greater toxicity, including proarrhythmic effects, these agents are used only for episodes of VT refractory to lidocaine. Supraventricular arrhythmias such as atrial fibrillation or flutter are common, generally occurring later in the perioperative course, the usual onset being several days after surgery. The best prophylaxis appears to be reinstitution of short-acting beta-blockers within 24 to 48 hours of surgery in patients whose ventricular function permits such therapy (generally, an ejection fraction of more than 25 to 30 percent). Treatment of atrial fibrillation or flutter is directed at gaining control of the ventricular rate, and subsequent restoration of sinus rhythm. Calcium channel blockers or digoxin (to control ventricular response) and procainamide or quinidine (to restore sinus rhythm) are used most often. Once sinus rhythm has been restored, therapy is generally continued for only 2 to 6 weeks, because recurrence beyond this period is rare in the absence of other risk factors for atrial fibrillation.

Overt pulmonary edema is an uncommon complication. It generally occurs within several days of surgery and is usually due to poor cardiac function, together with the increased capillary permeability associated with the postoperative state. Interstitial edema is also promoted by perioperative hormonal shifts that induce sodium and water retention. Several days after surgery, intravascular hypervolemia occurs when this excess interstitial fluid is mobilized but not excreted rapidly enough. This may lead to pulmonary edema. The complication of pulmonary edema and the need for prolonged respiratory support can often be avoided. Fluid administration can be reduced by appropriate use of colloid volume expanders, red blood cells, and inotropic agents to maximize cardiac performance. Beginning 24 to 48 hours after surgery, furosemide (Lasix) is administered to promote a diuresis sufficient to prevent intravascular hypervolemia and pulmonary edema.

Another cause of morbidity and mortality in the postoperative state is pulmonary infection. It is a frequent complication of prolonged intubation and ventilatory support (more than 24 to 48 hours). Avoidance of pulmonary edema, which itself requires prolonged support, reduces the risk of subsequent pulmonary infection. Maximizing pulmonary function early on by aggressive physiotherapy and pulmonary toilet allow for extubation within 12 to 24 hours for most patients, thus reducing a portal of entry for sepsis. Anesthetic techniques can be adjusted in stable patients with good cardiopulmonary function to allow for planned early extubation 3 to 5 hours after surgery.

An increasingly less frequent cause of respiratory failure is phrenic nerve injury resulting in diaphragmatic paresis or paralysis. Avoidable causes of this problem include freeze injury of the phrenic nerve (by ice saline slushes used for topical cardiac cooling) and excessive dissection of the proximal IMA pedicles. Prolonged ventilator dependence of any cause that has not resolved by 7 to 10 days after surgery should be considered an indication for prompt tracheostomy. This allows for more effective pulmonary toilet and greater patient comfort and mobility than that provided by endotracheal intubation, and often a more rapid resolution of the respiratory insufficiency.

In contradistinction to pulmonary complications that are closely tied to postoperative cardiac complications, neurologic complications may occur despite an uncomplicated cardiac recovery. There are numerous causes of intraoperative or postoperative stroke. Critical internal carotid artery (ICA) stenosis combined with the relative hypotension of cardiopulmonary bypass or transient postoperative hypotension may result in stroke. Simultaneous prophylactic carotid endarterectomy has not been clearly shown to reduce stroke rate, except possibly in the high-risk scenario of severe bilateral carotid stenosis or unilateral ICA occlusion with severe contralateral ICA stenosis. Atheroembolism from cannulation or clamping of the diseased ascending aorta can be minimized by using the no-touch techniques described earlier. Mural thrombus of the LV or left atrium can be a previously undetected source of perioperative or postoperative emboli. Prompt systemic anticoagulation with heparin may reduce the recurrence of thromboembolism. Recurrent paroxysmal or persistent atrial fibrillation or flutter may result in an embolic event several days to weeks after surgery. If sinus rhythm cannot be maintained consistently after several days of pharmacologic therapy or with electrical cardioversion, anticoagulation is advisable until sinus rhythm is restored. Air embolism can occur whenever the aorta or left cardiac cavities are opened to atmosphere during bypass or valvular surgery. Meticulous technique to clear air from vascular and cardiac structures minimizes the risk of stroke from this cause. Intracranial cerebrovascular disease due to either atherosclerosis or hypertensive vascular disease is a risk factor that may be reduced by maintaining greater mean perfusion pressures on cardiopulmonary bypass and by minimizing hypotensive or hypertensive events in the perioperative period.

An uncomplicated postoperative course usually allows for discharge home on the sixth or seventh postoperative day in most patients. Those with physical deconditioning secondary to a sedentary life style, or elderly patients over 70 years of age, frequently need a short interim stay in an inpatient rehabilitation facility in order to regain the strength and endurance necessary to return home and resume the usual activities of daily, semi-independent life. Early postoperative cardiopulmonary complications often result in prolonged intensive care and hospital stays. A more prolonged period of rehabilitation is commonly needed; however, a remarkable recovery generally results in a return to an active, independent life style.

SUGGESTED READING

Cameron A, Davis K, Green G, et al. Clinical implications of internal mammary artery bypass grafts: the Coronary Artery Surgery Study experience. Circulation 1988; 77:815–819.

CASS principal investigators and their associates. Coronary Artery Surgery Study (CASS): a randomized trial of coronary artery bypass surgery: survival data. Circulation 1983; 68:939–950.

CASS principal investigators and their associates. Coronary Artery Surgery Study (CASS): a randomized trial of coronary artery bypass surgery: quality of life in patients randomly assigned to treatment groups. Circulation 1983; 68:951–960.

European Coronary Surgery Study Group. Long-term results of prospective randomized study of coronary artery bypass surgery in stable angina pectoris. Lancet 1982; 2:1173–1180.

Kaiser G, Davis K, Fisher L, et al. Survival following coronary artery bypass grafting in patients with severe angina pectoris (CASS): an observational study. J Thorac Cardiovasc Surg 1985; 89:513–524.

Loop F, Lytle B, Cosgrove D, et al. Influence of the internal mammary artery graft on 10-year survival and other cardiac events. N Engl J Med 1986; 314:1–6.

Passamani E, Davis K, Gillespie M, et al. A randomized trial of coronary artery bypass surgery: survival of patients with a low ejection fraction. N Engl J Med 1985; 312:1665–1671.

Read R, Murphy M, Hultgren H, et al. Survival of men treated for chronic stable angina pectoris: a cooperative randomized study. J Thorac Cardiovasc Surg 1978; 75:1–16.

Takaro T, Hultgren H, Lipton M, et al. The VA cooperative randomized study of surgery for coronary arterial occlusive disease. II: Subgroup with significant left main lesions. Circulation 1976; 54(Suppl III):III-107–III-117.

The Veterans Administration Coronary Artery Bypass Surgery Cooperative Study Group. Eleven-year survival in the Veterans Administration randomized trial of coronary bypass surgery for stable angina. N Engl J Med 1984; 311:1333–1339.

ANTITHROMBOTIC THERAPY FOR ACUTE CORONARY SYNDROMES

JAMES H. CHESEBRO, M.D.
VALENTIN FUSTER, M.D.

The acute coronary syndromes of unstable angina, myocardial infarction, and sudden coronary death have a common underlying pathogenesis involving plaque rupture of chronic coronary lesions. Prior to plaque rupture more than half of the lesions are minor (less than a 50 percent luminal stenosis), and more than 80 percent of lesions are less than moderate (less than a 75 percent luminal stenosis). Plaque rupture occurs in lesions with an underlying lipid pool covered by a fibrous cap that is infiltrated with monocytes and macrophages, thinned, and weak. A delicate lattice work of collagen is present at the site where the fibrous cap tears.

Local factors contributing to thrombosis are substrates in the arterial wall and the rheology of blood flow.

A fissure or tear into the plaque and the lipid pool permits contact of flowing blood with thrombogenic substrates such as collagen (types I and III), tissue thromboplastin, lipid, and thrombin bound to arterial wall matrix. The other local factor contributing to thrombosis is the rheology of blood flow, which includes the severity of a stenosis (directly increases platelet deposition) and the shear force (directly related to flow velocity and inversely to the third power of the luminal diameter), which also increases platelet deposition. Systemic factors contributing to thrombosis include catecholamines, cholesterol, lipoprotein$_{(a)}$ (Lp$_a$), plasminogen activator inhibitor (PAI-1), and decreased HDL cholesterol (carries lipoprotein-associated coagulation inhibitor [LACI]).

The thrombus formed by plaque rupture (Fig. 1) begins in the fissure and often extends into the lumen to obstruct coronary blood flow. Progression of this process leads to unstable angina or to acute myocardial infarction with or without sudden death (Fig. 1A, B). Plaque rupture with organization of mural thrombus appears to be the leading cause of progression of coronary artery disease (Fig. 1D). Pharmacologic thrombolysis may recanalize the lumen but usually leaves residual thrombus, which may lead to reocclusion (Fig. 1B → A).

PATHOGENESIS OF ATHEROSCLEROSIS
Sequelae of Plaque Rupture

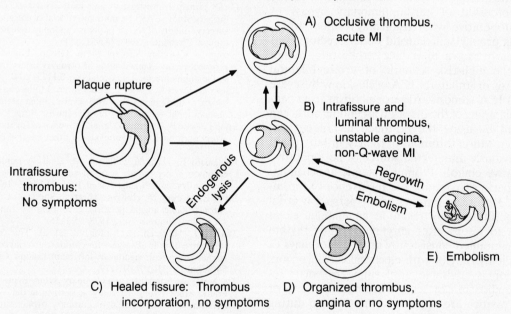

Figure 1 Diagram of plaque rupture and arterial thrombus. Plaque disruption leads to formation of a fissure. This allows flowing blood to contact thrombogenic intraplaque and medial tissue, resulting in thrombus within the fissure. This may be asymptomatic or may induce coronary spasm. The thrombus may progress to partially obstruct the lumen and cause unstable angina, non–Q-wave myocardial infarction (B), or total occlusion, which is often associated with transmural or Q-wave myocardial infarction (A). Intraluminal thrombus may undergo endogenous lysis with healing of the fissure and no progression of disease or symptoms (C). Intraluminal thrombus may organize and lead to progression of disease with or without subsequent symptoms (D). A portion of the thrombus may embolize (E) but may rapidly regrow (to B).

Occasionally, total inhibition of thrombosis and simultaneous endogenous thrombolysis may result in complete resolution of luminal thrombus and no significant obstruction to flow (Fig. 1*C*). Mechanisms of rethrombosis are shown in Figure 2.

Arterial thromboemboli may occur soon after a myocardial infarction. These originate from a left ventricular mural thrombus, usually in association with an anterior Q-wave myocardial infarction (90 percent), or with other Q-wave infarctions that involve the cardiac apex (10 percent), particularly those that result in akinetic or dyskinetic apical wall motion. Although left ventricular mural thrombus occurs in approximately 40 percent of these infarctions, thromboemboli are clinically manifested in only 10 percent of these patients. Most of these thrombi embolize to the brain (80 percent), occasionally to other organs (10 to 15 percent), and only rarely to the coronary arteries (5 to 10 percent). Prevention of thromboemboli is best accomplished by systemic anticoagulation to preclude the development of left ventricular thrombi, which are predominantly fibrin and related to stasis.

PRINCIPLES OF ANTITHROMBOTIC THERAPY

Goals

Antithrombotic therapy may involve antifibrin, antiplatelet, or both effects. These effects may depend on the antithrombotic agent, the dosage administered, and possibly two agents to provide both therapeutic effects. An anticoagulant effect may be present (heparin or warfarin) or absent (aspirin). The choice of antithrombotic therapies depends on the pathogenesis of thrombosis and the risk-benefit ratio of the therapy. Arterial thrombi are platelet rich and may require an anticoagulant (heparin or warfarin) plus an antiplatelet agent (such as aspirin). However, platelets are extremely sensitive to, and primarily activated by, thrombin. Therefore, they may be markedly inhibited by hirudin, which is a potent and specific thrombin inhibitor. Lower doses of specific thrombin inhibition inhibit fibrin formation, but considerably higher doses (blood levels approximately five to ten times higher) are required to limit in vivo platelet deposition to a single layer. When the goals of therapy are inhibition of predominately fibrin thrombi such as in venous thrombosis or large cardiac chambers with stasis, anticoagulant therapy with heparin (to activated partial thromboplastin time [aPTT] of 1.5 to 2.0 × control) or therapy with warfarin (International Normalized Ratio [INR] 2.0 to 3.0 or a prothrombin time ratio of 1.3 to 1.5 × control*) is usually sufficient to inhibit thrombus formation and growth. When these anticoagulants are used to protect against arterial thrombi and their growth, higher dosages of heparin (to an aPTT

*This ratio is therapeutic for prothrombin times generated by laboratories using thromboplastins with an International Sensitivity Index (ISI) of 2.2 to 2.6.

of 2.0 to 3.0 × control) or warfarin (to an INR of 3.0 to 4.5, or prothrombin time of 1.5 to 1.8 × control) are usually advised. In high-risk situations such as an arterial angioplasty procedure, administration of even higher doses of heparin (e.g., 10,000 to 20,000 U intravenous bolus plus a simultaneous infusion of 1300 U/h) combined with the platelet inhibitor aspirin is often employed.

Aspirin

Aspirin inhibits platelet function irreversibly and is cheap. It reduces the incidence of arterial thrombosis by 25 to 50 percent, mainly by inhibiting the central core of thrombus within the lumen of the artery and thus reducing the incidence of complete occlusion. Its effect may be incomplete because it does not totally inhibit the outer rim of mural thrombus, which is more rich in thrombin. Aspirin appears much less effective and often ineffective at preventing venous thrombi and stasis-related thrombi in cardiac chambers. Chronic aspirin therapy that is effective ranges in dosages of 80 to 325 mg per day. The minimal effective dosage is a loading dose of 160 mg and chronic therapy with 80 mg (possibly 50 mg) per day. This minimal but effective therapy is advised whenever aspirin is used with an anticoagulant so that side effects of bleeding are minimized. Aspirin dosages above this do not increase the antithrombotic effect. Aspirin dosages above 325 mg per day only increase the incidence of gastrointestinal side effects (indigestion and upper gastrointestinal bleeding).

Heparin

Heparin primarily acts as a catalyst of thrombin inactivation by antithrombin III. With a lower efficiency it also catalyzes inactivation of factors Xa, IXa, XIa, and XIIa. Immediate antithrombotic therapy with heparin is best achieved by administration of a bolus (5,000 to 10,000 U; the higher dose is used when there is ongoing thrombosis, because this is often associated with relative heparin resistance [see Fig. 2]), with a simultaneous infusion of 1,300 U per hour (goal approximately 31,000 U per day) to maintain the aPTT in therapeutic range. The heparin bolus serves to saturate all of the intravascular heparin-binding sites to achieve a therapeutic level maintained by the continuous heparin infusion. Starting and continuing therapy with only subcutaneous heparin delays the onset of therapeutic levels by as much as 2 days. If this approach is employed, one should begin with an initial dose of 20,000 U subcutaneously followed by the minimal therapeutic dosage of 12,500 U every 12 hours to achieve an aPTT of 1.5 to 2.0 × control at 8 to 12 hours after the initial dose. The subcutaneous dose often needs to be increased to maintain a therapeutic effect.

Heparin-induced thrombocytopenia may occur in 0.5 to 5.0 percent of patients given therapeutic levels of heparin. Paradoxically, it is more often associated with thrombosis rather than bleeding, and may lead to major

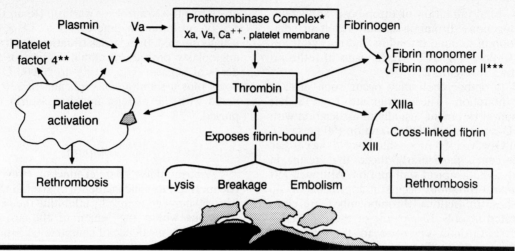

*Protects Xa from heparin-antithrombin III
**Neutralizes heparin
***Inhibits heparin-antithrombin III interaction with thrombin

Figure 2 Disturbance of thrombus by lysis (endogenous or exogenous), mechanical breakage (including coronary angioplasty), or spontaneous embolism exposes thrombin bound to fibrin. Thrombin activates platelets, and also activates factor V (which accelerates thrombin generation by 278,000 times via the prothrombinase complex $-\text{Ca}^{++}$ and factors Va and Xa assembled on a lipid membrane such as the platelet membrane). Thrombin converts fibrinogen to fibrin I and fibrin II, and activates factors XIII to XIIIa (which cross-link fibrin). These processes combine to produce rethrombosis. Heparin may only partially prevent rethrombosis because factor Xa within the prothrombinase complex is protected from heparin–antithrombin III. Furthermore, platelet factor 4 neutralizes heparin, and fibrin monomer II inhibits heparin–antithrombin III, the major inhibitor of thrombin.

venous or arterial occlusion, stroke, amputation, or death. Most episodes occur at least 7 days after exposure to heparin; this appear to be an immune-mediated phenomenon. Occasionally it does not recur with a rechallenge. It is twice as likely to occur with the use of bovine heparin as with porcine heparin, is not prevented by substituting low-molecular-weight heparin, and usually resolves uneventfully after discontinuation of heparin therapy. Because of the possibility of this side effect, platelet counts should be monitored in all patients when heparin is administered for longer than 7 days. In addition, if chronic anticoagulation is being considered for a heparinized patient, oral anticoagulants should be started expeditiously so as to achieve therapeutic oral anticoagulation quickly (i.e., within 3 days) to reduce heparin exposure.

Heparin also inhibits aldosterone synthesis. Rare cases of heparin-induced hypoaldosteronism with associated hyperkalemia and death have been reported in patients receiving heparin for more than several days. Hypersensitivity reactions are rare and may include urticaria, conjunctivitis, rhinitis, asthma, angioneurotic edema, and anaphylactic shock.

Warfarin

Warfarin inhibits the synthesis of the vitamin K–dependent coagulation proteins: factors II (prothrombin), VII, IX, and X and protein C and protein S.

Warfarin dosage to maintain therapeutic prothrombin time values (INR 3.0 to 4.5) averages 4.5 mg per day for individuals under age 75 and approximately 3.5 mg per day for those over age 75. A loading dose of approximately twice the expected daily dose may be used, followed by the expected daily dose. If patients are being switched from heparin to warfarin, an overlap of approximately 3 to 5 days is desirable to allow reduction of all vitamin K clotting factors before commencing warfarin alone. The dosage of warfarin will also depend on the patient's nutritional status and concomitant medical therapy. Antibiotic therapy may destroy vitamin K–producing bacteria in the gut and thus considerably reduce the therapeutic dosage of warfarin. Prothrombin times should be rechecked whenever concomitant medication is altered (added, deleted, or dosage changed). Routine rechecks of prothrombin times should be done at intervals of approximately 4 weeks.

Recent data suggest that increased variability of the prothrombin time increases the risk of thromboembolic events, particularly if the prothrombin time is periodically below therapeutic values. In addition, bleeding complications may result if the prothrombin time is too high. Bleeding during therapeutic prothrombin times (especially shortly after the initiation of therapy) might suggest an underlying latent disease process such as a tumor or gastrointestinal ulceration.

A rare and poorly understood complication of coumarin-type oral anticoagulants such as warfarin is hemorrhagic skin necrosis. Typically, these patients present with a discrete, painful, maculopapular eruption at a site with abundant subcutaneous adipose tissue such as the buttocks, thighs, and breast, usually after 4 to 10 days of therapy. These areas become hemorrhagic and bullous and proceed to necrosis. Warfarin necrosis occurs more frequently in females and is occasionally fatal. It is not usually associated with excessive anticoagulation, but may be associated with either protein C or protein S deficiency. Histologic studies of the lesion reveal thrombosis of the dermal capillaries and small venules. These thrombotic occlusions are thought to be due to a relative hypercoagulable state induced in the initial phase of anticoagulant therapy, during which protein C levels may decline faster than the other vitamin K–dependent proteins. (Unlike the other vitamin K–dependent proteins, protein C inhibits coagulation by cleaving with activated factors V and VIII.) However, this does not explain the localization of thrombosis to dermal vessels. It is unclear whether there is any effective therapy, but heparin may abort the development of skin necrosis in some patients (by inhibiting thrombosis) and thus should be tried along with discontinuation of warfarin. In cases in which life-long anticoagulant therapy may be required, such patients may be restarted on warfarin at a low dose such as 1 mg per day, while administering therapeutic doses of heparin and increasing warfarin gradually over several weeks. This would avoid abrupt falls in protein C levels before there is a reduction in levels of factors II, IX, and X.

THERAPEUTIC RECOMMENDATIONS

Unstable Angina or Non–Q-Wave Myocardial Infarction

The goals of antithrombotic therapy are to prevent the growth of thrombus and thus prevent recurrent ischemia, myocardial infarction, and death. An additional goal is to inhibit thrombosis so as to allow endogenous lysis of the residual mural thrombus. Optimal antithrombotic therapy would include intravenous heparin (100 U per kilogram bolus plus infusion to prolong the aPTT to 2 to 3 × control) plus platelet inhibition with aspirin (80 to 160 mg per day). Patients with unstable angina receiving no heparin therapy prior to coronary angioplasty have a lower success rate of angioplasty, increased incidence of thrombus in the coronary artery after percutaneous transluminal coronary angioplasty (PTCA), a higher incidence of acute occlusion with PTCA, and a higher risk of angioplasty-associated myocardial infarction, emergency coronary bypass surgery, or death. In medically treated patients without coronary revascularization, heparin should be converted to warfarin (INR 3.0 to 4.5 or prothrombin time 1.5-1.8 × control for thromboplastins with an ISI of 2.2 to 2.6) and continued on warfarin therapy for approximately 3 months along with aspirin 80 mg per day for maximal antithrombotic effectiveness. Nitrates and cal-

cium blockers may be used concomitantly to prevent coronary vasoconstriction or spasm that is associated with acute arterial injury (especially in the presence of thrombus) and may increase shear forces and platelet deposition.

When antithrombotic therapy is effective, patients with unstable angina may be treated medically without routine urgent coronary angiography. If there is no recurrence of symptoms on medical therapy, a predischarge exercise test may be performed to rule out residual ischemia. If there is no ischemia at a low work load, antithrombotic and antianginal therapy is continued to allow endogenous lysis of the residual mural thrombus. Improved antithrombotic therapy in the future may ultimately decrease the need for revascularization procedures, which are currently performed in approximately 40 to 50 percent of patients with unstable angina. Currently there are no data to support thrombolytic therapy in patients with unstable angina because emergency salvage of myocardium is not an issue, and systemic thrombolytic therapy carries a small but finite risk of cerebral bleeding. Effective antithrombotic therapy that promotes endogenous lysis may also prevent progression of coronary artery disease at the site of plaque rupture.

Acute or Evolving Q-Wave Myocardial Infarction

In patients presenting with prolonged ischemic myocardial pain of more than 30 minutes' duration who have no contraindication to anticoagulant therapy, heparin may be started with a bolus (100 U per kilogram) and a simultaneous infusion (1300 U per hour) titrated to prolong the aPTT to 2 to 3 × control.

Thrombolysis

Ninety-nine percent of patients with ST-segment elevation in two or more contiguous ECG leads and with chest pain as above will develop an acute myocardial infarction. Unless it is contraindicated, these patients may be treated with thrombolytic therapy, which may include recombinant tissue plasminogen activator (rt-PA), streptokinase, urokinase, or combined rt-PA–streptokinase or rt-PA–urokinase. With any of these thrombolytic therapies, simultaneous administration of heparin as described above appears optimal for the prevention of reocclusion and should be combined with aspirin, 160 mg per day as the loading dose and 80 mg per day thereafter. The intravenous heparin infusion is continued for 3 to 5 days and followed by subcutaneous heparin, 12,500 U every 12 hours (adjusting the aPTT to 1.5 to 2.5 × control, 6 to 12 hours after the previous dose) for approximately 5 days or until hospital discharge.

Adjunctive therapy with nitrates may be advantageous in reducing vasoconstriction at the site of the coronary lesion, since vasoconstriction increases local shear force and subsequent platelet deposition, a major contributing factor to rethrombosis. Nitrates produce an endothelium-independent vasodilation, which reduces shear force and also may enhance delivery of the thrombolytic agent to the site of thrombosis. Nitroglycerin may also reduce platelet deposition at the site of arterial injury and thus enhance thrombolysis. Intravenous nitroglycerin may be used empirically for approximately 24 hours. The calcium blocker diltiazem may be beneficial if there is good left ventricular function (ejection fraction greater than 40 percent).

Beta-adrenergic antagonists may be employed in the absence of contraindications (i.e., heart rate less than 55 beats per minute (bpm), systolic blood pressure less than 90 mm Hg, moist rales less than one-third of the lung fields, advanced atrioventricular block, or asthma). One regimen employs metoprolol, administered in three 5-mg intravenous injections at 5-minute intervals (observing closely the heart rate and blood pressure response) followed by oral metoprolol at 50 mg twice a day for the first day and 100 mg twice daily thereafter as tolerated. The intravenous bolus and subsequent oral dosage may be reduced if the target heart rate (approximately 60 bpm) and blood pressure (approximately 100 to 120 mm Hg systolic) are reached at lower doses. This therapy reduces myocardial demands, myocardial ischemia, and possibly necrosis. Beta-blocker therapy may also reduce the risk of intracerebral bleeding during thrombolytic therapy, as suggested by a retrospective analysis in Thrombolysis in Myocardial Infarction (TIMI) II in which none of over 600 patients on metoprolol had a cerebral bleed.

Coronary angiography may be considered if patients have recurrent ischemia, heart failure, or a positive exercise test at the time of discharge. Nearly 30 percent of patients may have recurrent chest pain during hospitalization.

During the first year after myocardial infarction treated with thrombolytic therapy, rehospitalization for recurrent ischemia or infarction has been required in nearly 30 percent of patients. Thus, patients who have incurred acute ischemic syndromes may benefit from oral warfarin therapy for approximately 3 months after the episode to encourage endogenous lysis of residual coronary thrombus. This approach may minimize coronary disease progression and recurrence of symptoms due to the infarct-related artery. Definitive trials to test this hypothesis are planned. The Warfarin Reinfarction Study (WARIS trial) has demonstrated the benefit of warfarin compared with placebo in the secondary prevention of myocardial infarction at rates comparable with those of aspirin therapy. The combination of warfarin and low-dose aspirin may be even more beneficial and requires further study. High-risk patients with a residual mural thrombus or a stenosis greater than 50 percent in the infarct-related artery may benefit most from this combined therapy.

Therapy Without Thrombolysis

Patients who arrive too late for thrombolytic therapy or in whom it is contraindicated may also benefit from the above antithrombotic therapy so as to encourage recanalization of the infarct-related artery. A persistently patent infarct-related artery appears beneficial for reducing future mortality and morbidity.

Prevention of Arterial Thromboembolism

Patients with acute anterior myocardial infarction or other infarction involving the left ventricular apex have a high risk of apical mural thrombosis and subsequent arterial thromboembolism. Subcutaneous heparin, 12,500 U every 12 hours, significantly reduces the incidence of left ventricular mural thrombus. However, the incidence (11 to 18 percent) of mural thrombus in the subcutaneous heparin group could probably be reduced even further with initial intravenous therapy so as to avoid the delay in reaching therapeutic levels. Thus, acute therapy with intravenous heparin and subsequent conversion to subcutaneous heparin may further reduce the incidence of mural thrombus. By meta-analysis of a number of studies, it is clear that heparin reduces the incidence of systemic embolism.

The peak incidence of embolism is during the first 7 to 10 days after infarction, and most of the remaining embolic events occur during the next 3 months. Mural thrombi and thus emboli are generally associated with persistent and severe left ventricular dysfunction and localized apical dyskinesis. Anticoagulation is most effective if started immediately, because emboli may occur before thrombus is visible on echocardiography. However, anticoagulation also appears to benefit patients with established thrombi.

The echocardiographic features of left ventricular mural thrombus frequently change spontaneously over time. Although many thrombi disappear during anticoagulation, some may recur soon after anticoagulants are stopped. Thus, it is advisable to continue therapy with oral anticoagulation for approximately 3 months after the acute myocardial infarction. Therapy should be continued indefinitely if there is diffusely abnormal left ventricular function with an ejection fraction under 30 percent. Patients with only localized apical dyskinesis have a long-term thromboembolic rate of less than 1 percent per year and do not appear to require chronic anticoagulation. Antiplatelet agents appear to be of little benefit in preventing left ventricular thrombi.

Venous Thromboembolism

All patients with acute myocardial infarction are at risk for venous thromboembolism, especially those with large infarcts or heart failure, those immobilized for more than 1 to 3 days, those over age 70, and those with a history of venous thrombosis. Early mobilization reduces venous thrombosis and embolism. Those patients not fully anticoagulated should receive low-dose heparin (5,000 U subcutaneously two or three times daily) prior to mobilization, which should be achieved as soon as possible.

SUGGESTED READING

Chesebro JH, Zoldhelyi P, Fuster V. Pathogenesis of thrombosis in unstable angina. Am J Cardiol 1991 (in press).

Fuster V, Badimon L, Chesebro JH. Coronary artery disease progression and acute coronary syndromes. N Engl J Med 1991 (in press).

Fuster V, Stein B, Ambrose JA, et al. Atherosclerotic plaque rupture and thrombosis: evolving concepts. Circulation 1990; 82(Suppl II):II-47–II-59.

Stein B, Fuster V, Halperin JL, Chesebro JH. Antithrombotic therapy in cardiac disease. An emerging approach based on pathogenesis and risk. Circulation 1989; 80:1501–1513.

Webster MWI, Chesebro JH, Fuster V. Antithrombotic therapy in acute myocardial infarction: enhancement of thrombolysis, reduction of reocclusion, and prevention of thromboembolism. In: Gersh BJ, Rahimtoola SH, eds. Acute myocardial infarction. Elsevier, 1991:333.

SILENT MYOCARDIAL ISCHEMIA

ALAN C. YEUNG, M.D.
ANDREW P. SELWYN, M.D.

Silent myocardial ischemia has long been recognized as an important clinical expression of coronary artery disease. However, only recently has clinical research demonstrated the important association with increased risk, thus raising important questions about management. In this chapter we consider the management strategy in patients with asymptomatic ischemia as detected by noninvasive testing, including exercise tolerance tests or ambulatory electrocardiographic (ECG) monitoring. We address the approach in patients with unstable angina, post–myocardial infarction ischemia, stable angina, and patients who are completely asymptomatic.

To grasp the implications of silent ischemia in particular, it is necessary to understand the pathophysiology of ischemia in general. Traditionally, ischemia is thought to occur when myocardial demand exceeds the fixed blood supply limited by coronary stenoses. Chierchia provided indirect evidence of a decrease in regional coronary blood supply preceding any hemodynamic or electrocardiographic changes in patients with rest angina. Thus, he implied that coronary stenoses may possess important dynamic functions and that this interaction with oxygen demand can precipitate ischemia. Studies using short-lived radioisotopes and provocative studies in the cardiac catheterization laboratory have shown that atherosclerotic stenoses constrict inappropriately, playing an important pathogenic role at the onset of transient ischemia. Studies out of the hospital in ambulatory patients have shown that ischemic episodes occur during physical and mental stress and are distributed over 24 hours in a circadian fashion; 75 percent of these events are asymptomatic.

APPROACH TO MANAGEMENT

The approach to patients with silent ischemia integrates the clinical characteristics of each patient derived from the history, physical examination, risk factor stratification, and noninvasive testing. The clinician must consider the method of detection, the setting in which it occurs, and the extent or severity of ischemia. Also, the presence of ischemia must be considered in the context of coronary anatomy and left ventricular function. Since there are no randomized studies that specifically address the management of silent ischemia, the clinician must individualize the synthesis of test results and devise a treatment plan for each patient.

The exercise test is the most frequent method for detection of ischemia, with or without radionuclide imaging of regional coronary blood flow or ventricular function. The important prognostic variables measured during the exercise test include exercise duration, maximal heart rate and blood pressure response, time to ST-segment depression, and degree of maximal ST-segment depression. Other noninvasive tests available include ambulatory ECG monitoring, which can provide the clinician with the number of ischemic episodes per 24 hours, the total duration of ischemia, the heart rate at which it occurs, and the activities that most often precipitate it. The presence or absence of symptoms during these studies should also be noted. In general, if the exercise test results are negative or strongly positive, ambulatory monitoring will provide little additional information. In patients whose exercise tests are mildly positive, ambulatory monitoring will help to further stratify their risks of future adverse events.

Unstable Angina

Patients with unstable angina are a heterogeneous group. The common theme is that they all have worsening symptoms of ischemia, those showing objective signs of ischemia at rest having the highest risk. It is clear from many clinical studies that routine medical therapy is highly effective in eliminating symptomatic ischemia, and that heparin or aspirin reduces coronary events. However, it is widely held that in patients with unstable angina who continue to be symptomatic on medical therapy, an early aggressive strategy should be followed by documentation of coronary anatomy and left ventricular function. It should be emphasized that randomized controlled trials comparing medical and surgical therapy have failed to demonstrate a survival benefit for all patients with unstable angina; benefit has been shown for subgroups such as those with left main or three-vessel disease, or multivessel disease and left ventricular dysfunction. There have been no equivalent randomized trials comparing coronary angioplasty with medical treatment, even though angioplasty has been shown to be effective in reducing ischemia and symptoms. The procedure itself is undertaken with increased risk of acute closure, presumably owing to the presence of intracoronary thrombus. It is generally agreed that a period of anticoagulation with intravenous heparin (3 to 7 days) should be initiated before the procedure. The risk and benefit of thrombolytic therapy (TIMI III) in unstable angina is being investigated; this strategy may reduce the need for emergent intervention in selected unstable patients. Thus, in patients whose symptoms continue despite medical therapy, an aggressive strategy is customary and acceptable practice.

The management strategy is less clear for patients with unstable angina whose symptoms resolve with medical therapy. Gottlieb and colleagues showed that silent ischemia documented on continuous ECG monitoring despite medical therapy conferred a worse prognosis, with an increased occurrence of myocardial infarction and death for up to 2 years. The implication is that these patients should undergo early invasive intervention. Conversely, those who have no further ischemic episodes can be considered at low risk, and early ambulation can be advised. An exercise test is then performed; if this test is positive for exercise-induced ischemia, invasive studies to evaluate coronary anatomy are pursued. Although this is the standard management strategy employed in these patients (Fig. 1), it has not been shown to reduce mortality, morbidity, or cost in controlled trials. In the future, success may be improved by better methods to identify patients requiring intervention such as real-time digital systems for ST-segment monitoring in the coronary care unit.

Post–Myocardial Infarction Ischemia

In the early hours of myocardial infarction with ST-segment elevation, extensive investigations support the use of thrombolytic therapy. The treatment of arrhythmias and heart failure and medical therapy for recurrent ischemia are standard in modern coronary care units. For patients who develop recurrent angina, persistent congestive failure, and complex arrhythmias, invasive investigations are customary, and revascularization procedures are performed according to the severity of the coronary disease. For patients who remain asymptomatic during the early postinfarct course, the treatment strategy hinges upon risk assessment, with the goal of preventing reinfarction or death. This involves the assessment of residual ischemia and left ventricular function. Studies have shown that if 100 patients are asymptomatic at discharge, 30 to 40 of them will have provocable ischemia on exercise stress testing (≥ 1 mm ST-segment depression). Thirty to 40 percent of these patients will have no symptoms. The literature and

clinical experience suggest that all patients with ischemia should be treated in a similar fashion regardless of symptoms. The current standard of care is for these patients to undergo coronary angiography and revascularization as necessary.

The use of ambulatory monitoring as an independent test after myocardial infarction is controversial. However, if the exercise test is equivocal, if the patient cannot exercise to a satisfactory degree, and if there is an adequate baseline ECG signal permitting interpretation of the ST segment, the literature supports the use of ambulatory monitoring to stratify the risk of adverse events. There is an increased risk of myocardial infarction and death when myocardial ischemia is detected by both exercise testing and ambulatory ECG monitoring. However, the latter test does not generally alter the approach in a patient with a positive exercise test, because invasive studies are usually initiated when strong evidence of ischemia is detected by exercise testing alone.

Patients whose ECG may obscure ischemic changes (left bundle branch block, left ventricular hypertrophy or

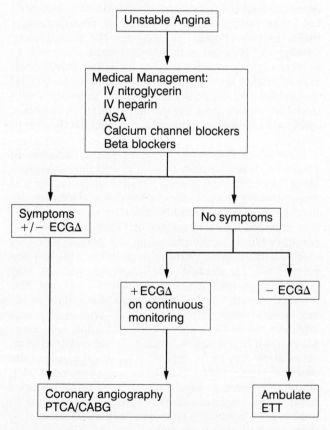

Figure 1 Management strategy for patients with unstable angina and silent ischemia. ECG, electrocardiographic evidence of myocardial ischemia during continuous ECG monitoring; ETT, exercise treadmill test; PTCA, coronary angioplasty; CABG, coronary artery bypass grafting; ASA, aspirin.

digitalis effect, extensive Q waves) are candidates for exercise testing with radionuclide studies. If a patient cannot exercise, intravenous or oral dipyridamole (Persantine) with thallium scintigraphy may be used. After myocardial infarction, evidence of ischemia by noninvasive testing should be aggressively evaluated and treated, regardless of symptoms. This approach is justified because postinfarction ischemia is a strong independent measure of increased risk, adding to the risk imposed by reduced left ventricular function and multivessel disease. Evidence of increased risk mandates aggressive management.

Stable Angina

Traditionally, management of patients with chronic stable angina has been shaped by the patient's symptoms and by information obtained from noninvasive testing such as exercise tolerance tests. Patients who have symptoms refractory to medical management, or who have markedly positive exercise test results, are referred for coronary angiography. On the basis of the angiographic results, medical therapy is continued or coronary bypass surgery or angioplasty advised. Obviously, opinions differ over when patients should undergo invasive investigation and therapy, but generally management strategy has been symptom driven. However, in the last few years it has become clear that in patients with stable coronary disease the lack of symptoms does not imply

decreased risk, because symptomatic anginal episodes represent less than one-third of their total ischemic episodes during daily life. Patients who have positive exercise test results and have episodes of asymptomatic ischemia on ambulatory ECG monitoring, on or off medical therapy, have a worse prognosis (death, myocardial infarction) in the succeeding 2 years (Fig. 2). This prognostic power is independent of the exercise test variables (total duration, time to ST-segment depression) and other clinical variables. It seems logical that the elimination of all ischemic episodes, whether symptomatic or not, will decrease the occurrence of adverse events. If this hypothesis is confirmed by future studies, it mandates a management strategy that is not exclusively driven by symptoms. This new strategy might include routine exercise testing and/or ambulatory monitoring to detect residual ischemia. If the patient has no further symptoms but continues to have objective evidence of ischemia, medical therapy is intensified. If ischemia continues to be present, invasive testing is considered. This proposed strategy seems to be a rational response to the new information regarding silent ischemia, although currently no clinical studies are available to support this approach. In 1991 the National Institutes of Health will conduct a multicenter trial, the Asymptomatic Cardiac Ischemia Pilot (ACIP), to address this issue. In the meantime, selection of patients for more aggressive evaluation and therapy will be based on symptoms or evidence of exercise-induced myocardial

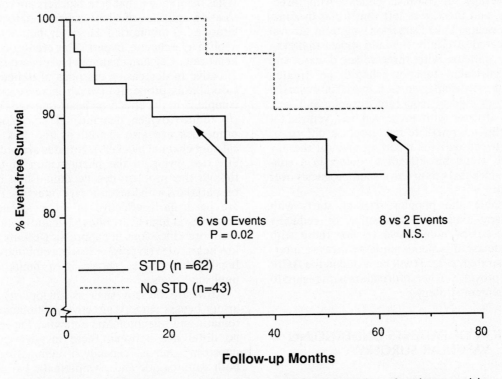

Figure 2 Kaplan-Meier curves comparing the cumulative proportion of patients surviving without cardiac death or infarction. All patients initially presented with stable angina and are divided into two groups based on whether or not ambulatory ECG monitoring revealed evidence of ST-segment depression (STD).

ischemia. In patients with stable angina who cannot exercise or in those with Prinzmetal's angina, ambulatory ECG monitoring, dipyridamole-thallium scan, or echocardiography can provide viable alternatives for risk stratification.

Asymptomatic Patients

In asymptomatic patients with no coronary risk factors, the prevalence of coronary artery disease is low and a search for silent ischemia will generate a significant number of false-positive results. Thus, routine screening is not justified. Patients with specific concerns (e.g., commercial airline pilots) and those with many risk factors may merit noninvasive testing. In this setting, negative or strongly positive tests are most useful; equivocal tests may require further evaluation, e.g., diagnostic angiography, to determine further management. Asymptomatic patients with strongly positive exercise tests pose a special challenge in management. Using the Coronary Artery Surgery Study (CASS) registry, Weiner and colleagues showed that patients who had exercise-induced ischemia, with or without symptoms, had a worse prognosis over 7 years than those without ischemia. Thus, it could be argued that ischemia, whether silent or not, should be treated in the same fashion. In a nonrandomized comparison in the CASS registry and the European Cooperative Study, the survival of patients with one- or two-vessel disease was not different whether they received medical or surgical therapy. In contrast, patients with three-vessel disease, and those with left ventricular dysfunction or severe ischemia, had superior long-term survival rates when treated surgically. It would appear that even asymptomatic patients with three-vessel disease and poor left ventricular function should be treated surgically; aggressive management is more controversial for patients with mild to moderate ischemia and one- or two-vessel disease with preserved left ventricular function. In this intermediate-risk group, a difference in survival between patients receiving medical therapy or angioplasty would be difficult to detect in a controlled study, since this group has a good prognosis over a long period.

A reasonable and popular strategy starts with medical therapy aimed at eliminating or reducing ischemia detected by noninvasive testing; those with continued evidence of ischemia undergo invasive intervention. This strategy (Fig. 3) will be tested in the ACIP study and will provide further information with regard to overall management strategy.

EVALUATION OF PATIENTS UNDERGOING VASCULAR SURGERY

Patients undergoing vascular surgery have a high pretest likelihood of coronary artery disease and are at risk of perioperative ischemia, myocardial infarction, and even death. A high percentage of these patients are asymptomatic and often cannot exercise, and thus pose a special problem in management. Raby and colleagues demonstrated that patients with evidence of ischemia on ambulatory monitoring exhibit a tenfold increase in the risk of postoperative unstable angina, myocardial infarction, or death. A study is currently under way to evaluate a management strategy for these patients. Patients with proven coronary artery disease or two risk factors, especially diabetes, will undergo ambulatory ECG monitoring. Those with no ischemia will undergo routine pre- and intraoperative care. Those patients with more than 120 minutes (cumulative) of ischemic episodes occurring over a 24-hour period will undergo invasive evaluation. Patients with 1 to 120 minutes of ischemia will have their antianginal medications increased and undergo further monitoring. If evidence of ischemia persists, patients will undergo a dipyridamole-thallium test and/or invasive studies, and revascularization will be considered. This strategy will be examined in a controlled study to determine whether it results in a reduction in perioperative morbidity and mortality.

THERAPEUTIC OPTIONS

As stated earlier, the pathogenesis of silent ischemia includes an increase in myocardial oxygen demand, and episodic coronary vasoconstriction. Thus, medical treatment should be aimed toward both supply and demand. It has been shown that beta-blockers are very effective in treating episodes of silent ischemia detected by ambulatory ECG monitoring. However, beta-blockers do not abolish all ischemia, in particular events occurring at low heart rate. Calcium channel blockers are somewhat less effective in decreasing episodes of ischemia, but their vasodilatory properties (which increase oxygen supply) complement the effects on heart rate and cardiac output (to reduce oxygen demand) of beta-blockers (which properties are also shared by the less vasoselective calcium channel blockers). Nitrates are only moderately effective owing to the phenomenon of tolerance, although this problem can be diminished by using oral preparations with longer dosage intervals. Beta-blockers are particularly effective in reducing silent ischemia occurring at high heart rates (demand), whereas nitrates are more efficacious in suppressing events that occur at low heart rates (supply). Clearly, combination therapy is highly effective, as shown in a limited number of published trials.

Invasive therapy such as angioplasty or coronary artery bypass surgery effectively eliminate both symptomatic and asymptomatic ischemia. There seems to be no difference between these invasive procedures in improving exercise capacity or eliminating ischemia in both symptomatic and asymptomatic patients. There is no definitive proof of improved survival rates in patients with silent ischemia undergoing bypass surgery or angioplasty.

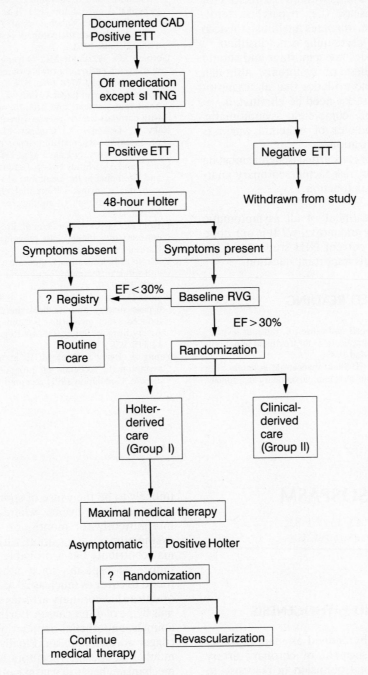

Figure 3 Management strategy for patients with stable angina and silent ischemia as proposed in the NIH-ACIP trial.

DISCUSSION

In the past decade, silent ischemia has been recognized and characterized as an important clinical concept. Many investigators have shown it to have prognostic significance in patients with unstable angina, postinfarction angina, and chronic stable angina, and even in asymptomatic men. However, studies addressing the specific management issues of silent myocardial ischemia are lacking. Thus, the current management of silent ischemia can be summarized as follows:

1. The absence of ischemia predicts an excellent prognosis.

2. In asymptomatic patients with no risk factors for coronary artery disease (i.e., hypercholesterolemia, hypertension, diabetes mellitus, tobacco use, family history), screening is not justified.
3. All ischemic episodes are important and should be treated regardless of symptoms, although currently there is no evidence that all asymptomatic ischemic episodes need be eliminated.
4. In patients who are completely asymptomatic, only profound evidence of ischemia warrants invasive revascularization.
5. The management of myocardial ischemia must be based on symptoms, risk factors, coronary anatomy, and ventricular function.

Will the effective treatment of all asymptomatic ischemia reduce morbidity and mortality? It is our hope and expectation that the current NIH studies (ACIP) will successfully answer this important question.

SUGGESTED READING

Deanfield JE, Selwyn AP. Character and causes of transient myocardial ischemia during daily life. Implications for treatment of patients with coronary disease. Am J Med 1986.
Gohlke C, Droste C, Roskamm H. Silent myocardial ischemia after bypass surgery and percutaneous transluminal coronary angioplasty.
In: Kellermann J, Braunwald E, eds. Adv cardiol: Silent myocardial ischemia: A critical appraisal. Basel: Karger, 1990:288.
Gordon J, Ganz P, Nabel E, et al. Atherosclerosis and endothelial function influence the coronary response to exercise. J Clin Invest 1989; 83:1946–1952.
Gottlieb SO, Weisfeldt ML, Ouyang P, et al. Silent ischemia as a marker for early unfavorable outcomes in patients with unstable angina. N Engl J Med 1986; 314:1214–1219.
McLenachan J, Weidinger F, Barry J, et al. The relationship between heart rate, ischemia and drug therapy during daily life in patients with coronary artery disease. Circulation 1991 (in press).
Raby K, Goldman L, Creager M, et al. Correlation between preoperative ischemia and major cardiac events after peripheral vascular surgery. N Engl J Med 1989; 321:1296–1300.
Stone P and ASIS Study Group. Comparison of propranolol, diltiazem, and nifedipine in the treatment of ambulatory ischemia in patients with stable angina: Differential effects on ambulatory ischemia, exercise performance, and angina symptoms. Circulation 1990; 82:1962–1972.
Tzivoni D, Gavish A, Zin D, et al. Prognostic significance of ischemia episodes in patients with previous myocardial infarction. Am J Cardiol 1988; 62:661–664.
Veterans Administration Cooperative Study. Comparison of medical and surgical treatment for unstable angina pectoris. N Engl J Med 1987; 316:977.
Weiner D, Ryan T, McCabe C, et al. Comparison of coronary artery bypass surgery and medical therapy in patients with exercise-induced silent myocardial ischemia: A report from the Coronary Artery Surgery Study (CASS) Registry. J Am Coll Cardiol 1988; 12:595–599.
Yeung A, Barry J, Bonassin E, et al. Time dependent effects of asymptomatic ischemia on prognosis in chronic stable coronary disease. Circulation 1991; accepted for publication.

CORONARY VASOSPASM

FILIPPO CREA, MD, F.A.C.C., F.E.S.C.
ATTILIO MASERI, F.R.C.P., F.A.C.C.

DEFINITION AND PATHOGENESIS

Coronary spasm can be defined as inappropriate, active constriction of a segment of coronary artery resulting in total or subtotal occlusion in response to stimuli that cause only minimal constriction in the adjacent segments. It is due to the variable interaction of two components: (1) a local alteration in a segment of epicardial coronary artery that makes it hyperreactive to constrictor stimuli and (2) a variety of constrictor stimuli that cause only mild coronary constriction in patients without variant angina and in the nonspastic coronary segments in patients with variant angina.

The precise causes of the hyperreactivity are as yet unknown. Certainly the syndrome of variant angina is too rare to be explained simply by those alterations, such as atheromatous plaques, frequently found in the coronary arteries. Plaque rupture or fissuring are also unlikely to be the cause of spontaneous spasm, because these are acute events, whereas variant angina occurs intermittently for months or even years. Endothelial dysfunction in association with atheromatous plaques may contribute but is probably not sufficient by itself to induce vasospasm, since atheromatous plaques are found to cover as much as 20 to 30 percent of the surface of epicardial coronary arteries of asymptomatic individuals dying of other causes. Furthermore, in experimental animals, endothelial denudation alone is insufficient to trigger coronary spasm. Finally, a local increase in the number of specific receptors has to be ruled out as a mechanism, because spasm can be triggered in the same patient by many unrelated stimuli, such as ergonovine, histamine, dopamine, hyperventilation, and exercise and cold pressor tests. A local alteration of postreceptor signaling pathways in vascular smooth muscle cells is a more likely explanation. The fact that coronary spasm can be induced by increasing the arterial blood pH with hyperventilation seems consistent with this hypothesis. In a minority of patients presenting with the clinical syndrome of vasospastic angina, diffuse constriction of all epicardial coronary branches severe enough to cause myocardial ischemia is observed, rather than localized occlusive or subocclusive coronary spasm. Whether this "diffuse spasm" results from mechanisms different from

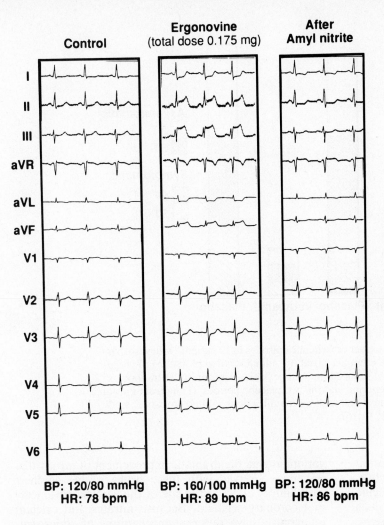

Figure 1 Typical electrocardiographic (ECG) response to ergonovine (total cumulative dose 175 μg) in a patient with coronary spasm of the right coronary artery. The patient developed severe chest pain and ST-segment elevation in inferior leads. The increase in heart rate and blood pressure is probably secondary to the stress caused by chest pain. The prompt administration of amyl nitrite resulted in a quick resolution of the vasospastic episode.

those responsible for occlusive segmental spasm remains to be established.

DIAGNOSIS

The clinical diagnosis of vasospastic angina should be considered when patients present with typical anginal pain recurring spontaneously, particularly at night and in the early morning, promptly relieved by sublingual nitrates, but with preserved or reasonably good effort tolerance. The presence during chest pain of palpitation or syncope is another important clue to the diagnosis of vasospastic angina. The electrocardiogram (ECG), however, is the key to the objective diagnosis of variant angina. Episodes of transient ST-segment elevation or pseudonormalization of negative T waves are pathognomonic of coronary spasm. In patients who have frequent anginal episodes, a 12-lead ECG recorded during chest pain, or ambulatory ECG monitoring, can usually identify the characteristic ischemic changes caused by coronary spasm. If anginal attacks are not frequent and ambulatory ECG monitoring does not provide objective evidence of episodes of transient myocardial ischemia, a maximal exercise test is mandatory (preferably after

discontinuation of antianginal therapy). If the exercise test is positive with typical ST-segment elevation and reproduces the symptoms, the diagnosis of vasospastic angina is documented.

Ergonovine may be used to establish the diagnosis of vasospastic angina in patients with episodes of a typical chest pain that are too rare to be investigated by ambulatory ECG monitoring (Fig. 1). Ergonovine can be infused intravenously (increasing doses of 25, 50, 100, 200, and 300 μg given at intervals of 5 minutes) during 12-lead ECG monitoring or selectively into the left or right coronary artery (increasing doses of 1, 2, 5, 10, and 20 μg) at the time of cardiac catheterization, followed by coronary angiography to document the presence of coronary spasm. The ergonovine test is potentially dangerous in patients with intense coronary hyperreactivity and should be performed only by experienced teams when appropriate.

THERAPY

In support of the hypothesis that vasospastic angina is due to a local hyperreactivity of vascular smooth muscle to all vasoconstrictor stimuli rather than a

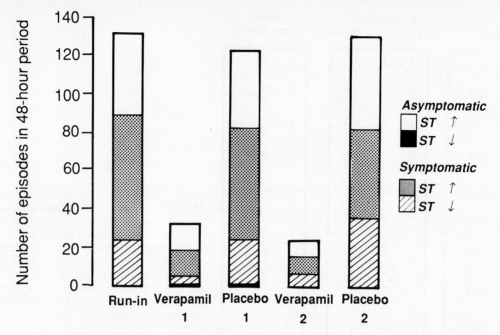

Figure 2 Effect of verapamil on the number of ischemic episodes in 12 patients with vasospastic angina. In this double-blind, double-cross-over trial the administration of 480 mg of verapamil per day (in both treatment periods) reduced the number of ischemic episodes by about 85 percent compared with both the run-in period and the two placebo periods. (Data from Parodi D, et al. Management of unstable angina at rest with verapamil: a double-blind cross-over study in a coronary care unit. Br Heart J 1979; 41:167–174.)

specific neurohumoral abnormality is the observation that specific vasoconstrictor antagonists are ineffective. Several clinical trials have demonstrated that specific blockade of adrenergic or serotoninergic receptors does not prevent vasospasm. Inhibition of thromboxane synthesis or action does not significantly affect the frequency and severity of coronary spasm. Conversely, drugs such as nitrates and calcium antagonists, which nonspecifically reduce the responsiveness of vascular smooth muscle to vasoconstrictor stimuli, are remarkably effective and represent the mainstay of therapy. Clinical trials have demonstrated that nitrates and calcium antagonists consistently and markedly reduce the frequency of spontaneous episodes of coronary spasm and improve prognosis in the vast majority of patients (Figs. 2 and 3). However, analysis of individual data shows that although near-total suppression of ischemic episodes is achieved in most patients, the beneficial effects in some are negligible. The reasons for these different responses in apparently similar patients are unknown.

Nitrates and Calcium Antagonists: Mechanism of Action, Dosage, and Therapy Monitoring

Both nitrates and calcium antagonists decrease intracellular calcium concentration, thus causing vasodilation of veins (in particular with nitrates), peripheral arterioles (in particular with calcium antagonists), and large epicardial coronary arteries. In patients with

variant angina the dramatic improvement of myocardial ischemia observed with these drugs is due to their vasodilatory effect at the site of the vasospastic epicardial coronary segment. Because nitrates and calcium antagonists have different mechanisms of action (nitrates reduce the intracellular release of calcium, whereas calcium antagonists block the entry of calcium into the cell), their vasodilatory actions may have additive effects.

In patients with variant angina who present with frequent and severe episodes of myocardial ischemia, especially if accompanied by threatening ventricular arrhythmias, the treatment of choice is intravenous administration of nitrates (nitroglycerin or isosorbide dinitrate [ISDN]). In fact, during the "hot" phases of the disease, the risk of myocardial infarction or sudden death is considerably high. ISDN is usually infused at a rate of 1 to 2 mg per hour; the dosage is then progressively increased until a pressure drop of 10 to 15 mm Hg is obtained. Oral administration of calcium antagonists is also recommended: verapamil, 240 to 480 mg per day; diltiazem, 180 to 360 mg per day; or nifedipine, 20 to 60 mg per day). This treatment controls the hot phase in the vast majority of patients with variant angina. Continuous ECG monitoring is important in determining the effect of the treatment. Once abolition of transient ischemic episodes has been achieved, oral treatment with slow-release nitrates (ISDN, 40 to 80 mg per day or isosorbide mononitrate, 20 to 40 mg per day, given intermittently to avoid tolerance) and a calcium

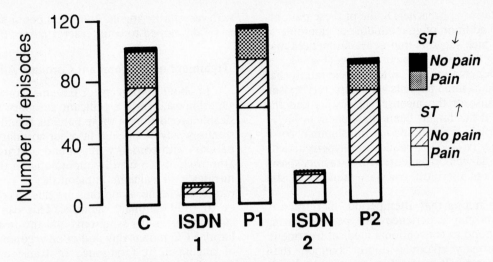

Figure 3 Effect of isosorbide dinitrate (ISDN) infusion on the number of ischemic episodes in 12 patients with vasospastic angina. In this double-blind, double-cross-over trial, ISDN administration at an infusion rate ranging between 1.25 and 5 mg per hour (periods 1 and 2) reduced the number of ischemic episodes by about 85 percent compared with both the run-in period (C) and the two placebo periods (P1 and P2). (Data from Distante A, et al. Management of vasospastic angina at rest with continuous infusion of isosorbide dinitrate: a double crossover study in a coronary care unit. Am J Cardiol 1979; 44:533–539.)

antagonist, at the dosages described above, is the treatment of choice. Sublingual nitrates (nitroglycerin, 0.25 mg or ISDN, 10 mg) or nifedipine (5 mg) can be used to relieve residual anginal attacks.

Nitrates may cause severe throbbing headache, which frequently spontaneously improves after the first few days of treatment. The development of tolerance, however, is the most important drawback of chronic treatment with nitrates. Intermittent administration of these drugs is appropriate in order to avoid the development of tolerance. Because patients with variant angina have many of their attacks at night and in the early morning hours, it is advisable to have the nadir of nitrate effect during the waking hours. Verapamil and diltiazem are the calcium antagonists of choice. Nifedipine, in association with nitrates, may cause excessive tachycardia and other unpleasant effects due to peripheral vasodilation such as headache and ankle swelling. Verapamil and diltiazem may cause P-R prolongation due to inhibition of calcium influx into the specialized myocytes of the conducting system. Therefore, their use is contraindicated in patients with sick sinus syndrome and atrioventricular conduction abnormalities; in these patients, nifedipine is preferable. Constipation is a frequent side effect of treatment with verapamil and diltiazem, although it is seldom severe enough to require interruption of the treatment.

Ambulatory ECG monitoring is an efficient, objective, and relatively inexpensive way to assess treatment efficacy, particularly when ischemic episodes are frequent. A confounding element is the frequent spontaneous variability of the symptoms. Therefore, ischemic episodes may disappear either in response to treatment or because of spontaneous waning of local coronary susceptibility to constrictor stimuli. Conversely, ischemic episodes may become more frequent, not because treatment is ineffective but because the susceptibility to spasm is increased by other factors as yet unknown. If the results of Holter monitoring are difficult to interpret, an ergonovine test on treatment may be useful. A positive response to the test indicates that the dosages of nitrates or calcium antagonists are insufficient and should be increased. When the therapy achieves the goal of persistently abolishing transient ischemic episodes over a period of several months, and the response to the ergonovine test on treatment is negative, gradual tapering of the drugs may be considered. At this stage a negative response to an ergonovine test performed off treatment is further evidence that the treatment can be tapered and perhaps even discontinued. However, as coronary spasm may recur, follow-up is mandatory.

Coronary Spasm Refractory to Treatment with Nitrates and Calcium Antagonists

As mentioned, in a small proportion of patients coronary spasm is refractory or becomes refractory to treatment with nitrates and calcium antagonists. This is indicated by the persistence of angina at rest (predominantly in the early morning hours) and episodes of ST-segment elevation or pseudonormalization of T waves during ambulatory ECG monitoring. In this case the dosage of nitrates and calcium antagonists may be considerably increased. We have used daily doses of verapamil and diltiazem up to 800 and 960 mg respectively, together with 80 mg of ISDN and 100 mg of nifedipine in the evening. If patients are refractory to these very high dosages, no consensus exists about the possible alternative approaches. Some of these patients respond to the addition of guanethidine or clonidine to the regimen, which suggests that neural influences may be contributing to spasm in these patients (Fig. 4).

Cardiac denervation or autotransplantation has been attempted in some patients with refractory spasm. However, because of the inconsistent results and the operative risk, it has largely been abandoned.

The potential of percutaneous transluminal coronary angioplasty (PTCA) to reduce the hyperreactivity of smooth vascular cells in patients with refractory spasm superimposed on a critical coronary stenosis is still unsettled.

It is worth noting that after periods of refractory angina, patients may experience long periods during which they respond to conventional medical treatment. Refractory coronary spasm is more common than previously suspected. It may play a critical role during the early phase of acute myocardial infarction. There is convincing evidence that coronary occlusion and myocardial infarction are often preceded or accompanied by periods of occlusion alternating with periods of reperfusion. Whereas permanent coronary occlusion is eventually caused by coronary thrombosis, the early phase of acute myocardial infarction may be characterized by transient thrombus formation and/or coronary spasm. This is suggested by experimental studies, as well as the clinical observation that in some cases intracoronary infusion of streptokinase may initially fail to achieve recanalization until administration of intracoronary nitrates. In this setting, coronary spasm may be refractory to intravenous administration of nitrates but respond to administration of nitroglycerin selectively into the infarct-related artery. Coronary spasm associated with acute myocardial infarction is more severe and refractory to therapy than that observed in most patients with vasospastic angina. New therapeutic strategies need to be developed to counteract it more effectively.

Treatment of Concomitant Coronary Atherosclerosis

In about 70 percent of patients, coronary spasm is superimposed on a significant coronary stenosis. In a sizable proportion of these patients significant coronary stenoses may be present in other coronary branches. If patients with coronary spasm and obstructive coronary atherosclerosis are still symptomatic on treatment with nitrates and calcium antagonists, it is important to establish whether symptoms are due to coronary spasm or to fixed coronary stenosis. This can be done by carefully assessing symptoms and the results of ambulatory ECG monitoring and of an ergonovine test. Lack of angina at rest, absence of transient ST-segment elevation or pseudonormalization of T waves during daily life, and a negative response to an ergonovine test strongly indicate that fixed coronary stenoses rather than coronary spasm are responsible for myocardial ischemia. A positive exercise test with ST-segment depression at low work load, performed on treatment with nitrates and calcium antagonists, will further confirm that myocardial ischemia is due to obstructive coronary atherosclerosis. If this is the case, any further medical or surgical management should be similar to that used in patients with chronic stable angina (see the three chapters on chronic ischemic heart disease, earlier in this section). It has been previously suggested that beta-blockers might be detrimental to coronary spasm because they allow unopposed alpha-receptor–mediated vasoconstriction. However, the observations that adrenergic agonists do not provoke coronary spasm, and that adrenergic antagonists do not prevent it, indicate that vasospasm is not a contraindication to the use of

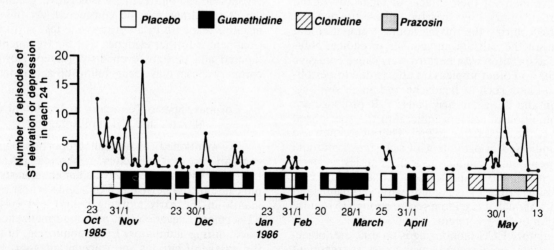

Figure 4 Number of ischemic episodes during intermittent ambulatory ECG monitoring over a period of 8 months in a patient with vasospastic angina refractory to treatment with nitrates and calcium antagonists. The addition of guanethidine or clonidine to treatment with nitrates and calcium antagonists (see text) resulted in an excellent control of ischemic episodes, whereas the addition of prazosin failed to produce any beneficial effect. (Data from Frennaux M, et al. Refractory variant angina relieved by guanethidine and clonidine. Am J Cardiol 1988; 62:832–833.)

beta-blockers. Furthermore, beta-blockers may also improve migraine (which is common in patients with variant angina and is often exacerbated by the use of vasodilators). With regard to PTCA, it is worth noting that dilatation of coronary stenoses associated with vasospasm is accompanied by a higher rate of acute complications and restenosis.

LIMITATIONS OF CURRENT APPROACH TO TREATMENT OF CORONARY SPASM

As outlined above, the fundamental abnormality in patients with vasospastic angina is a local hyperreactivity to vasoconstrictor stimuli in a segment of a coronary branch. The current treatment of coronary spasm is based on drugs that nonspecifically reduce smooth muscle tone and its reactivity to vasoconstrictor stimuli throughout the whole body. Although nitrates and calcium antagonists have been found to improve both symptoms and prognosis of vasospastic angina, they have systemic effects. An ideal therapeutic agent would specifically abolish the local coronary hyperreactivity without systemic effects.

The inability to target medical treatment with greater precision stems from the lack of knowledge of the mechanism of local coronary hyperreactivity. In-creased understanding of the mechanism of coronary vasospasm will allow us to develop more specific pharmacologic interventions without systemic side effects. This knowledge will also improve the treatment of coronary spasm, which is refractory to the agents currently available.

SUGGESTED READING

Distante A, Maseri A, Severi S, et al. Management of vasospastic angina at rest with continuous infusion of isosorbide dinitrate: a double crossover study in a coronary care unit. Am J Cardiol 1979; 44:533–539.

Frennaux M, Kaski JC, Brown M, Maseri A. Refractory variant angina relieved by guanethidine and clonidine. Am J Cardiol 1988; 62:832–833.

Hackett D, Davies G, Chierchia S, Maseri A. Intermittent coronary occlusion in acute myocardial infarction. Value of combined thrombolytic and vasodilatory therapy. N Engl J Med 1987; 317:1055–1059.

Maseri A, Chierchia S. Coronary artery spasm: demonstration, definition, diagnosis, and consequences. Progr Cardiovasc Dis 1982; 25:169–182.

Parodi O, Maseri A, Simonetti I. Management of unstable angina at rest with verapamil: a double-blind cross-over study in a coronary care unit. Br Heart J 1979; 41:167–174.

Severi S, Davies G, Maseri A, et al. Long-term prognosis of variant angina with medical treatment. Am J Cardiol 1980; 46:226–232.

CEREBROVASCULAR DISEASE

CAROTID ARTERY DISEASE: NONINVASIVE AND INVASIVE ASSESSMENT

JOSEPH F. POLAK, M.D.

The diagnostic assessment of carotid artery disease has focused mainly on the detection of significant narrowing of the internal carotid artery in symptomatic patients. The need to screen for patients who can possibly profit from surgical endarterectomy of the carotid has historically led to the development of noninvasive approaches that are used to triage patients. A smaller subset of patients then undergoes further evaluation with the more invasive approach, which is carotid angiography. Duplex sonography is the more useful screening test, since it can be used to detect significant carotid stenoses accurately and measure their severity. The technique is reproducible, making it possible to determine whether new lesions have developed in patients who have repeat examinations after endarterectomy. Serial studies can also be used to monitor for lesion progression in asymptomatic patients who have significant carotid artery stenoses, or to monitor patients who have lesions that are not hemodynamically significant. Since Doppler sonography cannot be used to measure serial changes in luminal diameter of noncritical stenoses, the progression or regression of atherosclerotic plaque is currently measured with the aid of high-resolution sonography. This approach is now being used to monitor the effects of medical therapies on the development of early atherosclerotic lesions. The treatment of early carotid atherosclerosis, before significant stenoses have developed, is now putting emphasis on high-resolution imaging of the carotids. Sonography and possibly magnetic resonance imaging (MRI) will probably take increasingly important roles in following the effects of such early interventions.

METHODS

Noninvasive Techniques

The establishment of a noninvasive vascular laboratory is motivated by the need to screen a large population base and to detect the presence of highly significant narrowing of the internal carotid artery. These patients are then referred for appropriate further evaluation by angiography. The noninvasive techniques are compared in Table 1.

Oculoplethysmography

The earliest and more basic approach focuses on the noninvasive measurement of pressure decreases in the ocular globe secondary to a narrowing of the internal carotid. The technique of oculoplethysmography (OPG) fills this need, and in fact has served for many years as a standard screening test to detect high-grade narrowing of the internal carotid. The technique can be used in one of two ways. The first is detection of a delay in the pulse arrival time (OPG/Zira) between both ocular globes. The second is the actual measurement of intraocular pressure (OPG/Gee), using negative pressure applied to the globe with a suction cup. Both techniques detect hemodynamically significant narrowing of the carotids and rely heavily on the presence of significant pressure decreases in the artery distal to the stenosis. They are highly accurate for the detection of stenosis above 75 percent narrowing of the luminal diameter (sensitivity of 80 percent, specificity of 90 percent). They do not, however, offer any spatial localization of the site of the stenoses and may fail in the presence of simultaneous bilateral high-grade carotid lesions.

Periorbital Directional Doppler Signals

Another technique still used today is the periorbital directional Doppler measurements performed on the periocular branches of the external carotid artery. Normal flow via collaterals between the external and internal carotid branches present around the orbit has a

Table 1 Comparison of Noninvasive Techniques

	Range of Stenosis Detected (Luminal Diameter)	Spatial Resolution	Limitations
Periorbital directional Doppler	Greater than 75%; best for greater than 90%	None	Operator dependent; depends on state of collateral branches
Oculoplethysmography	Greater than 75%	None	Possible damage to cornea; poor for bilateral lesions
High-resolution real-time sonography	Less than 50%	Excellent	Poor grading of stenosis greater than 50%; operator dependent
Continuous wave Doppler sonography	Greater than 50%	Good; does not image carotids directly but localizes site of lesion	Operator dependent; subtotal occlusion may be misinterpreted as total
Duplex (color Doppler) sonography	All ranges; can be used to grade stenoses	Excellent	Operator dependent; subtotal occlusion may be misinterpreted as total
MR angiography	All ranges	Excellent	Poor grading of stenoses; claustrophobia; metallic foreign objects in patient's body

preferential direction from the cranium outward. The development of retrograde or inward flow toward the cranium suggests a critical stenosis of the internal carotid artery. A high-grade lesion anywhere from the carotid bifurcation to the origin of the ophthalmic artery can cause such an abnormal result. The sensitivity of the technique is relatively poor for detecting lesions of 50 percent or greater luminal diameter narrowing (sensitivity 30 percent, specificity 98 percent). The technique performs better for narrowings above 75 percent (sensitivity 60 percent, specificity 96 percent).

With more chronic occlusions, the development of collateral pathways can cause these signals to return to normal.

Doppler Ultrasonography

Doppler ultrasonography has, over the last decade, become the "gold standard" for noninvasively detecting and quantitating internal carotid artery disease. The three principal applications of this technology are continuous wave (CW) Doppler ultrasonography, duplex sonography, and color Doppler flow sonography. Real-time imaging is a component of the latter two techniques.

These three approaches rely on the physics of the ultrasound beam interaction with moving blood. The frequency of the reflected ultrasound signal is shifted as a function of the velocity of the red cells. For example, blood moving away from the transducer causes a decrease in the frequency of the returning signal; blood moving toward the transducer causes an increase in that frequency. The shift in frequency of the reflected signals allows a calculation of the blood flow velocity. However, the frequency shift depends on the angle of interrogation between the motion of the red cells and the direction of the ultrasound beam. For example, an angle of 60 degrees results in a frequency shift half of that measured if the ultrasound beam is parallel to the moving red cells. The accuracy of blood velocity measurements is therefore critically dependent on correcting for the angle between the ultrasound probe and the blood vessel.

At the site of a stenosis the velocity of blood increases. This increase is measured as a frequency shift of the returning ultrasound signal. By measuring the amount of frequency shift, it is therefore possible to measure the severity of stenosis in a vessel.

CW Doppler Ultrasound. The simple continuous wave (CW) Doppler probe is a nonimaging device that is interfaced to a Doppler spectrum analyzer. It is used to measure the peak systolic frequency shifts across the length of the common, external, and internal carotid arteries. The technique requires a certain degree of sophistication and training. Spatial localization of significant lesions is coarse, yet possible. However, a major limitation is the sampling of collateral vessels or abnormal vascular channels associated with varied pathologic conditions. For example, the presence of enlarged thyroid in Graves' disease or of a hypervascular mass near the bifurcation causes high-frequency signals too easily ascribed to a significant narrowing of the internal carotid. Another limitation is the inability to standardize the angle between the CW Doppler probe and the vessel. Since this angle affects the measured frequency shift used to detect and grade stenoses, measurement variability is a problem.

Pulsed Doppler Sonography. Pulsed Doppler in combination with real-time ultrasound imaging is referred to as duplex sonography (Fig. 1). It is currently the standard noninvasive examination to detect internal carotid artery disease. Real-time sonographic imaging is used to detect and characterize atherosclerotic plaque within the branches of the carotid artery. Pulsed Doppler is then used to sample flow velocity at sites of significant atherosclerotic plaque. An increase in velocity measured by Doppler sonography and spectral analysis is used to grade the severity of the stenosis (Fig. 2). As with CW Doppler, pulsed Doppler is sensitive to the detection of stenosis above 50 percent narrowing of the luminal diameter. Lesions of less than 50 percent can cause a perturbation in the shape of the Doppler waveform, but no reliable criteria can be used to grade the suspected stenosis. The technique offers an accuracy over 90 percent for the detection of significant internal

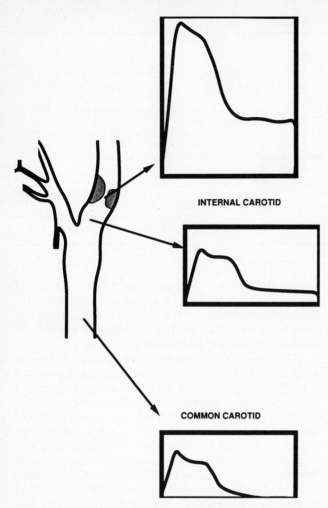

INTERNAL CAROTID

COMMON CAROTID

Figure 1 This diagram summarizes the diagnostic principle underlying the detection of significant internal carotid artery stenosis by duplex sonography. An increased velocity of blood flow is noted at the point of maximal narrowing in the internal carotid. This manifests itself by an elevation of both the peak systolic and the peak end-diastolic velocities of the Doppler waveform. The waveform proximal to the stenosis shows lower peak systolic and peak diastolic velocities. The common carotid waveform has a smaller component of antegrade diastolic blood flow than the internal carotid, a reflection of the higher vascular resistance of the external carotid system.

carotid artery narrowing of greater than 50 percent luminal diameter, using an increase in the measured peak systolic velocity of blood above 1.25 m per second as a diagnostic threshold. For the detection and characterization of lesions of less than 50 percent, a subjective grading of the extent and severity of the plaque is currently performed.

Color Doppler Flow Sonography. Color Doppler flow imaging is an improvement in sonography that permits the simultaneous display of moving blood as a color image superimposed on a real-time gray scale image. Velocity direction is normally encoded by color, i.e. red toward and blue away from the transducer. The

velocity is graded by the color saturation. The color image can be used to diagnose significant narrowing whenever a narrowing of the color lumen is perceived. The accuracy of this technique is slightly less than that of the more traditional duplex sonogram, because of the current limitation in the color Doppler processing algorithms that may cause an overestimation of luminal size. The most effective strategy is to combine color Doppler and duplex sonography, using the color image to rapidly localize areas of flow disturbance, and then perform the more quantitative spectral analysis to grade the stenosis. The examination is then as accurate as duplex sonography but less time-consuming.

The color image can also be used to grade stenosis of less than 50 percent by subjective evaluation of the size of the flow lumen. The reproducibility or accuracy of this approach has yet to be determined in any large published series.

Magnetic Resonance Angiography

Magnetic resonance (MR) angiography permits the detection of moving blood in a background of nonmoving tissues by means of selective radiofrequency pulse sequences. The technique is still under development, but offers the potential for objectively detecting and localizing the presence of significant stenosis (Fig. 3). A current limitation of this approach is the inability to grade stenosis above 50 percent. The turbulence in blood flow distal to the stenosis causes a loss of signal on the MR angiogram that is not necessarily proportional to the severity of the stenosis.

A major advantage of the technique is that it offers an impartial accurate projection of the anatomy of the carotid bifurcation, which is, in contrast to sonography, not operator dependent. This heavy reliance on the operator remains the major limitation of all the noninvasive techniques such as OPG, CW Doppler, and duplex sonography.

Invasive Techniques

The invasive techniques for assessing carotid artery disease are compared in Table 2.

Carotid Arteriography

Carotid arteriography remains the gold standard examination for the detection and grading of significant disease within the internal carotid artery.

In the early implementation of this technique, it was common practice to enter the common carotid artery directly and inject contrast material. Complications of this approach included local hematoma, carotid dissection, and adverse neurologic sequelae in up to 5 percent of patients.

This approach has been replaced by percutaneous entry of the femoral artery to permit placement of customized catheters at the origin of the common carotid

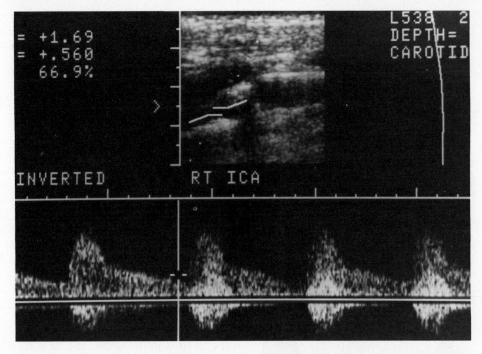

Figure 2 This Doppler spectral waveform of the right internal carotid artery of a patient with transient ischemic attacks shows a peak systolic velocity of 1.69 m per second. The peak end-diastolic velocity is also mildly increased at 0.56 m per second. This corresponds to a stenosis of approximately 50 percent luminal diameter narrowing.

artery. Subsequently, contrast material is selectively injected and films are taken (in at least two projections) using rapid film changer cassettes with high-resolution focal-spot x-ray tubes. This technique offers exact delineation of the anatomy of the carotid artery, from its origin in the aortic arch to the intracranial circulation. The complication rate includes stroke, transient ischemic attacks (2 to 5 percent), and local complications at the site of puncture such as arterial rupture or thrombosis (1 to 3 percent). Allergic reactions to the contrast material also occur, usually mild (5 to 10 percent) but occasionally life-threatening (0.1 to 1 percent).

Intravenous Digital Subtraction Angiography

This technique became popular in the late 1970s and was offered as a potential replacement to the use of intra-arterial carotid arteriography. The injection of high doses of contrast within the inferior vena cava, superior vena cava, or right heart generate a compact bolus of contrast that is subsequently imaged over the region of interest. These images are stored in a computer for specialized processing, using algorithms to "subtract out" non–contrast-containing background images and thus highlight the vessel of interest. The major disadvantage of this approach is the large amount of contrast necessary to visualize the vessels fully. Furthermore, despite the use of multiple projections, up to 15 percent

of cases yield unsatisfactory results. Large doses of contrast medium limit its use in patients with impaired renal function.

Intra-arterial Digital Subtraction Angiography

A new refinement is intra-arterial digital subtraction angiography (Fig. 4). This allows the use of small-caliber catheters and less contrast material. The time needed to perform the examination is reduced because x-ray films do not need to be developed, being replaced by a video playback of the digitized images. The arterial catheter may be removed sooner; this diminishes the likelihood of a local complication such as stroke or embolization. This technique has replaced most cut-film arteriography for the detection and grading of carotid artery disease.

LIMITATIONS

General Diagnostic Limitations

Carotid Ulceration

A limitation of both the invasive and noninvasive approaches is that they do not reliably and reproducibly assess ulcerated carotid plaques. Although ulceration may be accurately detected in 70 to 80 percent of cases,

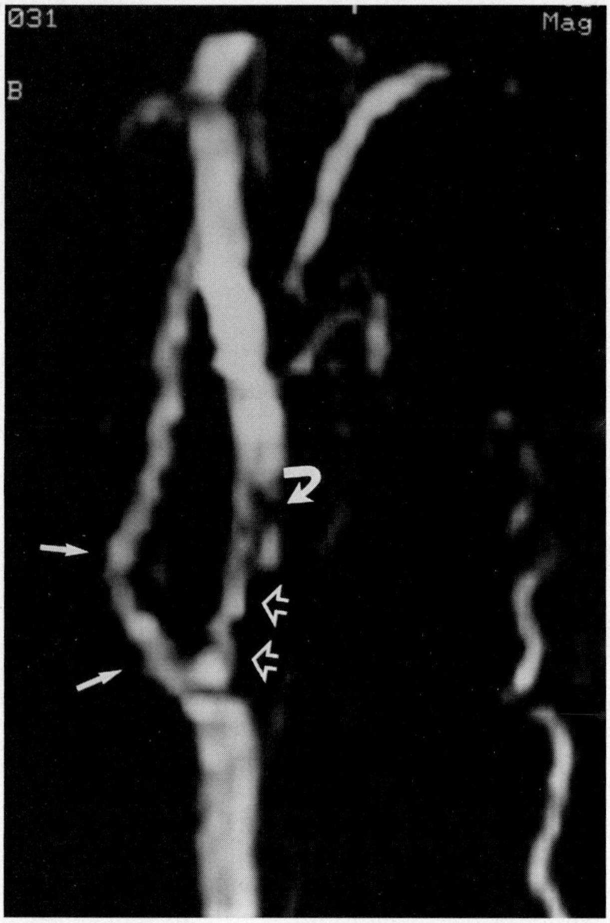

Figure 3 Same patient as in Figure 2. The corresponding magnetic resonance angiogram shows a narrowing in the lumen at the origin of the internal carotid artery *(open arrows)*. The external carotid artery is a smaller-diameter vessel to the left *(closed arrows)*. There is a zone of signal loss beyond the stenosis in the internal carotid due to turbulence *(curved arrow)*.

it cannot be reproducibly graded. Serial ultrasound examinations cannot be used to optimally determine the natural history of carotid plaque ulcerations. The accuracy of magnetic resonance imaging (MRI) has yet to be evaluated, but it may prove to be a more reliable means of evaluating such lesions.

Pseudo-Occlusion of Internal Carotid

All noninvasive techniques have significant failings when it comes to the detection of subtotal occlusions of the internal carotid. Narrowings of the internal carotid artery above 99 percent can reduce the blood flow velocity to the extent that Doppler signals may not be detected noninvasively: the so-called pseudo-occlusion. Likewise, the OPG and the periorbital Doppler signals cannot reliably differentiate total from subtotal occlusions. Thus, the noninvasive technique may misdiagnose subtotal occlusion. This is of clinical importance,

because endarterectomy of a subtotally occluded vessel has a high success rate and is the favored approach, whereas a totally occluded vessel is usually managed conservatively.

Specific Diagnostic Limitations

Sonography

The major limitation of Doppler sonography remains proper penetration of the ultrasound beam to the level of the carotid artery. Factors such as body habitus, skin thickness, or the presence of edema may perturb the quality of the diagnostic sonogram. In addition, bifurcations of the carotid artery high near the angle of the jaw make it difficult to sample within the distal carotid bifurcation and the more proximal internal and external branches. Calcified lesions may also mask the increased flow velocity associated with high-grade stenosis.

Magnetic Resonance Angiography

Magnetic resonance (MR) angiography can be very useful in confirming the site of a stenosis. Drawbacks include the inability to perform the test on claustrophobic patients and in patients who have had metallic implants such as aneurysm clips, cochlear implants, or metallic foreign bodies near the eyes. Although the technique cannot yet grade stenoses above 50 percent narrowing in a consistent fashion, newer developments in pulse sequences can overcome this current limitation.

Arteriography

Digital subtraction angiography has some additional weaknesses. Suboptimal technique or injection of over-concentrated contrast material may obscure lesions. Proper access and positioning of the intra-arterial catheters may not be possible or may be more difficult in patients with severe peripheral arterial disease.

Subtotal occlusion (pseudo-occlusion) may be misdiagnosed as total occlusion. This can be obviated by using standard cut-film technique and prolonged filming to detect the slow passage of contrast material through the high-grade stenosis.

APPLICATIONS

Noninvasive Screening

Duplex sonography is used for noninvasive screening of patients who present with an appropriate historical background or physical findings. Patients with high-grade narrowing of the internal carotid artery are therefore identified and undergo subsequent invasive evaluation with arteriography. The diagnostic efficacy of the test is reflected by the prevalence of disease in patients undergoing arteriography. Before the widespread use of sonography, significant carotid artery stenosis was detected in about 30 percent of the

Table 2 Comparison of Invasive Techniques

Technique	Range of Stenosis	Spatial Resolution	Advantages	Limitations
Intravenous digital subtraction angiography	All	Good	Outpatient procedure Venous puncture	Large amount of contrast needed Multiple views needed owing to vessel overlap; patient cooperation needed
Intra-arterial digital subtraction angiography	All	Good to excellent	Outpatient procedure; small catheters; short catheter residence times at origin of carotids	Patient cooperation needed; arterial puncture needed
Traditional angiography	All	Excellent	High resolution; distinguishes subtotal from total occlusions	Arterial puncture; longer residence time of catheter in artery

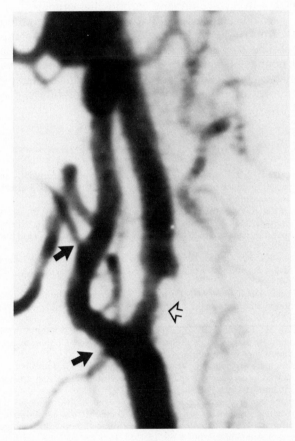

Figure 4 Same patient as in Figures 2 and 3. The corresponding intra-arterial digital subtraction arteriogram shows the corresponding 50 to 60 percent stenosis *(open arrow)*. The external carotid artery is recognized with its smaller side branches *(solid arrows)*.

population presenting for carotid angiography. With the increasing use of duplex sonography screening, about 90 percent of patients coming to arteriography are shown to have significant lesions. Duplex sonography is most effective as a screening technique when specific criteria are applied to diagnose a significant lesion. The two more commonly used criteria are (1) a peak systolic velocity of greater than 1.25 m per second within the internal carotid artery or (2) a peak systolic velocity ratio of greater than 1.5 between the internal and common carotid artery. The latter parameter is very useful in patients likely to show changes in cardiac output between repeat visits to the laboratory, or patients who have arrhythmias significant enough to perturb carotid blood flow velocities from beat to beat. Elevations in the peak end-diastolic velocity of blood above 0.8 m per second have more recently been used as a discriminator of severe carotid stenosis. Patients having velocities above this threshold are more likely to have greater than 75 percent narrowing of the luminal diameter of the internal carotid artery.

Follow-up Studies

Following Endarterectomy

Doppler sonography can be used to perform serial studies on patients after carotid endarterectomy. Significant residual lesions may occasionally be detected after surgery, although most centers perform an intraoperative arteriogram or a Doppler survey after the endarterectomy procedure to exclude any significant lesions before closure of the wound.

In the immediate postoperative period, localized areas of increased velocity are often present and may increase in severity for the first 3 to 6 months after the surgical procedure. This elevation of velocity most likely represents stenosis secondary to fibrointimal hyperplasia. These lesions tend to be self-limiting in extent and only rarely (5 percent) progress to cause a significant stenosis. If a lesion has progressed to a severity of greater than 75 percent narrowing, surgical intervention becomes more likely.

Asymptomatic Stenoses

Since carotid stenoses are often present bilaterally, the asymptomatic carotid opposite the endarterectomy should be followed to detect potential changes in the severity of the lesion. A measured increase in peak systolic velocity of more than 15 percent from the initial value is considered evidence of progression. Postoperative changes in flow dynamics secondary to a contralateral stenosis that has been corrected can be compensated for by the use of the internal to common carotid peak systolic velocity ratio. This parameter takes into consideration changes in common carotid blood flow due to the contralateral endarterectomy. The development of symptoms in the territory supplied by a carotid with a documented high-grade lesion would warrant surgical intervention.

A significant stenosis in the absence of symptoms generally does not warrant intervention. In this setting, once symptoms develop there is a high likelihood of a stroke in the ensuing few months, and endarterectomy should be performed.

The increased use of carotid sonography as a screening tool has led to the detection of many asymptomatic carotid lesions in the general population. Prevalence data suggest that hemodynamically significant stenoses are present in 5 to 10 percent of the population. A much larger percentage, approximately 30 percent, have lesions that narrow the luminal diameter by 25 to 50 percent. These patients are at potential risk for progression of the degree of stenosis and for stroke. Recent pathologic data suggest that nonobstructing plaque may hemorrhage, rupture, and serve as a nidus for thrombus formation. These lesions are now detectable noninvasively and can be followed serially to provide more information regarding their natural history.

Currently, lesions that are not hemodynamically significant are managed medically (i.e., with antiplatelet agents). If symptoms develop in association with progression of the lesion to greater than 50 percent narrowing of luminal diameter, more aggressive intervention (endarterectomy) is favored.

Epidemiologic and Outcome Studies

Duplex sonography has emerged over the last few years as an ideal tool for assessing the effects of surgical versus medical management. Serial monitoring of carotid lesions is more easily implemented by this noninvasive modality than by relying on repeat arteriography.

Recent studies using sonography will determine to what extent atherosclerotic plaque can regress with dietary or medical management.

There is also interest in documenting early atherosclerotic changes in the carotid. Thickening of the intima-media layer of the carotid wall has been detected in hypercholesterolemic patients, which may allow these more subtle changes to become a target for medical therapy.

DISCUSSION

The current therapeutic options for significant carotid artery disease have resulted in the development of a diagnostic strategy that relies heavily on duplex sonography to triage patients likely to have surgically correctable stenosis of the internal carotid artery. Arteriography is then used more selectively to define the anatomy preoperatively.

In the future, refinements in MR angiography may allow it to replace invasive carotid angiography.

As the emphasis shifts to study of the evolution of carotid atherosclerosis, the use of high-resolution real-time sonography is increasing. Serial monitoring of nonhemodynamically significant carotid plaque will gain in clinical importance and, as medical therapies improve, probably become the focus of future diagnostic work-ups.

SUGGESTED READING

Hobson RW II, Berry SM, Jamil Z, et al. Oculoplethysmography and pulsed Doppler ultrasonic imaging in diagnosis of carotid arterial disease. Surg Gynecol Obstet 1981; 152:433–436.

Johnston KW, Haynes RB, Douville Y, et al. Accuracy of carotid Doppler peak frequency analysis: results determined by receiver operating characteristic curves and likelihood ratios. J Vasc Surg 1985; 2:515–523.

Lusby RJ, Ferrell LD, Ehrenfeld WK, et al. Carotid plaque hemorrhage. Its role in production of cerebral ischemia. Stroke 1988; 19:1289–1290.

O'Leary DH, Clouse ME, Potter JE, Wheeler HG. The influence of noninvasive tests on the selection of patients for angiography. Stroke 1985; 16:264–267.

Polak JF, Dobkin GR, O'Leary DH, et al. Internal carotid artery stenosis: accuracy and reproducibility of color Doppler-assisted duplex imaging. Radiology 1989; 173:793–798.

Salonen R, Seppanen K, Ravramara R, Salonen JT. Prevalence of carotid atherosclerosis and serum cholesterol levels in Eastern Finland. Arteriosclerosis 1988; 8:788–792.

Weinberger J, Ramos L, Ambrose JA, Foster V. Morphologic and dynamic changes of atherosclerotic plaque at the carotid artery bifurcation: sequential imaging by real-time B-mode ultrasonography. J Am Coll Cardiol 1988; 12:1515–1521.

Wise B, Parker J, Burkholder J. Supraorbital Doppler studies, carotid bruits, and arteriography in unilateral ocular or cerebral ischemic disorders. Neurology 1979; 29:34–37.

CAROTID ARTERY DISEASE: MEDICAL MANAGEMENT

IRENE MEISSNER, M.D.

The most frequently evaluated carotid artery lesion is atherosclerotic occlusive disease, which often manifests for the first time as an acute stroke. Other less common pathophysiologic entities include fibromuscular disease and dissection. The clinician's approach to diagnosis and treatment in patients with stroke has changed dramatically during the past two decades. The nihilistic approach toward atherosclerotic risk factor and stroke management is no longer acceptable. With continuing progress being made in clinical and laboratory research toward defining mechanisms by which stroke occurs as well as risk factors associated with it, stroke is no longer viewed as the inevitable end result of a progressive, untreatable atherosclerotic condition. The recent development of sophisticated noninvasive diagnostic techniques for the evaluation of carotid artery disease is described in the preceding chapter, *Carotid Artery Disease: Noninvasive and Invasive Assessment.* This chapter focuses on the nonsurgical management of symptomatic and asymptomatic occlusive disease of the carotid system.

NATURAL HISTORY

Assessment of the efficacy and risk-to-benefit ratio of a particular treatment option requires an understanding of the natural history of the disorder in question. Population-based studies and clinical trials involving patients with symptomatic carotid occlusive disease have yielded stroke rate estimates of 10 percent in the first month after the initial transient ischemic attack (TIA) and 5 to 6 percent per year thereafter with antiplatelet or anticoagulant therapy.

With regard to asymptomatic carotid occlusive disease, the literature is confounded by a heterogeneous pool that includes patients symptomatic in one hemisphere with a contralateral asymptomatic vessel; truly asymptomatic patients with no previous carotid distribution symptoms in either hemisphere; patients with carotid bruits without a hemodynamic lesion; and patients with hemodynamically significant occlusive disease, with or without a bruit. Therefore, it is not surprising that confusion exists regarding the natural history and appropriate management of asymptomatic carotid occlusive disease. In a recent study at our institution that examined asymptomatic patients with and without pressure-significant carotid system lesions as defined by oculoplethysmography (OPG), an actuarial stroke rate of 3.4 percent per year over 4 years was observed regardless of the existence of an underlying

bruit. This finding suggests that the presence of a pressure-significant lesion may be a better predictor for future cerebral ischemic events than would be the presence of a bruit alone.

THE HEMODYNAMICALLY SIGNIFICANT LESION

The hemodynamically significant or pressure-significant stenosis varies directly with the effective cross-sectional area of an artery and inversely with velocity of blood flow. Hemodynamic studies have shown that a decrease in pressure may occur when the angiographically demonstrated luminal diameter is decreased by 50 percent, which corresponds to a cross-sectional decrease of 75 percent. Under routine conditions, normal blood flow may still be present; however, under conditions that require augmentation of blood flow, this degree of narrowing may act as a critical stenosis. This value defines the degree of luminal narrowing beyond which further small decrements in luminal area would result in abrupt decreases in pressure and flow rate distal to this stenosis. Significant compromise in the blood flow may occur when the luminal stenosis approaches 75 percent. Information regarding the presence or absence of pressure-significant carotid occlusive disease is useful in guiding patient management and selecting appropriate potential surgical candidates.

Clinical Diagnosis

The first step involves identifying the event as vascular, and if transient, distinguishing it from other mimickers of ischemic events, including migraine, seizures, labyrinthine disorders, and syncope. The temporal profile and duration of symptoms and signs will define the event as a TIA lasting less than 24 hours, a reversible ischemic neurologic deficit with symptoms lasting from 24 hours to 3 weeks, or a stroke lasting more than 3 weeks. Table 1 lists the pathophysiologic categories of TIA, important considerations when selecting the appropriate therapeutic manipulation. For example, the treatment of a hypertensive lacunar infarction is significantly different from that of a large-vessel thrombotic or embolic stroke.

Clinical clues are important in determining stroke mechanism and directing the appropriate diagnostic studies. For example, symptoms that involve multiple vascular distributions are suggestive of small vessel disease (hypertension, diabetes, vasculitis) or possibly a cardioembolic source. Alternatively, a single territory distribution would be more typical of focal atherosclerotic occlusive disease. Figures 1 and 2 outline appropriate diagnostic studies to be conducted based on the distribution of symptoms and signs. Evidence for a hemodynamic component would include postural TIAs or cardiac dysfunction (dysrhythmia, outflow obstruction) in the setting of a critical stenosis. Further support for a hemodynamic mechanism would include radiographic evidence of arterial border zone or "watershed" infarction. Watershed infarction refers to infarcts in portions of the brain where distal branches of the anterior, middle, and posterior cerebral arteries anastomose, regions that are vulnerable to marked decreases in flow.

The following are baseline laboratory studies that should be performed for all patients who have focal ischemic events; selected disorders that can be ruled out by the results are indicated in parentheses: hematology group, differential count (anemia, polycythemia, thrombocythemia), chemistry group (diabetes), lipid studies (hyperlipidemia), prothrombin time/partial thromboplastin time (coagulopathy, lupus anticoagulant), sedimentation rate (vasculitis), chest radiography (heart size), electrocardiography (arrhythmia, myocardial infarction), and urinalysis (hematuria, vasculitis). Numerous noninvasive studies are currently available that should be used selectively, such as the Holter monitor, OPG, ophthalmodynamometry (measurement of retinal artery pressures), transthoracic and transesophageal echocardiography, carotid ultrasonography, and trans-

cranial Doppler studies. A computed tomographic (CT) scan or magnetic resonance imaging (MRI) scan should also be done because, in approximately 5 percent of patients, other intracranial disease such as tumor may mimic a TIA. Invasive imaging techniques such as digital intravenous subtraction angiography or conventional arteriography ultimately may be necessary to perform for a definitive diagnosis. In the future, MRI angiography may emerge as a valuable diagnostic tool.

THERAPY

Currently, indication for the use of antiplatelet and anticoagulant therapy in patients with symptomatic and asymptomatic carotid occlusive disease is in dispute. This controversy is due, in part, to the following methodologic issues: 1) variable pathophysiologic mech-

Table 1 Pathophysiologic Categories of Transient Ischemic Attack

Large vessel extracranial atherosclerosis with or without ulceration
Large-to-medium vessel intracranial atherosclerosis with or without ulceration
Small vessel disease
  Accelerated atherosclerosis (diabetes, hypertension)
  Lipohyalinosis (hypertension)
Inflammatory arterial disease (vasculitis)
Nonatherosclerotic arterial disease
  Fibromuscular disease
  Dissection
Migraine (vasospasm?)
Cardiac disease
  Source of emboli
  Hemodynamic effects (decreased cardiac output)
    Dysrhythmia
    Congestive heart failure
    Valvular heart disease
      Native
      Prosthetic
    Left atrial lesion
      Appendage
      Septum
    Aortic atherosclerotic plaque
    Mural ventricular thrombus
Coagulopathies
  Dysproteinemias
    Waldenström's cryoglobulinemia
    Multiple myeloma
  Leukemia
  Thrombocythemia
  Polycythemia vera
  Sickle cell anemia
  Thrombotic thrombocytopenic purpura
  Lupus anticoagulant
  Antiphospholipid antibody syndrome
  Protein C and protein S deficiency
  Increased fibrinogen
  Disorders of fibrinolysis

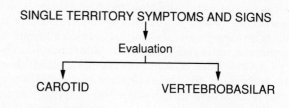

Figure 1 Outline of suggested tests in patients with focal cerebrovascular symptoms in a single (carotid or vertebral basilar) territory. TCD = transcranial Doppler echocardiography; ± = may or may not be appropriate depending on individual circumstance.

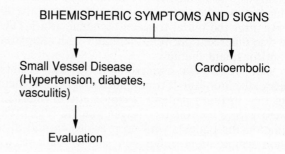

Figure 2 Mechanism and suggested initial evaluation in patients with focal or diffuse symptoms or signs, or both, of cerebrovascular disease affecting both hemispheres.

anisms of stroke and TIA — this makes it unlikely that all patients will respond uniformly to a given treatment; and 2) relatively low stroke incidence per year in patients with TIA (approximately 5 percent per year), which results in fewer patients for randomized clinical trials.

Platelet Antiaggregation Agents

There have been more than 30 trials of antiplatelet therapy involving approximately 30,000 patients with a history of TIA, minor stroke, unstable angina, or myocardial infarction. A meta-analysis of these data revealed that allocation to antiplatelet treatment decreased vascular mortality from stroke or myocardial infarction by 15 percent and nonfatal vascular events by 30 percent. Sulfinpyrazone and dipyridamole have not been shown to be of benefit in stroke prevention and the addition of dipyridamole to aspirin therapy for carotid occlusive disease is not advocated.

To date, no adequate data exist to compare low- and high-dose aspirin therapy. Pharmacologic studies suggest that cyclooxygenase-dependent platelet aggregation is inhibited just as effectively by 300 mg of aspirin as by higher doses and may, in fact, be preferable because of decreased dose-dependent gastrotoxicity. Thus far there is insufficient clinical evidence to support the superiority of low-dose over high-dose aspirin therapy. Some studies have reported a greater benefit of aspirin in men, although this finding has not been consistent. In general, women have fewer strokes and a lower rate of mortality than do men regardless of treatment. The issue of differing aspirin efficacy in men and women remains unresolved.

Ticlopidine is, to date, the only other platelet-antiaggregating agent that has been proved beneficial in initial and recurrent stroke prevention, as was found in two recently completed large multicenter North American trials. The mechanism of action of ticlopidine remains unclear, but, unlike aspirin, it does not involve arachidonic acid metabolism. This drug may become a future treatment option, particularly for patients who fail to respond to, or who are intolerant of, aspirin therapy. However, concerns regarding toxicity — including a significant reversible leukopenia — are still being assessed, and approval by the Food and Drug Administration is still pending.

Thromboxane synthetase inhibitors and thromboxane antagonists are being studied as potential future therapeutic options in stroke prevention. The mechanism of action of these compounds is the inhibition of thromboxane A2-mediated platelet aggregation, release, and vasoconstriction. Data are preliminary and further studies are necessary.

Anticoagulant Therapy

The value of anticoagulant therapy in the prevention of primary or recurrent stroke remains unclear. A critical review of the literature reveals methodologic flaws, including differing entry and endpoint criteria, small sample sizes, and patients having undergone previous revascularization procedures. Therefore, the use of anticoagulants has evolved empirically (Table 2). To illustrate, the following section outlines typical situations encountered by the clinician (excluding cardioembolic events) in which anticoagulant therapy may be considered.

1. Situation: Patient with a recent onset of progressive or crescendo TIAs who may be a candidate for carotid endarterectomy.
   Treatment: Heparin may be used during the presurgical evaluation period.
2. Situation: Patient with recent TIAs and a hemodynamically significant, surgically accessible carotid lesion who is, for medical reasons, not a surgical candidate and who has not responded to antiplatelet therapy.
   Treatment: A 3- to 6-month period of warfarin therapy followed by antiplatelet therapy.
3. Situation: Patient with recent TIAs and a hemodynamically significant or nonhemodynamically significant carotid lesion in which there is significant intimal irregularity and ulceration or a fresh thrombus.
   Treatment: Heparin administration during the evaluation followed by 3 to 6 months of warfarin therapy. Thereafter, aspirin may be used.
4. Situation: Patient with progressive or crescendo TIAs or cerebral infarction with a mild-to-moderate neurologic deficit and angiographically significant stenosis of a major intracranial carotid

Table 2 Indications for the Use of Heparin

| Variable | Heparin use | |
	More likely	Less likely
Symptoms	Typical	Atypical
Temporal profile	Progressing deficit	Stable deficit
Timing	Recent event	Remote event
Size of lesion	Small	Large
Functional deficit	Small (more salvageable)	Large
Overall	Potential benefit outweighs risk for hemorrhage	Risk for hemorrhage outweighs potential benefit

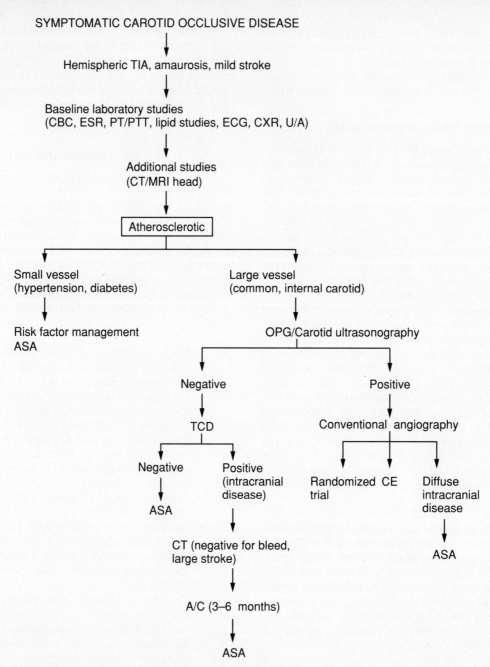

Figure 3 *A,* Simplified scheme for the evaluation and management of patients with symptomatic atherosclerotic carotid occlusive disease.

artery branch—i.e., the middle cerebral artery—who has not responded to antiplatelet therapy. Treatment: A 3- to 6-month period of warfarin therapy followed by antiplatelet therapy. In some cases, indefinite anticoagulation therapy may be appropriate.

5. Situation: Acute, angiographically defined occlusion of the internal carotid artery (ICA) *in the absence of* a major debilitating stroke. In all cases, a CT scan is mandatory at symptom onset and desirable within 24 to 48 hours thereafter to determine the radiographic extent of infarction and to rule out hemorrhagic transformation.

Treatment: Heparin therapy during the evaluation (first week), followed by warfarin therapy for 3 to 6 months. Antiplatelet therapy may be considered subsequently.

The major complication of short-term anticoagulation agents such as heparin and long-term agents such as warfarin is hemorrhage. Although the risk for bleeding with warfarin is directly proportional to the degree of anticoagulation as reflected by prolonged prothrombin time, other factors may also contribute to this increased risk including hemostatic defects (extensive trauma and surgical wounds), platelet dysfunction or thrombocy-

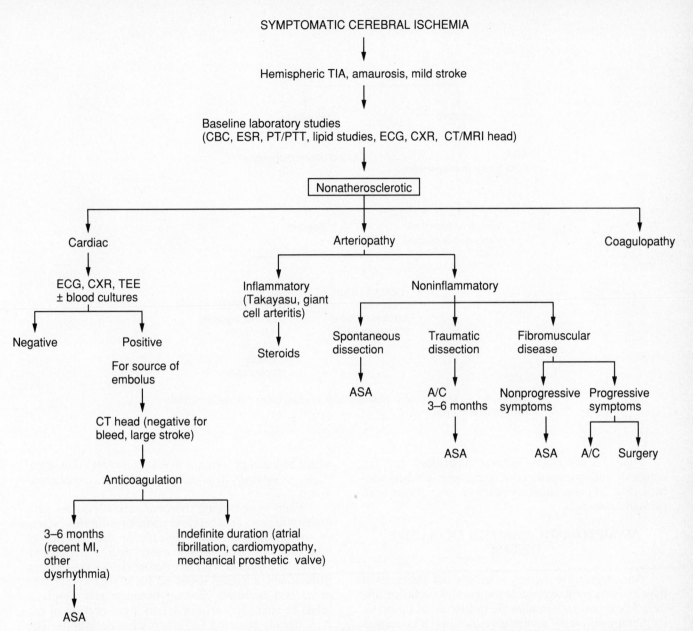

Figure 3, cont'd *B,* Similar scheme of evaluation and management for patients with nonatherosclerotic cerebrovascular disease. A/C = Anticoagulation; ASA = aspirin; CBC = complete blood cell count; CE = carotid endarterectomy; CT = computed tomography; CXR = chest radiograph; ECG = electrocardiography; ESR = erythrocyte sedimentation rate; MI = myocardial infarction; MRI = magnetic resonance imaging; OPG = oculoplethysmography; PT/PTT = prothrombin time/partial thromboplastin time; TCD = transcranial Doppler echocardiography; TEE = transesophageal echocardiography; TIA = transient ischemic attack; U/A = urinalysis.

topenia, synergistic drug interactions including the use of antiplatelet agents, and malabsorption syndromes or other coexisting morbid conditions that cause increased sensitivity to anticoagulants.

Reported overall bleeding complication rates for warfarin and heparin have ranged from approximately 2 to 10 percent, reflecting major and minor hemorrhage, respectively.

With regard to the administration of heparin, the 7,500 to 10,000 unit bolus dose is generally followed by a continuous infusion of 1,000 units hourly, adjusted to maintain the activated partial thromboplastin time

(aPTT) at 2 to 2.5 times the control value. The aPTT should be measured at 2 hours and at 4 to 6 hours for appropriate titration in the critical early hours after the ischemic event. In cases in which continued anticoagulation therapy is appropriate, warfarin therapy may be instituted with an initial loading dose of 10 to 20 mg followed by 5 to 10 mg daily until the optimal prothrombin time (PT), usually 1.5 to 2 times the control value, is attained. Daily PT measurements should be taken. Higher initial loading doses of 40 to 60 mg, although advocated by some investigators, generally are not recommended.

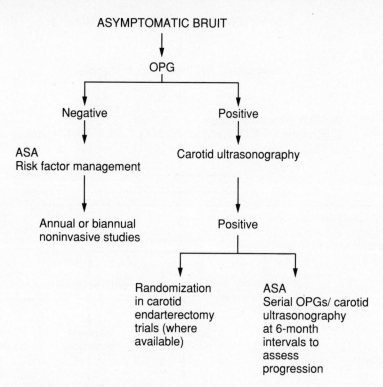

Figure 4 *A,* Outline of evaluation and management for patients with asymptomatic bruit.

Figure 3 illustrates general algorithms for the diagnosis and management of symptomatic atherosclerotic (Fig. 3*A*) and nonatherosclerotic (Fig. 3*B*) carotid occlusive disease.

ASYMPTOMATIC CAROTID OCCLUSIVE DISEASE

Anticoagulation therapy is usually not indicated in patients who have asymptomatic carotid occlusive disease. I generally recommend the institution of antiplatelet therapy with serial noninvasive studies (OPG, carotid ultrasonography, transcranial Doppler, echocardiography), as appropriate. Figure 4 outlines diagnostic and management schemes for the asymptomatic carotid bruit and stenosis.

NONATHEROSCLEROTIC DISEASE OF THE EXTRACRANIAL CAROTID ARTERY

Fibromuscular Dysplasia

Dysplasia of the cervical carotid artery is often incidentally found in an angiographic study performed for unrelated reasons. This entity, a segmental, non-atheromatous angiopathy of indeterminate cause, is thought to represent a developmental abnormality that affects primarily intermediate-sized muscular arteries. This disorder is thought to be autosomally dominant with a reduced penetrance in males; it is also thought to occur occasionally in association with intracranial aneurysms.

When symptomatic, fibromuscular dysplasia generally manifests as a cerebral ischemic event in a young or middle-aged woman, typically in the absence of atherosclerotic risk factors other than hypertension. Although a patient who has fibromuscular disease can present with a clinical stroke profile similar to that seen in carotid occlusive disease, fibromuscular dysplasia tends to spare the proximal 1 to 2 cm portion of the ICA usually reserved for atherosclerotic lesions. The frequency of subsequent cerebral ischemic events after diagnosis is low, reflecting a benign process in most cases. However, reported complications include aneurysm formation, rupture, and arterial dissection. Medical management initially involves the use of antiplatelet agents. Progressive symptoms may justify the use of anticoagulant therapy or, possibly, surgical intervention (see Fig. 3*B*).

Dissection of the Cervical Internal Carotid Artery

Dissection of the ICA occurs when circulating blood penetrates into the arterial wall, splits the media, and forms a false lumen. The true lumen of the ICA is often compressed and narrowed by the intramural hematoma. On occasion, the false lumen may extend toward the adventitia and form an aneurysmal dila-

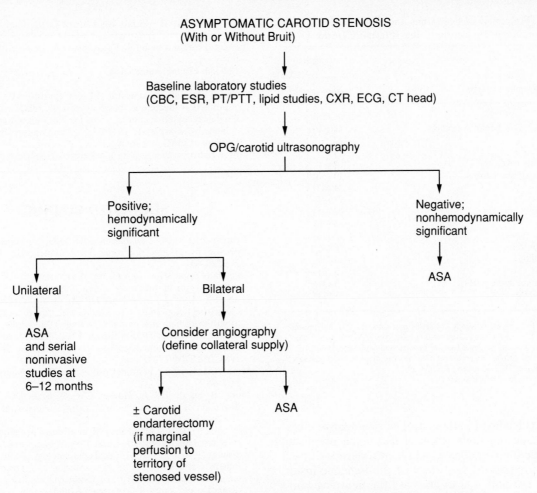

ASYMPTOMATIC CAROTID STENOSIS
(With or Without Bruit)

Baseline laboratory studies
(CBC, ESR, PT/PTT, lipid studies, CXR, ECG, CT head)

OPG/carotid ultrasonography

Positive;
hemodynamically
significant

Negative;
nonhemodynamically
significant

ASA

Unilateral

Bilateral

ASA
and serial
noninvasive
studies at
6–12 months

Consider angiography
(define collateral supply)

± Carotid
endarterectomy
(if marginal
perfusion to
territory of
stenosed vessel)

ASA

Figure 4, cont'd *B,* Outline of evaluation and management for patients with asymptomatic carotid stenosis, with or without an associated bruit. (See Figure 3 for abbreviations.)

tation called a *dissecting aneurysm.* ICA dissections may be "spontaneous," when no overt trauma is reported (although trivial trauma may be missed), or "traumatic," when there is a clear history of head or neck injury. Symptoms and signs in 80 patients with spontaneous ICA dissections are listed in decreasing order of frequency in Table 3.

The prognosis for patients with spontaneous carotid dissections is generally good; complete or partial resolution occurs in up to 90 percent of stenoses. More than 85 percent of patients have a satisfactory or complete clinical recovery. No standardized method of management has emerged; however, in view of the favorable natural history, I would recommend conservative management. The treatment of traumatic dissection depends on the clinical course. In patients with progressing neurologic deficits related to focal cerebral ischemia, thromboembolism, and distal embolization, anticoagulant therapy should be considered (see Fig. 3B). However, if there is evidence of cerebral or visceral trauma, anticoagulation therapy may be contraindicated. In post-traumatic situations in which patients have no

symptoms of focal cerebral ischemia, the use of antiplatelet agents may be sufficient.

FUTURE THERAPEUTIC APPROACHES TO FOCAL ISCHEMIA

At the basis of all forms of management of carotid artery disease is preventive therapy. No treatment focused on mitigating the ischemic insult will alter the natural history of the underlying disease process, particularly with regard to progression of atherosclerosis. Therefore, as mentioned earlier, risk factor management—that is, the treatment of hypertension, hyperlipidemia, and underlying cardiac disease—must not be overlooked.

Based on our current understanding of the pathophysiologic mechanisms of focal ischemia, medical therapeutic modalities can be divided into two major categories: those that increase cerebral blood flow and thus increase cerebral perfusion, and those that offer cytoprotection by decreasing the neuronal energy re-

Table 3 Frequency of Symptoms and Signs in 80 Patients With Spontaneous Dissection of the Internal Carotid Artery

Symptom or sign	Patients Number (%)
Headache	66 (83)
Focal cerebral ischemic symptoms	48 (60)
TIA	27
Stroke	14
TIA and stroke	7
Oculosympathetic paresis	40 (50)
Bruits	34 (43)
Neck pain	17 (21)
Lightheadedness	17 (21)
Syncope	8 (10)
Amaurosis fugax	11 (14)
Scalp tenderness	6 (8)
Neck swelling	3 (4)
Dysgeusia	3 (4)
Lower cranial nerve palsies	3 (4)
Asymptomatic	1 (1)

Updated from Mokri B, Sundt TM Jr, Houser OW, Piepgras DG. Spontaneous dissection of the cervical internal carotid artery. Ann Neurol 1986; 19:126–138; and Mokri B. Dissections of cervical and cephalic arteries. In: Sundt TM Jr, ed. Occlusive cerebrovascular disease: diagnosis and management. Philadelphia: WB Saunders, 1987:38–59.
TIA = transient ischemic attack.

quirements leading to attenuation of degradative metabolic cascade reactions. Table 4 lists some promising therapeutic interventions which, if introduced within a critical early period after onset of the ischemic insult, may have the potential to decrease the neurologic and functional deficit associated with acute stroke.

Table 4 Goals for Future Drug Therapy

Increased cerebral blood flow (vasodilation, increased collateral flow)
  Calcium channel antagonists
  Serotonin antagonists
  Tissue-plasminogen activator (t-PA) (reperfusion)
Cytoprotection (decreased metabolic cascade reactions)
  Excitatory amino acid antagonists (to block excitatory cell death):
    N-methyl-D-aspartate (NMDA), kainate, quisqualate receptors
  Calcium channel antagonists
  Free radical scavengers (to block oxidative cell damage)

SUGGESTED READING

Antiplatelet Trialists' Collaboration. Secondary prevention of vascular disease by prolonged antiplatelet treatment. Br Med J 1988; 296:320–331.
Canadian Cooperative Study Group. A randomized trial of aspirin and sulfinpyrazone in threatened stroke. N Engl J Med 1978; 299:53–59.
Haas WK, Easton JD, Adams HP Jr, et al. A randomized trial comparing ticlopidine hydrochloride with aspirin for the prevention of stroke in high-risk patients. N Engl J Med 1989; 321:501–507.
Meissner I, Wiebers DO, Whisnant JP, O'Fallon WM. The natural history of asymptomatic carotid artery occlusive lesions. JAMA 1987; 258:2704–2707.
Meyer FB. Ischemic neuronal protection. Prosp Neurol Surg 1990; 1:57–78.
Mokri B, Sundt TM Jr, Houser OW, Piepgras DG. Spontaneous dissection of the cervical internal carotid artery. Ann Neurol 1986; 19:126–138.
Sherman DG, Dyken ML, Fisher M, et al. Antithrombotic therapy for cerebrovascular disorders. Chest 1989; 95(suppl):140S–155S.
Whisnant JP, Wiebers DO. Clinical epidemiology of transient cerebral ischemic attacks (TIA) in the anterior and posterior cerebral circulation. In: Sundt TM Jr, ed. Occlusive cerebrovascular disease: diagnosis and surgical management. Philadelphia: WB Saunders, 1987:60–65.

CAROTID ARTERY DISEASE: SURGICAL MANAGEMENT

ANTHONY D. WHITTEMORE, M.D.

The surgical management of carotid artery disease is predicated on the ability to provide a more favorable alternative to the natural history of the disease process, and therein lies the basis for the current controversy surrounding carotid endarterectomy. This controversy is fueled by conflicting data with regard to the risks associated with significant carotid stenosis, both treated and untreated. As regards the natural history, the literature suggests an incidence of significant neurologic morbidity in patients symptomatic with transient ischemic attacks (TIAs) ranging between 20 and 60 percent over a period of 5 years. The risk of significant neurologic events in asymptomatic patients with stenotic lesions greater than 80 percent may range as high as 50 percent within 2 years, and individuals with carotid occlusion demonstrate an annual incidence of ipsilateral stroke of 6 percent, or 30 percent over 5 years. The goals of carotid endarterectomy, in essence, are to remove a prime source of thromboembolic events resulting in TIA and stroke and to prevent total internal carotid occlusion with its known sequelae. The operative mortality associated with carotid endarterectomy varies between 0.5 and 5 percent and the perioperative stroke rate ranges from 1 to 20 percent. It is clear, however, that most well-trained surgeons carrying out carotid endarterectomy on a routine basis have achieved a combined operative mortality and permanent neurologic morbidity rate of consistently less than 3 percent. Furthermore, the risk of significant neurologic events following carotid endarterectomy approximates 2 percent per year, substantially less than the rates associated with the natural history of the subpopulations previously mentioned. In the midst of continuing controversy and diverse recommendations, we as clinicians must advise these patients on a daily basis as best we can in the absence of compelling and conclusive data derived from well-controlled, randomized prospective studies. Within this context, then, carotid endarterectomy is indicated under several circumstances based on two primary considerations: the nature of the lesion and its associated symptoms.

PATIENT SELECTION

Patients with classic focal TIAs should initially undergo computed tomographic (CT) and carotid duplex scans. Patients with stenotic lesions of no hemodynamic significance, including those proved to have a simple atheroma with a shallow ulcer, may be managed with antiplatelet therapy and followed with serial noninvasive evaluations. If symptoms recur during appropriate antiplatelet therapy, or if the lesion progresses to a hemodynamically significant level (i.e., 80 percent stenosis), angiography and endarterectomy are advised. A CT scan should be obtained in all symptomatic patients, and the presence of ipsilateral focal infarcts prompts endarterectomy because antiplatelet therapy under these circumstances has not proved effective. Symptomatic patients with noninvasive evaluation indicating a hemodynamically significant carotid stenosis (Fig. 1) or a large, complex, multiulcerated plaque (Fig. 2) should clearly undergo angiography and subsequent endarterectomy as indicated.

The appropriate management of patients with asymptomatic lesions remains far more uncertain, reflecting the wide disparity in reported risks associated with the natural history. It is current policy to recommend endarterectomy for all patients who have developed lesions resulting in greater than 80 percent stenosis, and to manage those who have lesser degrees of stenosis with antiplatelet therapy and serial noninvasive examinations. Several observations form the basis for this policy. Recent evidence disputes the previously held reassuring maxim that prodromal TIAs precede a catastrophic stroke in the vast majority of affected patients. Second, patients with lesions documented to have progressed beyond 80 percent stenosis incur a risk of TIA or stroke that may approach 50 percent within 2 years. Patients with asymptomatic, nonhemodynamically significant lesions characterized by complex multiulcerated plaques also demonstrate a significant stroke rate approximating 8 percent annually, sharply contrasting with

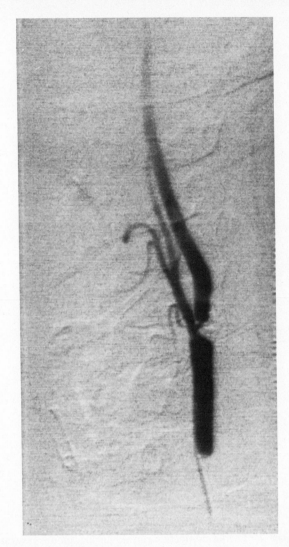

Figure 1 Digital subtraction carotid angiogram demonstrating a high-grade (80 percent) stenosis at the origin of the internal carotid artery, which was associated with transient ischemic attacks (TIAs).

the 1 percent annual stroke rate associated with lesions containing shallow, broad-based ulcers. Hypertensive patients, especially those over 70 years of age, appear to have an increased risk of neurologic sequelae approaching 6 percent per year. Finally, the definition of the asymptomatic state bears careful scrutiny. It is not infrequent that an initially asymptomatic patient on further reflection will admit to having sustained some of the more subtle focal neurologic events. Furthermore, the incidence of ipsilateral silent cerebral infarcts approaches 25 percent on CT scan in patients believed to be asymptomatic.

The role of carotid endarterectomy in patients with acute neurologic deficits is even more controversial than is the case for patients with TIAs or asymptomatic lesions. The basis for controversy lies in the high incidence of serious neurologic complications following

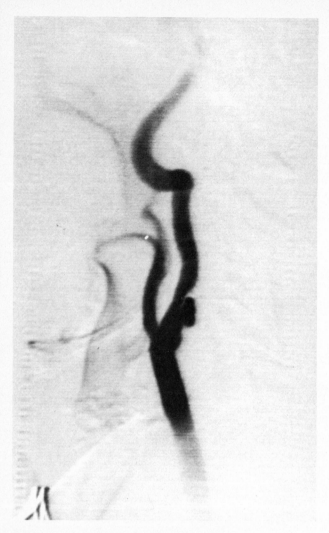

Figure 2 Digital subtraction carotid angiogram demonstrating a deeply ulcerated internal carotid artery atheroma responsible for TIAs refractory to antiplatelet therapy.

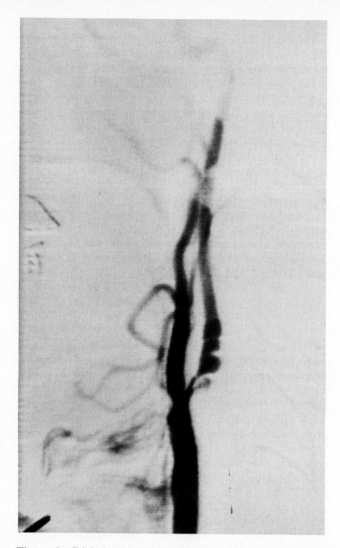

Figure 3 Digital subtraction carotid angiogram demonstrating a preocclusive high-grade stenosis resulting from a multiulcerated complex atheromatous plaque at the origin of the internal carotid artery associated with a mild contralateral upper extremity paresis.

endarterectomy in acute stroke patients reported in earlier series. Unfortunately, these patients represented a heterogenous group consisting of those with mass lesions and hemorrhage as well as ischemic infarcts of varying orders of magnitude. That early experience resulted in the teaching that a 4- to 6-week period of stabilization is required before angiography or surgical intervention. CT has eliminated much of this heterogeneity and allows angiography to be undertaken earlier in these patients' course. A group of individuals with high-grade, preocclusive stenotic lesions has emerged, and in spite of adequate anticoagulation, some have extended their infarcts and thus increased the magnitude of their disability (Fig. 3). For these patients with significant residual carotid territory at risk after the onset of a neurologic deficit of limited anatomic scope, endarterectomy should be considered.

Patients presenting with an acute neurologic deficit may be initially categorized as those with stable, fixed neurologic deficits and those with unstable or evolving

deficits (Fig. 4). After a complete neurologic examination and appropriate clinical stabilization, a CT scan is obtained along with noninvasive duplex evaluation. In the absence of evidence implicating acute intracerebral hemorrhage, contrast imaging is undertaken using intraarterial digital subtraction angiography to visualize both extra- and intracranial cerebral vasculature. Patients with fixed deficits may be further subdivided on clinical grounds on the basis of infarct size. For those with major infarcts clinically manifesting with a dense hemiplegia, with or without speech impairment, endarterectomy is not indicated, because little carotid territory remains at risk for further infarct. Patients with more limited deficits but no demonstrable ipsilateral carotid flow would also derive no benefit from a carotid endarterectomy. However, those with apparent angiographic occlusion at the origin of the internal carotid artery may demonstrate

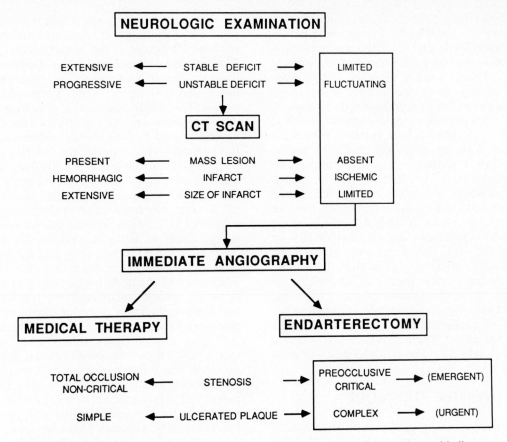

NEUROLOGIC EXAMINATION

| EXTENSIVE | ← STABLE DEFICIT → | LIMITED |
| PROGRESSIVE | ← UNSTABLE DEFICIT → | FLUCTUATING |

CT SCAN

PRESENT	← MASS LESION →	ABSENT
HEMORRHAGIC	← INFARCT →	ISCHEMIC
EXTENSIVE	← SIZE OF INFARCT →	LIMITED

IMMEDIATE ANGIOGRAPHY

MEDICAL THERAPY   **ENDARTERECTOMY**

| TOTAL OCCLUSION NON-CRITICAL | ← STENOSIS → | PREOCCLUSIVE CRITICAL → (EMERGENT) |
| SIMPLE | ← ULCERATED PLAQUE → | COMPLEX → (URGENT) |

Figure 4 Algorithm for evaluation of patients with neurologic deficits and carotid disease. (From Whittemore AD. Surgical treatment of carotid disease in patients with neurologic deficits. J Vasc Surg 1987; 5:910–916; with permission.)

a patent distal internal carotid artery on delayed films; these therefore may be appropriate candidates for urgent endarterectomy, since angiography may not adequately document a small residual lumen.

Patients with relatively limited neurologic deficits who retain significant ipsilateral carotid territory cerebral tissue at risk for recurrent infarct are indeed candidates for urgent endarterectomy, which can be undertaken within 24 hours of onset with no morbidity or mortality risks greater than those sustained as a consequence of elective endarterectomy.

Patients with coexistent carotid and coronary artery disease represent a special subcategory worthy of individual consideration. Patients with symptomatic coronary disease and concurrent significant carotid disease may be at increased risk for stroke associated with coronary bypass. Conversely, patients with significant carotid disease warranting endarterectomy may well harbor equally significant coexistent coronary artery disease. In both cases, the risk of postoperative cerebral and/or coronary events may well be higher than in the population without coexistent disease; therefore, simultaneous treatment for both conditions has been advocated. Once again, in the presence of conflicting data, I have taken the stand that, provided no additional morbidity is incurred, both lesions may be successfully man-

aged simultaneously. More commonly, patients with coronary insufficiency being prepared for bypass, who demonstrate significant carotid disease for which I would recommend endarterectomy independent of the coexistent coronary disease, are currently advised to undergo simultaneous carotid endarterectomy and coronary bypass. This policy is justified by the fact that no added morbidity is sustained, and a second hospitalization and general anesthetic is avoided. Similarly, patients for whom carotid endarterectomy has been advised, but who have significant and unstable angina increasing the risk of a postoperative cardiac event, should also undergo simultaneous repair.

PREOPERATIVE EVALUATION

The specific preoperative evaluation of patients being considered for carotid endarterectomy consists of CT and duplex scans. CT will rule out the presence of a mass lesion or hemorrhagic infarct, provide useful information with regard to the size of an infarct in patients with fixed deficits, and may supply evidence of silent cortical infarcts in patients previously thought to be asymptomatic. The duplex scan, particularly with the addition of color flow, provides adequate sensitivity and specificity for screening patients to determine the necessity for invasive arteriography. Patients with persistent TIAs on antiplatelet therapy without hemodynamically significant lesions on duplex scan may still warrant arteriography to determine the presence of significant ulceration. Similarly, since the duplex scan cannot reliably distinguish between a preocclusive, high-grade stenosis and total occlusion, arteriography for final differentiation is necessary in such patients. With these two exceptions, then, arteriography should be undertaken in patients with symptomatic carotid artery lesions resulting in greater than 50 percent stenosis, in asymptomatic patients whose lesions have progressed beyond 80 percent stenosis, and in individuals with fixed or evolving neurologic deficits of limited anatomic scope and with significant residual carotid territory at risk for further infarction. The recent addition of magnetic resonance imaging (MRI) may soon alter the routine preoperative management of these patients. MRI techniques to image the cerebral vasculature are improving, and MRI also provides the anatomic information for which CT is now required. In the near future, a single MRI will provide all the information currently obtained by angiography and CT, at less cost and inconvenience to the patient.

OPERATIVE TECHNIQUE

Once the decision to proceed with endarterectomy has been finalized, several options become available regarding the conduct of the operation. Satisfactory anesthesia may be administered with local, regional, or general techniques, and all three methods in experienced hands have proved satisfactory. Most surgeons and patients, however, prefer a general anesthetic, which has become increasingly more safe with the availability of intraoperative electroencephalographic (EEG) monitoring. Although most perioperative strokes are probably caused by embolization of atheromatous debris during the initial arterial dissection, rather than by hypoperfusion during the procedure, it seems prudent to provide sustained ipsilateral cerebral perfusion. Several methods of assessing the adequacy of such perfusion are available, primarily including the determination of stump pressure and EEG monitoring, but I prefer the selective approach using a multichannel EEG monitor. When a significant deviation from the baseline EEG is noted, a shunt may be expeditiously inserted to restore ipsilateral perfusion. I have noted that 16 percent of patients undergoing elective endarterectomy require intravascular shunting for reversal of such changes. It is significant to note that this shunt requirement increases to 27 percent in patients with a contralateral high-grade stenosis and to 40 percent in those with contralateral occlusion. A maximum of 67 percent of patients with fixed neurologic deficits and bilateral significant disease require the insertion of an indwelling shunt, which testifies to the substantial risk involved in endarterectomy in these patients operated on without appropriate cerebral protection.

The surgical procedure consists of the initial carotid artery dissection through an incision made along the anterior border of the sternocleidomastoid muscle. The common, internal, and external carotid arteries are dissected free of their companion structures, care being taken to avoid injury to the vagus and hypoglossal nerves. The major goal of this dissection is to ensure adequate distal exposure of the internal carotid artery beyond grossly evident disease. After intravenous anticoagulation with heparin, the arteries are occluded with atraumatic clamps, and a longitudinal incision is made in the distal common carotid artery and carried through the origin of the internal carotid artery with its stenotic atheroma until normal intima is clearly visualized in the distal internal carotid vessel (Fig. 5A). In the event of EEG changes at this point, an indwelling shunt is inserted (Fig. 5B). Endarterectomy is then undertaken by establishing a plane between the atheroma and the underlying residual media (Fig. 5C). It is of critical importance to remove the entire atheroma, including a posterior tongue of disease that extends a variable distance distally. The distal intimal cuff must also be firmly adherent to the underlying media, and on rare occasions fine tacking sutures are required. The orifice of the external carotid artery may also require endarterectomy to ensure the continued patency of this important collateral vessel. The arteriotomy is then closed primarily with fine suture material (Fig. 5D). Although I have not found it necessary, many surgeons prefer to close the arterial incision using an elliptical patch of vein or prosthetic material to minimize the impact of postoperative stenosis. After completion of the closure and restoration of cerebral perfusion, intraoperative arteriography and/or duplex scanning should be undertaken to ensure a technically satisfactory result. The incision is closed in routine fashion and the patient closely monitored in a recovery area until fully alert and normotensive. Approximately 25 percent of patients require some degree of intravenous antihypertensive agent for a short time postoperatively. This phenomenon does not appear to correlate with antecedent hypertension or with any other single variable. Most patients do not require admission to an intensive care unit and are routinely discharged on the second postoperative day.

POSTOPERATIVE COMPLICATIONS

Perioperative complications associated with carotid endarterectomy that result in death and significant neurologic morbidity are limited to less than 3 percent in my experience with more than 800 procedures during the past decade. This figure is representative of most series available in the current literature. It is important to differentiate between central and peripheral neurologic morbidity, since transient cranial nerve deficits may result in as many as 10 percent of patients from local manipulation during the dissection, and usually resolve within a few weeks. Difficulty in initiating swallowing

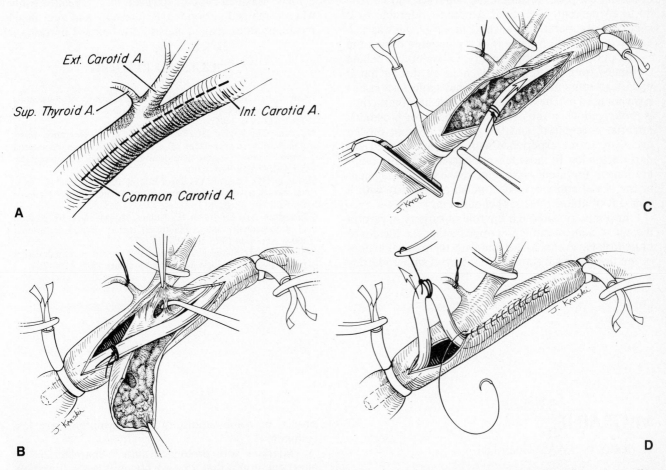

Figure 5 After a longitudinal arteriotomy through the origin of the internal carotid *(A)*, deterioration of baseline electroencephalographic tracing necessitated the insertion of an indwelling shunt as illustrated *(B)*. With cerebral perfusion re-established *(C)*, endarterectomy is carried out and the shunt removed *(D)* just before completion of the closure.

may accompany surgically induced cervical edema, but may also occasionally reflect dysfunction of the pharyngeal constrictors from manipulation of the glossopharyngeal nerve. A change in voice not infrequently results from cord edema associated with endotracheal intubation, but may also be produced by manipulation of the vagus or superior laryngeal nerves during operative dissection. The spinal accessory nerve is usually protected by the overlying sternocleidomastoid muscle and rarely becomes paretic. Adequate exposure of the distal internal carotid artery may require transection of the ansa hypoglossi and anteromedial reflection of the hypoglossal nerve. This maneuver may result in some degree of deviation of the tongue with associated paresthesias, which usually resolve within a few days. Retraction of the digastric muscle may be associated with trauma to the marginal mandibular branch of the cervical nerve. In this event, temporary paresis of the ipsilateral inferior orbicularis oris muscle should not be mistakenly attributed to a central facial deficit.

A second important distinction must be made with regard to postoperative neurologic deficits in patients operated on with earlier fixed deficits. Such patients often develop a temporary worsening of the deficit, with subsequent resolution after the first 48 or 72 hours. Whether this is a result of anesthesia or ischemia is unknown.

As with all arterial injuries, the initial phase of healing appears to be initiated by the adherence of platelets over the denuded surface. Smooth muscle cells are then stimulated to both proliferate and migrate to the luminal surface. Subsequent myointimal proliferation results in an unpredictable degree of recurrent stenosis. This restenosis appears to be progressive during the first 3 to 6 months and is almost inevitable, to a limited extent, in all patients. Only 2 percent of patients, however, develop symptoms referable to recurrent stenosis, and such lesions rarely become hemodynamically significant. Recurrent stenosis differs pathologically from an atheroma in that the lesion consists of a smooth, glistening white surface that is not conducive to the deposition of fibrin or platelets. Nevertheless, it has been my practice to monitor postendarterectomy patients with serial duplex evaluations every 4 months for the first 2 years in an effort to monitor the healing response and the status of the contralateral vessel, given the symmetry of the disease process. Should the vessel restenose to the 80 to 85 percent level, or if symptoms referable to it supervene, reoperation is advised; however, this was necessary in only 2 to 5 percent of my patients during the 5-year period after initial surgery. Considerable debate continues over the use of a vein patch during initial endarterectomy to minimize this inevitable response. I have not used patches routinely, because anesthesia time is prolonged when the use of a vein patch or prosthetic material is required, and the practice has not proved necessary in my experience with over 800 carotid endarterectomies. In those few patients who require reoperation, my preference is to reincise the stenotic segment of the vessel and carry out a patch angioplasty with a segment of autogenous saphenous vein.

In summary, although the role of surgery in carotid disease remains unsettled, it appears that the incidence of neurologic events associated with the natural history of the disease is substantially minimized with endarter-

ectomy. Maximal benefit, however, may be realized only when combined perioperative mortality and neurologic morbidity rates remain consistently below 3 percent.

SUGGESTED READING

Dixon S, Pais SO, Raviola C, et al. Natural history of nonstenotic, asymptomatic ulcerative lesions of the carotid artery. Arch Surg 1982; 117:1493–1498.

Mondeta GL, Taylor DC, Nicholls SC, et al. Operative versus nonoperative management of asymptomatic high-grade internal carotid artery stenosis: Improved results with endarterectomy. Stroke 1987; 18:1005–1010.

Roederer GO, Langlois YE, Jager KA, et al. The natural history of carotid arterial disease in asymptomatic patients with cervical bruits. Stroke 1984; 15:605–613.

Whittemore AD, Kauffman JL, Kohler TR, Mannick JA. Routine electroencephalographic monitoring during carotid endarterectomy. Ann Surg 1983; 197:707–713.

Whittemore AD, Mannick JA. Surgical treatment of carotid disease in patients with neurologic deficits. J Vasc Surg 1985; 2:250–254.

MIGRAINE

JERRY W. SWANSON, M.D.

Migraine is a chronic, idiopathic headache disorder that usually is manifested by attacks lasting for a few hours or up to 3 days. A typical headache involves half of the head, but not infrequently it can be bilateral. The pain usually is pulsatile and moderately severe in intensity. It is aggravated by physical activity and often is associated with nausea and sometimes with vomiting. The headache usually is accompanied by photophobia and intolerance to noise. Women are affected more commonly than men, and a family history is present in more than half of the patients. The onset of the disorder usually is during childhood or young adulthood, and a diagnosis of new-onset migraine after age 45 years should be made with care.

There are various clinical subtypes of migraine. Migraine without aura (common migraine) consists of attacks as described above without antecedent or accompanying neurologic symptoms. Migraine with typical aura (classic migraine) consists of attacks in which there are associated neurologic symptoms that reflect cerebral hemisphere dysfunction. They usually develop gradually over 15 to 30 minutes, and last not more than 60 minutes. The most common aura consists of a homonymous visual disturbance. Hemisensory symptoms, hemiparesis, dys-

phasia, or combinations of these symptoms are less common.

Migraine with prolonged aura is characterized by aura symptoms that exceed 60 minutes in duration. Migraine aura without headache has also been called "migraine equivalent" and can be difficult to differentiate from transient ischemic attacks of thromboembolic origin when they first begin in the elderly. Ophthalmoplegic migraine, retinal migraine, familial hemiplegic migraine, and basilar migraine are uncommon subtypes. The term "status migrainosus" (migraine status) refers to a migraine attack that persists for more than 72 hours.

The mechanisms of a migraine attack remain poorly understood. Changes in blood composition and platelet function, perhaps initiated endogenously or by environmental factors, may have a triggering role. The pathophysiology of the attack is presumed to reside in the brain, which, through the trigeminovascular and other systems, interacts with intracranial and extracranial vasculature and perivascular spaces. 5-Hydroxytryptamine (5-HT; also called serotonin) has been implicated in the genesis of migraine attacks, and a number of drugs that are thought to be beneficial in this disorder have an effect at 5-HT receptors. The mechanism of aura symptoms most likely reflects a local change in cerebral metabolism akin to the spreading cortical depression of Leão, although some authors have argued in favor of cortical arteriolar vasospasm with consequent ischemia. Precise delineation of the mechanism of migraine requires further investigation.

APPROACH TO THE MIGRAINE PATIENT

The primary goal in the management of a patient with migraine is to prevent attacks or, once an attack is initiated, to limit its duration and severity. Treatment of migraine can be considered to be of three general types: (1) avoidance of precipitating factors, (2) treatment of acute attacks, and (3) prophylactic (preventive) therapy. Typically, the initial approach includes the first two of these. Prophylactic treatment is used if the attacks are frequent, respond poorly to acute treatment, and have a significant impact on the patient's ability to function (e.g., produce frequent impairment at work or school). The foundation for treatment of these patients is the physician's genuine interest in alleviating their distress. The establishment of honest communication between physician and patient is important for successful treatment.

Avoidance of Precipitating Factors

Patients who recognize the precipitating factors of migraine can sometimes avoid them. Although this is uncommon, some foods trigger attacks in susceptible patients. Strong or aged cheeses, chocolate, alcoholic beverages, chicken livers, cured meats, pickled herring, canned figs, and pods of broad beans are some of the more commonly implicated substances. If there is a question regarding the role of a substance, it can be eliminated from the diet for a time to determine whether this decreases the frequency of headache. Persons who consume large amounts of caffeine sometimes benefit from decreasing or ceasing this intake.

Stress seems to be a potent trigger for migraines in some sufferers. Although the headache may emerge during a stressful period, it often emerges after a stressful event (the so-called let-down headache). Occasionally, biofeedback and stress management play a significant role in decreasing the severity of such headaches.

Changing sleep and waking times and missing meals may provoke a headache. Delayed awakening on weekends and holidays can be a potent headache precipitant. At least one study suggests that delayed awakening plus heavy caffeine intake during the week play synergistic roles in the precipitation of some weekend headaches. Patients should be encouraged to maintain stability in both meal and sleep patterns.

The previous wide use of high-estrogen-content oral contraceptives was associated with aggravation of migraine in a high percentage of women. Even the low-estrogen-content oral contraceptives now generally in use have been implicated in the aggravation of migraine in up to 5 percent of women migraine sufferers. When the headaches are troublesome, the oral contraceptives should be stopped. Interestingly, a small percentage of women with migraine note relief of their headaches with use of oral contraceptives.

Menopause may be associated with either alleviation or worsening of migraine. Estrogen replacement has been reported to be helpful in decreasing migraine headaches in some persons. Paradoxically, estrogen replacement sometimes aggravates migraine; decreasing the dosage may be of help in these patients.

Treatment of Acute Migraine Attacks

An acute migraine attack is more likely to be aborted if treated early. Mild analgesics such as aspirin (650 to 975 mg) or acetaminophen (1,000 mg) will provide many patients good relief from mild to moderate migraine attacks. Other nonsteroidal anti-inflammatory drugs such as naproxen sodium (825 mg, followed by another dose of 550 mg) or ibuprofen (400 to 800 mg) also can be effective.

Isometheptene mucate, a sympathomimetic agent, is available in the combination drug Midrin. Each Midrin capsule contains 65 mg of isometheptene mucate, 325 mg of acetaminophen, and 100 mg of dichloralphenazone, a mild tranquilizer. The combination is well tolerated with few side effects and is effective in the treatment of mild to moderate migraine attacks. The dosage is two capsules at attack onset, with repeat doses of one capsule at 30- to 60-minute intervals if needed but not to exceed five capsules per 12 hours.

The effectiveness of aspirin or acetaminophen appears to be enhanced in some patients by the addition of a mild barbiturate and caffeine; common combinations are aspirin (325 mg) or acetaminophen (325 mg) with caffeine (40 mg) and butalbital (50 mg). The dosage is one or two tablets every 4 hours as needed, not to exceed six tablets per day. The side effects include sedation and the potential for dependence; hence, these combinations are probably best avoided in most patients. These drugs, as well as Midrin, may predispose patients to chronic daily headaches and therefore should not be taken for more than 2 or 3 days a week.

Use of narcotics presents a significant risk for the development of dependence and should not be prescribed routinely for chronic headache disorders such as migraine.

Antiemetics

Nausea and vomiting are frequent accompaniments of migraine attacks. In addition, impaired gastric motility is common during migraine and is associated with impaired absorption of medications. Metoclopramide increases lower esophageal pressure and gastric motility. It can be given as 10- to 20-mg doses orally with or, preferably, 10 minutes before analgesics or ergotamine (see below). This drug is particularly worthwhile when the patient has significant nausea or has not responded to an antimigraine medication taken alone.

Metoclopramide should not be used whenever stimulation of gastrointestinal motility might be dangerous. It is also contraindicated in patients with pheochromocytoma or epilepsy, or patients receiving other drugs that are likely to cause extrapyramidal reactions. Extrapyramidal symptoms manifested primarily as acute dystonic reactions occur rarely. Restlessness, drowsiness, fatigue, and lassitude are fairly common side effects; insomnia, headache, confusion, and dizziness occur less frequently.

Domperidone also stimulates gastric motility and has a lower reported incidence of central nervous system side effects, presumably because it does not cross the blood-brain barrier in significant amounts. This drug is not yet available in the United States for general use.

Prochlorperazine, 5 to 10 mg orally or 20 mg by rectal suppository, is an alternative antiemetic. It can be sedating and may produce acute dystonic reactions.

Ergotamine Tartrate and Dihydroergotamine Mesylate

The acute treatment of severe migraine attacks with ergotamine tartrate is often successful, especially if used early in the attack. Ergotamine is an alpha-adrenergic blocking agent with direct stimulating effects on smooth muscle of blood vessels, and it has been held that this vasoconstrictor action accounts for its effectiveness in migraine. More recently, evidence has accumulated that its effect is mediated via action at 5-HT receptors. The drug is available in oral, rectal, and inhalant preparations; higher plasma concentrations usually are achieved with the latter two routes (Table 1). Preparations are available for sublingual administration, but ergotamine is poorly absorbed via this route. Ergotamine is often combined with caffeine, which increases its absorption and peak plasma level. Its use carries the disadvantage of a stimulant effect, which makes sleep difficult for patients in whom a period of sleep is necessary to terminate an attack. As noted above, the tolerance and effectiveness of oral administration of ergotamine can be significantly increased with coadministration of metoclopramide.

Relatively common side effects include nausea, vomiting, muscle cramps, and abdominal cramps. Less common effects include tremor, dyspnea, angina pectoris, and claudication. Angina or claudication requires discontinuation of the drug. Ergotism is the result of overuse of the drug, and its full manifestations include gangrene. Major vasoconstriction is usually preceded by lower limb paresthesias, coolness of the distal limbs, and the pain of claudication.

Ergotamine dependence with associated ergotamine-induced or ergotamine-withdrawal headaches can occur when the drug is used as infrequently as 3 days a week. Accordingly, this medication should not be used more often than 2 days a week on a regular basis.

Ergotamine is contraindicated in patients with peripheral vascular disease, impaired renal hepatic function, poorly controlled hypertension, ischemic heart disease, pregnancy, or sepsis.

Dihydroergotamine mesylate is available only in an injectable form and can be administered either intramuscularly or intravenously. It has a high affinity for a number of 5-HT receptors as well as a number of other biogenic amine receptors and is a potent vasoconstrictor, but it has a lesser effect than ergotamine on peripheral vessels. In patients who cannot tolerate other acute treatments or find them ineffective, self-administered intramuscular injection of dihydroergotamine is an alternative. The dose is 1 ml (1 mg) and can be repeated at 1-hour intervals to a total of 3 ml (3 mg) if needed. The maximal weekly dose is 6 ml (6 mg). Best results usually are attained by titrating the dose for a number of headache episodes to discover the minimal effective dose for the patient. This dosage should be used at the onset of subsequent attacks.

The most common side effect is nausea. This can be minimized by using dose titration or by adding metoclopramide, 10 to 20 mg orally, to the regimen. The use of a non-nauseating dose of dihydroergotamine is key if the drug is to be effective. Distal limb paresthesias and localized edema or itching are common. Leg weakness and precordial distress are uncommon side effects.

Dihydroergotamine is contraindicated in pregnancy, Prinzmetal's angina, or major organ failure. It has been used cautiously in patients with coronary artery disease.

Sumatriptan is an agonist at some 5-HT receptor subtypes. It has undergone clinical trials for use in the acute treatment of migraine attacks and appears to be effective by parenteral and oral routes. Intranasal and rectal preparations are being developed. It may be approved for general use in the United States in the future.

Treatment of Acute Migraine Attacks in the Emergency Room

A mixture of dihydroergotamine at 0.5 to 1 mg plus metoclopramide at 10 mg intravenously is effective in relieving acute migraine attacks in most patients. In addition to the side effects noted above, some patients experience a transient dysphoric effect when this combination is administered intravenously.

Intravenous injection of prochlorperazine edisylate

Table 1 Ergotamine Preparations

Preparation	Dosage
Oral Administration	
Ergotamine tartrate, 1 mg, with caffeine, 100 mg	One or two tablets initially; repeat one tablet each half hour, if needed, to maximum of 5 mg in 24 hr or 10 mg per wk
Ergotamine tartrate, 2 mg	One tablet initially; repeat dose every half hour, if needed, to maximum of 6 mg in 24 hr or 10 mg per wk
Rectal Suppository	
Ergotamine tartrate, 2 mg, with caffeine, 100 mg	One-fourth to one suppository; repeat in 1 hr, if needed, to maximum of 6 mg in 24 hr or 10 mg per wk
Inhalation Aerosol	
Ergotamine tartrate	Single inhalation (0.36 mg) initially; repeat at 5-min intervals, if needed, not exceeding six inhalations in 24 hr or 15 per wk

is another effective treatment for acute migraine attacks. The dosage is 10 mg given slowly over 2 minutes. The mechanism of action is uncertain. The most common side effect is drowsiness, and there is a risk of acute dystonic reactions and orthostatic hypotension. Contraindications include a history of hypersensitivity to phenothiazines, seizure disorder, pregnancy, lactation, hypotension, altered level of consciousness, and glaucoma. This drug can be combined with dihydroergotamine, 1 mg.

Chlorpromazine administered intravenously in a dosage of 0.1 mg per kilogram and repeated as needed every 15 minutes, up to a total of three doses, is another effective neuroleptic agent in the acute treatment of migraine attacks. It is best to first give the patient a bolus of isotonic saline, 5 ml per kilogram, to decrease the risk of orthostatic hypotension. The blood pressure should be monitored carefully. Mild drowsiness is the most common side effect; some patients also note dizziness, burning at the injection site, dry mouth, or nasal congestion. This drug should not be used in patients who have a history of allergy; are taking phenothiazines, monoamine oxidase inhibitors, or antidepressants; or have Parkinson's disease, a history of dystonic reactions, or a seizure disorder. It is also contraindicated in patients who are pregnant or nursing.

The combination of meperidine (75 to 100 mg) and hydroxyzine (50 to 75 mg) given intramuscularly has been widely used for acute treatment of migraine. This combination appears to be less effective than the other approaches described and carries the risk of possible narcotic abuse.

Treatment of Status Migrainosus

Status migrainosus is defined as an attack of migraine with a headache phase lasting longer than 72 hours despite treatment. Headache-free intervals may last less than 4 hours. Status migrainosus usually occurs in a background of chronic headaches and treatment with agents such as narcotics, hypnotics, tranquilizers, or ergotamine. An important part of therapy is discontinuation of or reduction in the use of these drugs, which may necessitate tapering of the medications and intravenous rehydration while the patient is hospitalized.

In addition, a regimen combining metoclopramide and dihydroergotamine has been described as helpful: 10 mg of metoclopramide intravenously, followed by 0.5 mg of dihydroergotamine intravenously. If significant nausea ensues after this dose or if the headache is absent within 1 hour, no more dihydroergotamine is given for 8 hours. After 8 hours, another 0.5-mg dose of dihydroergotamine is administered intravenously. If nausea occurs after the second dose, the dihydroergotamine dosage is decreased to 0.3 mg intravenously every 8 hours. If no nausea occurs after the first dose of medication but the head pain persists after 1 hour, an additional 0.5-mg dose of dihydroergotamine is given. Every 8 hours thereafter, another 1.0-mg dose is given for 2 days. The dihydroergotamine is then tapered over an additional 1 to 2 days in most cases, although some patients benefit by continuing its use intramuscularly at home. The metoclopramide is continued for at least the first 24 hours but often can be discontinued thereafter. This regimen is likely to be effective only if the dose-related nausea is minimized.

Prophylactic (Preventive) Treatment of Migraine

Prophylactic treatment of migraine is based on daily use of one or occasionally more medications to decrease the number or severity of attacks. This approach is reserved for patients whose frequency of migraine attacks exceeds the safety limitations for use of abortive or symptomatic medications and for patients in whom these medications are contraindicated or ineffective, circumstances that result in frequent interruptions of daily obligations such as work or school. Patients who experience more than two major attacks a month that respond poorly to abortive therapy often are candidates for such treatment. Most preventive agents should be used in therapeutic dosages for at least 6 to 8 weeks before it is assumed that they are not effective. Some agents are not tolerated by a patient and need to be discontinued sooner. If effective, preventive treatment should be used for 6 to 12 months, followed by a slow tapering of the medication to allow recognition of the natural remission of the headaches.

Beta-Adrenergic Blockers

These probably are the most widely used drugs for migraine prevention. Propranolol was the first found to have a beneficial effect incidental to its use for the treatment of angina. Other beta-adrenergic blockers that are useful in migraine treatment are nadolol, atenolol, metoprolol, and timolol. Propranolol is available in a slow-release form that allows administration only once or twice daily. Nadolol and atenolol have long half-lives, which also allows once-a-day administration. Each of these medications is best tolerated if started at a low dosage to minimize side effects; the dosage is slowly increased as tolerated and necessary. The dosage ranges are listed in Table 2.

The mechanism of action of these drugs remains open to speculation; not all of them appear to interact with 5-HT receptors. These drugs lack intrinsic sympathomimetic activity and antagonize $beta_1$-adrenergic receptors. Side effects include bradycardia, hypotension, decreased exercise tolerance, sedation, and depression. This group of drugs should be used with caution in patients with cardiac disease or insulin-treated diabetes mellitus. Nonselective beta-adrenergic blockers should not be used in patients with asthma, and even those with some selectivity should be used cautiously.

Calcium Channel Antagonists

There has been interest in this group of drugs for migraine therapy in recent years. They are potentially

Table 2 Beta-Adrenergic Blocking Agents

Preparation	Dosage Range (mg)
Propranolol	20 t.i.d. to 80 q.i.d.
Propranolol, long-acting	80 q.d. to 160 b.i.d.
Nadolol	20 to 160 q.d.
Atenolol	50 to 200 q.d.
Metoprolol	50 to 100 b.i.d.
Timolol	10 to 30 b.i.d.

useful when beta-adrenergic blockers are not tolerated or are contraindicated. This group of drugs may be especially effective in patients who have prolonged neurologic symptoms associated with migraine (migraine with prolonged aura) or when migraine is associated with Raynaud's phenomenon or Prinzmetal's angina. Some of these agents have affinity for the 5-HT$_2$ receptor, which may account for their usefulness, although their efficacy in migraine also has been attributed to their protective effects during hypoxia or their ability to block intracranial vasoconstriction. The following have been used for migraine prophylaxis: verapamil hydrochloride, 80 to 160 mg three times a day; nifedipine, 10 to 20 mg three times a day; and diltiazem, 30 to 90 mg four times a day.

Flunarizine also appears to be efficacious but is not available in the United States. Nimodipine has been studied for use in migraine prophylaxis but did not demonstrate activity significantly different from the placebo, although some workers in the field believe that the trial design was flawed. Occasional patients may benefit from its use. Potential side effects include headaches, vasomotor changes, heart block, heart failure, edema, constipation, and nausea.

Antidepressants

The tricyclic antidepressant amitriptyline is effective in the prophylactic management of migraine. The effective dosage, usually 25 to 150 mg per day, usually is given as a single dose at bedtime. The drug should be started at 10 or 25 mg and increased slowly to minimize side effects, especially sedation. Nortriptyline at 25 to 150 mg per day and doxepin at 25 to 150 mg per day also are efficacious in some cases. The potential mechanisms of action include the blockade of 5-HT uptake or 5-HT$_2$ receptor antagonism. Side effects include sedation, dry mouth, weight gain, constipation, orthostatic hypotension, palpitations, urinary retention, and confusion. These drugs should be used cautiously in patients with cardiac disorders, impaired renal or hepatic function, seizure disorders, benign prostatic hypertrophy, or angle-closure glaucoma.

The monoamine oxidase inhibitor phenelzine is an effective antimigraine drug. The starting dosage is 15 mg per day, which can be increased in increments of 15 mg per day every week until a total of 60 mg per day is given, divided into two or three doses. Occasionally, 75 mg per day is more effective than lower doses. Phenelzine's

efficacy as an antimigraine drug may be related to an increase in endogenous 5-HT levels. Common side effects include insomnia, anticholinergic symptoms, weight gain, orthostatic hypotension, decreased libido, and inhibition of ejaculation. Hypertensive reactions related to ingestion of tyramine-containing foods are a potential complication of therapy, and these substances must be eliminated from the patient's diet. They include (1) high-protein foods that have undergone aging, fermentation, pickling, smoking, or bacterial contamination; and (2) aged cheeses, red wine, fermented products, pods of broad beans, fava beans, and chocolate. Safe foods, when fresh and used in small amounts, include sour cream, yogurt, meat extracts, chopped liver, dry sausage, and alcoholic beverages (excluding red wine). Coadministration of meperidine, dextromethorphan, levodopa, anorexiants, amphetamines, ephedrine, phenylephrine, phenylpropanolamine, methylphenidate, or nonprescription drugs containing sympathomimetic agents is contraindicated.

Nonsteroidal Anti-inflammatory Drugs

Two drugs from this group have shown efficacy in the prophylactic management of migraine. Naproxen sodium has been used at a dosage of 550 mg twice daily and appears to decrease the severity, if not the frequency, of migraine headaches. Aspirin, 650 mg, has been useful in some patients. The side effects of the chronic use of aspirin are well known, and those of naproxen sodium are summarized earlier in this chapter. The mechanism of action of these agents is uncertain; it may involve prostaglandins and their antiplatelet effect.

Methysergide Maleate

Methysergide, a semisynthetic ergot alkaloid, is a very effective prophylactic agent for migraine. It has complex effects on serotonergic and other neurotransmitter systems. The dosage ranges from 2 to 8 mg per day in divided doses taken with meals. It should be started at 2 mg per day and increased slowly to avoid side effects. The usefulness of this drug is limited by its ability to produce retroperitoneal fibrosis, pleuropulmonary fibrosis, and endocardial fibrosis with prolonged administration. Fibrotic plaques simulating Peyronie's disease have also been associated with its use. Treatment with this drug should be interrupted after no more than 6 months to avoid fibrotic complications. Ideally, the dosage should be tapered at the end of a course to avoid rebound headache. This drug should be used only in patients with frequent and severe headaches that have failed to respond to most other agents.

Common gastrointestinal side effects include nausea, vomiting, abdominal pain, and diarrhea; these often can be controlled by gradual introduction of the medication and by administration of the drug with meals. Other side effects include muscle cramps, joint stiffness, peripheral vasoconstriction, limb claudication, tachycardia, angina pectoris, limb paresthesias, insomnia, drowsiness, euphoria, anxiety, vertigo, light-headedness, depression, facial flushing, weight gain, peripheral edema, neutropenia, and eosinophilia. It is contraindicated in pregnant or lactating women and in persons with peripheral vascular disease, severe arteriosclerosis, uncontrolled hypertension, coronary artery disease, thrombophlebitis, pulmonary disease, collagen disease or fibrotic disorders, impaired renal or hepatic function, valvular heart disease, debilitated state, or serious infections.

Cyproheptadine

This drug is an antihistaminic agent with strong blocking action at the 5-HT_2 receptors, which possibly explains its efficacy in migraine prophylaxis. It is not a markedly effective agent in adults but does seem to be effective in children. The dosage is 4 to 8 mg three times a day. The common side effects are sedation and weight gain; dry mouth, nausea, light-headedness, peripheral edema, diarrhea, and leg ache also can occur. It is contraindicated in pregnancy, nursing mothers, angle-closure glaucoma, stenosing peptic ulcer, symptomatic benign prostatic hypertrophy, bladder neck obstruction, and pyloroduodenal obstruction and in elderly, debilitated patients. It should be used with caution in patients with a history of bronchial asthma, increased intraocular pressure, hyperthyroidism, cardiovascular disease, or hypertension.

SUGGESTED READING

Belgrade MJ, Ling LJ, Schleevogt MB, et al. Comparison of single-dose meperidine, butorphanol, and dihydroergotamine in the treatment of vascular headache. Neurology 1989; 39:590–592.

Headache Classification Committee of the International Headache Society. Classification and diagnostic criteria for headache disorders, cranial neuralgias, and facial pain. Cephalalgia 1988; 8 Suppl 7:1–96.

Jones J, Sklar D, Dougherty J, White W. Randomized double-blind trial of intravenous prochlorperazine for the treatment of acute headache. JAMA 1989; 261:1174–1176.

Lane PL, McLellan BA, Baggoley CJ. Comparative efficacy of chlorpromazine and meperidine with dimenhydrinate in migraine headache. Ann Emerg Med 1989; 18:360–365.

Peroutka SJ. The pharmacology of current anti-migraine drugs. Headache 1990; 30 Suppl 1:5–11.

Raskin NH. Headache. 2nd ed. New York: Churchill Livingstone, 1988.

Raskin NH. Repetitive intravenous dihydroergotamine as therapy for intractable migraine. Neurology 1986; 36:995–997.

COMPLICATIONS OF INTRACRANIAL ANEURYSMS

EUGENE ROSSITCH, Jr., M.D.
JOHN P. COOKE, M.D., Ph.D.

In 1933 Egas Moniz demonstrated an aneurysm using cerebral angiography, and Dott performed the first planned operation for a saccular aneurysm. He placed muscle fragment against the aneurysm that had ruptured in the operating room, successfully stopping the bleeding and obtaining a good long-term result. Four years later, Dandy used a metal clip to isolate an aneurysm. He then desiccated the sac using electrocautery. Since these early days, much progress has been made in the technical aspects of aneurysm surgery. However, the management of cerebral vasospasm, a complication of subarachnoid hemorrhage due to aneurysm, remains difficult.

Intracranial aneurysms may be arteriosclerotic, mycotic, traumatic, or congenital. Arteriosclerotic aneurysms are fusiform, commonly originate from long segments of the internal carotid or basilar artery, and rarely rupture. Mycotic and traumatic aneurysms, however, frequently rupture. The most common intracranial aneurysm is the saccular (congenital) type, which most commonly arises from a vessel bifurcation at the circle of Willis. Most of these aneurysms have necks or stalks connecting them directly to the arterial lumen. In this respect, they differ from mycotic and traumatic aneurysms.

COMPLICATIONS

Approximately 5 million North Americans may have a saccular intracranial aneurysm. Most of these are small and associated with an uneventful course. However, about 30,000 of these individuals annually incur a subarachnoid hemorrhage from rupture of these lesions, and approximately one-third die immediately, never reaching medical care. Most victims are middle-aged, with a male predominance up to the fifth decade and a female predominance thereafter.

Headache is usually the most prominent feature of an aneurysmal subarachnoid hemorrhage. Its onset often marks the moment of vessel rupture. This often occurs with episodes of transient elevation in intracranial pressure such as during sexual intercourse or with the Valsalva maneuver. Most patients describe this as "the worst headache of my life." Aneurysms can also present as a focal neurologic deficit, e.g., a third nerve palsy. Meningismus, mental status changes, and autonomic disturbances can also be seen.

Subarachnoid hemorrhage can be traumatic or spontaneous. Spontaneous subarachnoid hemorrhage can be separated into primary or secondary types. In primary hemorrhages, the blood is deposited directly into the subarachnoid space. In secondary hemorrhages, the blood extends through brain parenchyma. Most primary hemorrhages are due to structural lesions of the blood vessels. Aneurysms account for 75 percent of primary subarachnoid hemorrhages, whereas 10 percent are due to arteriovenous malformations; the remaining 15 percent are of unknown cause. Subarachnoid hemorrhage secondary to an aneurysm rupture is most likely to result in intracranial vasospasm, probably because of the large amount of blood deposited in the subarachnoid space and its usual location at the base of the brain. Approximately 95 percent of aneurysms occur adjacent to the circle of Willis.

Morbidity and mortality from a ruptured aneurysm may be early or late. The early problems result from the local reaction to the initial hemorrhage as well as disturbances in the autonomic nervous system. These complications include acute hydrocephalus, labile hypertension, cardiac arrhythmias, and intraventricular extension of the blood. Late complications include rebleeding, delayed hydrocephalus, epilepsy, and cerebral vasospasm.

Cerebral vasospasm is the most feared complication of subarachnoid hemorrhage and causes symptoms in about 30 percent of patients who initially survive the bleed. Significant morbidity or mortality occurs in one-half of patients experiencing cerebral vasospasm. The pathophysiology of cerebral vasospasm remains enigmatic, but it is known that the cerebral vessels contain no vasa vasorum and depend on communication with the cerebrospinal fluid via the adventitia for oxygen, substrates, and waste disposal. The physical barrier of the subarachnoid blood may produce hypoxia of the vessel wall. In addition, a number of components of thrombus may have direct effects on blood vessel tone and growth. In animal models, the subarachnoid hemorrhage induces vasoconstriction, followed by structural alteration over a period of 48 hours; the first phase (vasoconstriction) is more difficult to demonstrate in humans, and symptoms are generally associated with the later phase of luminal narrowing owing to structural alterations. These changes in vascular structure begin with swelling of the endothelial cells and subintimal edema, followed by denudation of the endothelium and platelet adherence and aggregation. Subsequently, smooth muscle cell proliferation and infiltration of circulating blood cells (leukocytes and red cells) cause thickening of the vessel wall and further luminal narrowing. The reduction in cerebral blood flow may subsequently induce a transient neurologic deficit, a cerebrovascular accident, a disturbance of consciousness, or even death in severe cases.

The clinical manifestations of vasospasm are worsening headaches, nuccal rigidity, lethargy, fever, and deteriorating neurologic status. The electroencephalogram can show focal deficits, mostly consisting of a slow wave pattern that often correlates with the radiographic picture. Cerebral blood flow measurements by transcranial Doppler are not diagnostic, but a reduction in

cerebral blood flow to about half the normal value is a bad prognostic sign.

Arterial narrowing can be observed angiographically in almost 80 percent of patients with aneurysmal subarachnoid hemorrhage. It is rare to see angiographic vasospasm within 48 hours of the initial subarachnoid hemorrhage. The radiographic changes are delayed in onset and are most pronounced between days 5 and 14 after the subarachnoid hemorrhage. Patients with a significant amount of blood in the basal subarachnoid cisterns as seen on computed tomography (CT) are at greater risk for developing vasospasm. Intracranial arterial spasm affects mainly the anterior circulation, most often involving the distal internal carotid and proximal anterior and middle cerebral arteries (Fig. 1). The posterior circulation is not usually involved except in the case of basilar arterial aneurysms.

MANAGEMENT

Medical Therapy

General measures for patients suspected of harboring a ruptured intracranial aneurysm should be directed at prompt confirmation of the clinical diagnosis and hemodynamic stabilization. A CT scan should be per-

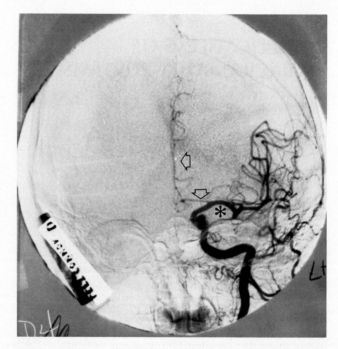

Figure 1 Digital subtraction angiography (anteroposterior view) performed in a woman who had incurred a subarachnoid hemorrhage 4 days earlier. The source of the bleed was an aneurysm of the anterior communicating artery. Note the marked luminal narrowing ("cerebral vasospasm") of the anterior cerebral artery and its branches *(arrowheads)*. Compare the dimension of the anterior cerebral artery to that of the middle cerebral artery *(asterisk),* which normally has about the same luminal diameter.

formed expeditiously; these are positive in over 90 percent of cases, but a negative scan does not rule out the diagnosis. Patients whose CT scan is negative should undergo a lumbar puncture to exclude a small hemorrhage. In patients with a positive CT or lumbar puncture result, cerebral angiography should be performed. Until surgery is performed, medical management is essential. This includes bed rest in a quiet, dark room; head elevation to 30 degrees; mild sedation; mild analgesics; stool softeners; and preoperative steroids. Blood pressure, fluid status, serum electrolytes, cardiac output, and hematocrit should be monitored. Antifibrinolytic agents were used in the past but are much less commonly employed today; they can lower the risk of rebleeding but also are associated with a rise in ischemic deficits from vasospasm. A greater emphasis on early surgery makes rebleeding less likely.

Hypertension is invariably associated with subarachnoid hemorrhages owing to increased sympathetic nervous outflow. In the absence of clinical or angiographic evidence of cerebral vasospasm, hypertension should be treated. However, autoregulation of cerebral resistance vessels is often disturbed, and overaggressive treatment of hypertension has been associated with evidence of cerebral ischemia, probably because of the reduced perfusion pressure. The hypertensive episodes are frequently severe, labile, and refractory to medical management. We find that the elevated blood pressure responds best to a combination of alpha- and beta-adrenergic blockade. Labetalol (which antagonizes both alpha- and beta-adrenoreceptors) may be given in intravenous boluses at 20 to 40 mg every 10 minutes up to a total dose of 300 mg or until the desired effect is obtained; a total dose of 200 mg is usually sufficient to attain an optimal blood pressure for these patients (range 150 to 170/80 to 90 mm Hg). Subsequently, oral doses of labetalol can be started in about 6 hours, usually beginning at 200 to 400 mg and titrating up to a maximal total dose of 1,200 mg twice daily. For patients with more labile blood pressure, a shorter-acting beta-blocker (e.g., intravenous esmolol) may be preferable. Frequently, we combine alpha- and beta-adrenergic blockade with a calcium entry antagonist for refractory hypertension. Sublingual nifedipine, 10 to 20 mg every 2 to 4 hours, has been our preferred agent. More vasoselective calcium entry antagonists are now available (e.g., nimodipine, nicardipine). There is some evidence that these agents may improve cerebral perfusion and perhaps reduce the incidence of cerebral vasospasm. Nimodipine has recently been approved by the Food and Drug Administration for treatment of cerebral vasospasm after subarachnoid hemorrhage. Use of nimodipine results in a decrease in morbidity and mortality and an improvement in neurologic deficits in patients with aneurysmal subarachnoid hemorrhage. Nimodipine therapy should be started within 96 hours of subarachnoid hemorrhage. The recommended dose is 60 mg every 4 hours for 3 weeks. The contents of these capsules can be administered through a nasogastric tube in patients who are unable to swallow.

Myocardial ischemia may be precipitated by the increase in sympathetic outflow that occurs with a subarachnoid hemorrhage. This is in part due to the increased myocardial oxygen demand brought about by the hypertensive state. In addition, increased coronary vasomotor tone may play a role in some patients, owing to excessive sympathetic outflow to the coronary vasculature. Indeed, electrocardiographic changes consistent with ischemia or coronary vasospasm may be observed in association with echocardiographically documented abnormalities of regional wall motion. Even young patients without a history of or risk factors for coronary artery disease may be affected. A combination of adrenergic and calcium channel blockade will serve to treat both the hypertension and the myocardial ischemia in these patients.

Cerebral vasospasm is a leading cause of morbidity in these patients and is second only to the devastating effects of the primary hemorrhage as a cause of death. The mainstay of therapy for cerebral vasospasm has been hypervolemia and induced arterial hypertension. At this point in the patient's course, the major concern is to sustain adequate cerebral perfusion, at the cost of systemic hypertension. Obviously this treatment is best suited to patients in whom the aneurysms have already been clipped. During this treatment it is necessary to monitor systemic arterial pressure, central venous pressure, pulmonary wedge pressure, and cardiac function. A Swan-Ganz catheter is placed to allow continuous evaluation of these parameters. Intracranial pressure, hemoglobin and hematocrit, serum electrolytes, serum osmolarities, blood gases, and fluid status are also closely observed.

Crystalloid solutions are employed to increase intravascular volume. Dopamine can be used if needed to elevate arterial pressure. Whole blood, packed cells, plasma fractionate, albumin, or low-molecular-weight dextran are used to expand intravascular volume. The central venous pressure should be elevated to about 15 cm of water. Fludrocortisone and vasopressin may also be useful to keep the intravascular volume and pressure high. If necessary, atropine can be used to counteract hemodynamically significant bradycardia. The hematocrit ideally should be kept in the low to middle 30s.

Removal of subarachnoid blood by early craniotomy has been advocated as beneficial by some authors, but this form of treatment is controversial and not generally employed. High-dose barbiturate therapy decreases the cerebral metabolic rate and appears to be theoretically useful, but current data have shown disappointing results. Recently, some have advocated balloon angioplasty for vasospastic cerebral vessels. However, evidence is very preliminary and it is likely that this technique will lead to a high rate of complications secondary to acute thrombosis or late restenosis, as observed after angioplasty for coronary vasospasm.

Epilepsy may develop in about 10 percent of patients after aneurysmal subarachnoid hemorrhage, mostly within the first year. It is prudent to treat these patients with anticonvulsants for at least 2 years after the rupture.

Surgical Measures

The timing of aneurysm surgery is still open to discussion, but a greater emphasis is now placed on early intervention. The advantages of early surgery are that the risk of rebleeding is reduced and that subsequent vasospasm can be more effectively treated. The disadvantage is that the brain is more edematous and difficult to handle. However, current neuroanesthesia and operative techniques can largely overcome this obstacle. Some surgeons prefer to wait until the patient is fully recovered from associated vasospasm or hydrocephalus. In general, early intervention is indicated if the patient is in good condition and not yet in vasospasm. There is more of a tendency to delay surgery in patients already in vasospasm who are doing poorly.

Surgery for anterior circulation aneurysms in patients in good condition preoperatively carries an operative risk of 5 percent or less. Patients in poor preoperative health, with aneurysms larger than 2.5 cm, or with posterior circulation aneurysms, represent a higher surgical risk. Smaller unruptured aneurysms can be operated on with a significant morbidity risk of less than 3 percent.

Acute hydrocephalus should be treated as an emergency with external ventricular drainage. This allows for monitoring of intracranial pressure. A delayed hydrocephalus is best treated with a ventriculoperitoneal shunt.

SUGGESTED READING

Kassell N, Drake C. Timing of aneurysm surgery. Neurosurgery 1982; 10:514–519.

Kassell NF, Peerless SJ, Drake CG. Cerebral vasospasm: acute proliferative vasculopathy? I. Hypothesis. In: Wilkins RH, ed. Cerebral vasospasm. Baltimore: Williams & Wilkins, 1980:85.

Liszczak TM, Varsos VG, Black PM, et al. Cerebral arterial constriction after experimental subarachnoid hemorrhage is associated with blood components in the arterial wall. J Neurosurg 1983; 58:18–26.

Sundt TM, Davis DH. Reactions of cerebrovascular smooth muscle to blood and ischemia: primary versus secondary vasospasm. In: Wilkins RH, ed. Cerebral vasospasm. Baltimore: Williams & Wilkins, 1980:244.

Weir B, Grace M, Hansen J, et al. Time course of vasospasm in man. J Neurosurg 1978; 48:173–178.

DISORDERS OF THE AORTA AND THE VISCERAL ARTERIES

ACUTE AORTIC DISSECTION

JOHNNY BIRBE
D. CRAIG MILLER, M.D.

INCIDENCE AND PATHOGENESIS

Acute aortic dissection is the most frequent lethal disease involving the aorta, and its incidence is probably increasing in the industrialized world; tertiary referral cardiovascular surgical centers encounter more than 30 cases annually. The estimated occurrence of aortic dissection is 10 to 20 cases per million population per year, and the condition is lethal if not diagnosed early and managed appropriately. It is estimated that 50 percent of patients die within the first 48 hours. Therefore, a high clinical index of suspicion is imperative in order to make the correct diagnosis early. Increased clinical suspicion and earlier diagnosis will be the most important keys in the future to increase overall patient salvage rates.

Although most patients are middle-aged or elderly men, aortic dissection does affect women, including young women in the third trimester of pregnancy or during labor and delivery, frequently resulting in death of both mother and fetus. Children can also be affected. Both of these latter groups include patients with Marfan's and Ehlers-Danlos syndromes (who have a propensity for type A dissection caused by elastic tissue degeneration in the aortic media) as well as "normal" individuals without any known congenital propensity for aortic dissection. In older patients, who tend to have hypertension and generalized atherosclerosis, type B dissection is more likely.

The primary event leading to acute aortic dissection is a tear in the aortic intima allowing blood to enter the aortic wall. The direction of hematoma propagation usually extends distally from the intimal tear; however, proximal propagation of the dissecting hematoma may also occur. The extent of the distal dissection is variable and unpredictable, as one or more re-entry tears ("fenestrations") typically occur. Along its path the dissection can affect the origin of any aortic branch and

therefore cause ischemia by compression of the true lumen of important arterial tributaries. Significant end-organ ischemia or infarction, e.g., of kidney, bowel, or brain, can portend a lethal outcome and is an important clinical manifestation.

CLASSIFICATION SYSTEMS AND PATHOANATOMIC DIVERSITY

Over the years, many different classification schemes have been devised in attempts to represent the various types of aortic dissection by using general descriptive features. The Stanford classification system was created by Daily and colleagues to simplify categorization according to the predicted biologic behavior of the dissection, the most important factor being involvement of the ascending aorta. Using the Stanford criteria, dissections involving the ascending aorta are termed *type A,* regardless of the site of primary intimal tear and irrespective of the distal extent of propagation. If the ascending aorta is not involved, the dissection is called *type B.* A Stanford type A dissection is synonymous with the terms *proximal* (Massachusetts General Hospital), *ascending* (University of Alabama), *anterior* (Najafi and colleagues), and *type I* (DeBakey classification). A Stanford type B dissection is equivalent to a *distal, descending, posterior,* or *type III* dissection, respectively. The type of dissection connotes specific treatment methods (medical versus medical plus surgical) as well as the specific surgical approach (i.e., sternotomy and total cardiopulmonary bypass (CPB) in type A versus left thoracotomy and partial femorofemoral CPB in patients with type B dissections). An additional advantage of such a practical terminology approach is the fact that computed tomography (CT), magnetic resonance imaging (MRI), transesophageal echocardiography (TEE), angiography, and digital subtraction angiography (DSA) can discern involvement of the ascending aorta by the dissection more readily and accurately than the actual site(s) of tear(s) and the exact extent of distal dissection. Aortic dissections are also classified arbitrarily as acute or chronic; they are considered to be acute if less than 14 days old. Although patients with chronic dissections have a better prognosis, the cardinal feature of all classification systems today is whether the ascending aorta is involved by the dissecting process.

In the Stanford experience (a 20-year historical series consisting of both acute and chronic dissections), two-thirds of the patients had type A dissections and about one-third type B; the majority (58 percent) had acute dissections. Approximately two-thirds had the primary intimal tear in the ascending aorta, one-tenth had an arch tear, and slightly less than one-third had a tear in the descending thoracic aorta. In patients with type A dissections, 89 percent had an ascending aortic tear, 6 percent had an arch tear, and 5 percent had a descending aortic tear (with retrograde propagation). Eighty-five percent of patients with type B dissections had the tear in the descending thoracic aorta, and 15 percent had an arch tear.

CLINICAL PRESENTATION AND NATURAL HISTORY

Acute aortic dissection has been called the "great clinical masquerader" since the clinical manifestations are protean; therefore, many patients with dissections are initially misdiagnosed. This is partly due to the unpredictable perturbations that occur in end-organ blood supply as the dissecting process propagates distally, resulting in various pathoanatomic consequences at each major aortic tributary. Clinically, it is helpful to suspect the diagnosis of aortic dissection when the constellation of physical signs and symptoms simply does not add up, i.e., when simultaneous involvement of multiple, diverse organ systems does not appear to have any common explanation. Thus, a high clinical index of suspicion is imperative. One common incorrect diagnosis is acute myocardial infarction (MI); to complicate matters further, the increasing use of early intravenous thrombolytic therapy for patients with suspected MI (without angiographic confirmation) can be rapidly fatal if they actually have an acute type A aortic dissection or if the MI is secondary to a dissection. The cardinal symptom of acute dissection is sudden onset of severe, lancinating pain (typically, "The worst pain I've ever had"), usually starting in the anterior chest or interscapular region of the back; the pain commonly migrates, either initially or later. Unlike a typical MI, the pain is worse at onset, and the blood pressure is either normal or elevated despite a shocklike clinical appearance. Very rarely, however, some patients present months or years later with a chronic dissection without any recall of an acute painful event. Other classic signs and symptoms of acute dissection include a normal electrocardiogram (ECG) in combination with hypertension, ischemia, or neurologic changes in one or more extremities (paresthesia or motor weakness, pallor, and pulselessness) and a chest x-ray film revealing mediastinal widening, rightward deviation of the trachea, pleural or pericardial effusion, and separation of luminal aortic calcification from the lateral aortic shadow. These classic findings in an otherwise healthy patient would make a correct diagnosis very likely, but this is not always the case. A careful physical examination may frequently be unrevealing; however, careful (serial) palpation of all peripheral pulses, blood pressure measurement in both arms, and cardiac auscultation (listening for a diastolic murmur associated with aortic insufficiency) may provide additional clues.

Acute aortic dissection can be misdiagnosed as almost any other acute medical or surgical disorder. It can mimic very different medical conditions including acute MI, unstable angina, pericarditis, acute aortic and/or mitral valve regurgitation, congestive heart failure, heart block, acute hypertensive crisis, pulmonary embolism, esophagitis, peptic ulcer disease, acute cholecystitis, biliary colic, pancreatitis, appendicitis, ureteral colic, "acute surgical abdomen," incarcerated hernia, pyelonephritis, acute renal failure, hematuria, renal colic, pancreatitis, musculoskeletal back pain, sciatica, stroke, syncope, paraplegia, transient ischemic attack, acute arterial embolism or thrombosis, esophagitis, esophageal spasm, esophageal rupture, pleurisy, pleurodynia, and thoracic neoplasm.

Undiagnosed (or misdiagnosed and untreated) acute type A aortic dissection is rapidly fatal; the untreated mortality rate for patients with acute type A dissections is 1 to 3 percent per hour during the first 24 to 48 hours, and over 90 percent of patients die within 3 months. Even in the last two decades, 11 to 35 percent of patients admitted to the hospital have died without the correct diagnosis being made; this figure may be as high as 55 percent for patients with acute type A dissections.

DIAGNOSTIC METHODS

Owing to the lethal nature of untreated acute aortic dissection, it is crucial to make the correct diagnosis early. Thus, the most rapid and definitive test available is usually best. Diagnostic methods used today include electrocardiography (ECG), chest radiography, CT, cine-CT, aortography, MRI, TEE (preferably with Doppler color flow mapping), DSA, and biplane cineangiography.

CT scanning with intravenous contrast infusion is a valuable screening procedure because it is rapid and relatively accurate (Fig. 1), but TEE may play a more major screening role in the future. CT is an accurate method to detect the proximal and distal extent of the dissection, but can fail to define the actual site of intimal entry tear in approximately 50 percent of cases. CT can also provide valuable information regarding flow dynamics by assessing flow in the true and false lumens. If the intimal flap is moving rapidly, e.g., in the ascending aorta in cases of type A dissection, CT may miss the flap or differential opacification of the two lumens; the likelihood of a false-negative scan is much less with cine-CT scans (imaging at 20 to 50 Hz) owing to the increased temporal sampling resolution. Differentiating a concentric layer of laminated thrombus from a small, thrombosed false lumen can be exceedingly difficult. The sensitivity of CT ranges from 88 to 100 percent, and

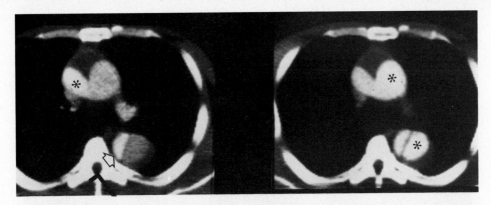

Figure 1 Example of a contrast computed tomographic (CT) scan illustrating an acute type A aortic dissection. Note in the left-hand panel the deformed true lumen in the ascending aorta *(asterisk)* and the narrowed true lumen in the descending aorta *(arrowhead),* which are both densely opacified by contrast material; later in this dynamic CT scan *(right-hand panel)* the false lumen *(asterisks)* of the descending thoracic aorta is also opacified. The flap or septum between the two channels is clearly visible as a linear lucency.

specificity from 92 to 100 percent. Therefore, if a high-quality CT scan is negative but a strong clinical suspicion of aortic dissection still exists, additional diagnostic examinations must be performed.

Large-film aortography and cineangiography have been the classic diagnostic "gold standards," but either of these must be performed using simultaneous or sequential biplane techniques (Fig. 2). The diagnosis is clear if an intimal flap or double lumen can be identified; indirect signs can also be important, including thickening of the aortic wall as well as a true lumen that is extrinsically narrowed. The site of primary entry tear can usually, but not always, be identified. Aortography reveals the degree of aortic valve insufficiency that is present. Combined with left ventriculography, global and regional left ventricular wall motion abnormalities can be defined. Aortography can also reveal involvement of important aortic tributaries. However, with this technique it may be difficult to differentiate a thrombosed false lumen from a laminated thrombus in a dilated, ectatic thoracic aorta or an atherosclerotic thoracic aneurysm. This problem also pertains to CT, MRI, and TEE eco-imaging to various degrees. Aortography has a sensitivity rate similar to that of CT (80 to 90 percent), although the specificity is somewhat higher. An excellent diagnostic approach is to employ biplane cineangiography of the thoracic aorta, which can demonstrate blood flow in the false lumen and aortic branches more readily than large-film, biplane aortography. Since the temporal imaging rate is higher (typically 30 to 60 Hz), this technique is more accurate in detecting rapidly moving intimal flaps and primary entry sites. Intra-arterial DSA can also provide important information in patients with aortic dissection; DSA, when readily available, is worthwhile as an initial screening test if CT cannot be performed immediately.

Making the correct diagnosis earlier by means of one of these diagnostic techniques is the main key to improving the overall mortality rate in patients with acute aortic dissection. In this regard, TEE (with Doppler color flow mapping) will probably have a larger role in future years as more experience is gained and the transducers are refined. One advantage of TEE is that it can be performed rapidly at the bedside, including examination in the emergency room or intensive care unit requiring less than 15 minutes. TEE can confirm or exclude the diagnosis of aortic dissection; the diagnosis is clear if two lumens separated by an intimal flap can be visualized within the aorta; in addition, biphasic flow in systole and diastole through fenestrations (e.g., sheared-off tributaries, including intercostal arteries) can be visualized between the two aortic lumens. If the false lumen is thrombosed, central displacement of intimal calcification distinguishes dissection from aneurysm with mural thrombus. Pericardial effusion (found in roughly 20 percent of patients), aortic insufficiency (seen in about 35 percent), segmental left ventricular wall motion abnormalities, mitral regurgitation, and pathologic involvement of the great vessels can also be assessed with TEE. Bronchospasm, atrioventricular block, ventricular ectopy, and bradycardia may occur during the introduction of the TEE probe, but these complications are usually transient and easily reversible. Air in the trachea limits TEE visualization of the proximal aortic arch and distal ascending aorta to some extent, but this limitation is largely obviated by biplane TEE transducers. Overall, the European cooperative study showed that TEE had sensitivity and specificity rates exceeding those of angiography and CT in the diagnosis of aortic dissection.

Unlike TEE, the diagnostic accuracy of transthoracic echocardiography is limited owing to many conditions (abnormal chest wall configuration, narrow intercostal space, obesity, emphysema, and artifacts due to mechanical ventilation) associated with technically suboptimal studies. The sensitivity and specificity of transthoracic echocardiography are 77 to 80 percent and 93 to 96 percent, respectively; therefore, a negative transthoracic echo is not helpful, and transthoracic echocar-

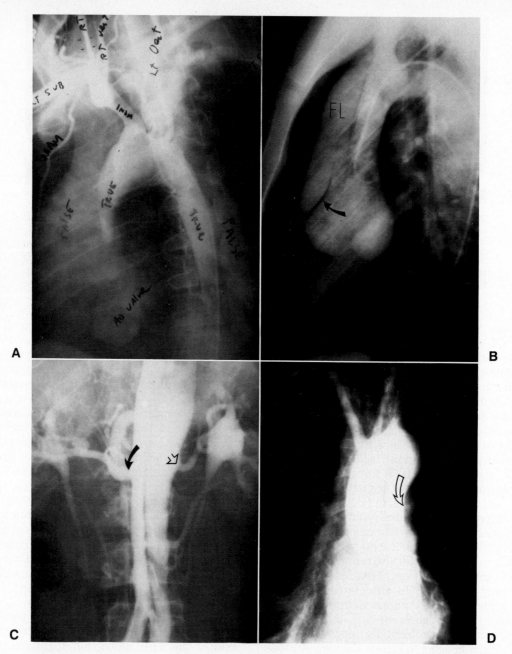

Figure 2 *A,* Thoracic aortogram demonstrating an acute type A aortic dissection. The true and false lumens are labeled. *B,* Another example of an acute type A dissection in a young patient with Marfan's syndrome. Here the aortogram shows the flap arising from the anterior sinus of Valsalva *(arrow).* FL = false lumen. *C,* Abdominal aortic aortogram demonstrating the classic "double-barrel" aorta. The narrowed true lumen *(closed arrow)* is perfusing the right renal artery, but the false lumen *(open arrow)* is filling the left renal artery. *D,* Example of an aortogram in a patient with an acute type B aortic dissection. Here the findings are more subtle; the true lumen *(open arrow)* is extrinsically compressed by the (nonopacified) false lumen. Despite the relatively benign appearance of this dissection and satisfactory medical therapy, the descending thoracic aorta of this patient ruptured.

diography is not a reliable screening test for aortic dissection.

MRI is a good diagnostic tool, but is currently too time-consuming to be considered as a first-line screening procedure for patients with acute aortic dissections; at present, it also is not practical to image critically ill patients receiving intravenous infusions. MRI can provide precise pathoanatomic information, however, in patients with chronic dissections during late postoperative follow-up surveillance (Fig. 3). Also, with "cine-

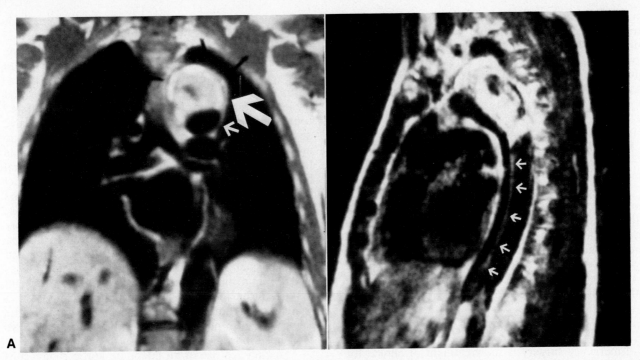

Figure 3 Magnetic resonance imaging (MRI) scans of a patient with a chronic type B aortic dissection complicated by formation over time of a large false aneurysm in the distal arch and proximal descending thoracic aorta. *A,* In this anteroposterior image the large arrow indicates the false lumen component with slow flow and/or thrombus and a calcified rim; the true lumen *(small arrow)* is the black channel below the false lumen. The distal main pulmonary artery is the other vessel *(black lumen)* immediately below the true aortic lumen. *B,* This lateral MR image of the same patient illustrates both the true (anterior, small) and false (posterior, larger) lumens in addition to the longitudinal flap (outlined by multiple small arrowheads) that separates the two channels. The localized false aneurysmal component involving the distal arch and proximal descending aorta is also apparent.

loop" and "VINNIE" postprocessing software, MRI can provide unique information concerning aortic blood flow in the true and false lumens. Such MR images can help determine the source of blood flow to various important aortic tributaries (e.g., celiac axis, superior mesenteric artery, renal arteries) and characterize evolution of the hematoma in the false lumen over time (using methemoglobin spin-echo signals). However, on the basis of cost considerations alone, the use of serial MRI (compared with CT) may be hard to justify for routine follow-up in most patients.

MEDICAL STABILIZATION PROTOCOL

The initial goal in patients with acute dissection is to control mean arterial pressure (MAP) in the range of 60 to 70 mm Hg while simultaneously providing adequate coronary, cerebral, and renal blood flow. Aortic dP/dt (i.e., aortic shear stress) and mean arterial pressure are the major determinants of progression of the acute dissection, regardless of type. Antihypertensive treatment should be instituted immediately after the diagnosis is suspected; this involves admission to an intensive care or coronary care unit for hemodynamic monitoring of central venous, pulmonary arterial, and systemic arterial pressures; ECG; monitoring of urinary output,

and assessment of level of consciousness. The drugs of choice include negative inotropic medications (beta-blockers and/or calcium antagonists) and short-acting vasodilators (e.g., sodium nitroprusside). Incremental doses of intravenous propranolol (0.5 to 1.0 mg every 5 to 10 minutes) can be titrated to obtain the targeted response in conjunction with a nitroprusside drip; the propranolol is then continued at a dose of 2 to 5 mg IV every 1 to 2 hours as needed. Newer beta-blockers have also proved effective and easier to administer, including metoprolol (intermittent IV bolus, 5 to 15 mg every 4 to 6 hours), labetalol (IV bolus followed by continuous infusion), and esmolol (IV bolus followed by continuous infusion). An intravenous infusion of nitroprusside is usually also required with beta-adrenergic antagonists (0.5-5.0 μg per kilogram per minute). If the patient remains hypertensive despite higher doses of beta-blocker plus sodium nitroprusside, an intravenous drip of trimethaphan camsylate or intravenous boluses of verapamil can be added. Because nitroprusside actually increases aortic shear stress secondarily to its arteriolar dilating effect, concomitant beta-blockade is crucial to reduce aortic dP/dt. If surgical intervention is undertaken, strict blood pressure control is continued in the operating room and maintained postoperatively. When clinically appropriate, oral medications are then started. The beta-blockers and/or calcium antagonists are continued indefinitely thereafter, even if the patient is normotensive. Medically treated patients (e.g., elderly individuals with uncomplicated type B dissections) should remain in the intensive care setting until their pain and hypertension have completely resolved, they have been weaned from intravenous medications, and appropriate oral therapy has been instituted.

INDICATIONS, GOALS, AND TECHNIQUES OF SURGICAL TREATMENT

It is important to understand that surgical treatment does not "cure" this disease; the main therapeutic goal is to prevent the most common causes of death, which are (1) intrapericardial rupture and tamponade (80 to 90 percent) and extrapericardial rupture (5 to 10 percent) in patients with acute type A dissections and (2) rupture of the descending thoracic aorta (60 to 70 percent) in patients with acute type B dissections.

Acute Type A Dissections

Emergency surgery is the treatment of choice for patients with acute type A dissections, because the mortality rate for patients treated medically exceeds 90 percent. This aggressive approach is justified by the highly lethal nature of acute type A dissections and the relatively low operative risk (15 to 20 percent or less today). Furthermore, the long-term prognosis is satisfactory; in the Stanford series, 75 percent of survivors of surgery were alive at 5 years and 49 percent at 10 years. There are no absolute contraindications to surgical repair of patients with acute type A dissection, but exceptions based on individual judgment may include the very elderly or patients with other severe chronic illness or neoplasm. The old tenet that patients with a thrombosed false lumen have an excellent prognosis with medical therapy is now known to be fallacious. If these patients are treated medically, close clinical follow-up and frequent serial assessment of the aorta with MRI, CT, or TEE is essential. The main surgical goals are replacement of the ascending aorta (using total CPB with femoral arterial cannulation), resection of the primary intimal tear (if exposed), preservation of the native aortic valve whenever possible (unless the patient has Marfan's syndrome), reconstitution of distal flow into the true lumen, and repair of damage to contiguous aortic branches, e.g., the coronary, innominate, and left carotid arteries.

More than 60 percent of patients with an acute type A dissection may have aortic regurgitation, and the question of routine aortic valve replacement (AVR) has been controversial; we believe that universal AVR is justified only in individuals with Marfan's or Ehlers-Danlos syndrome or with gross annuloaortic ectasia. There may be a worldwide trend toward routine AVR, however. At Stanford University the aortic valve was preserved in over 82 percent of patients with acute type A dissections (and 50 percent of those with chronic

dissections). In a recent retrospective database study from Stanford-Duke by Fann and colleagues, only 30 percent of patients with an acute aortic dissection required AVR; the remainder underwent concomitant valve resuspension or required no direct valvular procedure. Analysis of the results of this study revealed that the long-term outcome in terms of survival, valve-related complications, late AVR, and residual aortic valve disease was similar in all three subgroups. There is no prosthetic, bioprosthetic, or allograft valve available today that is superior to even a slightly abnormal, natural human aortic valve. On the other hand, to reconstruct the aortic root and resuspend the aortic valve safely and adequately is considered by some surgeons to be a more difficult technical procedure (and certainly a more time-consuming one) than simple insertion of a composite valve graft. The results of the study by Fann and colleagues, coupled with the theoretical advantages inherent in avoiding a mechanical prosthetic valve and the need for indefinite anticoagulation, represent a compelling argument in favor of saving the native aortic valve whenever possible if the patient does not have Marfan's syndrome.

The key feature of an adequate aortic root reconstruction (with valve resuspension) is the middle layer of Teflon felt, which is custom tailored to fit into all the irregular niches of the false lumen within the proximal aortic root, extending down to the level of the aortic annulus. Also, to ensure that the external layer of Teflon felt incorporates full-thickness bites of the aortic wall in the sinuses of Valsalva and that the proximal suture line will be sound, the bulk of the aortic root below the level of the sinotubular ridge must be dissected free from the main pulmonary artery, the pulmonary annulus, and the right ventricular outflow tract. After the proximal and distal aortic cuffs are reinforced, a short, tubular Dacron interposition graft is anastomosed in an end-to-end fashion using full-thickness suture bites. We prefer to use woven velour grafts autoclaved in 25 percent albumin because these grafts are soft, conform to the fragile aorta well, and are quite hemostatic. Extreme care and gentle techniques are key in any operation for aortic dissection.

The management of patients with a dissection due to a tear in the transverse arch is another controversial surgical area. Patients with arch tears are a very-high-risk subset whether or not the arch tear is resected. In this regard, it should be clarified that "location of the tear" is not synonymous with "tear resection." In the Stanford series, the tear was in the arch in 4 percent of patients with type A dissections, in the descending aorta in 9 percent, and in the ascending aorta in 87 percent. Long-term analysis demonstrated that inability or unwillingness to resect the tear (when in the arch or descending aorta) was not associated with any statistically significant increase in operative risk or likelihood of late death. On the other hand, the location of the tear was an incremental risk factor in terms of operative mortality (when all 175 patients with either a type A or type B dissection were considered; see below) and late aortic reoperation. In patients with the tear in the arch, the reoperation rate was 27 percent after 1 year; however, only 24 percent of these repeat operations involved the transverse arch. Therefore, it cannot be imputed directly that the presence of an arch tear means that all patients will eventually need arch replacement if the tear is not resected during the initial procedure. Moreover, it was interesting that the site of the tear had no important bearing on late survival. In patients with severe, dissection-induced damage to the arch resulting from a tear in the arch (which fortunately is rare), an aggressive approach is warranted to resect the intimal tear. On the basis of the results of another recent Stanford-Duke study by Yun and colleagues, we also feel that an arch tear should be resected simultaneously in young, low-risk patients when the ascending aorta is being replaced, provided that the surgeons have extensive experience with aortic arch surgery. Concomitant arch or semiarch replacement is also the only option if the arch has ruptured in a patient with an acute type A or type B dissection, even if the tear is not actually in the arch. In such dire circumstances, however, the operative risk is higher (20 to 25 percent or more).

When total aortic arch replacement must be performed, circulatory arrest using profound systemic hypothermia (15°C) is employed. More commonly, even in cases of acute type A dissection in which the tear is in the ascending aorta, the distal aortic anastomosis (and/or hemiarch replacement) is performed by means of an "open technique" during a short period of circulatory arrest (10 to 15 minutes at about 20 to 23°C). This approach enables a more secure and technically sound distal aortic anastomosis to be performed and minimizes clamp injuries to the fragile dissected distal ascending aorta.

Acute Type B Dissections

In most institutions, conventional management of patients with type B aortic dissections has reserved surgical intervention for those with major complications such as rupture, acute expansion, intractable pain, or ischemia of distal vascular beds. In the last decade, however, the operative mortality rate for patients with acute type B aortic dissections has declined; several institutions report mortality rates as low as 10 percent in large series. Nonetheless, no data currently exist comparing the results of medical and surgical therapy in a prospective, controlled fashion. In patients with acute, uncomplicated type B dissection, long-term medical and surgical therapy was associated with similar long-term survival rates and incidence of late operation in a retrospective Stanford-Duke database investigation by Glower and colleagues. The only significant, independent predictors of overall (early or late) mortality were age, dissection complications, and the presence of other medical problems. Glower and colleagues suggested that medical management should be the primary form of treatment for most patients with uncomplicated acute type B dissection, with surgical therapy reserved for

patients with serious complications or other worrisome pathoanatomic problems. At Stanford, emergency surgical intervention is the treatment of choice for selected patients with acute type B dissections, even if these are uncomplicated; specifically, younger patients without serious cardiac or pulmonary disease are initially approached as potential surgical candidates. The rationale for this strategy is that these particular patients have a low surgical risk and may do better in the long term after early replacement of the proximal descending thoracic aorta. Relative contraindications to early, elective surgical treatment include a systemic medical disorder; major cardiac, pulmonary, renal, or cerebrovascular disease; and advanced age; such individuals probably have a better prognosis if treated medically. On the other hand, when surgical treatment is reserved for patients with acute type B dissections who acutely fail medical management, the operative mortality rate in this subset can be expected to be about 75 percent. Furthermore, such a management philosophy produces the paradoxical and illogical situation in which the indications for operation are the same factors that portend an increased likelihood of operative death. Type B dissections are approached through a left thoracotomy incision using partial femorofemoral CPB to replace the most severely damaged segment of the descending thoracic aorta with a double-velour woven Dacron graft. If more extensive lengths of the descending aorta, or even the entire thoracoabdominal aorta, are replaced, the risk of paraplegia becomes excessive; replacement of only a conservative, short segment of the proximal descending aorta was associated with a 4 percent rate of new paraplegia at Stanford using partial CPB. Circulatory arrest and profound hypothermia (also using femorofemoral CPB) can be employed in patients with or without previous surgery who present with a large distal arch dissection component. In these patients, it may be technically impossible to open the left chest safely or to gain proximal control at the level of the transverse arch for cross-clamping owing to the size of the dissection and/or attendant periaortic scarring. However, the added risks inherent in resorting to profound hypothermia and circulatory arrest to replace the arch and/or proximal descending aorta via a left thoracotomy are substantial. Cardiovascular disease and residual aortic pathology are significant causes of late death and morbidity in these patients; this mandates careful long-term follow-up and serial imaging of the aorta in patients with type B aortic dissection.

RESULTS OF SURGICAL TREATMENT

Operative Morbidity

The incidence of surgical complications has declined over the years but remains substantial. Major early postoperative complications for patients with type A dissections in the Stanford experience were, in order of frequency, tracheostomy, reoperation for hemorrhage, hemodialysis, visceral infarction, and MI. For individuals with acute type B dissections, they were tracheostomy, reoperation for hemorrhage, hemodialysis, visceral infarction, MI, and new paraplegia.

Long-Term Survival (Discharged Patients Only)

There were no differences in long-term survival rates based on type and acuity of dissection in the 15-year Stanford analysis. The overall actuarial survival rates were 82 percent at 5 years and 64 percent at 10 years (78 percent for type A dissection and 88 percent for type B dissection at 5 years).

Operative Mortality Risk

Patients with acute type A dissection had an operative risk of 7 percent at Stanford between 1977 and 1982. For acute type B dissection the risk was 13 percent. Similar figures have been established in other European and North American centers with extensive surgical experience.

Independent Predictors of Operative Death

In a retrospective analysis from Stanford, the following factors were significant, independent predictors of operative mortality (in declining order of predictive power) for patients with type A dissection: acute renal failure, renal and/or visceral ischemia, cardiac tamponade, and (earlier) operative date. Although the operative date is not amenable to modification, it is hoped that earlier diagnosis will reduce the frequency of the other dissection-related complications, which theoretically should translate into further reductions in operative risk. Earlier diagnosis and surgical referral of patients with acute dissection before irreversible major end-organ ischemia and/or infarction occur was probably responsible, at least in part, for the substantially improved results over time.

For patients with type B dissections, rupture, renal or visceral ischemia, and (older) age were the only significant multivariate determinants. The adverse clinical impact of aortic rupture and renal or visceral ischemia was substantial; therefore, earlier correct diagnosis should reduce the incidence of these risk factors and lower the overall operative risk for these patients. Unfortunately, these two complications represent compelling indications for operation, so that realistically surgical intervention cannot be avoided in these patients, despite the obvious high surgical risk.

For all 175 patients in the Stanford study (type A or type B dissections), renal dysfunction, renal or visceral ischemia, site of tear (ascending ≤ descending ≤ arch), tamponade, (earlier) operative date, and pulmonary disease emerged as the significant, independent determinants indicating an increased likelihood of operative death. This information allows calculation of any individual patient's operative risk, which is helpful in discussing the options with the family preoperatively in patients with acute type A dissections and in medical-

surgical decision making for patients with acute type B dissections.

Independent Determinants of Long-Term Prognosis

In another retrospective investigation from Stanford the following factors were shown to be significant, independent determinants of late death: earlier operative era, stroke, remote MI, and renal dysfunction. Although stroke had an adverse effect on long-term prognosis, it is not considered a contraindication to surgery at Stanford because one cannot predict with certainty which patients have an irreversible neurologic deficit. Marfan's syndrome per se did not have a significant independent effect, but the actuarial survival rate was slightly lower for these individuals than for those without Marfan's syndrome. With stroke as the exception, no dissection complication or intraoperative factor significantly influenced late survival.

Independent Predictors of Late Reoperation

After initial surgical treatment of acute aortic dissection in patients treated medically, late reoperations may be necessary. The rate of late postoperative aortic reoperation related to the dissection was 3.1 percent per patient per year at Stanford; the actuarial incidence of reoperation was 13 percent at 5 years and 23 percent at 10 years. These procedures can be subdivided into two categories: (1) treatment failure and (2) late aortic sequelae. In the first group the initial operation either was inadequate or failed postoperatively; this type is associated with a high reoperative mortality risk. On the other hand, in the second group, late reoperation represents the favorable consequences of more intensive postoperative aortic surveillance and medical follow-up, i.e., detection of a problem in the remaining aorta prior to catastrophic rupture. The operative risk for patients in this second category is relatively low compared with those in the "treatment failure" category.

The independent significant predictors of late thoracic or abdominal aortic or aortic valve reoperation were younger age, site of tear (aortic arch ≥ descending aorta ≥ ascending aorta), and cardiac tamponade. The presence of one or more of these factors significantly increased the likelihood of late reoperation. Inspection of reoperation in the context of age showed that patients over 55 years old had a higher probability of avoiding repeat surgery irrespective of whether they had Marfan's syndrome. Patients with Marfan's syndrome were more likely to require reoperation, but this parameter per se did not attain statistical significance in the multivariate analysis. Patients with an arch tear had a relatively high incidence of reoperation within the first postoperative year. On the other hand, only a few of these reoperative procedures involved arch replacement; more often, the procedure was replacement of the descending, ascending, or abdominal aorta. Therefore, relatively few reoperations could have theoretically been avoided if concomitant arch repair had been performed at the time of the initial operation. Nevertheless, arch tear probably is still a clinically important portent of high early and late risk.

POSTOPERATIVE LONG-TERM CONSIDERATIONS

Fifteen percent of late postoperative deaths in our experience, and 29 percent of those in the 20-year study of DeBakey and colleagues, were due to late aortic rupture, usually in another portion of the aorta. The proportion of late deaths due to rupture in individuals with type B dissections was lower (8 percent) than that in patients with type A dissections (18 percent). On the other hand, 32 percent of late deaths were sudden or unexpected in the subgroup with type B dissections (versus 18 percent in type A patients). Since autopsies were not available in all patients, some of these sudden unexplained deaths could also have been due to aortic rupture. This sobering point emphasizes how important it is to ensure that long-term, close medical follow-up of these patients is provided by a combined cardiology–cardiac surgery–radiology team, including serial surveillance imaging of the aorta. Excellent follow-up communication between the surgeon and the primary cardiologist or vascular internist is mandatory. This facet of care includes negative inotropic therapy (beta-blockers or calcium antagonists), strict control of hypertension, and serial imaging of the remaining portions of the thoracic and abdominal aorta with CT, MRI, or TEE. In our opinion, all patients should be treated with negative inotropic medications and/or vasodilators after operation, even if they are normotensive. The minimal risk and inconvenience and relatively small costs associated with indefinite beta-blocker, calcium antagonist, or angiotensin-converting enzyme inhibitor therapy justify the potential reduction in the incidence of acute redissection or rupture of another portion of the aorta.

For follow-up surveillance imaging of the remainder of the aorta, TEE is a promising approach that is less costly than CT or MRI, but another test (CT or MRI) is necessary for the abdominal aorta. Earlier detection of localized false aneurysmal aortic segments and other aortic pathology will enable elective surgical treatment to be carried out prior to rupture, helping to reduce this major late problem. The current recommendations at Stanford for follow-up include CT or MRI scans or TEE before the patient leaves the hospital, and 3 months later. If there is no change in the caliber of the aorta and if no clinical symptoms occur, the next imaging study should be performed 6 months later. If the dissected aorta is again stable and no new symptoms have arisen, the time interval between scans or TEE examinations can be extended to 12 months. Studies thereafter should be conducted no less often than annually. The entire aorta, including the ascending and descending thoracic aorta, the transverse arch, and the abdominal aorta, should be examined. Whichever method is used for follow-up, the study must be performed frequently, serially, and indefinitely.

SUGGESTED READING

Acute aortic dissection (editorial). Lancet 1988; 2:827–828.

Bachet J, Teodori G, Goudot B, et al. Replacement of the transverse aortic arch during emergency surgery of type A acute aortic dissection (26 cases). J Thorac Cardiovasc Surg 1988; 96:878–886.

DeBakey ME, McCollum CH, Crawford ES, et al. Dissection and dissecting aneurysms of the aorta: twenty-year follow-up of five hundred twenty-seven patients treated surgically. Surgery 1982; 92:1118–1134.

DeSanctis RW, Doroghazi RM, Austen WG, Buckley MJ. Aortic dissection. N Engl J Med 1987; 317:1060–1967.

Doroghazi RM, Slater EE, eds. Aortic dissection. New York: McGraw-Hill, 1983.

Erbel R, Engbergbing R, Daniel W, et al. Echocardiography in the diagnosis of aortic dissection. Lancet 1989; 1:457–461.

Fann JI, Glower DD, Miller DC, et al. Preservation of the aortic valve in patients with type A aortic dissection complicated by aortic valvular regurgitation. J Thorac Cardiovasc Surg 1991; 101 (in press).

Glower DD, Fann JI, Speier RH, et al. Comparison of medical and surgical therapy for uncomplicated descending aortic dissection. Circulation 1990; 82(Suppl IV):39–46.

Haverich A, Miller DC, Scott WC, et al. Acute and chronic aortic dissections – determinants of long-term outcome for operative survivors. Circulation 1985; 72(Suppl II):22–34.

Lansman SL, Raissi S, Ergin MA, Griepp RB. Urgent surgery for acute arch dissection. J Thorac Cardiovasc Surg 1989; 97:334–341.

Miller DC, Mitchell RS, Oyer PE, et al. Independent determinants of operative mortality for patients with aortic dissections. Circulation 1984; 70(Suppl I):153–164.

Mohr-Kahaly S, Erbel R, Rennollet H, et al. Ambulatory follow-up of aortic dissection by transesophageal two-dimensional and color-coded Doppler echocardiography. Circulation 1989; 80:24–33.

Roberts CS, Roberts WC. Aortic dissection with entrance tear in the descending thoracic aorta: analysis of 40 necropsy patients. Ann Surg 1991; 231:356–368.

Svensson LG, Crawford ES, Hess KR, et al. Dissection of the aorta and dissecting aneurysms: improving early and long-term surgical results. Circulation 1990; 82(Suppl IV):24–38.

Yun KL, Glower DL, Miller DC, et al. Aortic dissection due to transverse arch tear: is concomitant arch repair warranted? J Thorac Cardiovasc Surg 1991; 101 (in press).

AORTIC ANEURYSM

ALAN SINGER, M.D.
JOHN P. COOKE, M.D., Ph.D.

Given the fact that aortic aneurysm is largely a disease of the elderly, its incidence can be expected to increase as the proportion of the U.S. population over the age of 50 increases. Aortic aneurysm will therefore be an increasingly common cause of potentially preventable death in the United States.

An aneurysm is any persistent, localized, pathologic dilatation of an artery. Aneurysms can be divided into three types: (1) a true aneurysm is a dilatation involving all three layers of the vessel, (2) a false aneurysm occurs when the media is disrupted and the luminal contents are confined only by the advential layer of the vessel, and (3) a dissecting aneurysm occurs when blood enters the wall of the vessel and dissects through the planes of the media.

True aneurysms of the aorta are due to degeneration of the media, the cause of which is not well understood in most cases. These aneurysms are most often associated with atherosclerosis, although the role of atherosclerosis in their etiology and pathogenesis is not yet understood. Any proposed etiology must account for the well-documented familial clustering of aortic aneurysms. There is evidence that in some cases aortic aneurysms are due to transmission of a single gene locus, and recently a family has been identified in which abdominal aortic aneurysm is associated with a single point mutation in type III collagen.

Well-known causes of true aneurysms of the aorta include tertiary syphilis, Marfan's syndrome, Ehlers-Danlos syndrome, and vasculitis (e.g., giant cell arteritis). Discussion of all of these entities is beyond the scope of this chapter, which is largely limited to descriptions of true aneurysms in association with atherosclerosis or due to degeneration of the aortic media of unknown etiology. Aneurysms resulting from, or in association with, aortic dissection are discussed in the chapters *Acute Aortic Dissection* and *The Marfan Syndrome*.

The natural history of aortic aneurysms, regardless of location, is to increase in size. By Laplace's law, wall stress increases proportionally as the vessel diameter increases. Laminated thrombus develops within the aneurysm, but this does not decrease the stress on the vessel wall. Recruitment of collagen fibers may strengthen the expanding aortic wall, but eventually even this adaptation fails and the aneurysm ruptures.

ABDOMINAL AORTIC ANEURYSMS

Presentation

Abdominal aortic aneurysms are more common in men, and their prevalence increases with age. The prevalence in men aged 50 to 60 years has been estimated at 0.7 percent, whereas it is about five times more prevalent in men over 70. In women the prevalence is about half that of age-matched men until the age of 70, when the prevalence is almost equal. Abdominal aortic aneurysms present in a variety of ways. Most often they are asymptomatic and detected only by a careful examiner, or by a radiologic procedure performed for an unassociated disorder. When they are symptomatic, pain in the abdomen or back is the most common feature. Symptoms also occur from compression of adjacent structures, and patients may complain of abdominal fullness and weight loss. Patients may first present with blue toes, abdominal pain, and nausea, or sudden deterioration of renal function and exacerbation of hypertension; all of these are potential manifestations of atheroembolism originating from the aneurysm. More unusual presentations include obstructive uropathy due to ureteral compression, aortocaval fistula, and consumptive coagulopathy. The initial presentation of aortic abdominal aneurysm is often abdominal pain and syncope due to rupture. About half of these patients die before reaching medical care.

A careful physical examination can detect most abdominal aortic aneurysms and allow an estimation of size. Palpation of the aorta is particularly important in individuals at higher risk: elderly and middle-aged males with a history of hypertension, hyperlipidemia, or tobacco use or a family history of aneurysmal disease. In high-risk individuals in whom obesity precludes palpation of the aorta, ultrasonography or computed tomography (CT) should be considered. Another high-risk group includes patients with peripheral arterial aneurysms or arteriomegaly: 50 percent of patients with a popliteal aneurysm also have an aortic aneurysm (and 15 percent of patients with aortic aneurysm have a popliteal aneurysm). Therefore, attention to the rest of the vasculature may provide additional clues. Abdominal tenderness with palpation is worrisome in these patients and may signify impending rupture, an inflammatory process involving the aorta, or an unrelated process. This finding should accelerate the diagnostic evaluation and surgical consultation.

Evaluation

Accurate radiologic methods to diagnose and evaluate an abdominal aortic aneurysm include ultrasonography, CT, magnetic resonance imaging (MRI), and angiography. When an abdominal aortic aneurysm is suspected from the history or physical examination, ultrasonography is generally the study of choice for initial evaluation. Ultrasonography is noninvasive, rapid, and extremely sensitive and specific in confirming the diagnosis. Measurements of aneurysm size by ultrasonography correlate very closely with findings at surgery. Although ultrasonography can demonstrate thrombus within the aneurysm and demonstrate perianeurysmal structure, it is often suboptimal in eval-

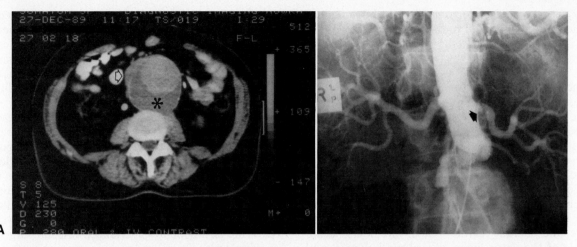

Figure 1 *A,* Computed tomographic (CT) scan reveals a large infrarenal aneurysm of the abdominal aorta *(arrowhead).* Note the laminated thrombus *(asterisk)* within the lumen of the aneurysm. An aortogram of this aneurysm would underestimate its size, because the luminal diameter is reduced by the laminated thrombus. *B,* Aortogram of the same patient. An infrarenal aortic aneurysm is visualized. Note the additional finding of a hemodynamically significant stenosis of the left renal artery *(arrowhead).* This case illustrates the complementary nature of CT and aortography.

uation of associated renal artery disease. Ultrasonography may be technically difficult in obese patients.

CT is also a highly accurate aid in the diagnosis and sizing of aneurysms (Fig. 1*A*). It visualizes intraluminal thrombus, perianeurysmal structures, and retroperitoneal hematoma. Optimal visualization by CT requires administration of both oral and intravenous contrast material. Assessment of the renal arteries is not always accurate with CT, especially when multiple renal arteries are present.

Experience with the use of MRI is still being gained, but it appears to be a highly accurate diagnostic tool. It demonstrates the extent of the aneurysm, intra-aneurysmal thrombus, perianeurysmal structures, and involvement of branch vessels, without requiring contrast agents. It may also give hemodynamic information (i.e., the presence or absence of flow in vascular structures) not provided by CT. The primary limitations of MRI are availability, cost, and acquisition time. MRI is not feasible for patients who are unstable and require close monitoring.

Angiography has been considered the gold standard for evaluation of the abdominal aorta (Fig. 1*B*). It best evaluates patency of the mesenteric, renal, and other branch vessels. However, angiography frequently underestimates the size of aneurysms owing to the presence of mural thrombus that prevents opacification of the entire lumen. Nevertheless, many surgeons prefer to have an angiographic study before abdominal aortic aneurysm repair in order to assess technical difficulty and surgical approach. Other surgeons use arteriography only in selected patients, such as those with suspected suprarenal extension, those with suspected renovascular hypertension, those showing evidence of iliofemoral occlusive disease, and those with mesenteric ischemia.

Prognosis

As discussed above, the natural course of abdominal aortic aneurysms is to increase in size and eventually to rupture. The mean rate of expansion is 2 to 4 mm per year, but this can be highly variable. The risk of rupture correlates with aneurysm size, but even small aneurysms can rupture.

As the size of the aneurysm increases, so does the risk of rupture: 60 to 80 percent of aneurysms 7 cm or larger in diameter rupture if surgery is not undertaken, and 95 percent of aneurysms over 10 cm in diameter rupture. Smaller aneurysms also rupture; in one autopsy series, 18 percent of ruptured abdominal aortic aneurysms were 5 cm in diameter or smaller. Pain or aneurysmal tenderness usually indicates aneurysmal expansion and therefore represents a significant risk of rupture regardless of the size of the aneurysm. Life expectancy is only about 6 months in patients with unruptured but symptomatic aneurysms, if elective surgery is not undertaken. Poorly controlled hypertension is also a risk factor for rupture.

There may be an increased risk of abdominal aortic aneurysm rupture after unrelated surgery. This issue is especially relevant, because patients with abdominal aortic aneurysm have a high incidence of coronary and cerebrovascular disease, and revascularization surgery may be considered before repair of the aneurysm. Although one prospective study failed to find an inordinately high incidence of rupture with unrelated surgery, the study sample size was small. There remains reason for concern, especially in patients with large aneurysms who are undergoing major abdominal or thoracic surgery unrelated to the aneurysm.

Management

The decision whether to repair an abdominal aortic aneurysm surgically depends on two issues: (1) the relative risk of repair versus the risk of waiting and (2) the medical condition of the patient. The most common medical conditions that require careful consideration in these patients are coronary, cerebrovascular, and chronic obstructive pulmonary disease. In patients selected for elective repair, the hospital mortality rate is generally under 5 percent. Major complications occur in an additional 5 percent of patients undergoing surgery and include cardiovascular accidents, acute ischemia of the lower limbs, mesenteric ischemia, and renal failure.

Contrary to the results of elective aneurysm repair, the results of emergent repair of ruptured abdominal aortic aneurysm remain poor. Rupture is generally a catastrophic event, and 25 to 50 percent of these patients die before reaching medical care. Of patients who do present to medical care with a ruptured abdominal aortic aneurysm, in-hospital mortality is as high as 70 percent in some series.

In view of this evidence, it is clear that the way to decrease mortality and morbidity from abdominal aortic aneurysm is to identify and repair the aneurysm before rupture, and preferably before the onset of symptoms. This can be done by screening asymptomatic patients at high risk for abdominal aortic aneurysm. As mentioned, the groups known to have a relatively high prevalence of abdominal aortic aneurysm are (1) first-degree relatives of patients with known abdominal aortic aneurysm who are over the age of 55; (2) males over the age of 55 who have a history of hypertension, hyperlipidemia, or tobacco use; and (3) patients with peripheral arterial aneurysms.

In nonobese patients, physical examination of the abdomen is usually adequate for screening. However, this examination must be specifically directed toward finding an abdominal aortic aneurysm and, if suggestive, must be followed up with abdominal ultrasonography. Because of the decreased sensitivity of physical examination in obese patients, ultrasonography or CT should be performed to screen for abdominal aortic aneurysm. Screening should be repeated every 3 to 5 years as long as it is negative.

Since even small aneurysms carry some risk of rupture, surgical repair of aneurysms 4 to 5 cm in diameter should be considered in young, healthy patients. An alternative approach, especially in patients who are at mild to moderately increased surgical risk owing to comorbid conditions or advanced age, consists of ultrasonographic follow-up every 3 to 6 months. Surgery can then be performed if there is a significant increase in aneurysmal size. Hypertension, if present, should be controlled, preferably with a beta-adrenergic blocking agent (to reduce aortic shear stress as well as mean arterial pressure). Verapamil or diltiazem are reasonable alternatives. An abdominal aortic aneurysm over 5 cm in diameter should be resected unless the surgical risk is high because of comorbid conditions. Patients with a symptomatic abdominal aortic aneurysm should undergo urgent surgical repair regardless of aneurysmal size.

Because abdominal aortic aneurysm repair results in significant physiologic stress, and because these patients frequently have coronary artery disease, aggressive hemodynamic monitoring is indicated in the perioperative period. This includes intra-arterial pressure monitoring, pulmonary arterial catheterization, and intraoperative transesophageal echocardiography to monitor left ventricular function. Elective aortic aneurysm repairs are best done by experienced vascular surgeons in hospitals with specialized vascular units, because surgical success is highly dependent on the level of experience with this surgery. A retroperitoneal approach combined with postoperative epidural anesthesia reduces respiratory complications in patients with significant chronic pulmonary disease.

THORACIC AORTIC ANEURYSMS

Presentation

As with abdominal aortic aneurysms, symptoms associated with thoracic aortic aneurysms are due to rapid enlargement of the aneurysm, compression of adjacent structures by the aneurysm, rupture of the aneurysm, or embolization from thrombus within the aneurysm. An additional presentation unique to ascending aortic aneurysms is stretching of the aortic valve ring with secondary aortic insufficiency.

Most often the patient is asymptomatic and the aneurysm is detected incidentally during a radiologic study. Occasionally the initial presentation reveals rupture of the aneurysm, which is frequently fatal. When patients present with symptoms, anterior chest pain or interscapular back pain is most frequent. The pain may be described as a mild and fleeting ache or as a severe "tearing" or lancinating pain (usually with a dissecting aneurysm). Anterior chest wall pain often reflects involvement of the ascending thoracic aorta, whereas disease of the descending thoracic aorta is often referred to the midscapular region. Less commonly, dysphagia, hoarseness, or stridor are associated with compression of the esophagus, left recurrent laryngeal nerve, or trachea, respectively. The same mechanism is responsible for superior vena caval syndrome in association with a large ascending aortic aneurysm. These patients describe a sensation of fullness in the head and neck, exacerbated by bending over or coughing, and they present with jugular venous distention without respiratory variation, a suffused head and neck, and prominent superficial collateral veins of the upper trunk and neck. Finally, hematemesis or hemoptysis may result from rupture into the esophagus or trachea, respectively.

Evaluation

Chest radiography is usually the first screening examination for a patient with a suspected thoracic aortic aneurysm. Widening of the mediastinum is a common finding. Other chest x-ray findings may include displacement of the trachea or esophagus and pleural effusion due to leaking or rupture of the aneurysm. All of these findings on chest radiography, however, are nonspecific. Often the aorta is clearly seen to be aneurysmal.

MRI or CT accurately sizes the aneurysm, identifies adjacent structures, visualizes mediastinal hematoma, and images intraluminal thrombus. MRI is becoming increasingly useful for evaluation of branch vessels and aortic insufficiency; in addition to being noninvasive, it has the advantage of not requiring intravenous contrast material. The primary disadvantage of both CT and MRI is the inability to evaluate the coronary arteries. Neither technique is suitable for unstable patients who require close monitoring. Both MRI and CT are ideal for serial evaluation of thoracic aortic aneurysms.

Transesophageal echocardiography is highly accurate for diagnosing and evaluating thoracic aortic pathology, including intraluminal thrombus. For aneurysms involving the ascending aorta, transesophageal echocardiography is especially useful for assessing left ventricular function and aortic insufficiency. Its primary limitation is inability to evaluate coronary arteries, other branch vessels, and structures adjacent to the aorta.

Angiography remains the "gold standard" for evaluating the coronary arteries, the branch vessels, aortic valve insufficiency, and left ventricular function. It is also the test of first choice in unstable patients in whom emergency surgery is planned. The size of the aneurysm, however, is often underestimated owing to intra-aortic mural thrombus; also, adjacent anatomy is not visualized. With improvements in noninvasive imaging techniques, angiography is often unnecessary for evaluation of stable patients. It is an inappropriate technique for serial evaluation of thoracic aortic aneurysms.

Prognosis

Like abdominal aortic aneurysms, the natural history of thoracic aortic aneurysms is to enlarge and eventually to rupture. In large published series, 1-year survival in patients with thoracic aortic aneurysms without dissection is less than 60 percent, and 5-year survival about 20 percent. About half of these deaths are due to aneurysm rupture. Determining which thoracic aortic aneurysms are most likely to rupture is difficult. The most important risk factors for rupture include aneurysmal diameter greater than 10 cm, rapid expansion of the aneurysm, or symptomatic aneurysm. It is important to note, however, that most ruptured aneurysms are less than 10 cm in size. A recent review revealed that in 117 cases of ruptured aneurysms of the thoracic and thoracoabdominal aorta, the aneurysmal size was 5 to 6 cm in 14 percent, 6 to 8 cm in 36 percent, 8 to 10 cm in 39 percent, and greater than 10 cm in only 12 percent. The median diameter of ruptured aneurysms due to chronic dissection was 8 cm, whereas aneurysms due to degenerative disease (primarily atherosclerosis) had a median diameter at rupture of 9 cm.

Patients undergoing elective resection of the aneurysm have a higher survival rate than those not undergoing surgery. Five-year (Kaplan-Meier) survival is about 70 percent. However, morbidity and mortality rates for repair of thoracic aortic aneurysms vary widely depending on the patient population being studied. The most important determinant of surgical outcome is whether the repair is urgent or elective. Most patients with rupture of a thoracic or thoracoabdominal aorta die before reaching the hospital. Of those who receive urgent operation, 20 to 60 percent die in the postoperative period, compared with 5 to 10 percent mortality for elective surgery. There is also a much higher incidence of postoperative complications, such as paraplegia and renal failure, after urgent surgery. Five-year (Kaplan-Meier) survival after urgent repair is only 30 percent. Another major determinant of perioperative mortality is patient age: hospital mortality is 50 percent for patients over 75 years of age but only 7 percent for younger patients. Pre-existing renal dysfunction or congestive heart failure also significantly increase the risk of postoperative death. Finally, surgical results are highly dependent on the experience of the surgeon and the center.

Significant operative complications occur in approximately 40 percent of patients undergoing elective repair. Important early complications include postoperative hemorrhage, renal failure, cerebrovascular accident, atrial and ventricular arrhythmias, myocardial infarction, congestive heart failure, prolonged respiratory insufficiency, rupture of a distal aneurysm, and infection. Approximately 15 percent of patients are left paraplegic after the operation. Late complications of thoracic aortic aneurysm repair include false aneurysm, prosthetic valve endocarditis, and prosthetic valve failure. However, most late deaths after thoracic aortic aneurysm surgery are due to associated cardiovascular or cerebrovascular disease. This underscores the importance of aggressive medical follow-up of these patients by the vascular internist, with particular attention to the diagnosis and treatment of coronary and carotid artery disease, hypertension, congestive heart failure, and aneurysmal disease of the remaining aorta.

Management

The decision whether to repair a thoracic aortic aneurysm surgically is based on (1) the relative risk of the repair versus the risk of aneurysmal rupture and (2) the medical condition of the patient. Since survival risk varies among patients as described above, management must be individualized. Generally, surgery should be strongly considered in patients with a symptomatic thoracic aortic aneurysm (regardless of size) or an asymptomatic aneurysm in the range of 6 to 8 cm in transverse diameter. Enthusiasm is diminished for resecting an asymptomatic aneurysm in patients older than 75 years, or in patients with significant myocardial or renal dysfunction. However, even in these patients, large (10 cm) or symptomatic aneurysms are usually resected. If the aneurysm is not associated with symptoms and is less than 6 cm in diameter, conservative management is indicated, except in patients with Marfan's syndrome, in whom ascending aortic aneurysms greater than 5.5 cm are usually resected and replaced with a valved conduit. Unrestricted aneurysms should be followed with serial CT or MRI every 3 to 6 months, and surgery reconsidered if there is evidence of progression.

Penetrating Aortic Ulceration

This is a recently recognized clinical entity affecting the thoracic (usually descending limb) or the abdominal aorta that must be differentiated from aortic aneurysm or dissection. The aortic ulceration is thought to be secondary to rupture of atherosclerotic plaque, exposing the underlying media to the shear stress of pulsatile flow. These hemodynamic forces may induce fissuring of the media and intramedial hematoma, or may promote progression of the ulcer through the media, resulting in rupture or containment by the adventitia (pseudoaneurysm).

This disorder usually afflicts elderly hypertensive males with a history of hyperlipidemia and/or tobacco use. Patients typically present with anterior chest or interscapular back pain that is usually described as "aching" and is usually intermittent. Occasionally the presentation mimics a classic aortic dissection.

The diagnosis is difficult to make. Occasionally one notes an irregularity of the aortic contour on a chest radiograph (Fig. 2), representing a pseudoaneurysm. CT or MRI is probably more sensitive than aortography, because the ulcerations may be partially filled with thrombus (Fig. 3).

Treatment of this entity remains controversial. Our practice is to recommend surgery for aortic ulcerations that have progressed to the stage of pseudoaneurysm formation. Aortic ulcerations associated with medial hematoma, without pseudoaneurysm formation, have been managed conservatively. Aggressive control of blood pressure with agents that lower pressure and shear stress often relieves symptoms. Risk factor modification (treatment of hyperlipidemia and tobacco use) is also recommended.

PREOPERATIVE EVALUATION OF PATIENTS WITH AORTIC ANEURYSMS

Atherosclerotic disease, including coronary artery and cerebrovascular disease, is common in patients with aortic aneurysms. Myocardial infarction is the most common cause of late death after aortic aneurysm repair. Since aneurysm repair is associated with significant physiologic stress, these patients require careful preoperative evaluation and perioperative management.

Because of the high incidence of coronary disease in

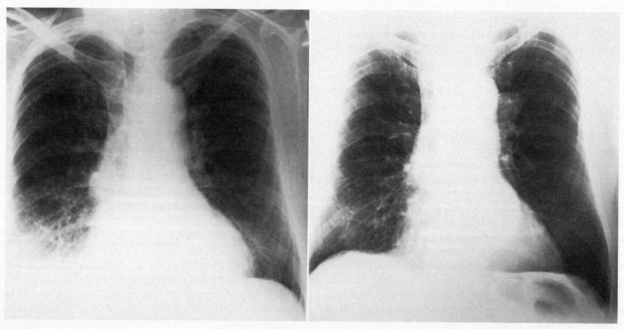

A   B

Figure 2 Chest radiograph of a patient with a penetrating aortic ulcer. *A,* At time of presentation with back pain. Note the mass density projected along the superior aspect of the left hilum. *B,* Routine film taken 2 years before presentation. The mass was not present at that time. (From Cooke JP, Kazmier FJ, Orszulak TA. The penetrating aortic ulcer: pathology, diagnosis and management. Mayo Clin Proc 1988; 63:718–725; with permission.)

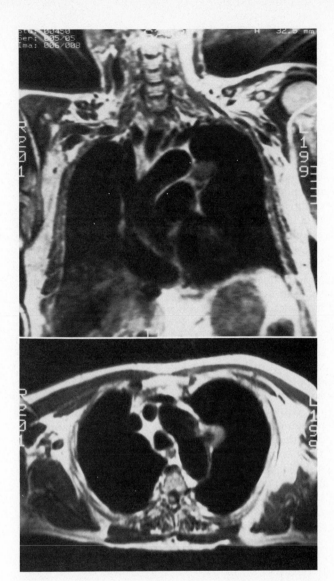

Figure 3 Magnetic resonance image of the chest; same patient as in Figure 2. Sagittal *(A)* and transverse *(B)* images reveal ulceration and penetration of the wall of the proximal descending thoracic aorta. (From Cooke JP, Kazmier FJ, Orszulak TA. The penetrating aortic ulcer: pathology, diagnosis and management. Mayo Clin Proc 1988; 63:718–725; with permission.)

patients with abdominal and thoracic aortic aneurysms, use of the Goldman index of cardiac risk is not adequate for the preoperative evaluation of these patients. Relatively young, active patients without symptoms of coronary disease, and with normal treadmill exercise test results, are at low risk for perioperative myocardial infarction and do not require preoperative coronary angiography. At the other end of the spectrum, patients with accelerating angina, or angina at rest, should undergo coronary angiography and, if possible, revascularization prior to repair of descending aortic aneurysms

or simultaneously with repair of ascending aortic aneurysms. Patients with stable angina should be evaluated noninvasively with exercise treadmill testing. If they are unable to exercise adequately owing to arterial occlusive disease affecting the lower extremities, dipyridamole thallium myocardial scanning should be used. Patients with a positive stress test or reperfusion on dipyridamole thallium testing have a higher risk of a cardiac event during vascular surgery. Therefore, preoperative coronary angiography should be considered in this group. A fixed thallium defect on the dipyridamole thallium study signifies a previous myocardial infarction. This latter finding does not increase the surgical risk unless it is associated with significant left ventricular dysfunction. If left ventricular dysfunction is suspected, echocardiography should be considered to evaluate ventricular function.

Hypertension is present in most of these patients and needs to be aggressively treated in the perioperative period, and chronically. Beta-adrenergic antagonists, verapamil, or diltiazem are all reasonable choices because of their ability to reduce systemic pressure and aortic shear stress. Chronic obstructive pulmonary disease is a frequent comorbid condition, and pulmonary function testing provides valuable information in these patients. Preoperative treatment with bronchodilators, and antibiotics if indicated, as well as discontinuation of tobacco use, will reduce pulmonary complications.

SUGGESTED READING

Cooke JP, Kazmier FJ, Orszulak TA. The penetrating aortic ulcer: pathology, diagnosis and management. Mayo Clin Proc 1988; 63:718–725.

Crawford ES, Hess KR, Cohen ES, et al. Ruptured aneurysm of the descending thoracic and thoracoabdominal aorta: analysis according to size and treatment. Ann Surg 1991; 213:417–426.

Crawford ES, Svensson LG, Coselli J, et al. Surgical treatment of aneurysm and/or dissection of the ascending aorta, transverse aortic arch, and ascending aorta and transverse aortic arch: factors influencing survival. J Thorac Cardiovasc Surg 1989; 98:659–674.

Durham SJ, Steed DL, et al. Probability of rupture of an abdominal aortic aneurysm after an unrelated operative procedure: a prospective study. J Vasc Surg 1991; 13:248–252.

Frist WH, Miller DC. Aneurysms of ascending thoracic aorta and transverse aortic arch. Cardiovasc Clin 1987; 17:263–287.

Johansen K, Kohler TR, et al. Ruptured abdominal aneurysm: the Harborview experience. J Vasc Surg 1991; 13:240–247.

Lederle FA, Walker JM, Reinke DB. Selective screening for abdominal aortic aneurysms with physical examination and ultrasound. Arch Intern Med 1988; 148:1753–1756.

McEnroe CS, O'Donnell TF, et al. Comparison of ejection fraction and Goldman risk factor analysis to dipyridamole-thallium 201 studies in the evaluation of cardiac morbidity after aortic aneurysm surgery. J Vasc Surg 1990; 11:497–504.

McFarlane MJ. The epidemiologic necropsy for abdominal aortic aneurysm. JAMA 1991; 265:2085–2088.

Moreno-Cabral CE, Miller DC, et al. Degenerative and atherosclerotic aneurysms of the thoracic aorta. J Thorac Cardiovasc Surg 1984; 88:1020–1032.

Webster MW, Ferrell RE, et al. Ultrasound screening of first-degree relatives of patients with an abdominal aortic aneurysm. J Vasc Surg 1991; 13:9–14.

AORTOILIAC OCCLUSIVE DISEASE

JOHN W. HALLETT, Jr., M.D.

Aortoiliac atherosclerosis remains a common pattern of highly treatable arterial occlusive disease. When arterial reconstructive surgery began in the 1950s, aortoiliac occlusive disease was primarily a disease of men with a male predominance of 10:1. Recent surgical series reveal an alarming increase in affected women, who now make up 40 percent of operated patients. This dramatic change is related to the increased number of women smokers. Most of these men and women are still in their active and productive years (40 to 65 years) and present with life style and work-limiting claudication. Adequate relief of symptoms frequently requires invasive therapy, e.g. percutaneous transluminal angioplasty (PTA) or surgical revascularization. Excellent therapeutic results continue to justify an aggressive diagnostic and therapeutic approach to aortoiliac occlusive disease.

This chapter reviews the approach to the diagnosis and management of these patients. Because of the insidious onset of symptoms, diagnosis is often delayed. Once it is suspected from a careful history taking and physical examination, the diagnosis can be confirmed by noninvasive vascular testing and arteriography in selected patients. Choosing the appropriate patients for intervention, the safest techniques for revascularization, and the ideal time for angioplasty or operation is obviously critical to a good outcome.

CLINICAL PRESENTATIONS

Aortoiliac occlusive disease can present with a remarkable spectrum of clinical symptoms and signs. Classically, claudication is the first symptom, but the muscle tiring is occasionally attributed to simple deconditioning or other more common musculoskeletal conditions. Classic aortoiliac claudication affects the buttock and thigh muscles, but such proximal lower extremity symptoms usually do not occur until the disease is advanced. Other patients present with ambulatory low back pain radiating into the hips and thighs and are mistakenly thought to have neurogenic lumbar spine or disk disease. A few such patients have already had back surgery for concomitant lumbar disk abnormalities before the true vascular origin of their claudication is recognized. Men who present with bilateral lower extremity claudication and impotence should be suspected of having Leriche's syndrome (claudication, impotence, and absent femoral pulses due to aortoiliac occlusive disease).

Although some form of claudication is the principal presentation in 75 percent of patients with aortoiliac disease, 25 percent present with threatened limb loss. They complain of ischemic rest pain, nonhealing foot sores, or early gangrene. They are usually elderly (over 65 years) and often have multiple medical risks, includ-

TYPE I

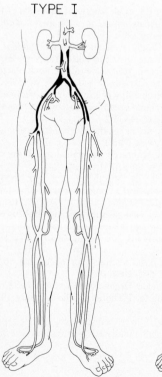

II

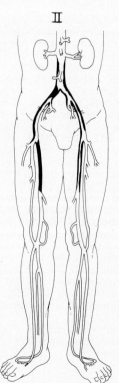

III

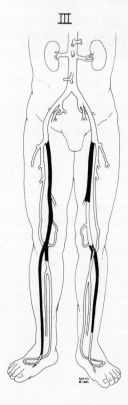

Figure 1 Patterns of aortoiliac and femoropopliteal arterial occlusive disease. Type I is limited to the distal abdominal aorta and common iliac arteries. Type II is a combination of aortoiliac and femoropopliteal disease. Type III involves primarily the superficial femoral, popliteal, and tibial arteries. (From Hallett JW Jr, et al. Patient care in vascular surgery. 2nd ed. Boston: Little, Brown, 1987; with permission.)

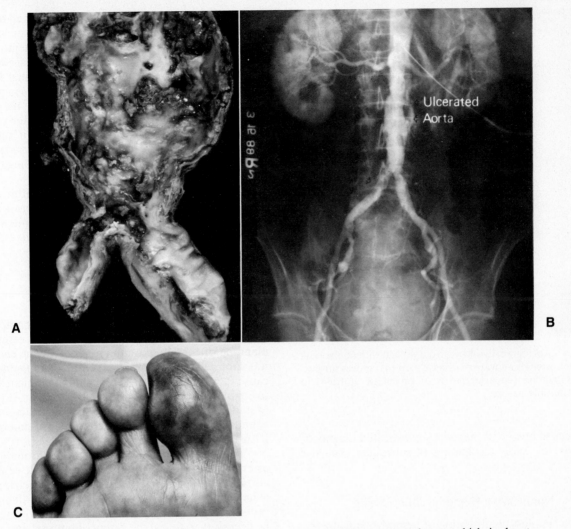

Figure 2 Ulcerative aortoiliac disease *(A, B)* can result in blue toe syndrome, which is due to atheroembolism in the feet *(C).*

ing hypertension, adult-onset diabetes mellitus, coronary and carotid artery disease, and chronic lung disease. Typically, they have multilevel aortoiliac and femoropopliteal occlusive disease (Fig. 1).

One variant of threatened limb loss is the blue toe syndrome, which is due to atheroembolism from an ulcerated aortoiliac atheroma (Fig. 2). These patients have painful blue toes and lower limb skin mottling. They frequently still have palpable pedal pulses and occasionally an elevated serum creatinine level if the ulcerated aorta extends above the renal arteries. A clinical pearl associated with renal atheroembolism is eosinophilia.

DIAGNOSIS

When the clinical symptoms suggest aortoiliac occlusive disease, the diagnosis can often be made by physical examination. Relatively simple Doppler pres-

sure measurements can then be used to confirm the clinical impression. A subsequent aortogram remains the diagnostic "road map" for intervention.

Physical Examination

Patients with early aortoiliac disease usually still have palpable femoral and pedal pulses. At this stage of disease, bruits over the abdominal aorta or femoral arteries may be the only positive physical finding at rest. Further evidence of significant aortoiliac disease can be generated by exercising the patient at the bedside (e.g., gentle jogging for 30 to 60 seconds). Abdominal and femoral bruits will be augmented and pedal pulses diminished. Advanced aortoiliac disease, of course, may be recognized by absent femoral pulses. Aortoiliac disease can also be distinguished from lumbar neurogenic disease or orthopedic hip disorders in many patients by bedside back and hip maneuvers plus a basic neurologic assessment. A thorough physical examination

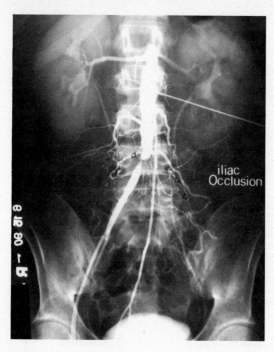

Figure 3 Aortogram in a 40-year-old woman with nonhealing left foot ulcers. This advanced disease pattern requires surgical revascularization (endarterectomy or prosthetic grafting) to achieve durable patency.

continues to be one of the most sophisticated diagnostic methods for early recognition of aortoiliac occlusive disease.

Noninvasive Hemodynamic Testing

The simplest confirmation of hemodynamically significant lower limb arterial occlusive disease is a diminished ankle-brachial blood pressure index (ABI). The ABI, however, may be normal (ABI = 1.0) *at rest* when the arterial disease is in an early stage of development. More advanced occlusive disease is usually associated with a resting ABI of 0.5 to 0.8, which falls dramatically to 0 to 0.2 after treadmill exercise. Treadmill exercise also reveals the onset and location of symptoms (e.g., buttocks, thighs, calves) and the walking distance. If electrocardiographic (ECG) monitoring is used, significant coronary artery disease may also be revealed.

Patients with threatened limb loss usually have an ABI less than 0.50 and transcutaneous oxygen tensions of the foot less than 20 to 30 torr. Since the blue toe syndrome is embolic and not occlusive in nature, the ABI may be relatively normal despite extensive microemboli of the toes and feet.

The primary limitation of Doppler pressures is difficulty in localizing the precise anatomic point of the lesion. This is a real problem in patients with multilevel aortoiliac and femoropopliteal occlusive disease. Although femoral waveform analysis and segmental thigh and leg pressures are helpful, they are not infallible.

Recently, duplex ultrasonography and newer magnetic resonance (MR) scanning are providing data that may allow more accurate localization of the hemodynamically significant lesions in multilevel occlusive disease.

If impotence is present, a penile-brachial Doppler pressure index (PBI) less than 0.70 is highly suggestive of vasculogenic erectile dysfunction. When the PBI is borderline, it should be measured again after treadmill walking exercise, when it is likely to fall if significant aortoiliac disease is present. Penile duplex sonography is also useful in differentiating between venogenic and arteriogenic impotence.

In essence, a normal ABI at rest and after exercise rules out significant aortoiliac occlusive disease. An ABI that falls with exercise adds validity to the initial clinical impression of aortoiliac disease and justifies the next diagnostic step: an aortogram with runoff.

ARTERIOGRAPHY

Standard or digital intra-arterial arteriography with runoff views of the lower extremities is essential to planning of therapeutic interventions. Intravenous digital subtraction aortograms are not recommended because they frequently lack sufficient anatomic resolution to enable unequivocal decisions to be made. At the time of standard aortography, several technical factors ensure adequate imaging, hemodynamic measurements, and PTA in selected patients.

To provide complete anatomic information, the arteriogram should demonstrate the entire abdominal aorta, including the renal, mesenteric, and pelvic arteries (Fig. 3). Biplane aortography via a transfemoral or transaxillary catheter is ideal. Oblique pelvic views may be necessary to reveal the extent of internal iliac disease. In addition, the lateral aortogram is essential for clear visualization of the origins of the celiac and superior mesenteric arteries (Fig. 4). The lateral aortogram is also necessary to visualize adequately the posterior aortic surface where ulcerated "coral-reef" atheromas frequently originate. These posterior wall atheromas may not be clearly seen on the standard anteroposterior aortic view. If renal atheroembolism is suspected, visualization of the descending thoracic aorta should also be obtained, since the offending ulcerated aortic lesion may be at this level.

If femoral catheterization is difficult and the transaxillary approach is not desired, a high translumbar injection can also provide an excellent aortographic view with runoff (Fig. 5). The lower extremity runoff views should demonstrate both the thigh and leg arteries. In particular, one should search for any evident stenosis at the origin of the profunda femoris artery, a common site of critical distal occlusive disease in patients with aortoileofemoral disease. Another common distal lesion is superficial femoral stenosis or short occlusion. These stenoses often require correction in addition to the aortoiliac disease if the patient is to achieve satisfactory relief of claudication.

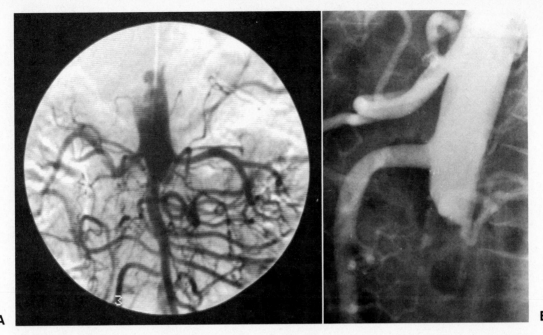

A   B

Figure 4 *A,* Transaxillary aortogram in a man with Leriche's syndrome (see text) due to juxtarenal aortic occlusion. *B,* Lateral aortogram in the same patient. There are patent celiac and superior mesenteric arteries.

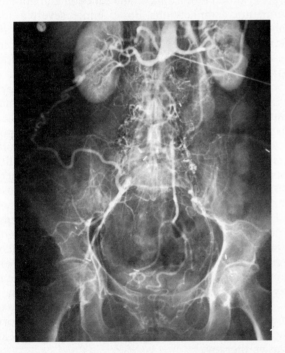

Figure 5 Translumbar aortogram demonstrating chronic juxtarenal aortic occlusion amenable to transaortic thromboendarterectomy and a bifurcated infrarenal aortic graft.

If the hemodynamic significance of the aortoiliac disease is questionable, pressure gradients across stenoses should be measured at the time of arteriography (Table 1). Generally, a resting gradient of more than 10 mm Hg indicates a hemodynamically significant lesion. If the gradient increases after reactive hyperemia, the stenosis must be considered significant and corrected to improve aortofemoral flow.

INITIAL MANAGEMENT

Long-term attention to reduction of risk factors is important whether the patient is initially given a walking program or more invasive therapy. Such patients benefit from evaluation and follow-up in a vascular clinic where hyperlipidemia, hypertension, diabetes mellitus, and any coagulopathies can be managed. Some form of intervention for tobacco dependence should also be offered, although the long-term results of such smoking cessation programs are debatable.

If the presenting symptoms are not incapacitating, a walking program has a 70 to 80 percent chance of stabilizing or improving claudication. Although the details of such a program vary, the essential ingredients should include walking at a comfortable pace at least 3 to 5 days a week for a specified time (15 to 30 minutes). Patients should be asked to keep a record of their walking days, time, and distance to review with their physician. Most patients can comfortably increase their walking time to 30 to 60 minutes a day and double to quadruple their walking distance after 6 to 8 weeks. An exercise program should be supplemented by avoidance of tobacco. Whether the hemorrheologic agent Trental adds much to exercise and smoking cessation remains debatable.

To evaluate this initial management plan, the physician and patient must discuss the outcome after 6

Table 1 Aortofemoral Graft (AF) for Multilevel Occlusive Disease: Predictors of Success and Need for Distal Bypass

Emphasis of Evaluation	Predictors of Good Result with AF Bypass Alone	Predictors of Need for Distal Bypass
Proximal disease	Absent or severely reduced femoral pulse Severe stenosis/occlusion (arteriogram) (+ femoral artery pressure study)*	"Normal" femoral pulse Mild–moderate inflow disease (arteriogram) (− femoral artery pressure study)
Distal disease	Good outflow tract (arteriogram) Index runoff resistance† less than 0.2	Poor outflow tract (arteriogram) Index runoff resistance ≥ 0.2
Intraoperative	Improved pulse volume recorder amplitude	Unimproved/worse pulse volume recorder amplitude
Clinical	Nonadvanced ischemic symptoms (i.e., claudication, rest pain)	Advanced ischemia (necrosis/sepsis)

From Brewster DC, Perler BA, Robison JG, Darling RC. Aortofemoral graft for multilevel occlusive disease: predictors of success and need for distal bypass. Arch Surg 1982; 117:1593; with permission

*Femoral artery pressure study. An iliac stenosis is significant when the resting pressure gradient across the iliac segment is greater than 10 mm Hg or falls more than 15 percent after reactive hyperemia or papaverine injection.

†Index runoff resistance = $\dfrac{\text{thigh-ankle pressure difference}}{\text{brachial pressure}}$

to 8 weeks. If the patient is not satisfied or is worse, more invasive therapy must be considered. Patients must have confidence that the primary vascular physician or surgeon will stay with them until the condition is relieved.

INDICATIONS FOR INVASIVE THERAPY

The initial walking program for early aortoiliac disease is sufficient for many patients but is often inadequate for those with more advanced disease. Consequently, indications for invasive therapy include

1. Threatened limb loss (rest pain, foot sores, gangrene or blue toe syndrome)
2. Work-limiting progressive claudication
3. Severe, life style–limiting claudication in a good-risk patient
4. Vasculogenic impotence

Relative contraindications or cautions for invasive therapy are

1. *Stable* claudication in the presence of diffuse multilevel aortoiliac and femoropopliteal tibial occlusive disease in a poor-risk patient
2. Other life-limiting medical conditions such as congestive heart failure
3. Purulent infection at some other site that could result in contiguous or hematogenous spread to a synthetic aortic graft. In such a patient, percutaneous angioplasty or endarterectomy may suffice for limb-threatening ischemia.

Timing of invasive therapy is essential to achieving the best long-term relief of aortoiliac disease. Some of

these patients are more durable than the results of an angioplasty or operation. Thus, invasive therapy must be carefully timed to maximize limb function and minimize therapeutic complications. For example, severe atheroembolism from balloon angioplasty or graft infection after aortofemoral bypass can be more limb- and life-threatening than the initial two-block claudication. Patients must understand these risks.

Another aspect of timing for invasive therapy is planning that 15 to 30 percent of patients will eventually require multiple interventions. Initially, an iliac balloon dilatation may palliate the condition enough to postpone an aortic operation for some years. Likewise, an aorto-iliac endarterectomy may be sufficient for localized disease and may avoid placement of a synthetic Dacron graft until later in life. Initiation of any type of invasive therapy "sets the clock ticking" for arterial restenosis and late graft complications or failure. Consequently, patients should have unequivocal indications for the initiation of invasive therapy, whether it be percutaneous angioplasty or surgical revascularization. In the end, stepwise increases in the magnitude of invasive therapy may offer the best chance of durable limb function.

In day-to-day practice, positive "yes" answers to the following key questions usually indicate that the aorto-iliac disease is severe enough to justify angiography and invasive therapy:

1. Is the limb at risk of amputation if foot perfusion is not improved?
2. Does the claudication keep the patient from adequately taking care of self, job, or family?
3. Is the claudication rapidly progressive over the previous few months (indicating a critical stenosis or occlusion)?
4. Is the patient ready to undergo an operation if angioplasty is not possible or fails?

5. Is the patient expected to have a low operative mortality risk (< 5 percent) and a reasonable life expectancy (> 12 to 18 months)?

ASSESSING OPERATIVE RISK

Surgical procedures to alleviate aortoiliac disease place the patient at increased risk of cardiopulmonary complications and occasional associated death. Severe coronary artery disease is present in approximately 15 percent of patients presenting with focal aortoiliac disease. Those patients with more advanced, multilevel aortoiliac and femoropopliteal disease have twice the risk (30 percent) of severe coronary atherosclerosis. Most postoperative morbidity and mortality occur in these patients with multisegmental disease. Other medical factors that increase operative risk are chronic congestive heart failure (ejection fraction < 35 percent), obstructive lung disease (FEV_1 < 1 liter), and chronic renal insufficiency (serum creatinine > 3.0 mg per deciliter). Such patients are more likely to have an operative mortality rate of 7 to 10 percent in contrast to the usual 2 to 3 percent rate for patients in better health.

Since coronary artery disease is the primary cause of operative and late death after aortoiliac operations, preoperative evaluation must focus on detection of any severe coronary insufficiency. *Patients with progressive or unstable angina pectoris need coronary angiography and revascularization before elective aortoiliac intervention for claudication.* Patients with a history of myocardial infarction or stable angina pectoris generally should undergo some type of cardiac stress test. Since claudication may prevent adequate exercise levels, dipyridamole thallium scans are one method to identify ischemic reperfusion zones of the heart. Positive thallium scans justify coronary angiography and selective revascularization. Another useful noninvasive method of assessing cardiac risk is ambulatory 24-hour ECG monitoring for ischemic ST-segment changes. Finally, patients with no clinical evidence of cardiac disease and with good exercise tolerance can usually undergo aortoiliac arterial reconstructive surgery without further cardiac testing.

Controversy continues over the management of concurrent carotid artery disease. Patients with transient ischemic attacks (TIAs) or recent strokes obviously need a complete neurologic evaluation and operative correction of any causative ulcerated or occlusive extracranial arterial lesions. In patients with asymptomatic cervical bruits there should be noninvasive ascertainment of the hemodynamic significance of the carotid bruits. Patients with hemodynamically significant internal carotid arterial lesions are at increased risk of future TIAs or strokes. In selected patients, especially those with bilateral stenosis of the internal carotid arteries exceeding 80 percent, elective repair of one lesion before major aortic surgery is reasonable. Asymptomatic, nonhemodynamically significant carotid disease should be followed for progression or symptoms.

SPECIFIC INVASIVE THERAPIES

Percutaneous Angioplasty

Percutaneous transluminal angioplasty (PTA) has become the treatment of choice for a focal common iliac artery stenosis. At the present time, the Gruntzig balloon catheter is the essential tool for PTA (Fig. 6). Occasionally, a short period of intra-arterial thrombolytic infusion may be necessary to lyse recent thrombus in an occluded iliac artery stenosis before angioplasty. Additional use of a hot-tip laser or an atherectomy device does not appear currently to change the basic results of a simple balloon dilatation. Whether the addition of intra-arterial stents will ensure better long-term patency rates requires more investigation.

The best results for iliac PTA are obtained in claudicants with focal (< 3 cm) common iliac stenosis and good runoff. Initial success is 90 percent, with 60 to 70 percent good results at 5 years. Less favorable results are achieved in stenotic lesions in the aorta and internal and external iliac arteries. Although iliac balloon angioplasty may improve claudication, postexercise Doppler ankle pressures may not show complete hemodynamic improvement and should be followed periodically to detect restenosis.

Aortoiliac Surgical Reconstruction

Some type of direct aortoiliac endarterectomy or bypass grafting will be necessary for most patients with advanced aortoiliac disease (Figs. 7 and 8). In experienced hands, the operative mortality and morbidity rates are low (2 to 3 and 5 to 10 percent, respectively). The most common cause of perioperative and late death is heart disease. Excellent symptomatic relief of chronic lower extremity ischemia is achieved in 95 percent of patients. Early results are best for claudication in the absence of distal femoropopliteal disease. The perioperative (95 to 98 percent), 5-year (80 to 90 percent), 10-year (70 to 80 percent), 15-year (70 percent), and 20-year (60 to 70 percent) cumulative patency rates for aortofemoral bypass are highly satisfactory and document the durability of this operation. It is unlikely that any percutaneous method of transluminal angioplasty can be expected to equal the durability of replacing the diseased aortoiliac segment with a prosthetic graft or performing a surgical thromboendarterectomy of the entire atheroma (Fig. 9).

Early postoperative graft thrombosis (3 to 8 percent) and infection (0.8 to 1.0 percent) are uncommon. Femoral anastomotic pseudoaneurysm remains one of the most common late graft problems (5 percent). Amputations are eventually necessary in only 3 to 5 percent of patients with claudication and in 15 percent with rest pain. Successful limb function is maintained in 80, 70, and 60 percent at 10, 15, and 20 years, respectively. However, coronary artery disease takes its toll as late survival rates decline rapidly for the entire surgical cohort: 50, 30, and 15 percent at 10, 15, and 20

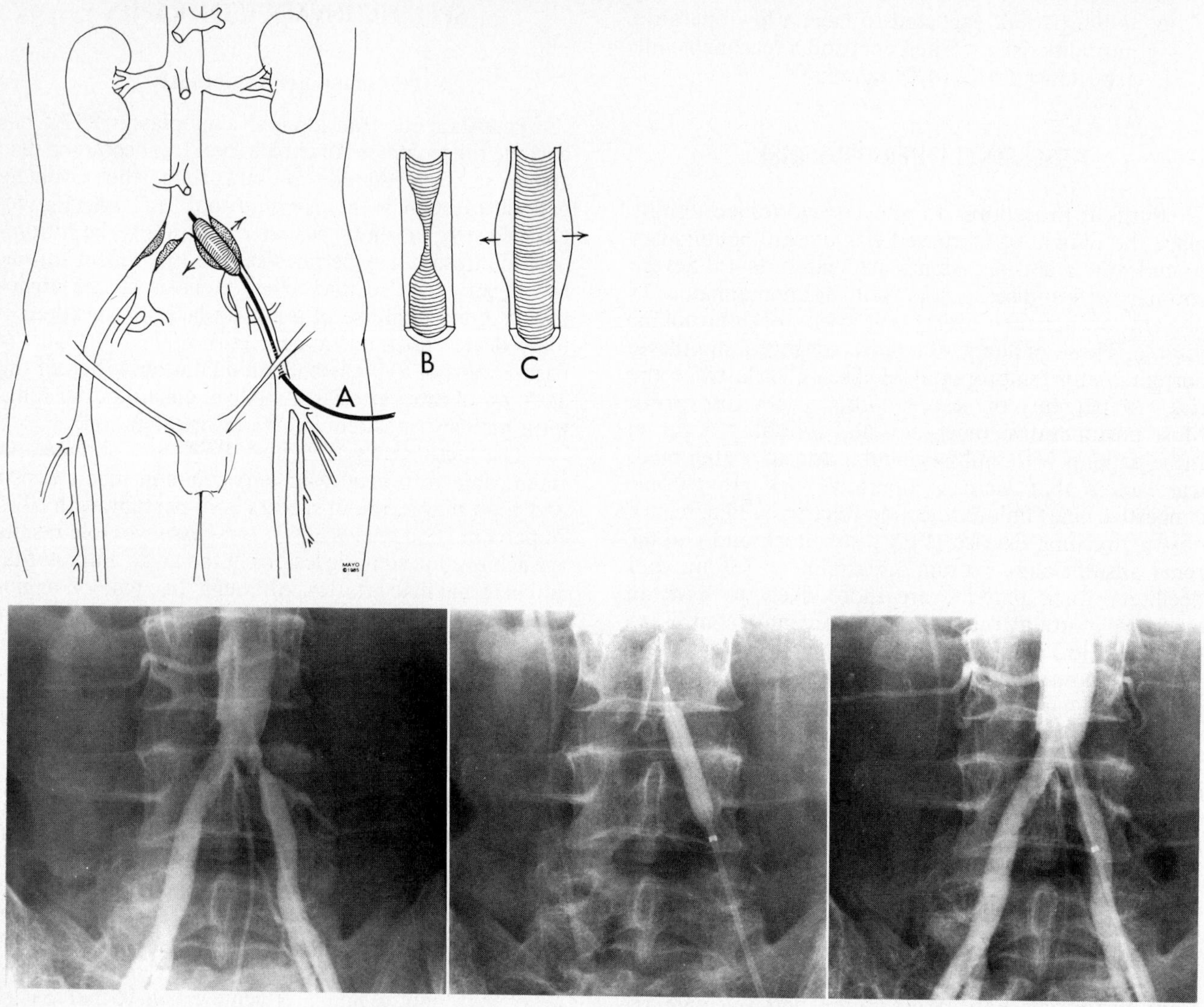

Figure 6 Percutaneous transluminal balloon angioplasty is the treatment of choice for a focal (<3-cm) common iliac stenosis. *A, B, C,* Transfemoral approach and mechanism of percutaneous balloon angioplasty. *D,* Focal left common iliac stenosis. *E,* Inflation of a Gruntzig angioplasty balloon in the left common iliac artery. *F,* Postangiography improvement in iliac stenosis.

years, respectively. In contrast, 5-year survival is more encouraging for patients without evident coronary disease (80 to 85 percent) and those who have undergone coronary bypass surgery (70 to 75 percent).

Associated Renal and Visceral Occlusive Disease

An occasional patient with symptomatic aortoiliac disease also has significant lesions of the renal and intestinal arteries. These lesions are usually orificial stenoses or occlusions that extend from the aortic atheroma. They can be managed by either transaortic endarterectomy or bypass grafting. Combined aortic and renal or visceral revascularization does increase operative mortality (7 to 10 percent). The increased risk is due primarily to underlying cardiopulmonary disease and not to the operation itself.

Extra-anatomic Surgical Procedures

Extra-anatomic bypasses, such as axillofemoral or femorofemoral grafts, should play a limited role in the surgical management of aortoiliac occlusive disease. Although they may be associated with lower operative morbidity and mortality than direct intra-abdominal aortic grafting, extra-anatomic grafts carry a high likelihood of eventual and repetitive thrombosis.

Nonetheless, a femorofemoral cross-over bypass is a reasonable option for unilateral iliac occlusion associated with a normal contralateral inflow, or for chronic occlusion of one limb of an aortofemoral graft. The 5-year patency is 70 to 80 percent if secondary repeat operations for thrombosis are included.

Axillofemoral bypasses are reserved for situations in which abdominal aortic reconstruction is contraindi-

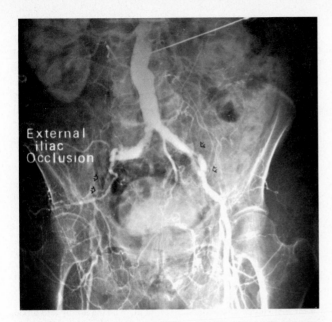

Figure 7 Translumbar aortogram showing extensive aortoiliac disease with right external iliac artery occlusion and high-grade left external iliac artery stenosis. This disease pattern requires aortofemoral bypass grafting.

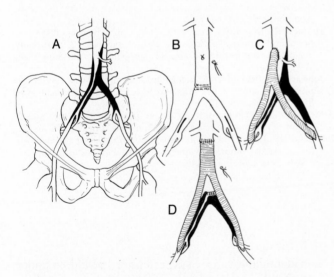

Figure 8 Types of aortoiliac reconstruction. Aortoiliac endarterectomy *(B)* is one good option for occlusive disease localized to the distal abdominal aorta and common iliac arteries *(A)*. Most patients, however, need an aortofemoral bypass *(C, D)* for extensive aortoiliac disease. (From Hallett JW Jr, et al. Patient care in vascular surgery. 2nd ed. Boston: Little, Brown, 1987; with permission.)

cated or excessively risky. Examples include infected aortic grafts, a history of severe intestinal adhesions, irradiation complications of the abdomen, or marginal cardiorespiratory reserve. In some of these situations, the aorta can still be approached safely by an extraperitoneal incision. The 5-year patency for axillofemoral

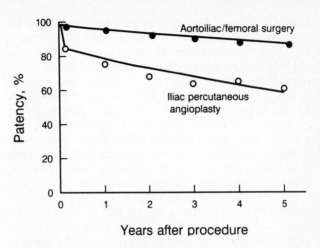

Figure 9 Limb patency rates among survivors of surgical procedures or percutaneous transluminal angioplasty (PTA) for aortoiliac disease during a 5-year period. (Modified from Doubliet P, Abrams HL. The cost of underutilization: percutaneous transluminal angioplasty for peripheral vascular disease. N Engl J Med 1984; 310:95; with permission.)

bypass grafts depends on femoropopliteal runoff: 70 to 80 percent for good runoff but only 50 percent for poor runoff.

Concomitant Nonvascular Abdominal Pathology

Elective aortoiliac synthetic grafting should generally not be combined with other nonvascular operations. The most common dilemma is whether to perform cholecystectomy for asymptomatic gallstones or inguinal herniorrhaphy for a chronic groin hernia. Combined procedures potentially increase mortality compared with aortic grafting alone (6 to 9 percent versus 3 percent) and involve more complications (60 percent versus 15 percent). Occasionally, concomitant cholecystectomy is indicated if the aortic grafting and retroperitoneal closure proceed smoothly and the cholelithiasis is associated with signs of chronic cholecystitis that may recur in the early postoperative period. Incidental discovery of a gastrointestinal tumor (e.g., a colonic or pancreatic mass) is best managed at a later operation after adequate evaluation and bowel preparation.

LONG-TERM FOLLOW-UP

Patients who have undergone PTA or reconstructive arterial surgery remain at risk for recurrent occlusive disease or late graft failure for the rest of their lives. Consequently, they need lifelong, periodic reexamination. It is unfortunate that many patients ignore the need for such follow-up and return only when problems occur.

To ensure adequate long-term follow-up, patients need to be informed of its importance at the time of angioplasty or surgery. Generally, they should be reexamined 6 to 8 weeks after invasive therapy to evaluate wound healing and relief of symptoms. In addition, the hemodynamic result of the angioplasty or operation should be documented by resting and postexercise ankle Doppler pressures. Subsequent follow-up visits depend on patient progress, but yearly check-ups will detect most late problems. Patients must be instructed to return immediately if recurrent ischemic symptoms or signs of incisional or systemic infection are noted. Because graft infection may follow a bacteremia, prophylactic antibiotics are recommended for all dental work, other operations, or superficial skin abrasions and infection. Since late anastomotic false aneurysm is a common late graft complication, it seems reasonable to perform ultrasonography or CT of aortofemoral grafts at least every 5 years or whenever physical examination detects pseudoaneurysms of the groin or abdomen.

The leading cause of late death remains myocardial infarction with subsequent arrhythmias or heart failure. Long-term follow-up therefore must include close monitoring for new or progressive cardiac symptoms. During periodic treadmill exercise tests to check lower extremity pressures, continuous ECG monitoring will occasionally detect new ST-segment changes. Such exercise ECG abnormalities are associated with an increased risk of eventual cardiac events and should be further evaluated. Patients must also be instructed to report any new angina, limiting dyspnea, or orthopnea.

FUTURE CHALLENGES

Continued widespread tobacco abuse and atherogenic life styles are likely to perpetuate the development of aortoiliac arterial occlusive disease. An increased number of women smokers has reduced the male predominance of this pattern of atherosclerosis. Fortunately, exercise programs and modification of risk factors can benefit many patients with early aortoiliac disease. In addition, PTA offers excellent palliation for focal common iliac artery stenoses. With over 30 years of follow-up, aortoiliac endarterectomy and bypass grafting have repeatedly demonstrated excellent and durable relief of more advanced aortoiliac disease. Coronary artery disease remains the main threat to late survival and must receive more attention and better management if the late outcome in aortoiliac disease is to be improved.

Acknowledgments. The author gratefully acknowledges the editorial assistance of Gail Prechel and the illustrations by John Desley.

SUGGESTED READING

Brewster DC, Perler BA, Robison JG, Darling RC. Aortofemoral graft for multilevel occlusive disease: predictors of success and need for distal bypass. Arch Surg 1982; 117:1593–1600.

Carter SA, Hamel ER, Paterson JM, et al. Walking ability and ankle systolic pressures: observations in patients with intermittent claudication in a short-term walking exercise program. J Vasc Surg 1989; 10:642–649.

Freeman WK, Gibbons RJ, Shub C. Preoperative assessment of cardiac patients undergoing noncardiac surgical procedures. Mayo Clin Proc 1989; 64:1105–1117.

Hallett JW, Greenwood LH, Robison JG. Lower extremity arterial disease in young adults: a systematic approach to early diagnosis. Ann Surg 1985; 202:647–652.

Hertzer NR, Beven EG, Young JR, et al. Coronary artery disease in peripheral vascular patients: a classification of 1000 coronary angiograms and results of surgical management. Ann Surg 1984; 199:223–224.

Johnston KW, Rae M, Hogg-Johnston SA, et al. Five-year results of a prospective study of percutaneous transluminal angioplasty. Ann Surg 1987; 206:403–413.

McDaniel MD, Cronenwett JL. Basic data related to the natural history of intermittent claudication. Ann Vasc Surg 1989; 3:273–277.

Szilagyi DE, Elliott JP Jr, Smith RF, et al. A thirty-year survey of the reconstructive surgical treatment of aortoiliac occlusive disease. J Vasc Surg 1986; 3:421–436.

COARCTATION OF THE AORTA

DAVID J. DRISCOLL, M.D.

Coarctation of the aorta is a congenital vascular malformation consisting of an obstruction of the aorta, usually discrete and near the aortic origin of the ductus or ligamentum arteriosum (Fig. 1). The usual obstruction is caused by a crescent-shaped ledge of tissue projecting into the lumen of the aorta. The condition makes up 5 to 8 percent of all congenital cardiovascular defects. Two-thirds of cases are in males. Coarctation and congenital renal abnormalities are the most common identifiable cause of hypertension in children under 5 years old.

Although the location of the usual coarctation has been described as pre- or postductal, the vast majority are juxtaductal. Rarely, the area of aortic obstruction can occur in the aortic arch or the abdominal aorta. The cause of aortic arch or abdominal aortic obstruction is presumably different from that of a juxtaductal or periductal coarctation.

In the fetus, blood flow from the pulmonary artery traverses the patent ductus into the descending thoracic aorta. As the patent ductus arteriosus closes, the lumen of the aorta is compromised further because of contractile ductal tissue that extends onto the aorta. As the ductus constricts, the aorta is narrowed. This phenomenon explains, to some extent, the onset of congestive

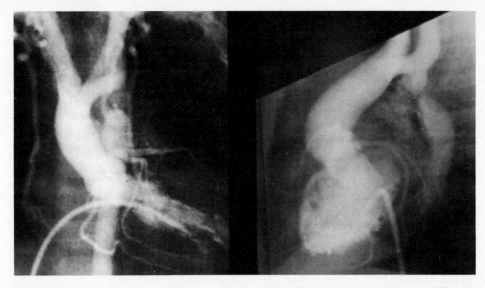

Figure 1 Left ventricular angiogram demonstrating coarctation of the aorta. Collateral vessels are apparent.

heart failure in neonates, with coarctation of the aorta, at the time of ductal closure.

ASSOCIATED ANOMALIES

Coarctation of the aorta frequently is associated with other malformations. Bicuspid aortic valve coexists in up to 85 percent of cases. Coarctation can occur in a variety of combinations with aortic stenosis, mitral stenosis, and ventricular septal defect. Patients with Turner's syndrome have a higher than expected incidence of coarctation of the aorta, and in these the aorta may be more friable than normal.

Associated abnormalities of the subclavian arteries may affect the clinical recognition of coarctation. The orifice of the left subclavian artery may be compromised or may originate distally to the coarctation site. The right subclavian artery may arise aberrantly from the descending thoracic aorta distally to the area of coarctation. Because of these abnormalities, it is important to measure blood pressure in both arms and a leg, and to assess the quality of both the carotid and femoral pulses when assessing patients for coarctation.

In most clinically significant cases of coarctation, collateral vessels form to provide a route for blood to bypass the coarcted site (Figs. 1 and 2). These vessels include the subclavian, internal mammary, intercostal, scapular, and epigastric vessels. The presence of dilated tortuous intercostal vessels produces the classical rib notching noted on chest radiograms (Fig. 3). This notching rarely occurs in infants but is present in most older children and adults. If blood flow to a subclavian artery is compromised, collaterals may form only contralateral to the compromised subclavian artery.

CLINICAL PRESENTATION

When presenting in infants with severe congestive heart failure, coarctation of the aorta usually is associated with other significant intracardiac defects such as aortic stenosis or ventricular septal defect. When associated with congestive heart failure and poor cardiac output, pulses in *all* extremities may be reduced or absent, and the diagnosis of severe coarctation may be inapparent or the condition may be misdiagnosed as hypoplastic left heart syndrome (or aortic or mitral atresia). After appropriate therapy with prostaglandin and/or digitalis and diuretics, cardiac output improves, the upper extremity pulses return, and the discrepancy between upper and lower extremity pulses becomes apparent.

In children, adolescents, and adults, coarctation presents with upper extremity hypertension or a cardiac murmur. Less commonly, the diagnosis is made only after a cerebrovascular accident or an episode of infective endocarditis. Reduced femoral pulses, an abnormal chest radiogram (rib notching, dilated aorta, or cardiomegaly), or left ventricular hypertrophy noted on an electrocardiogram (ECG) are frequent supportive findings.

PHYSICAL EXAMINATION

Appearance

Except for patients with coarctation of the aorta associated with Turner's syndrome, the general physical appearance of patients with this condition is normal. Rarely, infants with coarctation (and associated patent

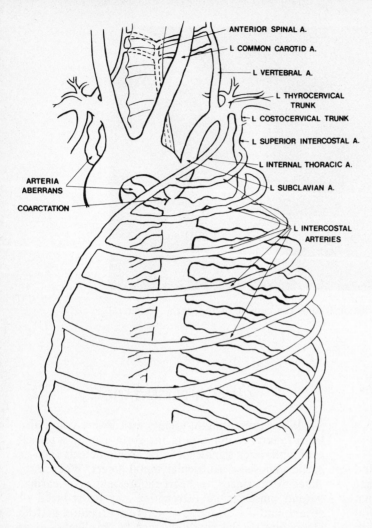

ANTERIOR SPINAL A.
L COMMON CAROTID A.
L VERTEBRAL A.
L THYROCERVICAL TRUNK
L COSTOCERVICAL TRUNK
L SUPERIOR INTERCOSTAL A.
L INTERNAL THORACIC A.
L SUBCLAVIAN A.
ARTERIA ABERRANS
COARCTATION
L INTERCOSTAL ARTERIES

Figure 2 Diagrammatic representation of collateral blood supply. (From Morriss M, McNamara D. Coarctation of the aorta and interrupted aortic arch. In: Garson A, Bricker J, McNamara D, eds. The science and practice of pediatric cardiology. Philadelphia: Lea & Febiger, 1990; with permission.)

ductus arteriosus) may have differential cyanosis, the lower extremities being cyanotic and the upper acyanotic.

Palpation

Palpation of all major pulses and potential sites of collateral vessels is critical in the evaluation for suspected coarctation. There is a reduction of the pulse volume in the lower extremities. There may be a delay in the femoral pulse relative to the brachial pulse, and upper extremity and carotid pulses may be increased in amplitude. As noted above, the relative quality of upper and lower extremity pulses depends on the location and presence or absence of stenosis of the subclavian arteries.

Abnormalities of the pulses will be reflected in abnormalities of blood pressure in the upper and lower extremities. The systolic blood pressure in vessels that originate proximal to the coarctation site will be higher than in vessels arising below the area of coarctation. However, diastolic blood pressure is usually similar.

The difference between the upper and lower ex-

tremity pulse volume and blood pressure reflect, to some degree, the severity of the aortic obstruction. However, in the presence of well-developed collateral vessels, the severity of the aortic obstruction may be underestimated by the difference between upper and lower extremity blood pressure and pulse volume. One should search for evidence of collateral vessels. In most older children and adults, the collateral vessels can be felt and murmurs heard in the parascapular regions. Also, upper extremity hypertension results not only from the mechanical obstruction of the aorta, but also from changes in the renin-angiotensin system presumably caused by abnormal renal perfusion and renal artery pulse pressure.

A palpable thrill over the carotid arteries or in the suprasternal notch suggests the association of aortic stenosis. A prominent left ventricular impulse reflects left ventricular hypertension and hypertrophy.

Auscultation

The first heart sound is normal. The second heart sound usually is normal, but the pulmonary component

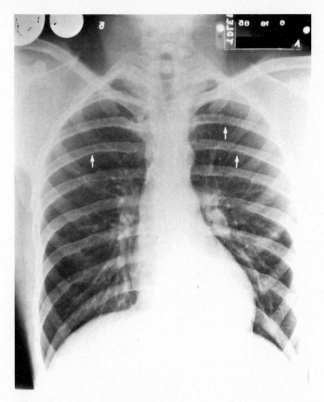

Figure 3 Chest radiogram of a patient with coarctation of the aorta, demonstrating rib notching.

may be increased in infants with associated congestive heart failure and pulmonary hypertension. The aortic component of the second heart sound may be increased in adolescents and adults with significant systemic hypertension. An aortic ejection click usually is audible in patients with a bicuspid aortic valve or aortic valve stenosis.

A systolic ejection murmur may be heard at the cardiac apex and presumably results from flow through the area of coarctation. This also may produce a systolic murmur audible over the back and abdomen. A systolic ejection murmur located more medially and basally and carotid bruits may result from an abnormal aortic valve. Precordial murmurs and murmurs over the back (especially near the scapula) may result from collateral vessels; these murmurs may be continuous or heard only in systole.

Diastolic murmurs may occur in infants because of congestive heart failure. In patients of all ages, a diastolic murmur may result from associated mitral valve abnormalities, aortic valvular insufficiency, or flow through collateral vessels.

CHEST ROENTGENOGRAM

The classic appearance of the chest roentgenogram includes rib notching, the "3" sign, a dilated ascending aorta, and occasionally cardiomegaly (Fig. 3). Rib notching results from dilated tortuous intercostal arteries and usually is limited to the upper three or four ribs. The "3" sign results from dilatation of the aorta immediately proximal and distal to the area of coarctation.

ELECTROCARDIOGRAM

Infants with coarctation and congestive heart failure exhibit right ventricular or biventricular hypertrophy on ECG. Infants without congestive heart failure, children, adolescents, and adults may have a normal ECG or evidence of left ventricular hypertrophy.

ECHOCARDIOGRAM

Although the presence of coarctation of the aorta is determined by clinical examination, echocardiography is useful to localize the area of coarctation, exclude the presence of an atypical coarctation (i.e., a long segmental rather than discrete coarctation, or an "abdominal coarctation"), and to define the presence or absence of associated cardiovascular abnormalities. With Doppler technology, the pressure drop across the coarctation can be estimated.

MAGNETIC RESONANCE IMAGING

Magnetic resonance imaging (MRI) provides a useful noninvasive means of displaying the coarctation. This is particularly helpful in assessing the anatomy of the aorta after coarctation repair.

CARDIAC CATHETERIZATION AND ANGIOGRAPHY

Diagnostic cardiac catheterization and angiography is unnecessary for patients with strong clinical evidence of coarctation (i.e., pulse and blood pressure difference between the upper and lower extremities, and clinical and/or chest radiographic evidence for collateral vessels). In such patients one may noninvasively delineate the location and length of the coarctation, and detect associated abnormalities using MRI or echocardiography.

Catheterization and angiography may be necessary to assess the presence or absence of collateral vessels in patients for whom operation is planned and in whom there is no other clinical evidence of collateral vessels. Also, invasive studies may be necessary to differentiate pseudocoarctation from true coarctation of the aorta. Pseudocoarctation of the aorta consists of infolding and tortuosity of the aorta without obstruction. Patients with pseudocoarctation do not have significant differences between arm and leg blood pressures or pulses and have no evidence of collateral vessels on clinical examination or chest radiography.

MANAGEMENT

Infants

The initial management of infants with coarctation of the aorta and significant congestive heart failure is medical and includes correction of acidosis and administration of oxygen, digitalis, and diuretics. Prostaglandin E_1 to reopen or to maintain patency of the ductus arteriosus is particularly useful and may be life-saving for the neonate with severe congestive heart failure and acidosis. As a general rule, if significant congestive heart failure persists despite 24 hours of aggressive medical decongestive therapy, surgery or perhaps balloon dilatation is indicated. For infants who respond to decongestive therapy, who resume normal feeding and growth, and who do not have significant upper extremity hypertension, surgery can be delayed. Because of the significant incidence of recoarctation in infants operated on at under 1 year of age, operation should be delayed, if possible, until the patient reaches 1 to 4 years of age.

Children and Adolescents

Surgery or balloon dilatation is indicated for all children and adolescents with significant coarctation of the aorta. This condition is significant when associated with upper extremity hypertension and a significantly lower systolic blood pressure in the lower than in the upper extremities (a difference of greater than 10 to 15 mm Hg). In the presence of significant collateral vessels, the coarctation may be significant despite minimal differences between upper and lower extremity systolic blood pressure and, in some cases, normal upper extremity blood pressure. However, the absence of collateral vessels should raise the suspicion of pseudocoarctation and make one wary of the need for repair.

The ideal age for repair of significant coarctation is between 1 and 4 years, when the operative risk and likelihood of persistent or repeat coarctation is low. Repair after the age of 6 years is associated with a higher incidence of persistent hypertension than when the repair is performed before that age.

Adults

The indications for repair of coarctation of the aorta in adults are similar to those in children and adolescents. Because of increased friability of the aorta of adults, excessive bleeding can occur during the operation. Because of this, many surgeons elect to perform repair of coarctation of the aorta in adults using cardiopulmonary bypass, or at least are ready to use cardiopulmonary bypass should surgical difficulties arise.

OPERATIVE TECHNIQUES AND RESULTS OF OPERATION

There are three commonly used surgical techniques: (1) end-to-end anastomosis, (2) patch aortoplasty, and

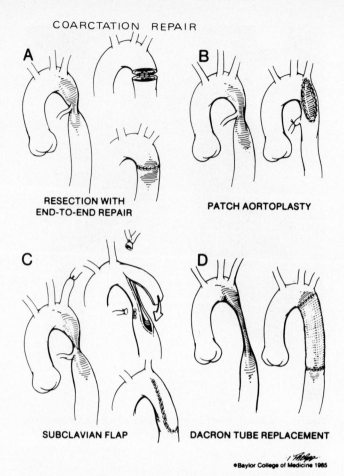

COARCTATION REPAIR

A — RESECTION WITH END-TO-END REPAIR

B — PATCH AORTOPLASTY

C — SUBCLAVIAN FLAP

D — DACRON TUBE REPLACEMENT

●Baylor College of Medicine 1985

Figure 4 The three types of surgical repair of coarctation of the aorta. (From Morriss M, McNamara D. Coarctation of the aorta and interrupted aortic arch. In: Garson A, Bricker J, McNamara D, eds. The science and practice of pediatric cardiology. Philadelphia: Lea & Febiger, 1990; with permission.)

(3) subclavian flap repair. In addition, interposition of a synthetic tube graft may be necessary for patients with an atypical long segmental coarctation (Fig. 4). End-to-end anastomosis usually is performed in children, adolescents, and adults. Subclavian flap repair is preferred by some surgeons for infants. Patch aortoplasty also is used in infants but is associated with aneurysm formation in the area of the repair. Potential operative complications include recurrent laryngeal or phrenic nerve injury, chylothorax, and spinal cord ischemia, which can result in lower body paralysis. Fortunately, the last-named complication is rare.

Early postoperative problems include persistent systemic hypertension and mesenteric ischemia. Most episodes of postoperative hypertension can be treated effectively with afterload-reducing agents or beta-blocking agents. Postrepair hypertension may persist for several weeks. Maintenance of normal blood pressure after surgery seems to reduce significantly the incidence of postoperative mesenteric ischemia.

If coarctation of the aorta remains unrepaired, life expectancy is considerably shorter than normal, most

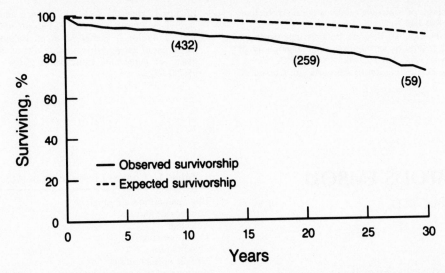

Figure 5 Survival curve of patients undergoing repair of coarctation of the aorta. (Based on data by Cohen M, Fuster V, Steele P, et al. Coarctation of the aorta: long-term follow-up in prediction of outcome after surgical correction. Circulation 1989; 80:840–845.)

patients dying before the age of 40. Causes of death include stroke, heart failure, ruptured aorta, and infective endocarditis.

Cohen and associates reported the long-term results of coarctation repair in 646 patients operated on at the Mayo Clinic between 1946 and 1981. The 10- and 30-year survival rates for these patients were 91 and 72 percent, respectively (Fig. 5). The mean age of patients who died was 38 years. Most deaths resulted from coronary artery disease, and the mean age of fatal myocardial infarction was 48 years. Six patients died from a cerebrovascular accident and all were over 25 years old at the time of coarctation repair. Older age at the time of operation, male gender, and higher postrepair systolic blood pressure were significantly related to death. The best survival was in patients operated on at under 9 years of age. Twenty-year survival for patients operated on at under 14 years of age was 91 percent, but for those operated on at 14 years of age or over survival was only 79 percent. Eighty-one of the initial operative survivors required reoperation. Operation for recurrent or persistent coarctation was necessary for 17 (3 percent) of the patients. However, of patients operated on at less than 1 year of age, 26 percent required reoperation for persistent or recurrent coarctation. Aortic valve replacement was necessary for 40 (7 percent) of the 571 initial operative survivors, and mitral valve replacement was necessary for 12 (2 percent). Six patients (1 percent) underwent repair of an aortic aneurysm.

The average systolic and diastolic blood pressure decreased from 159 to 131 and 91 to 77 mm Hg, respectively, after surgery. Depending on the definition of persistent hypertension, it was noted in 8 to 25 percent of the patients. Persistent hypertension occurred in 7 percent of patients initially repaired at under 1 year of age but in 38 percent of those repaired at over 14 years of age.

BALLOON DILATATION

Tynan and colleagues reported the results of dilatation of native coarctation for 140 patients aged 3 days to 29 years. The pressure gradient across the area of coarctation decreased from 48 ± 19 to 12 ± 11 mm Hg and the diameter of the aorta increased from 3.9 ± 2.2 to 8.8 ± 3.8 mm. Late results were not reported.

For 200 patients who had balloon dilatation for recurrence of coarctation after surgical repair, the pressure gradient across the area of coarctation decreased from 41.9 ± 19.6 to 13.3 ± 12.1 mm Hg and the diameter of the aorta increased from 5.2 ± 3 to 8.9 ± 3 mm. There were five deaths.

Because of the technical difficulties of surgically repairing recoarctation, balloon dilatation may be more advantageous than surgery for treatment of recoarctation. The relative efficacy of balloon dilatation and surgical repair of both native coarctation and recoarctation is still unclear.

SUGGESTED READING

Beekman R, Rocchini A, Behrendt T, Rosenthal A. Reoperation for coarctation of the aorta. Am J Cardiol 1981; 48:1108–1114.

Clarkson P, Nicholson M, Barratt-Boyes B, et al. Results after repair of coarctation of the aorta beyond infancy: a 10- to 28-year follow-up with particular reference to late systemic hypertension. Am J Cardiol 1983; 51:1481–1488.

Cohen M, Fuster V, Steele P, et al. Coarctation of the aorta: long-term follow-up in prediction of outcome after surgical correction. Circulation 1989; 80:840–845.

Hellenbrand W, Allen H, Golinko R, et al. Balloon angioplasty for aortic recoarctation: results of valvuloplasty and angioplasty of congenital anomalies registry. Am J Cardiol 1990; 65:793–797.

Morriss M, McNamara D. Coarctation of the aorta. In: Garson A, Bricker J, McNamara D, eds. Science and practice of pediatric cardiology. Philadelphia: Lea & Febiger, 1990:1353.

Tynan M, Finley J, Fontes V, et al. Balloon angioplasty for the treatment of native coarctation: results of valvuloplasty and angioplasty of congenital anomalies registry. Am J Cardiol 1990; 65:790–792.

ATHEROMATOUS EMBOLI

JAY D. COFFMAN, M.D.

CLINICAL PROBLEM

Patients with atheromatous emboli present with unilateral or bilateral cyanotic and painful toes. Ulcers and gangrene of the toes may occur. Patchy areas of cyanosis may also be present on the feet, usually on the soles or lateral aspects. Skin surrounding the discolored areas generally appears normal. Livedo reticularis, skin plaques, and petechiae may be seen on the lower legs and feet. There may also be calf muscle pain, or only tenderness on palpation. The dorsal pedis and posterior pulses are usually normal. Systolic bruits may be present over the femoral arteries or abdominal aorta. In some patients, this embolic syndrome may involve many organs in the body, producing renal failure, transient ischemic attacks or strokes, hemorrhagic pancreatitis, ischemia or ulceration of the gastrointestinal tract, and upper extremity lesions.

Atheromatous emboli originate from the aorta or more peripheral vessels severely involved with atherosclerosis, although aneurysms are sometimes the source. Cholesterol crystals and amorphous atherosclerotic material from the shaggy lining of the vessels embolize to the limbs or body organs. Embolization may be spontaneous or instigated by catheterization of blood vessels. Coumarin has been associated with this syndrome but is not a proved cause.

The diagnosis can be made from the typical picture of blue and painful toes, livedo reticularis, petechiae, skin plaques, tender calf muscles, and normal pulses, usually in a male over 50 years of age (Table 1). However, other causes of a blue toe syndrome must be considered (Table 2). Echocardiography will help rule out thrombi in the heart. Suitable blood studies will ascertain whether there are thrombocytosis, polycythemia, cryoglobulins, macroglobulins, or antiphospholipid antibodies. A careful history and physical examination will help diagnose Raynaud's phenomenon and the connective tissue diseases. A definitive diagnosis can often be made from a biopsy of skin or muscles. Skin biopsies cause the least trauma and should be done first; the ischemic toes must be avoided, or the biopsy site may become an ulcer. Characteristic needle-shaped clefts are seen in small arterial vessels. If the skin biopsy fails to show the pathologic picture, a muscle biopsy is indicated. Even if the biopsies fail to show the cholesterol crystals, they will help rule out other causes of a blue toe syndrome. Angiography is usually necessary to find the source of the emboli.

Table 1 Clinical Presentation of Atheromatous Emboli

Blue, painful toes or gangrene
Tender calf muscles
Petechiae
Livedo reticularis
Skin plaques
Usually normal pulses
Acute renal failure or insufficiency
Mesenteric ischemia

Table 2 Differential Diagnosis of Blue Toe Syndrome

Emboli from the heart
Primary or secondary Raynaud's phenomenon
Polycythemia or thrombocytosis
Connective tissue diseases
Polyarteritis or vasculitis
Antiphospholipid antibodies
Malignancy with or without cryoglobulins or macroglobulins

THERAPEUTIC ALTERNATIVES

The preferred treatment is surgical exclusion of the source of the emboli from the circulation. However, in many patients there are contraindications to major surgery, and heparin or antiplatelet agents may be successful.

Surgical Treatment

The most logical approach to the treatment of atheromatous emboli is to eliminate the source by surgery (Fig. 1). Most emboli originate in an atherosclerotic or aneurysmal aorta. In patients with normal cerebral, cardiac, and renal function, an aortoiliac bypass to exclude the abdominal aorta or iliac arteries is the surgery of choice and should be performed as soon as possible. A stress test for myocardial ischemia is usually necessary before such major surgery. In patients unable to undergo extensive surgery, an axillofemo-

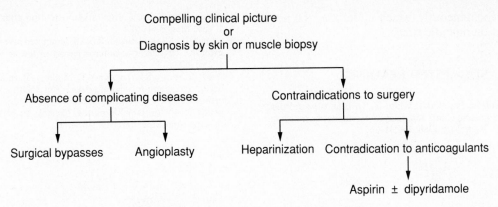

Figure 1 Treatment of atheromatous emboli.

rofemoral bypass with ligation of the iliac arteries is an option, but will not prevent atheroembolism to visceral arteries. These bypasses may last 2 to 10 years, but if they undergo thrombosis, thrombectomy can often be performed. Occasionally the grafts deteriorate or become aneurysmal at the anastomotic sites and must be replaced. When the femoral arteries are the sources of emboli, femoropopliteal bypasses can be performed. If renal emboli are occurring, transaortic endarterectomy and aortoiliac bypass is the usual approach. In patients with emboli from the thoracic aorta to many organs, the definitive therapy is replacement of the involved thoracic aorta. Reconstruction of the thoracic aorta is associated with considerably more morbidity and mortality than procedures involving the abdominal aorta, and these risks must be weighed against the high mortality associated with atheroembolic events originating from the thoracic aorta.

These surgical procedures are usually successful in preventing further embolic events. However, the postoperative course is often complicated by myocardial infarctions and strokes despite careful screening of the patients. The previously common complication of pulmonary edema with aortic surgery has been reduced by careful fluid control monitored by a Swan-Ganz catheter.

Because of the morbidity and mortality resulting from surgical approaches, transluminal angioplasty with balloon dilatation of the iliac or femoral arteries has been used with successful cessation of the embolization in a few patients. However, the iliac or femoral stenoses must be the sources of the emboli for this approach to be successful. Angioplasty has been reported to induce atheroembolism acutely, although I have not seen significant embolization caused by the procedure. Patients are treated with heparin for 24 hours after angioplasty and then aspirin, 600 mg a day.

Medical Treatment

In many patients with atheromatous emboli there are contraindications to major surgery owing to complications from atherosclerosis in other organs of the body. Renal failure, myocardial ischemic syndromes, and cerebrovascular disease are often present. My approach to these patients is the immediate institution of therapeutic anticoagulation with heparin. However, heparin cannot be used in patients with gastrointestinal ulcers or bleeding, hemorrhagic strokes, or vascular tumors. Patients must also be capable of self-administering subcutaneous heparin or be in a setting where it can be given for long-term therapy as necessary. Heparin is given intravenously with a 5,000 unit bolus and then 1,000 units per hour. In 4 hours the heparin dosage is adjusted by a partial thromboplastin time (PTT) to one and one-half to two times control level. During heparin therapy the platelet count is carefully monitored; a decreasing platelet count to below 100,000 mandates discontinuation of heparin before arterial or venous thrombosis develops. During intravenous heparin therapy the patient is carefully observed for signs of new emboli. If none occur after 5 days, subcutaneous heparin injections are instituted at a dosage (usually 8,000 to 12,000 units every 12 hours) that will maintain a therapeutic PTT. After the patient is taught to self-administer the heparin and instructed not to pinch or rub the skin with the injections, he or she can be followed on an ambulatory basis. The PTT should be monitored at least every 3 weeks. Therapy is continued for 1 year if embolization does not recur. Cholesterol emboli often cease spontaneously within this time. Heparinization has been successful in my experience in about 50 percent of patients. I have avoided warfarin therapy because of the alleged relationship to the development of atheromatous emboli and because some patients are already on the drug at presentation. However, in an occasional patient, I have used warfarin with success when other therapy was contraindicated or had failed.

If anticoagulation cannot be used, antiplatelet agents can be tried. Aspirin is used empirically at a dosage of 600 mg daily. If embolization continues, dipyridamole, 25 mg three times a day, can be added. Despite successful reports in the literature, I have not had patients respond to antiplatelet agents.

Large controlled treatment studies have not been performed for this disease. Cholesterol embolization often ceases spontaneously, which underlines the need for controlled therapeutic trials.

SUGGESTED READING

Brewer ML, Kinnison, Perler BA, White RI Jr. Blue toe syndrome: treatment with anticoagulants and delayed percutaneous transluminal angioplasty. Radiology 1988; 166:31–36.

Coffman JD. Clinical Forum: atheroembolism after cardiac surgery. J Vasc Med Biol 1989; 1:37–41.

Kaufman JL, Stark K, Brolin RE: Disseminated atheroembolism from extensive degenerative atherosclerosis of the aorta. Surgery 1987; 102:63–69.

Lee BY, Brancato RF, Thoden WR, Madden JL. Blue digit syndrome: urgent indication for digital salvage. Am J Surg 1984; 147:418–422.

Morris-Jones W, Preston FE, Greeney M, Chatterjee DK. Gangrene of the toes with palpable pulses: response to platelet suppressive therapy. Ann Surg 1981; 193:462–466.

MESENTERIC ISCHEMIA

PETER C. SPITTELL, M.D
JOHN P. COOKE, M.D., Ph.D.

Mesenteric ischemia is most commonly due to occlusive arterial disease, caused by embolism or thrombosis, usually with evidence of pre-existing atherosclerosis of the mesenteric arteries (Table 1). Despite the frequent finding of atherosclerotic narrowing of one or more of the visceral arteries, the clinical syndrome of intestinal angina is relatively uncommon owing to the development of extensive and efficient mesenteric collateral vessels. Although mesenteric ischemia is infrequently seen by most clinicians, awareness of its clinical features is important, because its frequency is likely to increase as the general population continues to age. A high index of suspicion of mesenteric ischemia, the routine use of early angiography, and prompt intervention are of paramount importance, as the morbidity and mortality rates associated with intestinal infarction are high.

ACUTE MESENTERIC ISCHEMIA

Acute mesenteric ischemia most commonly results from either embolic occlusion of one or more visceral arteries, or from nonocclusive mesenteric vascular dis-

Table 1 General Classification of Causes of Mesenteric Ischemia

Occlusive arterial disease
  Major artery stenosis or occlusion
    Chronic
    Acute
  Mesenteric arterial compression
  Small artery disease
  Angiographic procedures
  Surgical procedures
  Medication
Nonocclusive arterial disease
  "Low-output" states

ease seen in conditions associated with a markedly diminished cardiac output. Thrombotic occlusion of one or more mesenteric arteries in the setting of occlusive or aneurysmal visceral arterial disease is a less common cause of acute mesenteric ischemia. Prompt diagnosis of acute mesenteric ischemia and early intervention is important, because mortality rates associated with intestinal infarction and gangrene are high.

Mesenteric Artery Embolism

Embolic occlusion of the superior mesenteric artery is the most common cause of acute mesenteric ischemia. Most patients with visceral arterial emboli are middle aged or older and have associated cardiovascular disease (Table 2). An embolic event to the extremities or cerebrum often precedes a mesenteric embolus, and up to 20 percent of patients have simultaneous embolization to other arteries at the time acute mesenteric ischemia develops. Angiography also predisposes to mesenteric artery embolization, especially in patients with a severely atheromatous aorta.

Symptoms of mesenteric artery embolism are variable, but most patients present with sudden onset of severe abdominal pain, vomiting, and a change in bowel habits, in association with few findings on abdominal examination. In an elderly person with underlying cardiovascular disease, the acute onset of abdominal pain warrants consideration of acute mesenteric ischemia. Early diagnosis with angiography is essential, because mortality is high when the diagnosis of acute mesenteric ischemia is delayed to the point where intestinal infarction has occurred.

Initial treatment of patients with suspected mesenteric artery embolism includes aggressive fluid resuscitation and correction of predisposing or precipitating factors. Prompt correction of hypotension, hypovolemia, congestive heart failure, and cardiac

Table 2 Clinical Features of Visceral Artery Embolism

Middle-aged or older person
Cardiovascular disease (± recent angiography)
Acute abdominal process
Vomiting and change in bowel habits
Few signs on abdominal examination

arrhythmias is required before and during subsequent diagnostic studies.

Early in the course of acute mesenteric ischemia, many clinical laboratory abnormalities may be seen. Leukocytosis occurs in 75 percent of patients, and elevations of hemoglobin and hematocrit often occur owing to fluid shifts within the intestinal wall and resultant hemoconcentration. Metabolic acidosis with elevation of the serum lactate level is present in 50 percent of patients; elevation of serum inorganic phosphate is also commonly seen. With prolonged ischemia and subsequent intestinal infarction, elevations of the serum glutamic oxaloacetic transaminase (SGOT), serum glutamic pyruvic transaminase (SGPT), serum lactic dehydrogenase (LDH), serum creatine kinase (CK), and serum amylase occur. Although these laboratory abnormalities are relatively nonspecific, their presence in a middle-aged or older person with acute abdominal pain and cardiovascular disease should suggest the diagnosis of acute mesenteric ischemia.

Plain x-ray films of the abdomen, although not diagnostic of acute mesenteric ischemia, can help to exclude other abdominal conditions. With acute mesenteric ischemia, progressive dilatation of large and small bowel loops, loss of haustral marking, "formless loops," intramural air, or air in the portal venous system may be seen. Duplex ultrasound scanning of the mesenteric arteries has recently provided a means for rapid and noninvasive assessment of persons with acute mesenteric ischemia due to visceral artery embolism. Unfortunately, results may be negative in proximal embolism, and the presence of air can give misleading results, making it difficult to rule out more distal embolization.

Angiography remains the best modality for a definitive diagnosis of acute mesenteric ischemia due to mesenteric artery embolism. It can identify the sites of emboli and also provide invaluable information when revascularization is indicated. It also provides access to the superior mesenteric artery for intra-arterial infusion of the vasodilator papaverine. An initial view in the left posterior oblique plane is first obtained to eliminate the possibility of ostial embolization, to exclude other causes of acute mesenteric ischemia, and to determine the extent and location of the emboli. A "meniscus sign" is often seen several centimeters from the origin of the involved mesenteric artery. Major emboli are those that occlude the superior mesenteric artery proximal to the orgin of the iliocolic artery, whereas minor emboli are limited to branches of the superior mesenteric artery or to the superior mesenteric artery distal to the orgin of the iliocolic artery.

After angiographic confirmation of acute mesenteric ischemia due to mesenteric artery embolization, the catheter is secured in the orifice of the involved artery, and a continuous infusion of papaverine (30 to 60 mg per hour) is given to alleviate associated vasospasm. Systemic arterial pressure, heart rate, and cardiac rhythm must be monitored, as papaverine can cause peripheral vasodilation, increased myocardial oxygen demand, and cardiac arrhythmias. The duration of time papaverine is infused depends on the clinical and angiographic response in each patient.

Medical therapy may be considered in patients with minor emboli distal to the fourth jejunal artery and good perfusion of the vascular bed distal to the embolus, when clinical findings are not life-threatening. Aggressive fluid and hemodynamic management and intra-arterial papaverine infusion, combined with systemic anticoagulant therapy to prevent extensive thrombosis, are the mainstays of therapy. The selective intra-arterial infusion of thrombolytic agents has been used with success when started within 10 hours after the onset of ischemia, but the risk of intestinal hemorrhage with these agents is unpredictable. Thrombolysis may provide an effective alternative to surgery in some critically ill patients, but the routine use of thrombolysis in mesenteric artery embolism requires further study.

Early laparotomy with embolectomy and revascularization is indicated in most patients with mesenteric artery embolism. The goals of surgical therapy are to restore intestinal arterial flow and to resect any irreparably damaged bowel. Revascularization should precede any evaluation of intestinal viability, because bowel that appears infarcted initially may show significant recovery after restoration of blood flow. Early in the course of mesenteric artery embolism, a simple embolectomy without the need for intestinal resection may suffice. After embolectomy, if pulsations in the distal mesenteric arcade are diminished, intraoperative assessment of intestinal blood flow can be done using laser Doppler flowmetry. Doppler studies can provide substantial information on tissue viability and help determine the need for revascularization. Intravenous injection of fluorescein (10 to 15 mg per kilogram), followed by examination of the bowel with ultraviolet light, is also helpful in determining bowel viability. When intestinal infarction is found, wide intestinal resection is needed so that intestinal anastomosis can be performed in healthy tissues. With distal mesenteric artery embolism, short segmental intestinal ischemia, and a patent superior mesenteric artery, isolated resection of the infarcted intestinal segments without associated embolectomy can often be performed. With current surgical techniques and methods to determine bowel viability, routine "second-look" operations are generally not indicated unless dictated by the intra- or postoperative course.

Papaverine infusion is generally continued for 12 to 24 hours postoperatively, at which time angiography is performed. If signs of mesenteric vasospasm are absent, the infusion is discontinued and the catheter removed. If mesenteric vasospasm is still evident, the papaverine infusion is continued until angiographic signs of mesenteric vasospasm have resolved.

Aggressive perioperative management of fluid balance and maintenance of optimal cardiac indices are essential to a successful outcome. Both systemic and topical antibiotics help to treat associated sepsis and improve the viability of compromised bowel. Antibiotics effective against enteric organisms, such as a second- or third-generation cephalosporin and an aminoglycoside, are generally used. Persistent sepsis in the postoperative setting should prompt further evaluation to exclude pyogenic liver abscess, which is known to occur after revascularization for acute mesenteric ischemia. Postoperative anticoagulation is recommended for patients with acute mesenteric ischemia without intestinal infarction. When intestinal infarction has occurred, anticoagulants should be delayed for 48 to 72 hours postoperatively until bowel function has resumed and signs of bleeding are absent.

Although mesenteric artery embolism is the most treatable of conditions causing acute mesenteric ischemia, the current postoperative morbity and mortality rates remain high. This emphasizes the need for early diagnosis and intervention aimed at preventing intestinal infarction and its devastating consequences.

Mesenteric Artery Thrombosis

Mesenteric artery thrombosis is a less common cause of acute mesenteric ischemia and is usually seen in patients with severe, diffuse atherosclerosis and a history of coronary, cerebral, or peripheral arterial disease. A history of intestinal angina is often present. Typically, patients present with periumbilical, colicky abdominal pain in association with few findings on abdominal examination. Unrecognized, mesenteric artery thrombosis can progress to intestinal infarction and gangrene with associated hemorrhage, volume depletion, and eventual sepsis and cardiovascular collapse. Awareness of the clinical features of mesenteric artery thrombosis is important to allow for early diagnosis and intervention. Unfortunately, many patients come to medical attention hours after the onset of symptoms, when intestinal infarction has already occurred.

Laboratory findings in mesenteric artery thrombosis are similar to those previously described for acute mesenteric ischemia due to mesenteric artery embolism, and are nonspecific. X-ray films of the abdomen soon after mesenteric artery thrombosis may reveal air-fluid levels and bowel distention. Barium examination of the small intestine reveals nonspecific dilatation, poor motility, and evidence of thick mucosal folds ("thumbprinting").

Emergent angiography is indicated when mesenteric artery thrombosis is suspected, in order to establish the diagnosis and to help plan the surgical intervention. Angiography most commonly shows evidence of chronic arterial occlusive disease involving one or more of the mesenteric arteries in their proximal portions, with associated thrombosis of variable degrees (Fig. 1).

Medical therapy with thrombolysis, when used early in the course of mesenteric artery thrombosis, may help to improve mesenteric perfusion in some patients, but the overall efficacy of thrombolytic therapy and the risks of bleeding complications require further study. Surgery remains the treatment of choice for mesenteric artery thrombosis. As with acute mesenteric ischemia due to mesenteric artery embolization, thrombectomy and re-

vascularization precede assessment of bowel viability. If areas of compromised bowel or intestinal infarction are present after revascularization, resection is then performed.

The postoperative management of patients with mesenteric artery thrombosis is similar to that described for persons with mesenteric artery embolism. Associated cardiac and cerebrovascular disease continue to contribute to the increased postoperative morbidity and mortality. Postoperative anticoagulation is also routinely used to maintain graft patency and prevent reocclusion.

Nonocclusive Mesenteric Ischemia

Nonocclusive mesenteric ischemia is a common cause of acute mesenteric ischemia in conditions associated with a reduced cardiac output. It results from splanchnic vasoconstriction and decreased splanchnic perfusion in response to the so-called low-flow states often complicated by pre-existing atherosclerotic lesions of the mesenteric vessels. Conditions that predispose to this condition include myocardial infarction, congestive heart failure, aortic regurgitation, renal and hepatic disease, and major abdominal or cardiac operations. Other contributory factors include hypovolemia, hypotension, shock states, diabetic ketoacidosis, vasopressor agents, digitalis, and nitroglycerin therapy. A recent decline in nonocclusive mesenteric ischemia has been attributed to the increased use of vasodilator therapy in the management of ischemic heart disease, as well as more aggressive management of cardiogenic shock with left ventricular assist devices that prevent prolonged periods of hypotension after myocardial infarction.

The clinical features of nonocclusive mesenteric ischemia are similar to those seen with other causes of

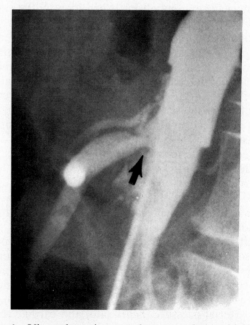

Figure 1 Visceral angiogram demonstrating a high-grade atheromatous stenosis in the origin of the celiac axis (arrow).

acute mesenteric ischemia, except that a history of intestinal angina is often lacking and abdominal pain at the time of evaluation is absent in up to 25 percent of patients. In fact, abdominal distention and gastrointestinal bleeding may be the only clues to the diagnosis of nonocclusive mesenteric ischemia in the critically ill patient.

Angiography is virtually diagnostic in nonocclusive mesenteric ischemia, revealing patency of the major mesenteric arteries, and vasospastic changes of more peripheral intestinal arteries. In addition, angiography helps exclude other causes of acute mesenteric ischemia.

Treatment of nonocclusive mesenteric ischemia consists of vasodilator therapy and correction of the cause of the low-flow state. Selective intra-arterial infusion of papaverine is useful to decrease vasoconstriction of the distal mesenteric vessels. Aggressive correction of fluid and electrolyte imbalance, optimization of cardiac indices with vasodilator and inotropic support, and close observation are crucial in order to improve the chance of survival and prevent intestinal infarction. If intestinal infarction occurs, surgical intervention is the treatment of choice unless the risks are prohibitive. The risks involved in surgical revascularization are generally increased in patients with nonocclusive mesenteric ischemia owing to their advanced age, associated dehydration, sepsis, and other serious medical conditions. The surgical risks need to be evaluated in the individual patients.

Ischemic Colitis

Ischemic colitis, spontaneous or iatrogenic, most commonly affects middle-aged or elderly persons. Spontaneous ischemic colitis is often due to low colonic blood flow in association with diseases causing diminished cardiac output. Iatrogenic ischemic colitis most commonly follows ligation of the inferior mesenteric artery during abdominal aortic surgery for aneurysmal or occlusive atherosclerotic disease. Iatrogenic ischemic colitis can generally be avoided by documentation of colonic viability at the time of initial surgery.

The clinical features of ischemic colitis depend on the degree of ischemia and the rate of its development. Most patients present with subacute ischemic colitis characterized by mild abdominal pain and bloody diarrhea occurring over several days or weeks. Barium enema examination reveals edema, cobblestoning, thumbprinting, and occasionally superficial ulceration. Angiography is not generally recommended unless the ischemia involves the right colon, because this is thought to predict hemodynamically significant superior mesenteric artery disease.

The therapy for subacute ischemic colitis is medical and includes optimization of cardiac indices and treatment of predisposing and precipitating factors. Most cases of subacute ischemic colitis resolve with conservative therapy in 2 to 4 weeks. Occasionally, surgical treatment for obstruction secondary to postischemic stricture formation may be necessary.

Acute fulminant ischemic colitis is a less common and more serious form of ischemic colitis. Patients present with severe lower abdominal pain, rectal bleeding, and hypotension. Peritoneal signs may be present in severe cases. Plain abdominal films may reveal thumbprinting, but barium enema examination should be avoided in the acute setting because of the increased risk of perforation. Sigmoidoscopy or

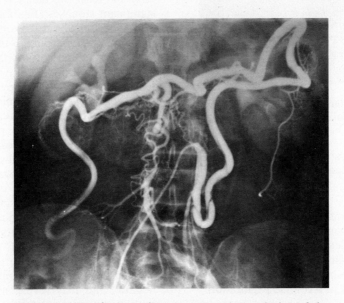

Figure 2 Visceral angiogram demonstrating occlusion of the superior mesenteric artery (SMA) and marked enlargement of the inferior mesenteric artery, the latter giving rise to a gigantic collateral vessel (the arc of Rilon), which supplies branches to the distal SMA.

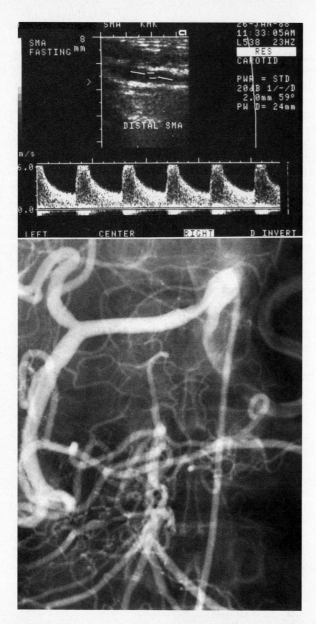

Figure 3 Doppler and color flow Doppler ultrasound examination demonstrating an occlusion of the proximal superior mesenteric artery (SMA) with patency of the distal SMA *(A)*. A visceral angiogram of the same patient demonstrated occlusion of the proximal SMA, with collateral circulation to the distal SMA via the gastroduodenal artery and its pancreatic branches *(B)*.

colonoscopy can show ulceration, friability, and bulging folds due to submucosal hemorrhage. Angiography is usually performed, but a lesion amenable to surgical therapy is rarely found. Surgical resection is reserved for patients with persistent symptoms, for removal of gangrenous bowel, or for repair of a colonic perforation.

CHRONIC MESENTERIC ISCHEMIA

Chronic mesenteric ischemia, usually caused by atherosclerosis, is relatively uncommon, but its fre-

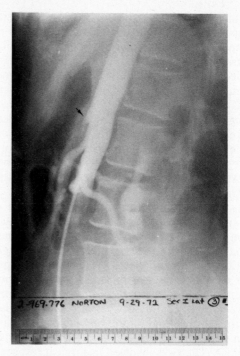

Figure 4 Visceral angiogram showing a high-grade (almost complete) stenosis *(arrow)* of the celiac axis and a moderate stenosis at the origin of the superior mesenteric artery.

quency is likely to increase as the general population continues to age. Despite frequent atherosclerotic narrowing of the proximal portions of one or more visceral arteries, symptoms of intestinal angina are rare. The rich potential for the development of extensive mesenteric collaterals decreases the likelihood of intestinal angina, unless at least two major vessels have hemodynamically significant stenoses (Fig. 2).

The clinical expression of mesenteric ischemia is intestinal angina, which is usually present for months to years in up to one-half of the patients who later die from intestinal infarction. The predominant symptom of intestinal angina is crampy epigastric or periumbilical pain, beginning 15 to 30 minutes after eating. The pain may last several hours after meals, and over time may progress in severity and occur sooner after smaller meals. Significant weight loss occurs owing to a decrease in food intake and malabsorption; in the absence of significant weight loss, mesenteric ischemia is unlikely in the differential diagnosis of abdominal pain. Physical examination frequently discloses one or more abdominal bruits that support (but do not confirm) the diagnosis of intestinal angina. Patients should be evaluated for coronary, cerebrovascular, and peripheral arterial occlusive disease, which is present in up to one-third.

Evaluation with gastrointestinal x-ray films is usually negative but may reveal signs of decreased intestinal motility, thumbprinting, or flocculation and segmentation of barium in the small intestine. More recently, duplex ultrasonography has permitted the rapid, noninvasive diagnosis of chronic mesenteric ischemia. By imaging the abdominal aorta and origins of the major

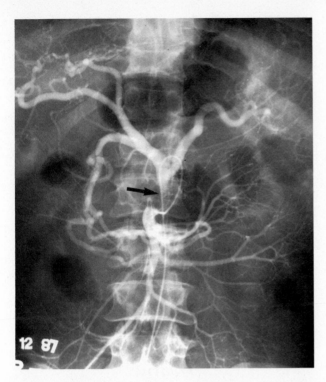

Figure 5 Visceral angiogram in a patient with the median arcuate ligament syndrome. Note the occlusion at the origin of the celiac artery *(arrow),* with collateral filling of the celiac artery branches by a large pancreaticoduodenal arcade.

visceral arteries, disturbances in mesenteric artery flow velocities can be detected. Abnormalities in the spectral display, including an increase in peak systolic velocity at the origin of the visceral artery and abnormalities on color flow imaging, are particularly useful (Fig. 3). The sensitivity of Duplex ultrasonography is increased by giving a provocative high-calorie meal (240 ml of Ensure Plus) followed by repeat assessment of superior mesenteric artery flow. The finding of increased turbulence, or a failure of superior mesenteric artery flow to increase, signifies a significant stenosis. Future potentially useful techniques for noninvasive assessment of mesenteric perfusion include reflectance spectrophotometry and tonometric measurement of mucosal pH.

Visceral angiography remains the gold standard for establishing a definitive diagnosis of chronic mesenteric ischemia. Standard biplane aortography with selective mesenteric artery views is usually performed. The anteroposterior views demonstrate the origin of the inferior mesenteric artery; the lateral views most clearly reveal the origins of the celiac and superior mesenteric arteries. Marked stenosis or occlusion of the superior mesenteric artery is characteristically seen, usually together with occlusive disease of the proximal portion of at least one of the other two mesenteric arteries (Fig. 4). If the proximal portions of the visceral arteries are normal, selective visceral artery injections may reveal more distal small artery disease.

Treatment of chronic mesenteric ischemia is most

commonly surgical, but medical therapy has been successful in some patients. Percutaneous transluminal balloon angioplasty (PTA) has been used to dilate discrete, proximal stenoses with good initial results, and it may be useful as an alternative to surgery, especially in patients with other serious medical conditions. Long-term results of PTA require further study. Continuous enteral nutrition and pentoxifylline (Trental), 400 mg orally three times a day, have been reported to alleviate symptoms of intestinal angina in some patients, but their usefulness is limited.

Surgical intervention remains the most definitive treatment for chronic mesenteric ischemia. Indications for surgery depend on the severity of symptoms and the arteriographic findings in the individual patient. Transaortic endarterectomy and antegrade aortomesenteric grafting are the current techniques most commonly used, with good initial and long-term results. Recurrent postoperative symptoms can be reduced by revascularization of as many stenotic or occluded arteries as possible at the initial surgery. Recurrence of intestinal angina has been reported to be as low as 10 percent with this approach.

CELIAC ARTERY COMPRESSION SYNDROME

The celiac artery compression syndrome, first described in 1963, remains a controversial cause of chronic mesenteric ischemia for numerous reasons. Extrinsic compression of the celiac artery by the median arcuate ligament, or less commonly the celiac ganglion, or both, occurs in 12 to 49 percent of asymptomatic persons. Also, the symptoms of the celiac artery compression syndrome are usually atypical of small bowel ischemia, and there is a poor correlation between the severity of symptoms and the degree of celiac artery compression. The presence of significant celiac artery compression in a patient with atypical or vague abdominal symptoms warrants a thorough evaluation for other causes of abdominal pain before surgical therapy to relieve the celiac artery compression is considered.

Most patients with celiac artery compression are young, although persons of any age can be affected. Typically, there is epigastric abdominal discomfort that is chronic and refractory to treatment. An epigastric bruit is often heard and may be the only clue to the diagnosis.

Duplex ultrasonography of the visceral arteries often confirms compression and stenosis of the celiac artery. It provides important information about the collateral circulation and can help to identify patients who may require angiography. Visceral angiography is usually diagnostic, as shown in Figure 5.

In patients with postprandial abdominal pain and significant weight loss in whom a thorough examination reveals only celiac artery compression, surgery is probably indicated. At laparotomy, extensive abdominal exploration is performed to exclude other possible causes of abdominal pain. If exploration is negative, surgical excision of the median arcuate ligament can be performed. After excision, intraoperative measurement of the pressure gradient between the aorta and celiac artery may help to identify patients who require an additional revascularization procedure. This should also help to decrease recurrent symptoms due to residual celiac artery stenosis, which often occurs after excision of the median arcuate ligament alone.

SUGGESTED READING

Batellier J, Kieny R. Superior mesenteric artery embolism: eighty-two cases. Ann Vasc Surg 1990; 4:112–116.

Hallet JW, James ME, Ahlquist DA, et al. Recent trends in the diagnosis and management of chronic intestinal ischemia. Ann Vasc Surg 1990; 4:126–132.
Stanton PE Jr, Hollier PA, Seidel TW, et al. Chronic intestinal ischemia: diagnosis and therapy. J Vasc Surg 1986; 4:338–344.
Watson WC, Sadikali F. Celiac axis compression: experience with 20 patients and a critical appraisal of the syndrome. Ann Intern Med 1977; 86:278–284.
Wilson C, Gupta R, Gilmour DG, Imire CW. Acute superior mesenteric ischaemia. Br J Surg 1987; 74:279–281.

PUDENDAL INSUFFICIENCY AND IMPOTENCE

YASUSHI F. SHIBUTANI, M.D.
VICTOR L. CARPINIELLO, M.D.

Since 1940, when Leriche described a syndrome involving symptoms of ischemia of the lower extremities accompanied by erectile impotence, sexual dysfunction in the male with occlusive disease of the aortoiliac segment has been widely recognized. However, little attention was centered specifically on surgical correction of vasculogenic impotence until the 1950s. Advances in the comprehension of the mechanism, physiology, and pharmacology of erection have provided new strategies for the clinician managing the patient with impotence.

ETIOLOGY

Impotence may have psychogenic, hormonal, neurologic, or vasculogenic causes. Insufficiency of the arterial blood supply during sexual stimulation, resulting in erectile dysfunction, is usually caused by arteriosclerosis of the vessels leading to the erectile tissue. Indeed, impotence may be the first and only sign of this form of vascular disease. Other causes of vascular impotence are arterial dysplasias, sequelae of reconstructive surgery of the abdominal aorta, venous insufficiency, and arterial occlusions after pelvic trauma. Recently, attention has been drawn toward occlusive disease involving the internal pudendal artery and its penile tributaries. A phenomenon called the femoral artery steal syndrome has been described in which collateral flow to the ischemic extremity derived from the hypogastric artery impedes erectile ability. The choice of treatment for vasculogenic impotence depends on the cause of the disturbance and the overall condition of the patient.

ANATOMY

The penis is composed of two corpora cavernosa and a single ventral corpus spongiosum. The paired corpora cavernosa communicate in the penile shaft. The arterial supply of the penis originates in the paired internal pudendal arteries, branches of the right and left internal iliac or hypogastric arteries. The internal pudendal artery becoming the penile artery branches to supply the penis in three terminal vessels: (1) dorsal artery, (2) cavernous (deep or central) artery, and (3) bulbourethral artery. The venous drainage of the penis is formed through the interconnection of three systems: (1) superficial (superficial dorsal vein), (2) intermediate (deep dorsal and circumflex veins), and (3) deep (cavernous and crural veins). Many anastomotic channels connect these three venous systems.

ERECTILE PHYSIOLOGY

A complex interaction of vascular, neurologic, hormonal, and psychological components is required in the normal physiology that constitutes penile erectile function. Briefly, baseline constriction of arterioles and sinusoids results in a high-pressure, low-flow vascular environment reflected in the flaccid state. Induction of the erectile response results in relaxation of the smooth muscle in the cavernous arterioles and sinusoids. Increased arterial inflow and sinusoidal dilatation results in mechanical compression of emissary veins. This veno-occlusive mechanism traps and maintains blood within the corpora cavernosa, resulting in tumescence and rigidity of the penis. Disruption of any point in this cascade of events may result in erectile dysfunction.

CLINICAL EVALUATION

In searching for a cause and site of vasculogenic impotence, a thorough history is the first and most important step. When screening these patients for impotence, it is imperative to note whether they can obtain and sustain an erection for satisfactory intercourse, and if not, whether the impairment is constant or episodic. Classically, organic dysfunction is recognized by the gradual onset of an inability to achieve firm erections in the setting of an otherwise satisfactory relationship. Failure to diagnose organic impotence can be devastating to both partners and can quickly lead to psychological sequelae. Therefore, the clinician should be alert for the risk factors of arteriosclerotic disease that may play a role in impotence, such as smoking, hypertension, hyperlipidemia, and diabetes. A review of the patient's medications often reveals offending agents. True dysfunction often begins with the complaint of an increase in the time needed to initiate and obtain a full erection. Morning and spontaneous erections become weaker and less frequent. The patient often complains of an inability to maintain an erection over a prolonged period, producing flaccidity before ejaculation. Progressively, erections weaken and finally disappear. This is usually a slow process spanning several years. As already stated, vascular erectile dysfunction may be the presenting sign of severe vascular disease.

Vasculogenic impotence and pudendal insufficiency may be investigated with numerous noninvasive diagnostic tests. Suitable candidates may require more sophisticated and invasive diagnostic imaging to elucidate specific defects before surgical reconstruction of the arterial or venous system.

Penile Brachial Index

By measuring the pressures found in the cavernosal artery compared with the brachial systolic blood pressure, one can determine the penile-brachial index (PBI). Generally, PBI values between 0.85 and 1.0 are considered normal. If the ratio falls below 0.6, the diagnosis of vascular insufficiency may be suspected. Disadvantages of this test include the inability to measure the cavernosal artery flow consistently, interference from background Doppler signals of other vessels, and inconclusive interpretations over a wide range of PBI. Also, the test does not provide information regarding the hemodynamics of the erect state.

Penile Plethysmography

Penile plethysmography is a noninvasive test used to assess penile blood flow. By means of a pneumatic cuff with a transducer around the base of the penile shaft, arterial waveforms are measured. Unfortunately, this test is nonspecific and cannot isolate a specific lesion. It has largely been replaced by duplex ultrasonography with Doppler analysis.

Intracavernous Injection

Intracavernous injection of vasoactive agents such as papaverine or prostaglandin E_1 (PGE_1) is increasingly being used in the diagnostic evaluation of vasculogenic erectile impotence. When the agent is injected into the corpora cavernosa of a patient with normal erectile ability, the response is usually one of erection and rigidity for approximately 30 minutes. Pharmacologic erection is used to discriminate between organic disease and psychogenic impotence. Critics of this diagnostic evaluation point to the lack of standardized drug dosing, variation between repeat examinations, and the test's susceptibility to uncontrollable factors such as environment and patient anxiety. However, in concert with radiologic imaging, these vasoactive agents have provided a valuable means of studying the erectile tissue in a more physiologic state.

Nocturnal Penile Tumescence

Nocturnal penile tumescence (NPT) monitoring helps differentiate psychogenic from organic impotence. Patients with organic impotence have disturbances in erections during the rapid-eye-movement (REM) phase of sleep; normal patients or those with psychogenic impotence have three to five erections per night. This overnight sleep study measures changes in penile circumference but does not necessarily record rigidity. Other methods to detect nocturnal erections include the stamp test, the Snap Gauge, and the Rigiscan device.

Duplex Ultrasonography with Doppler Analysis

In 1985 Lue and colleagues introduced the use of a high-resolution ultrasound probe and pulsed Doppler analysis to evaluate vasculogenic impotence. High-resolution duplex ultrasound scanners and Doppler analysis, in conjunction with vasoactive compounds such as papaverine or PGE_1, are a highly effective means of obtaining anatomic and physiologic data about the penile vascular system. Intracorporeal injection of vasoactive agents with ultrasound imaging provides the clinician with qualitative and quantitative information on cavernous artery diameter and dilatation, blood velocity (centimeters per second), flow volume (milliliters per second), and peak systolic velocity (centimeters per second). Currently, a normal response to intracavernous vasoactive drug injection is an increase in luminal diameter of the cavernous artery by approximately 75 percent above the preinjection dimension, with a change in peak flow velocity of greater than 25 cm per second. The recent addition of color Doppler sonography will make vessel detection and Doppler angle correction easier and more accurate. This noninvasive diagnostic tool has rapidly established its place in the evaluation of vasculogenic impotence. Duplex ultrasonography with Doppler analysis and dynamic infusion cavernosometry are the current tests of choice in the evaluation of cavernous artery insufficiency.

Arteriography

The tremendous progress in noninvasive diagnostic imaging has not outmoded the use of invasive vascular procedures in the ultimate evaluation of arterial anatomy. Arteriography, in combination with selective pudendal pharmacoarteriography and dynamic cavernosometry-cavernosography, provides anatomic and physiologic detail crucial to the surgical approach to vasculogenic impotence. The limitations of arteriography are its inability to discern whether an obstructive lesion is functionally significant and whether stenosis is not in fact vasospasm. Our relative inexperience with the accepted norms for potent men in this age group make interpretation of this subset of patients more difficult. Penile angiography is performed in an outpatient setting under local anesthesia with intravenous sedation in most centers.

Cavernosometry-Cavernosography

Evaluation of the penile venous system is made by using the techniques of dynamic infusion pharmaco-cavernosometry-cavernosography developed by Goldstein. In patients suspected of venous impotence, it is the definitive study to demonstrate insufficiency of the corpora cavernosa. A full erection and the physiologic vascular changes accompanying it are induced through intracavernous injection of saline and supplemental administration of intracavernosal vasoactive agents. The intracavernosal pressures and flow rates required to sustain the erect state vary with the competence of the veno-occlusive mechanism. A low venous outflow resistance, subnormal clinical response to papaverine, and high maintenance flow rates (>10 ml per minute) are suggestive of venous insufficiency. Physiologic evidence of venous leakage provided by pharmacocavernosometry is a valuable adjunct to the anatomic map of venous insufficiency seen on pharmacocavernosography. Further standardization and experience with these techniques will enable surgeons to improve their efforts in venoablative surgery.

MEDICAL THERAPY

The introduction of penile intracavernous injection of vasoactive agents has revolutionized the diagnosis and treatment of erectile dysfunction. The induction of erection by papaverine was reported by Virag in 1982. Papaverine hydrochloride, alone or in combination with phentolamine mesylate and PGE_1, is the agent most commonly used. In clinical settings, common dosage ranges are 30 to 60 mg of papaverine, 0.5 to 1.0 mg of phentolamine, and 1 to 30 μg of PGE_1. The addition of manual genital stimulation or a vacuum constriction device has been found to improve response to dosage.

Patients with organic, nonhormonal, or psychogenic impotence are candidates for therapy. Patients with sickle cell disease, and those unable to tolerate the possible hemodynamic side effects of intracavernosal injection secondary to cerebrovascular or cardiovascular disease, are not suitable candidates. A clear understanding by the patient and physician of the risks, benefits, and potential complications is crucial if this therapy is chosen. A tuberculin or insulin syringe with a 30-gauge needle is used to inject the drug(s) into the lateral aspect of one corpus cavernosum. Responses must be carefully dose titrated and monitored in the office before self-injection at home. Follow-up examination is important to monitor for possible complications.

The complications of intracavernous injection therapy are rarely systemic and mostly localized to the penis. Priapism, hematoma, corporeal fibrosis, urethral injection, local induration, and paresthesia are local complications noted. Priapism remains one of the most serious complications and can be avoided by careful dose titration and patient selection. Should priapism result, detumescence may be achieved by careful irrigation and injection of diluted alpha-adrenergic agents into the corpora cavernosa. Continued application and experience with vasoactive intracavernous pharmacotherapy will be necessary to determine its long-term efficacy and morbidity.

ARTERIOGENIC IMPOTENCE

Vascular impotence is the most common cause of organic erectile dysfunction. Pioneering work by Michal and associates in the early 1970s showed that it was possible to re-establish penile arterial supply surgically and thus restore erectile potential. Exact diagnosis through careful arteriogenic study and selection of patients is critical to success. Duplex ultrasonography, in combination with vasoactive agents such as papaverine or PGE_1 and dynamic cavernosometry-cavernosography, enables the surgeon to better isolate the vascular defect involved. Less sensitive diagnostic modalities, lack of recognition of the venous contribution to erectile dysfunction, and limited study design and follow-up make interpretation of the early revascularization literature difficult.

This early procedure referred to as Michal I involved direct anastomosis of the inferior epigastric artery to the corpus cavernosum. A short-term erectile success was reported in nearly 60 to 70 percent, but follow-up revealed a significant incidence of postoperative priapism and subsequent arterial thrombosis. The Michal II is an end-to-side anastomosis of the inferior epigastric artery to the dorsal penile artery. This operation depends on good runoff into the smaller penile arteries and is therefore not suitable in patients with distal arteriosclerotic disease. Patients with isolated internal pudendal or common penile artery occlusion are revascularized via the retrograde flow from the dorsal penile artery to the cavernous arteries. Most arteriosclerotic patients would not be good candidates for this approach to revascularization, however; Goldstein reported success in approximately 74 percent of young men with impotence secondary to pelvic and perineal trauma.

A direct microsurgical approach to the cavernous artery using direct anastomosis of the inferior epigastric artery to the cavernous arteries was reported by Konnak and Ohl. The procedure is technically difficult because of the size discrepancy between anastomotic vessels and the small luminal diameter of the cavernous artery, approximately 0.5 to 1.0 mm. Patient selection is again difficult.

Some patients with vasculogenic impotence are affected by both arterial and venous insufficiency. The Virag procedures attempt to address this combined defect in one operation by shunting blood into the corporeal body via arterialization of the deep dorsal vein. The most common variations include Virag 2 and Virag 5. In Virag 2, the inferior epigastric artery is anastomosed end to side to the deep dorsal vein, tying the vein both proximally and distally. Virag 5 is similar to the Virag 2 operation except that it incorporates a shunt between the dorsal vein and cavernous body. Conceptually, venous arterialization reduces the component of venous leakage by impeding drainage via the deep dorsal vein. At arterial pressures the venous valves are no longer competent and therefore do not impede flow. The corpora cavernosa are supplied by additional arterial supply via the retrograde flow through dorsal and emissary veins. Analysis of the clinical success of these procedures remains uncertain.

Advantages of the surgical approach include the ability to bypass proximal vessel disease with a physiologic approach to erectile dysfunction. Disadvantages include the technical difficulty, the poorly documented long-term success, and the lack of clear-cut patient selection criteria. The current short-term success rate of these procedures is between 40 and 90 percent. Complications include postoperative priapism, hyperemia of the glans penis, postoperative venous leakage, and penile edema. Nevertheless, as diagnostic methods, patient selection, and understanding of surgical failure improve, it is hoped that revascularization operations may become more reliable.

VENOUS INSUFFICIENCY

Normal erectile function depends on sufficient arterial inflow and a competent veno-occlusive mechanism. Improved understanding of the hemodynamic changes of erectile physiology, and diagnostic tests directed at venous insufficiency such as dynamic pharmacocavernosometry and pharmacocavernosography, have heightened our awareness of this entity. Isolated venogenic impotence is probably less common than initially thought; however, in combination with arteriogenic disease, as a mixed phenomenon, it accounts for a large portion of the population with a vasculogenic basis for impotence.

A surgical approach to the problem of venogenic impotence was unknowingly identified by Wooten in 1902 when he described ligation of the dorsal penile vein for impotence, with an approximately 50 percent cure rate. Since the turn of the century, imaging modalities such as pharmacocavernosography have enabled surgeons to improve patient selection for venogenic surgery. Suitable candidates have undergone intracavernous injection testing and analysis of arterial insufficiency by duplex ultrasonography with pulsed Doppler analysis. Pharmacocavernosometry-cavernosography with papaverine-type agents may demonstrate venous leakage in a "physiologic" manner. Venous leakage is not always restricted to the deep dorsal vein, and therefore surgical technique varies from mere ligation of the deep dorsal vein to more extensive ligation and excision of all abnormal penile veins (dorsal, cavernous, and crural). Infrapubic horizontal and oblique, vertical scrotal, and circumferential circumcision incisions are used. Once the abnormal draining veins are identified and ligated or excised, artificial erection and intraoperative corporeal pressure measurements are used as a means to assess the adequacy of venoablative interventions. Success rates reported by various investigators vary between 40 and 75 percent. Penile edema is common and resolved within 2 weeks postoperatively. Other complications include scrotal bruising, penile numbness, and scar contracture with shortening of the penis. Hematomas are rare.

The improved means for detecting venous leak as a single entity or in combination with arteriogenic impotence enable surgeons to select the most suitable patients for appropriate surgery. Treatment failure may arise from residual abnormal venous drainage, subsequent collateralization, or a primary cavernous sinusoidal smooth muscle myopathy. Further investigation into the pathogenesis of veno-occlusive dysfunction will yield new strategies to identify and treat this subset of patients.

SURGICAL TREATMENT

Prosthesis

Implantation of a prosthetic device into the penis is a viable and popular surgical alternative for vasculogenic impotence. The inflatable penile prosthesis has been in use for more than two decades and is associated with low morbidity, satisfactory cosmetic results, reliable function, and high patient satisfaction. Rigid and semirigid devices are also used with comparable results but are cosmetically less appealing. Improvements in technique and mechanical reliability have reduced the incidence of infection and device malfunction requiring reoperation.

REMARKS

Clinicians and patients dealing with vasculogenic impotence are faced with a vast array of diagnostic and management strategies. Improved understanding of erectile mechanism, physiology, and pharmacology have enhanced our ability to study the penile vascular system in great anatomic and physiologic detail. Intracavernous penile injection as a diagnostic and therapeutic modality has renewed interest in nonprosthetic approaches to vasculogenic impotence. Strides in elucidating the basic defects of arteriogenic and venogenic impotence will continue to have a positive effect on the medical and surgical management of pudendal insufficiency and impotence.

SUGGESTED READING

Benson G, Boileau M. The penis: sexual function and dysfunction. In: Gillenwater J, Grayhack J, Howard S, Duckett J, eds. Adult and pediatric urology. Chicago: Year Book, 1987:1407.

Bookstein JJ. Angiography of the genitourinary tract: techniques and applications. In: Pollack HM, ed. Clinical urography. Philadelphia: WB Saunders, 1990:477.

Goldstein I. Penile revascularization. Urol Clin North Am 1987; 14:805–813.

Impotence. Urol Clin North Am 1988; 15:000–000.

Lue T, et al. Vasculogenic impotence evaluated by high resolution ultrasound and pulsed Doppler spectrum analysis. Radiology 1985; 155:777–781.

Lue TF. Penile venous surgery. Urol Clin North Am 1989; 16.

Lue T, Takamura T, Schmidt R, et al. Hemodynamics of erection in the monkey. J Urol 1983; 130:1237.

Lue T, Tanagho E. Physiology of erection and pharmacologic management of impotence. J Urol 1987; 137:829–836.

PERIPHERAL ARTERIAL DISEASE

ARTERIAL DISEASE: NONINVASIVE ASSESSMENT

THOM W. ROOKE, M.D.

ROLE OF THE NONINVASIVE VASCULAR LABORATORY

Patients with arterial disease may require noninvasive studies of the arterial system for a variety of reasons, including those listed below.

To Confirm the Diagnosis of Occlusive Disease. Usually the history and physical examination provide sufficient information to confirm the diagnosis of arterial occlusive disease, but occasionally they may be so atypical that the diagnosis is left in question. When this occurs, the noninvasive vascular laboratory can be used to establish the diagnosis.

To Assess Severity. Often the issue is not whether arterial disease exists, but how severe it is. The noninvasive vascular laboratory provides a means for accurately quantifying the extent and severity of disease.

To Provide Documentation. In this age of increasing pressure from government agencies and third-party payers to justify invasive evaluations or therapies, the noninvasive vascular laboratory provides accurate, cost-effective documentation of arterial disease.

To Follow Disease Progression and Assess Response to Therapy. Because noninvasive studies may be performed serially, they can be used to follow the progression of disease in patients over time, or to assess the benefits produced by specific therapies such as revascularization and exercise.

CLASSIFICATION OF NONINVASIVE TESTS

Noninvasive tests can generally be divided according to the type of information they provide about arterial disease.

Anatomic

These tests are used to identify and localize stenotic or occluded regions of the artery; in some cases they can also be used to estimate disease severity on the basis of the morphologic findings. Examples of anatomic studies include arteriography (invasive, but still the gold standard) and two-dimensional real-time ultrasonic imaging. Increasing usefulness is also being reported for traditional radiologic tests such as computed tomography (CT) and magnetic resonance imaging (MRI), but these tests are not usually considered to be within the realm of the noninvasive vascular laboratory. Tests that are primarily hemodynamic, such as segmental pressures and continuous wave Doppler analysis, also yield some data about the location of diseased arterial segments and therefore provide information that is at least partly anatomic.

Hemodynamic

These tests give information about the hemodynamic significance of particular lesions. A good example of this kind of testing is the continuous wave Doppler examination (especially when used in conjunction with two-dimensional ultrasonic imaging, i.e., duplex scanning). With duplex scanning the Doppler shift across a specific stenotic lesion can be measured, and from this the hemodynamic significance of the lesion can be estimated.

Functional

Sometimes, information provided by anatomic and hemodynamic testing is insufficient to explain the patient's symptoms or impairment. In this situation a functional test may be necessary. Functional tests are those that evaluate the impact of arterial disease on the limb. For example, treadmill testing can be used to assess walking distances and claudication thresholds. The value of this type of information can be appreciated by considering a hypothetical situation in which two patients present with similar degrees of obstruction in the major lower extremity arteries (based on assessments made with anatomic and/or hemodynamic studies). However, one patient is well conditioned and has well-developed collateral arteries, while the other is poorly conditioned and has poorly developed collaterals. Functional testing will identify and quantify the differences between these two patients and enable the clinician to make appropriate choices of therapy.

Arterial disease may affect any artery in the body. For purposes of illustration, I will confine the discussion of testing to the evaluation of lower extremity and carotid disease.

LOWER EXTREMITY ARTERIAL ASSESSMENT

The algorithm in Figure 1 outlines the usual steps taken to evaluate patients referred to the Mayo Clinic Noninvasive Vascular Laboratory with known or suspected lower extremity arterial disease. In most situations, the initial studies are performed at rest and include continuous wave Doppler assessment, segmental pressures, and pulse volume recordings.

Continuous Wave Doppler

The hand-held continuous wave Doppler (Fig. 2) is used to study the arterial flow signal at multiple levels along the limb. Signals are normally bi- or triphasic (consisting of a rapid forward flow component during systole and flow reversal during diastole). However, at sites of evaluation distal to a hemodynamically significant arterial stenosis, the flow signal becomes monophasic. This monophasic signal typically shows reduced (and delayed) forward flow during systole, and sustained forward flow during diastole (i.e., the normal diastolic flow reversal is lost). This component of the resting examination identifies and localizes arterial segments with occlusive disease; unfortunately, it is relatively insensitive as a method of quantifying disease severity.

Segmental Pressures

Segmental pressures are obtained by placing inflatable blood pressure cuffs at multiple levels around the leg (usually the thigh, calf, and ankle) and then sequentially inflating and deflating each to determine the arterial blood pressure at the different levels (Fig. 3). The pressure at which flow resumes during cuff deflation is determined by Doppler analysis at a site distal to the cuff. Segmental pressures are typically divided by a reference pressure (usually the brachial artery pressure), thus creating an "index"; e.g., the ankle-brachial index (ABI).

Segmental pressure analysis is a simple, inexpensive, reproducible, and accurate method of determining (1) whether arterial obstruction is present, (2) how severe it is, and (3) in which segment the obstruction is located. When necessary, arterial obstructions that are too minor to produce pressure drops at rest can be made apparent by exercising the patient. This form of testing has the added advantage of providing quantitative information about the walking distance. The major drawback of segmental pressure measurement is encountered in the patient with noncompressible blood vessels. This condition is most common in diabetics and usually reflects calcium deposition in the arteries. If the arteries cannot be occluded by externally applied cuff pressure, the true arterial pressure cannot be measured accurately.

Pulse Volume Recording (PVR)

The PVR provides an index of limb arterial pulsatility. It is obtained by encircling the limb at a given level

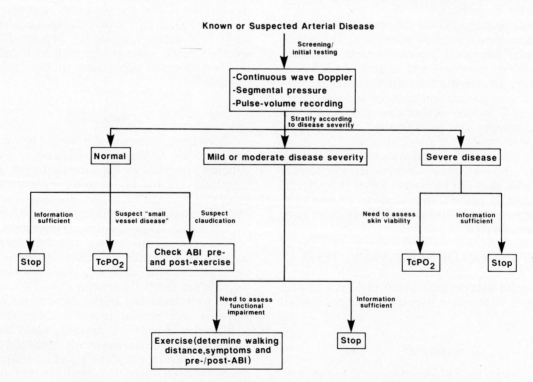

Figure 1 Noninvasive assessment of lower extremity arterial occlusive disease.

with a pneumatic pressure cuff, which is inflated (typically with a relatively low pressure such as 40 to 70 mm Hg) and connected to a pressure transducer. During systole, blood is ejected from the heart and enters the limb, causing the limb to become slightly larger. The increase in limb volume compresses air within the cuff, thus changing the cuff pressure; this allows "pulsatile" changes to be assessed. Although PVR provides quick information about the location and severity of arterial occlusive disease, there are two major drawbacks to its use: (1) the reproducibility is poor and (2) flow that is nonpulsatile (such as that which has been dampened by passage through small collateral vessels) cannot be assessed.

Transcutaneous Oximetry

Transcutaneous oxygen (TcPO$_2$) measurement represents a significant new advance in the assessment of

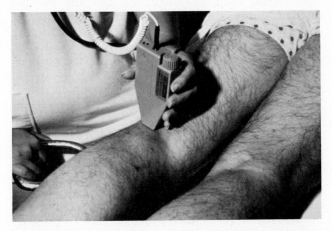

Figure 2 Hand-held continuous wave Doppler. With this device, the arterial waveform can be evaluated at multiple sites and the level of arterial blockage can be determined.

cutaneous blood flow, particularly when arterial insufficiency is present. Transcutaneous oximetry uses oxygen-sensing Clark-type electrodes attached to the skin at the desired sites by means of adhesive rings. These rings form an airtight seal with the skin, and thus the oxygen entering the electrode is limited to that which diffuses from the skin itself. In order to ensure that skin blood flow is not limited by cutaneous vasoconstriction, the surface of the electrode is warmed with the heating element to 45° C; this has been shown to produce a maximal vasodilation in the underlying cutaneous vasculature. Under these conditions, skin blood flow is determined by the patency of the proximal arteries.

Oxygen diffusion from the skin depends on a number of factors, including arterial PO$_2$, skin blood flow, and cutaneous oxygen consumption. When the skin blood flow and oxygen delivery are high (relative to the oxygen consumption by the skin), the TcPO$_2$ approaches arterial PO$_2$; in contrast, during low-flow states the TcPO$_2$ is reduced. TcPO$_2$ measurement is therefore an index of skin blood flow. More important, the oxygen that reaches the electrode reflects the ratio between oxygen delivery and consumption, and thus TcPO$_2$ is an excellent indicator of the adequacy of skin blood flow.

Transcutaneous oximetry has proved most useful in the following settings:

1. *Evaluation of severe ischemia.* Although it is often easy to diagnose arterial occlusive disease on clinical grounds or with basic noninvasive testing, it may be more difficult to assess its functional impact on the limb. This is especially true in patients with severe arterial occlusive disease. For example, one patient with an ABI of 0.4 may have adequate distal skin perfusion because of a well-developed collateral circulation, while another patient with an identical 0.4 ABI and poorly developed collaterals may have severe ischemia.

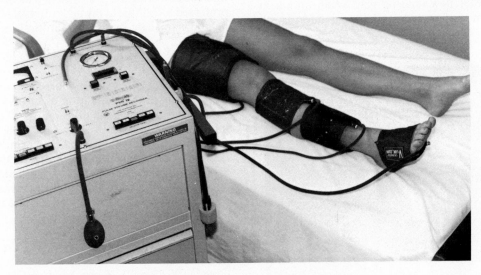

Figure 3 Segmental pressure measurement. By inflating and deflating the various pressure cuffs, the arterial pressure can be measured at multiple levels.

A functional assessment of the adequacy of skin blood flow provides information to help the clinician decide whether revascularization is indicated.

2. *Determination of amputation level.* By defining the adequacy of skin blood flow, the $TcPO_2$ can be used to determine whether an amputation will heal at a given site (Fig. 4). Typically, values greater than 40 mm Hg heal, whereas those less than 20 mm Hg do not; values between these form a "gray zone."

3. *Assessment of the microcirculation.* Some diseases affect the small, distal vessels while leaving the larger vessels relatively intact. When this occurs, the continuous wave Doppler, segmental pressures, and pulse volume recordings may be normal despite the fact that small vessel occlusion has made the limb ischemic.

4. *Patients with diabetes.* Diabetic limbs have two characteristics that often make transcutaneous oxygen assessment useful:
   a. The larger vessels may be noncompressible, rendering segmental pressures impossible to measure or interpret.
   b. There is frequently an associated small vessel abnormality in the skin of the limb.

Duplex Scanning

Real-time two-dimensional ultrasonic imaging combined with continuous or pulse-wave Doppler is referred to as duplex scanning. This technique provides both anatomic and hemodynamic information about vascular stenosis or occlusion; for example, specific lesions can be identified and localized by the two-dimensional imaging component, and the hemodynamic severity of specific lesions can be evaluated by using the Doppler to determine the change in blood flow velocity across the lesion(s). In cases of arterial occlusion, no flow signal will be detected. Color flow imaging may be an option in some equipment and provides additional information that can improve examination quality or reduce examination time.

Widespread application of duplex scanning to assess peripheral vascular disease has been limited by several factors: (1) adequate images cannot always be obtained in patients who are obese or have other abnormalities of body habitus, (2) the studies are time-consuming and relatively expensive, and (3) pelvic and infrapopliteal vessels are often poorly seen. These and other factors have kept duplex scanning from replacing arteriography in many situations. Improvements in technique and additional experience may lead to more widespread applicability in the future.

CEREBROVASCULAR ASSESSMENT

Oculoplethysmography (OPG)

OPG is a noninvasive test for assessing cerebral arterial perfusion. Several techniques for its performance have been advocated; we currently use the method described by Gee. With this method, pressure is applied to the globe of the eye and transmitted to the retinal vessels, causing ocular blood flow to cease. The pressure at which this occurs is noted, and comparisons are made between the left and right eyes as well as between the eyes and the brachial pressure. A decreased ocular pressure suggests the presence of arterial occlusive disease in the carotid system.

The OPG provides valuable information about the hemodynamic status of the intra- and extracranial circulation. Some authors dismiss it as an insensitive screening study because patients with high-grade carotid occlusive disease may have normal OPG examination results. However, it can be argued that the significance of these lesions (even when a total occlusion is present) is questionable if the OPG is normal, since collateral flow must be very good. OPG is therefore a tool that is more useful for determining the significance of disease than for detecting the presence of disease. It remains the preferred technique at my institution of screening for the hemodynamically significant carotid lesion.

Carotid Duplex Scan

Arterial duplex scanning currently enjoys its greatest applicability in the evaluation of carotid disease. Many studies have verified its ability to provide outstanding information about the presence, location, and severity of carotid occlusive lesions. In some centers, surgery has been performed on the basis of carotid duplex scanning alone, although in my practice (and most others) angiography is required before surgery in order to assess the proximal brachiocephalic vessels and the intracranial circulation.

SUGGESTED READING

Cossman DV, Ellison JE, Wagner WH, et al. Comparison of contrast arteriography to arterial mapping with color-flow duplex imaging in the lower extremities. J Vasc Surg 1989; 10:522–529.

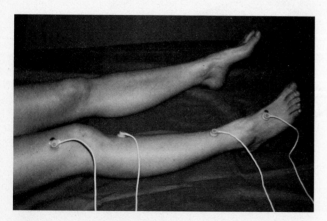

Figure 4 Transcutaneous oximetry. $TcPO_2$ can be measured at multiple limb sites to determine the amputation level.

Creager MA. Intermittent claudication. In: Decision making in cardiovascular disease. New York: HP Publishing, 1990.

Lewis BD, James EM. Current applications of duplex and color ultrasound imaging: abdomen. Mayo Clin Proc 1989; 64:1158–1169.

Lewis BD, James EM, Welch TJ. Current applications of duplex and color Doppler ultrasound imaging: carotid and peripheral vascular system. Mayo Clin Proc 1989; 64: 1147–1157.

Rooke TW, Osmundson PJ. The influence of age, sex, smoking, and diabetes on lower limb transcutaneous oxygen tension in patients with arterial occlusive disease. Arch Intern Med 1990; 150:129–132.

Strandness DE Jr. Duplex scanning in vascular disorders. New York: Raven Press, 1990.

CHRONIC ARTERIAL OCCLUSIVE DISEASE: MEDICAL MANAGEMENT

JOHN P. COOKE, M.D., Ph.D.

Arterial occlusive disease of the lower extremities is manifested by intermittent claudication, rest pain, or ischemic ulceration. The most common etiology is atherosclerosis. This is a common problem in the Western hemisphere, with a prevalence of approximately 2 percent in all individuals 40 to 60 years of age, increasing to 6 percent in those over age 70. In these age groups, intermittent claudication is more common than diabetes mellitus.

In over 75 percent of patients the disease does not progress and does not require invasive intervention. Medical therapy, including modification of risk factors and treatment of associated conditions, is the mainstay of therapy and is all that is necessary in most patients. This is not to say, however, that intermittent claudication is a benign disease. It is associated with a doubling of the age-specific risk of death, usually due to significant coronary artery or cerebrovascular disease. A recent study even suggests that intermittent claudication is an additional risk factor for coronary artery disease, independent of the accepted risk factors of hypercholesterolemia, diabetes mellitus, tobacco use, and hypertension. Unfortunately, only a minority of these patients receive medical care for their condition. The vascular internist therefore plays a critical role in the preoperative evaluation, management, and postoperative care of these patients. He or she must diligently modify associated risk factors, maintain vigilance for evidence of significant arterial disease in other circulations, evaluate the severity of the disorder, and decide whether further invasive studies or interventions are needed.

EVALUATION

Chronic arterial occlusive disease of the lower extremities, in its mildest symptomatic form, is manifested by intermittent claudication. Patients describe cramping or fatigue of the leg with walking. Occasionally this pain is limited to cramping in the foot (as with isolated infrapopliteal arterial disease). Most often, however, symptoms involve the calf (with stenosis of the superficial femoral artery) and may even involve the thigh and buttocks (as with iliofemoral arterial disease). In any patient, the pain is reproducible after walking a certain distance; symptoms are exacerbated by walking uphill, by carrying additional weight, or by increasing the pace. The pain of claudication abates when the patient simply stands still. This is in contrast to the leg pain induced by spinal stenosis, also known as pseudoclaudication. The aching discomfort of pseudoclaudication mimics that of intermittent claudication, but relief can be obtained only by sitting down or leaning against a support. In addition, these patients often have low back pain or a history of back trauma and may have some manifestations of neurologic damage (paresthesias or a broad-based gait).

As the disease progresses, the patient becomes increasingly limited. It is important to gauge the effects of the disease on life style, because this will affect the choice of therapeutic options. A 60-year-old mailman may feel significantly limited by three-block claudication, whereas an 80-year-old retiree may feel unencumbered by claudication occurring at 100 yards. One would be more inclined to pursue angiography and intervention in the former case than the latter. The indication for more aggressive intervention becomes clear when the patient presents with rest pain or an ischemic ulcer. Generally, these patients undergo angiography and revascularization if possible. Rest pain may be described as a severe ache (similar in quality to a toothache) or numbness, which may be associated with intermittent episodes of lancinating pain and is often worse at night. These patients obtain some relief by placing the legs in a dependent position.

It is important to determine whether there are symptoms reflecting arterial disease in other circulations, i.e., coronary or carotid. One should also determine the presence of risk factors predisposing to these conditions, such as tobacco use, hyperlipidemia, hypertension, diabetes mellitus, and family history. Approximately 75 percent of these patients use tobacco; those that do not generally have disorders of lipid or carbohydrate metabolism. In patients without obvious risk factors for atherosclerosis, less common causes of chronic arterial occlusive disease should be considered:

vasculitides, disorders of coagulation, homocystinemia, popliteal entrapment, and less well characterized lipid disorders, such as elevated levels of Lp(a) lipoprotein.

Physical Examination

The physical examination includes an evaluation for disease in other arterial circulations, as well as associated conditions predisposing to atherosclerosis. Blood pressure should be taken in both arms to detect evidence of subclavian stenosis; a pressure difference of more than 20 mm confirms the diagnosis. When asked, a minority of these patients describe claudication of the upper extremity with use. Most patients are asymptomatic, but subclavian stenosis is a worrisome finding because of its frequent association with significant carotid artery disease. Elevated blood pressure not only is a risk factor for progression of atherosclerosis, but also may signify renovascular stenosis. An irregular pulse may provide a clue to the origin of a peripheral arterial embolism; most of these cases occur in elderly patients with atrial fibrillation.

"Cigarette-paper facies" (fine diffuse wrinkling of the facial skin) and tobacco staining of the teeth and fingers are common stigmata in this patient population, most of whom are smokers. Xanthelasmas and xanthomas are specific, but not sensitive, indicators of hypercholesterolemia. Examination of the fundus may reveal "copper-wiring" and arteriovenous nicking characteristic of patients with diffuse atherosclerosis, or may reveal the retinopathy of diabetes or hypertension. The carotid arteries are always auscultated before palpation, to avoid compromising a high-grade stenosis. A clue to the latter condition is a bruit extending into diastole; this finding indicates a hemodynamically significant lesion (75 percent or greater luminal obstruction).

An increased anteroposterior diameter of the chest and reduced breath sounds denote chronic obstructive pulmonary disease, which is not uncommon in this group and may warrant further evaluation with spirometry for patients in whom vascular surgery is considered. Another common auscultatory finding in these patients is a fourth heart sound, reflecting diastolic dysfunction, usually due to long-standing hypertension. A third heart sound denotes more significant ventricular dysfunction, as with an ischemic cardiomyopathy. The abdomen is always auscultated for the presence of bruits that may signify aortoiliac, mesenteric, or renal artery occlusive disease. The astute examiner will carefully palpate the abdomen for the presence of an aortic aneurysm. Most often these are palpated in retrospect after their incidental detection on a radiologic study for another condition, but a careful examination should reveal these earlier. Occasionally, patients' obesity may preclude palpation of the aortic aneurysm; in these individuals, especially if they are at increased risk for aneurysm (if they are hypertensive or hyperlipidemic or have a family history of aortic aneurysms), computed tomographic (CT) or ultrasonic examination of the abdomen should be performed.

Careful palpation of the peripheral pulses often establishes the level of significant disease. A reduced femoral pulse (often with a bruit) denotes aortoiliac occlusive disease. A popliteal pulse cannot be obtained in patients with superficial femoral arterial occlusion. One should carefully palpate the popliteal region so as not to miss the opportunity of detecting a popliteal aneurysm; these aneurysms have a tendency to thrombose, often with drastic sequelae. Furthermore, 50 percent of these patients also have an abdominal aortic aneurysm. Absence of the dorsalis pedis pulse may be seen as an anatomic variant in about 5 percent of normal individuals. This condition is almost always bilateral. By contrast, absence of the posterior tibial pulses is always an indication of a pathologic process. An occasional patient has no pulses in the lower extremities but admits to only mild claudication. These patients almost always have an aortic occlusion and have developed a rich supply of collaterals circumventing the obstruction. Also, an occasional patient may complain of intermittent claudication but has a normal arterial examination at rest. These patients should be asked to walk to the point of claudication and then be re-examined; many of these will now demonstrate a reduction in ankle pulses (or pressures); they have an isolated iliac artery stenosis and are often good candidates for balloon angioplasty.

The hand-held Doppler probe is a very useful tool in the office. The probe is placed over the artery to be examined, and the quality of the signal is evaluated. In normal young individuals the signal will be strong and clearly biphasic (and in some cases triphasic); with progression of atherosclerosis the signal becomes less biphasic and eventually monophasic. With severe arterial occlusive disease the signal is faint and monophasic, or absent entirely. To further quantitate the severity of arterial occlusive disease, one may obtain an ankle-brachial index (ABI) test. This is done by obtaining a simultaneous ankle and brachial systolic blood pressure, and expressing this as a ratio. One simply places the blood pressure cuff above the ankle, positions the Doppler probe over the dorsalis pedis or posterior tibial artery, and inflates the cuff to suprasystolic pressures. Upon deflation of the cuff, the pressure at which the signal returns is the ankle pressure. The ABI is useful in quantitating the severity of the obstruction, as well as in following patients in the long term (Table 1). However, in a subset of patients the ABI is not helpful owing to arterial calcification. Elderly patients, and those with diabetes, often have substantial calcification of the infrapopliteal vessels. These vessels are resistant to compression by the blood pressure cuff, and the systolic pressures obtained are artifactually elevated. In these patients there is a discordance between ankle pressures and other clinical clues regarding tissue perfusion (i.e., elevation pallor, dependent rubor, and nutritive changes secondary to ischemia).

Elevation pallor is detected by raising the extremity to an angle of 30 degrees and observing the digits. Pallor occurring within 60 seconds denotes mild ischemia; within 30 seconds, moderate ischemia; and within 15

Table 1 Ankle-Brachial Index (ABI) for Determination of the Severity of Arterial Occlusive Disease

ABI Value (Patient Resting)	Severity of Stenoses
1–1.1	Normal
0.85	Mild
0.70	Moderate
0.50	Severe

The ABI is the systolic pressure measured at the ankle divided by the systolic pressure measured in the arm.

seconds, severe ischemia. If pallor is noted at rest, the extremity is in jeopardy. Subsequently, the lower extremities are placed in a dependent position, the venous filling time determined, and the patient observed for dependent rubor. Normally the superficial veins of the foot fill within 15 to 20 seconds with dependency. A filling time of 20 to 30 seconds denotes mild ischemia; 30 to 45 seconds, moderate ischemia; and over 45 seconds, severe ischemia. Dependent rubor is also noted in patients with significant arterial occlusive disease. Additional evidence of reduced tissue perfusion may be obtained by observing the capillary refill time. A digit is pinched lightly so that it blanches: in a normal individual the color will return almost immediately upon release of the digit; conversely, with significant arterial occlusive disease (or vasospasm) the return of normal color (capillary refill) is sluggish.

Nutritive changes are also seen in patients with significant long-standing ischemia. The subcutaneous tissues atrophy, lending a shiny appearance to the skin. Hair loss is evident. With severe ischemia, cutaneous ulcerations form, invariably at sites of pressure (the heel, malleoli), and at sites of contact between the digits ("kissing" ulcers). The ischemic ulcer may be differentiated from others because of its location, because it is covered with a thick black eschar, and because the periphery of the ulceration is painful to touch. Generally the ulcer is round and well circumscribed; if the eschar is removed, the base of the ulcer is noted to be pale and will bleed less than expected.

One may also detect evidence of a recent atheroembolic event that has precipitated or exacerbated the patient's symptoms. A cyanotic toe or livedo reticularis of the foot, calf, thigh, or buttocks is a clue to significant proximal occlusive or aneurysmal disease (the source of the atheroembolism). If these findings are bilateral, the patient has an aortic aneurysm, or a severely atherosclerotic, ulcerated ("shaggy") aorta, which is the source of the atheroembolism. If the findings are unilateral, the patient most likely has an ipsilateral ulcerated iliac artery plaque, or a popliteal aneurysm, serving as the nidus of thromboembolism. Evidence of atheroembolism is an indication for angiography and surgical intervention, since these patients may be at risk of recurrent embolic events leading to renal failure, mesenteric insufficiency, or peripheral arterial occlusion.

Moreover, they may be at risk for rupture of an aortic aneurysm or thrombosis of a popliteal aneurysm.

Laboratory Studies

The seasoned clinician recognizes arterial occlusive disease of the extremities, and laboratory studies are not necessary for a diagnosis of intermittent claudication, rest pain, or ischemic ulceration. However, noninvasive vascular laboratory studies are helpful in quantitating the severity and progression of the disorder. These tests are also useful in patients in whom spinal stenosis is responsible for a component of their symptoms. In such patients, CT of the spine and electromyography help determine the extent to which spinal stenosis is contributing to their disability.

Noninvasive vascular laboratory studies routinely used include segmental pressure measurements, pulse volume recordings, and ABIs at rest and after exercise. Segmental pressure measurements are performed by placing blood pressure cuffs at the thigh, above the knee, below the knee, and above the ankle; these allow for detection of systolic pressure gradients at the iliofemoral, superficial femoral, popliteal, and infrapopliteal levels, respectively. A pressure decrement of 15 percent from one level to the next denotes a hemodynamically significant lesion between those levels. These measurements at rest are supplemented by measurements of ankle systolic pressure before and after exercise. Treadmill exercise using a modified Bruce protocol is practical for many patients. This test should include continuous monitoring of a 12-lead electrocardiographic (ECG) record during exercise to detect evidence of exercise-induced myocardial ischemia. Exercise is discontinued at the point of significant claudication, and supine ankle and brachial systolic blood pressures are taken for calculation of a postexercise ABI. Blood pressure measurements and ECG records are taken every 3 minutes until these values have returned to baseline. Severe claudication is characterized by a marked drop in the ABI, occurring at a low level of exertion and persisting well into the rest period.

Pulse-volume recordings are obtained simultaneously. With significant arterial occlusive disease, the amplitude of the pulse volume is reduced and its contour altered from a biphasic wave form, with a clearly evident dicrotic notch, to a monophasic wave form.

As mentioned, the systolic pressure measurements and ABI readings may be artifactually elevated owing to arterial calcification in the elderly and in diabetics. By contrast, in these patients the pulse-volume recordings are markedly abnormal. However, this is only a qualitative observation. To further quantitate tissue perfusion, some laboratories use transcutaneous oximetry (see the preceding chapter) or laser Doppler spectroscopy. The latter is a semiquantitative technique in which a probe affixed to the skin delivers a low-energy infrared laser light to illuminate the underlying cutaneous microcirculation (with a hemispheric sampling volume of approximately 1 mm). The laser light is reflected back to the probe with a Doppler shift in its frequency, which is related to the average velocity of the red cells coursing through the microvasculature. The intensity of the reflected signal is inversely proportional to the volume of red cells in the microvasculature, because the laser light is absorbed by the heme moiety of the red cells. Therefore, an estimate of the red cell volume and velocity can be obtained, allowing for a semiquantitative estimation of microvascular flow. The advantage of this technique is that it exclusively reflects cutaneous blood flow, with a short time constant. A disadvantage is that the sampling volume is small and the measurements are only semiquantitative.

Color flow Doppler ultrasonography is increasingly used in the noninvasive vascular laboratory. This technique allows for direct visualization of the major conduit vessels and an estimation of the flow through them. It is particularly good in the postoperative assessment and long-term follow-up of saphenous vein bypass grafts in the lower extremity. Here it is useful in detecting technical problems (retained valve leaflets, arteriovenous anastomoses, misplaced sutures, and thrombus). Detection of these abnormalities can allow for early correction, and therefore prevention, of graft thrombosis. Disadvantages of the technique include its dependence on the skill of the operator and the time required to perform a careful examination.

MANAGEMENT

General Measures

Ischemia limits wound healing and the response to infection. These patients must therefore be advised to protect the ischemic extremity from trauma. Approximately 75 percent of amputations in this patient population result from a nonhealing wound due to preventable trauma (poorly fitting shoes, inadvertent injury during clipping of the nails, puncture wound incurred while ambulating). Ambling about in bare feet is a luxury these patients can ill afford. Emollients applied twice daily after a bath or shower maintain the skin in a supple and hydrated condition to prevent drying and fissuring, which can create a portal of entry for bacteria. For the same reason, fungal infections should be aggressively treated. Lamb's wool placed between adjacent toes prevents pressure necrosis and "kissing" ulcers.

Reducing the load that the exercising leg muscles must bear can increase walking distance. The symptoms of claudication can be markedly improved in obese patients by weight loss. Modifications in the workplace may allow patients to adjust to their limitations; for example, the heavy tool belt of a maintenance worker may be replaced by a push cart.

The most potent conservative measure in the treatment of claudication is an exercise program. Most patients can double their walking distance within 3 months with a daily exercise routine. If they understand that surgery and angioplasty are not curative and are only meant to extend the walking distance, they may choose a more conservative approach, knowing that a significant improvement in walking distance can be expected. Exercise in the treatment of intermittent claudication is described in detail in the chapter *Chronic Arterial Occlusive Disease: Exercise Rehabilitation.*

Risk Factor Modification

The use of tobacco is the most prevalent risk factor, with 80 to 90 percent of claudicants acknowledging a history of smoking. The continued use of tobacco is also a predictor of a poor long-term result. In a study from the Mayo Clinic, claudicants who abstained from tobacco did not incur any tissue loss over a 5-year period; of those who continued to smoke, approximately 10 percent underwent amputation for ischemic gangrene over the same period. Saphenous vein bypass grafts (in the coronary or peripheral circulations) are more likely to fail if the patient continues to smoke. When claudication is due to thromboangitis obliterans, approximately 50 percent of the patients who continue to smoke will suffer tissue loss, whereas only 5 percent of those who desist will incur this complication. A simple admonition from the physician will be sufficient stimulus for a minority of patients. A recent study revealed that a written contract between the physician and the patient, stating that the patient will discontinue the use of tobacco before the next office visit, significantly increases the number of patients who abstain. These simple counseling techniques, combined with the use of nicotine, produce long-term success in 30 percent of patients.

There is increasing evidence that aggressive reduction of serum cholesterol can reduce the progression, and even induce regression, of atherosclerotic plaque. In an angiographic study, Blankenhorn and colleagues demonstrated that this approach was successful in inducing regression of atherosclerotic disease in the superficial femoral artery (see the chapter *Hyperlipidemia in Patients with Vascular Disease*). A number of studies have confirmed this work and have extended it to the coronary circulation. Hypertension is also a risk factor for atherosclerotic arterial occlusive disease. Treatment of severe hypertension limits its vascular complications (stroke, myocardial infarction). No studies have yet been performed to determine whether treatment of hypertension reduces the progression of peripheral arterial occlusive disease. Hypertension in the patient with claudication should alert the physician to the possibility of renovascular stenosis (see the chapter *Renovascular Hypertension*). Therefore, if such a patient requires angiographic evaluation of the peripheral vessels, consideration should be given to aortography and possibly selective renal arteriography during the same procedure. Diabetes mellitus is another risk factor for atherosclerotic arterial occlusive disease. Patients with diabetes are more likely to have distal (infrapopliteal) disease that is difficult to correct surgically or with catheter techniques. In these patients there is also a higher incidence of amputation (approximately four times that in nondiabetics). It is not known if aggressive control of diabetes mellitus will reduce the progression of disease in the peripheral vasculature.

Antiplatelet Treatment

Antiplatelet treatment reduces the thrombotic complications associated with many vascular disorders. It reduces acute closure of saphenous vein bypass grafts and substantially decreases the incidence of acute thrombosis after coronary angioplasty. It has similar beneficial effects in patients with unstable angina and in those with an acute myocardial infarction. It therefore is not unreasonable to extrapolate this clinical experience to the peripheral vasculature. The same processes that induce unstable angina or an acute myocardial infarction (plaque rupture followed by luminal thrombosis) can exacerbate claudication, precipitate rest pain, or produce an acute occlusion jeopardizing the viability of the limb. The minimal dose of aspirin required to have a significant beneficial effect on these processes is not known, but one baby aspirin daily is probably sufficient.

Eicosapentanoic acid and docahexanoic acid are omega$_3$ unsaturated fatty acids with antiplatelet activity. Marine lipids are rich in these fatty acids. It is likely for this reason that populations consuming large amounts of marine lipids (e.g., Greenland Eskimos) manifest alterations in platelet activity (i.e., increased bleeding time). These populations have a reduced prevalence of cardiovascular disease. Experimentally, fish oil reduces the progression of atherosclerosis in animal models and improves endothelial function. These observations have led to the use of fish oils, and/or their omega$_3$ fatty acid constituents, in the treatment of various vascular diseases. However, the beneficial effects of fish oil appear to be only modest in humans. In addition, large amounts of omega$_3$ fatty acids (approximately 10 g) are required to equal the effect of one aspirin; these large doses are often associated with gastrointestinal side effects. Nevertheless, on the basis of the experimental and epidemiologic data, it seems rational to advise patients to increase the amount of fish in their diet.

Hemorrheologic Therapy

Pentoxiflyline is often used to treat claudicants. This is a hemorrheologic agent that is purported to increase red cell deformability and thereby reduce blood viscosity. Since blood flow is inversely proportional to blood viscosity, a reduction in blood viscosity theoretically should increase flow. In a major double-blind, placebo-controlled study, pentoxiphylline increased the duration of treadmill exercise time by 40 percent. In my experience, pentoxiphylline has minimal or no benefit in most patients; a minority of patients claim significant relief.

Vasodilator Therapy

The use of vasodilators in intermittent claudication has been disappointing. Many clinical trials have been carried out using a variety of vasodilators without any beneficial effect. This lack of effect extends to all classes of vasodilators, including alpha-adrenergic antagonists, beta-adrenergic agonists, calcium entry antagonists, serotonergic antagonists, angiotensin converting enzyme inhibitors, and so-called direct-acting vasodilators such as hydralazine. Recent evidence suggests that prostacyclin or more stable analogs may be of benefit in patients with severe arterial occlusive disease secondary to thromboangiitis obliterans; whether this therapy will have any utility for other claudicants is not known. It is not yet approved for this use in the United States. Potentially, vasodilators that act specifically on the collateral circulation would be of benefit in these patients; such an agent is not yet available.

Medical Treatment of Ischemic Ulcers

Rest pain or an ischemic ulceration is absolute indication for angiography. Occasionally, the angiogram reveals that the disease is not correctable surgically or with catheter techniques. These patients are more likely to be elderly and diabetic. Patients with vasculitis, or those with thromboangiitis obliterans, often have noncorrectable distal disease. Most often these patients require an amputation, but about 30 percent of ischemic ulcers may heal with conservative medical therapy. The same therapeutic measures mentioned previously apply, with a few changes and additions. First, ambulation should be limited, since this reduces perfusion to an area of severe arterial insufficiency. If the ulcer is infected, oral antibiotics are insufficient, and intravenous administration must be used to achieve therapeutic levels locally. Wet-to-dry soaks are used to debride the thick black eschar from these ischemic ulcerations. The foot should be kept protected in a bulky, warm dressing or in a thermal boot (a Rooke boot). Patients should be cautioned not to apply a warming pad to the extremity; because of the markedly reduced blood flow, local thermoregulation is grossly impaired, and the skin is vulnerable to a burn if a heating pad is applied. Conversely, a surgical sympathectomy (as opposed to thermal sympatholysis) should be considered; this often allows healing of a cutaneous ulcer. There is ongoing investigation of the usefulness of various epidermal growth factors in the treatment of ulcerations. This approach appears to have some benefit for venous stasis ulcers; whether this can be successfully applied to ischemic ulcerations remains to be seen.

This conservative approach is not without its risks. The ischemic ulceration limits the activity of the patient, particularly the elderly, and predisposes to muscle atrophy, deep venous thrombosis, and pneumonia. Furthermore, the chronic ischemic pain can have a denervating effect on the most stolid patient. Sometimes the wisest course is amputation. This is occasionally a difficult decision, and transcutaneous oximetry may be used to determine the likelihood of healing of an ischemic ulceration. Typically, cutaneous PO$_2$ values greater than 40 mm Hg are associated with healing, whereas those less than 20 mm Hg will not heal.

SUGGESTED READING

Blankenhorn DH, Brooks SH, Selzer RH, et al. The rate of atherosclerosis change during treatment of hyperlipoproteinemia. Circulation 1978; 57:355.

Coffman JD. Vasodilator drugs in peripheral vascular disease. N Engl J Med 1979; 300:713–717.

Porter JM, Cutler BS, Lee BY, et al. Pentoxifylline efficacy in the treatment of intermittent claudication: multicenter controlled double-blind trial with objective assessment of chronic occlusive arterial disease patients. Am Heart J 1982; 104:66–72.

Radack K, Wyderski RJ. Conservative management of intermittent claudication. Ann Intern Med 1990; 113:135–146.

Smith GD, Shipley MJ, Rose G. Intermittent claudication, heart disease risk factors, and mortality: the Whitehall study. Circulation 1990; 82:1925–1931.

Steering Committee of The Physicians' Health Study Research Group. Final report on the aspirin component of the ongoing physicians' health study. N Engl J Med 1989; 321:129–135.

CHRONIC ARTERIAL OCCLUSIVE DISEASE: EXERCISE REHABILITATION

WILLIAM R. HIATT, M.D.
MELANIE E. HARGARTEN, M.S.
JUDITH G. REGENSTEINER, Ph.D.

In an aging population, the manifestations of atherosclerosis are among the leading causes of morbidity and mortality. Atherosclerotic peripheral arterial disease (PAD) of the lower extremities produces exercise-induced muscle aching or cramping secondary to ischemia in the calf, thigh, or buttocks. This exercise-induced ischemic pain is referred to as intermittent claudication. Most patients are symptomatic only during walking, but with more severe forms of the disease there is pain in the limb at rest, ischemic ulceration, or gangrene.

As with all forms of atherosclerosis, the prevalence of PAD increases with age. Studies done in large populations have shown that the prevalence, as defined by noninvasive testing, is 6 percent at ages 50 to 55 but increases to 12 to 16 percent at age 65 and to 20 percent over age 75. Clearly, PAD affects a large number of individuals, who are at increased risk for walking disability as well as other cardiovascular events.

Clinically, PAD is an important cause of impaired exercise capacity, because symptomatic patients typically can walk only one to three blocks before having to stop and rest. The limited ability to ambulate leads to disability as patients are unable to meet the personal, social, or occupational demands of daily life. This disability is particularly detrimental to quality of life, since both leisure and work activities are often severely curtailed. For example, job activities that involve walking short distances, shopping, stair climbing, and outdoor recreation may be limited. Thus, a major focus of therapy for these patients is to relieve the symptom of intermittent claudication and the disability that ensues.

Patients with PAD have an increased mortality rate from other cardiovascular diseases, but a relatively stable natural history of symptoms of intermittent claudication. In contrast to patients with coronary artery disease, in whom there is often a spontaneous recovery of function after a myocardial infarction or cardiac surgery, patients with PAD may remain at the same level of walking impairment for years if not treated. This stable natural history influences treatment decisions so that, for most patients, the primary goals are to modify the risk factors for the disease and to improve walking ability.

CURRENT FORMS OF TREATMENT

In comparison to patients with coronary artery disease, there are fewer treatment options to improve functional capacity in patients with PAD. The major forms of treatment are discussed below.

Modification of Risk Factors

Risk factors for PAD include diabetes, cigarette smoking, hypertension, and hyperlipidemia (particularly disorders in the metabolism of triglycerides and high-density lipoprotein [HDL] cholesterol). Aggressive treatment of these risk factors may slow or stabilize the progression of atherosclerotic disease in the peripheral vessels and may favorably influence cardiac mortality, but does not directly relieve the symptom of intermittent claudication or improve exercise performance.

Invasive Interventions

In patients with severe forms of the disease who manifest ischemic rest pain, ulceration, or gangrene, surgery or angioplasty may be necessary for the relief of symptoms and limb preservation. Also, patients with severe claudication that limits home, leisure, or occupational activities and is unresponsive to other medical therapies may be candidates for revascularization. However, most patients with intermittent claudication can be managed without a surgical procedure. Bypass surgery or angioplasty is indicated for only 10 to 20 percent of the population of patients with PAD. Surgery has the potential to restore the circulation but is associated with a morbidity of approximately 10 percent and a mortality rate of 2 to 4 percent, depending on the type of procedure, the age of the patient, and the presence of diabetes and other concomitant medical disorders. The morbidity and mortality rates for angioplasty are less than for surgery, but the patency rates are also less. Interestingly, the functional benefits of surgery or angioplasty for intermittent claudication have not been rigorously studied in terms of improved walking ability, community activity, or quality of life.

Pharmacology

Several classes of drugs have been evaluated in patients with PAD. Vasodilators were once commonly used, but in controlled clinical trials these agents did not increase peripheral blood flow or relieve claudication symptoms. Antiplatelet and anticoagulant drugs are also ineffective in treating claudication. Pentoxifylline, a hemorrheologic agent that decreases blood viscosity, is the only approved drug for treating intermittent claudication. In controlled clinical trials the drug is associated with a 50 to 100 percent improvement in treadmill walking ability, particularly in patients with moderately severe disease. Carnitine, an experimental drug, appears to increase exercise performance by improving ischemic muscle metabolism, but currently is not approved for this purpose. The role of drug therapy in improving blood flow in these patients is currently minimal.

Exercise Rehabilitation

Walking exercise has been recommended for over 40 years as a means to help patients with PAD improve their walking ability. In 1966 the first randomized, controlled trial of exercise training in patients with PAD demonstrated a marked improvement in treadmill walking ability from an exercise program. Since this first controlled study, there have been numerous reports of the benefit of exercise training for walking ability in patients with PAD. However, to date, few institutions offer formal programs specifically designed for patients with vascular diseases. This is in sharp contrast to the numerous free-standing and institution-based cardiac rehabilitation programs that are available for patients who have undergone cardiac surgery or experienced a myocardial infarction, or who have angina or congestive heart failure.

It is important to contrast exercise rehabilitation for patients with PAD with rehabilitation programs for patients with coronary artery disease. Some patients who suffer a myocardial infarction or undergo coronary artery bypass surgery spontaneously recover a significant amount of functional capacity. The benefit of cardiac rehabilitation for these patients is questioned because they often do not have cardiovascular impairment, defined as an exercise performance of less than 9 METs.

A MET is the multiple of the resting oxygen consumption (3.5 ml per kilogram per minute) that defines exercise capacity and the energy expenditure of certain tasks. In contrast, patients with PAD often have a chronic impairment that does not spontaneously improve and a peak exercise capacity of only 3 to 4 METS. Thus, the average patient with PAD typically has a greater degree of functional impairment than the average patient with coronary artery disease. In addition, other major interventions are frequently used in the treatment of coronary disease, including coronary artery bypass surgery, coronary angioplasty, and a number of clinically important drugs (nitrates, beta-adrenergic blockers, and calcium channel blockers). In patients with PAD, surgery and angioplasty are used less frequently and there are fewer drugs available than for patients with coronary artery disease.

Results of Exercise Rehabilitation

All studies of exercise conditioning in patients with PAD have reported an increase in treadmill exercise performance, and a lessening of claudication pain severity during exercise. This consistent finding demonstrates that exercise training programs can have a clinically important impact on functional capacity in patients for whom other treatment options are limited and for whom spontaneous recovery does not occur. Twenty-six trials of exercise conditioning in this population have been conducted to date, of which 17 were not controlled trials and nine employed a controlled (sometimes randomized) design. Most of the studies evaluated changes in walking ability with a constant-load treadmill protocol. The improvement in pain-free walking time (defined as the time or distance walked before the onset of claudication) ranged from 44 to 290 percent, with an average increase of 134 percent. The peak walking time increased from between 25 percent to 183 percent, with an average of 96 percent. Thus, the ability to sustain walking exercise for longer durations with less claudication pain is improved by training. In addition, studies that employ a graded exercise protocol have evaluated changes in submaximal exercise performance. At a given submaximal workload, exercise training leads to a decrease in heart rate, ventilation, and oxygen consumption. These changes may contribute to the ability to sustain walking exercise for a longer time before claudication pain limits the activity. Improvements in peak exercise performance and oxygen consumption are also important because patients are able to perform activities of higher intensities such as climbing stairs, gardening, and dancing.

Clinical predictors of the response to a rehabilitation program have also been evaluated. The severity of the arterial disease does not appear to affect the training response. In one study, patients with ischemic rest pain improved as much as those who were either mildly or moderately affected by claudication. Other studies confirm this observation, in that the ankle-arm index at rest (a measure of disease severity) could predict only 10 percent of the increase in walking distance on the treadmill after an exercise program. Finally, disease location and associated conditions such as coronary artery disease do not limit the ability to receive benefit from a training program. Therefore, patients should not be excluded from consideration for a training program simply on the basis of disease severity or other illnesses.

We recently completed a randomized, controlled trial of exercise conditioning for patients with PAD. On entry, patients could walk an average of only 6 minutes on our standard treadmill protocol (see below) to a peak oxygen consumption (VO_2) of 12.8 ml per kilogram per minute. After the initial evaluation, patients were randomized into treated and control groups. Those in the treated group were enrolled in a supervised, progressive treadmill walking program of 12 weeks' duration (36 1-hour sessions). Control subjects were asked to maintain their usual level of activity. Testing was performed on entry and at 6 and 12 weeks after enrollment. Treated subjects increased their maximal walking time by 7.5 minutes (123 percent) and peak VO_2 by 3.7 ml per kilogram per minute (30 percent). The control group had a 1.1-minute (20 percent) increase in walking time and no change in peak VO_2. Importantly, in treated patients only, pain-free walking time on the treadmill increased by 165 percent and there was an even greater relief in the amount of mild, moderate, and severe claudication pain during treadmill walking.

As a result of the program (assessed by means of a walking impairment questionnaire), treated subjects could walk a greater distance at a faster speed and thus perform activities that were considered difficult to impossible before the treatment (e.g., return to work, dancing, outdoor activities, and shopping). Control subjects had no change in their walking ability (from treadmill testing or questionnaire) or level of disability (from questionnaire) during the course of the study. The mechanism of improvement in treated subjects was associated with a change in skeletal muscle metabolism and not with a change in skeletal muscle blood flow.

Thus, a progressive walking exercise program can improve exercise performance, relieve the pain of intermittent claudication, and facilitate the ability to perform personal, social, and occupational activities. Critical to the development of a training program is an understanding of the methods of exercise testing and training of patients with peripheral arterial disease.

ASSESSMENT OF PERIPHERAL CIRCULATION AND FUNCTIONAL CAPACITY

A number of methods are available to evaluate changes in both the hemodynamic and functional status of patients with PAD as the result of an intervention.

An evaluation of the peripheral circulation is focused primarily on measurement of peripheral blood pressure and flow. These hemodynamic measures are routinely used to evaluate patency rates after peripheral vascular surgery and angioplasty. Although reperfusion

is the goal of vascular surgery or angioplasty, a change in the hemodynamic status of patients does not necessarily translate into a change in their functional status. Therefore, other measures of functional capacity must be employed in the complete evaluation of persons undergoing a therapeutic intervention.

Our current approach is to evaluate hemodynamic end points before and after treatment, as well as to assess walking impairment by treadmill testing and by specific questionnaires developed for these patients. In this way, we wish to evaluate the impact of a therapeutic program on quality of life and community-based activities.

Evaluation of Hemodynamics

The peripheral circulation is generally evaluated at rest and immediately after exercise by measurement of ankle and arm systolic blood pressures with a Doppler ultrasonic instrument. At rest, the ratio of ankle to arm systolic blood pressure is an index of the severity of the underlying vascular disease. After exercise, pressure in the ankle typically falls in patients with PAD. Factors that influence this drop in ankle pressure include the extent of arterial occlusive disease, the amount of vasodilatation distal to the obstruction, and the amount of shunting of blood away from the distal vessels in the extremity toward more proximal muscles. Measurements of blood flow can be made using plethysmographic or pulsed Doppler techniques. In addition, measurement of the pulse volume at different locations on the extremity provides complementary data about the location and degree of occlusion of the peripheral arterial system. Taken together, these noninvasive measures of pressure, flow, and pulse volume can be used as a substitute for angiography in following the vascular disease status of the patient.

Evaluation of Functional Capacity

The traditional treadmill protocol for patients with PAD has generally been conducted at a constant workload, at a slow speed of 1 to 2 mph, with the grade ranging from 0 to 12 percent. Despite the constant workload, most patients reach a maximal level of claudication pain at which point they stop walking. During the exercise test, the time (or distance) at which claudication pain first begins is recorded, as well as the maximal, claudication-limited walking time. A drawback is that this type of treadmill test often is not reproducible and patients do not always reach maximal claudication as an end point.

We have recently developed and validated a graded treadmill exercise protocol specifically for patients with PAD. Walking speed is held constant at 2 mph, which is well tolerated by all patients. Every 3 minutes there is an increase in grade of 3.5 percent until the patient reaches maximal claudication pain and can exercise no further. Perceived exertion is evaluated every 30 seconds throughout the treadmill test on a 1 to 5 scale: 1 = no claudication pain, 2 = onset of pain, 3 = mild pain, 4 = moderate pain, and 5 = maximal pain. All patients are able to attain a symptom-limited peak performance as defined by the maximal walking time and the peak oxygen consumption measured by indirect calorimetry. These measures of peak performance have proved to be more reproducible than the patients' rating of claudication pain severity during exercise. When used in our training study, this protocol made it possible to detect changes in claudication pain severity and peak exercise performance in patients with PAD as a result of the intervention.

Questionnaires are used to determine the benefits of exercise training in terms of the activities of daily living. Walking is a fundamental activity that when impaired may limit the ability to perform many essential tasks. With training, it is assumed that improvements in treadmill exercise performance will allow patients to better meet the physical demands of home, occupational, and leisure-time activities. To determine the impact of training programs on community function and quality of life, questionnaires that evaluate walking ability and quality of life should be used in addition to questionnaires that specifically assess activities that are curtailed by PAD. In our studies, we have used a walking impairment questionnaire that evaluates walking speed, distance, and symptoms leading to impairment. This instrument showed that treated patients were able to walk further and faster in the community setting.

Assessment of Gait and Strength

Other functional aspects that may be evaluated are gait and muscle strength, because both of these factors may affect the ability to walk. Changes in patients' walking speed, step frequency, and other aspects of gait have not been measured in training studies, yet it is possible that a problematic gait may be a factor that makes walking more difficult. Rehabilitation physicians may be consulted if an evaluation of gait abnormalities is desired.

Muscular strength has been little evaluated in the population with PAD. However, since a basic level of strength is required to enable a person to walk, we are currently carrying out studies involving strengthening the lower limbs to determine the role of strength in the rehabilitation of PAD patients. As with gait analysis, rehabilitation medicine physicians may be consulted to evaluate strength in the lower extremity and to design a treatment plan when appropriate.

METHODS OF EXERCISE REHABILITATION

Many of the basic principles of exercise rehabilitation in diseased populations were developed in patients with coronary artery disease. However, the specific methods used to train patients with PAD differ from those used in cardiac rehabilitation. For all patients with cardiovascular diseases, rehabilitation programs are designed to optimize and maintain the highest degree of functional capacity. In addition, a rehabilitation program is *longitudinal* in that the formal, supervised exercise sessions last an average of 3 months, with a maintenance program of exercise recommended for an extended period. The service is *individualized* in that the exercise prescription uniquely meets each patient's needs and is upgraded at regular intervals. The program is *participatory* and requires an active involvement by the patient in regular, structured exercise sessions. Finally, the program is *preventive* and is designed to favorably affect or modify many of the risk factors for cardiovascular disease.

The most utilized mode of exercise therapy for PAD to date has been treadmill walking exercise. A patient is enrolled in an exercise rehabilitation program after entry assessment has been completed. Exercise sessions are typically held three times a week for approximately 1 hour each, and 3-month periods of training are customary. On the initial visit the patient is instructed in the use of the telemetry monitors if monitoring is desired to evaluate heart rate response, or required, as in the case of the subgroup who have coronary artery disease in addition to PAD. A 5-minute warm-up period precedes every class, and a 5-minute cool-down follows it to minimize risk of injury. The warm-up period is designed to increase the heart rate slowly and promote flexibility, and should involve the use of large muscle groups, especially the muscles used for walking. The cool-down period is designed to return the heart rate to baseline value and primarily involves stretching of the large muscle groups, particularly those in the legs.

The initial training workload is determined from the symptom-limited maximal treadmill test on entry, so that the intensity of the treadmill exercise is set to the workload that initially brings on claudication pain in the patient. In subsequent visits the speed or grade is increased if the patient is able to walk for 10 minutes or longer at the lower workload without reaching moderate claudication pain. Either speed or grade can be increased, but in our program we increase grade first if the patient can already walk at 2 mph. If the patient's initial speed of walking is less than 2 mph, we increase speed first. One of the goals of our program is to increase patient walking speed up to the normal 3 mph, from the average PAD patient walking speed of 1.5 to 2 mph.

The initial training session lasts 35 minutes, with subsequent increases of 5 minutes each session until a 50-minute session is possible. During the exercise sessions, rest periods (induced by claudication) are interspersed between bouts of treadmill walking. The patient walks on the treadmill until a mild or moderate level of pain is reached (scored as 3 or 4 on the 1 to 5 scale described above). At that point, the patient sits and rests until the pain abates. After the pain is gone, the patient resumes walking until a mild or moderate level of pain is reached again, and this is followed by another rest period. This process is repeated until the 50-minute exercise period has elapsed. Our experience, after patients become somewhat conditioned, has been that out of the 50-minute period, walking on the treadmill takes about 35 minutes and rest periods total about 15 minutes.

Gait abnormalities can be treated through the attention of a physical therapist, who works with the patient to normalize gait. Muscular weakness can be treated by strengthening exercises, also with the help of a physical therapist.

PRECAUTIONS

In our previous experience of aerobic training, no patients have suffered any adverse effects, including a cardiovascular complication or musculoskeletal injury. However, the potential for an adverse event exists in any exercise program, especially one in which a diseased group of individuals is involved. There are two main types of problems to consider. First, a cardiovascular complication is possible in PAD patients, a group that has a high rate of cardiac disease as well as peripheral arterial disease. To promote safety, all patients are monitored by telemetry during exercise sessions to evaluate heart rate and cardiac rhythm during exercise, and blood pressure is recorded before and after each training session. In addition, safety concerns dictate the use of warm-up periods before and cool-down periods after exercise sessions to increase heart rate slowly, return the heart rate to a resting value slowly, and prevent muscle soreness due to training by increasing flexibility.

REMARKS

The benefit of walking exercise training for patients with PAD has been consistently demonstrated. There-fore, exercise training constitutes an important form of therapy for this disabling disease, which affects over 5 million older people. Only the 10 to 20 percent most severely afflicted are surgical candidates, and drug therapies are currently limited. Thus, most patients with PAD may not be optimally treated. The large numbers of people affected by PAD makes it likely that their disability will be costly, both in monetary terms, as patients require medical care and help with activities of daily life, and in terms of decreased quality of life and ability to maintain employment. Therefore, dissemination of exercise training methods specifically formulated for PAD patients may prove to be highly useful. The use of reproducible testing methods and proved training programs will ensure that patients receive the greatest benefit possible.

Supported by Grants #G008635118 and #H133G90114 from the National Institute on Disability and Rehabilitation Research.

SUGGESTED READING

Hiatt WR, Nawaz D, Regensteiner JG, Hossack K. The evaluation of exercise performance in patients with peripheral vascular disease. J Cardiopulm Rehabil 1988; 12:525–532.

Hiatt WR, Regensteiner JG, Hargarten ME, et al. Benefit of exercise conditioning for patients with peripheral arterial disease. Circulation 1990; 81:602–609.

Larsen O, Lassen N. Effect of daily muscular exercise in patients with intermittent claudication. Lancet 1966; 2:1093–1095.

Radack K, Wyderski RJ. Conservative management of intermittent claudication. Ann Intern Med 1990; 113:135–146.

Regensteiner JG, Steiner JF, Panzer RJ, Hiatt WR. Evaluation of walking impairment by questionnaire in patients with peripheral arterial disease. J Vasc Med Biol 1990; 2:142–152.

CHRONIC ARTERIAL OCCLUSIVE DISEASE: PERCUTANEOUS INTERVENTIONAL TREATMENT

ROBERT A. GRAOR, M.D.
BRUCE H. GRAY, D.O.

Most claudicating patients with symptomatic atherosclerotic occlusive disease of the iliac or femoropopliteal arterial segments have been treated nonoperatively. This nonoperative treatment includes reduction of risk factors, smoking cessation, weight loss, and treatment of associated diseases such as hypertension, hyperlipidemia, and diabetes. It also should include a daily walking program so as to enhance collateral formation and to accelerate conditioning of the muscles distal to the arterial obstructions.

Kannel and McGee reported the annual age-adjusted incidence of intermittent claudication in the Framingham population survey to be 0.3 percent in men and 0.1 percent in women. Claudication is approximately five times more common among diabetics, and the incidence of serious coronary events is approximately five times higher than those without claudication, even in the absence of diabetes. McDaniel and Cronenwett conducted an extensive review of the literature and found that claudication occurs in about 1.8 percent of patients under 60 years of age, in 3.7 percent of those aged 60 to 70 years, and in 5.2 percent of those over the age of 70. They also concluded that claudication is more likely to be caused by aortoiliac occlusive disease (53 percent) in patients under 40 years of age, whereas femoropopliteal disease (65 percent) is usually responsible for claudication symptoms in older patients.

Approximately 20 percent of each of these two groups have multisegmental arterial involvement.

It is also important to note that many patients who have lower extremity occlusive disease experience no symptoms whatsoever. The absence of popliteal or pedal pulses caused by segmental lesions in the superficial femoral artery or in isolated tibial arteries is often an incidental finding on physical examination in those who have developed compensatory collateral circulation or otherwise lead sedentary lives. Since functional disability is a prerequisite for any type of intervention, such patients customarily require no treatment.

Juergens and colleagues provided late information concerning the incidence of severe ischemia or urgent operative intervention for a series of patients with claudication (Table 1). Conceding an inherent selection bias, a number of subsequent surgical reports suggested that such acute events occur in 19 to 27 percent of claudicants within 4 to 7 years after the diagnosis of lower extremity arterial disease. McDaniel and Cronenwett in their collective review found that sudden complications appear to be slightly more prevalent among patients whose diagnosis has been confirmed by noninvasive testing or angiography, which is not altogether surprising because such patients might have had more impressive evidence of lower extremity ischemia at the time of initial presentation. The amputation rate potential among these patients ranges from 4 to 8 percent, compared with a 3 percent risk for all patients with claudication who were evaluated at the Mayo Clinic before arterial reconstruction became available.

Since it is clear that not all patients with a simple finding of claudication, absence of pulses, or abnormal noninvasive study results progress to severe ischemia, not all patients will choose, or should be provided, a percutaneous treatment or surgical reconstruction of their arterial disease. Only those with socially or economically disabling claudication or limb-threatening ischemia should be considered for treatment either percutaneously or surgically.

MORPHOLOGIC CHANGES INDUCED BY ANGIOPLASTY

Angioplasty may be attended by acute or chronic complications and is thus reserved for patients with disabling claudication or limb-threatening ischemia. The acute complications of angioplasty have already been discussed in the chapter *Chronic Ischemic Heart Disease: Angioplasty and Other Catheter-Based Revascularization Techniques.* Chronic morphologic and histologic changes that may be associated with angioplasty include (1) fibrocellular intimal proliferation (restenosis) and (2) accelerated atherosclerosis.

The most widely accepted theory for the development of fibrocellular intimal proliferation involves responses from the damaged vessel endothelium and media. Major participants in this response appear to be smooth muscle cells in the media and diseased intima, together with adherent platelets. With plaque disruption, localized deposition of platelets occurs with subsequent release of thromboxane A_2, further platelet deposition, and subsequent release of growth factors such as platelet-derived growth factor. Vessel endothelium also releases various growth factors such as endothelial and fibroblast growth factors. This process appears to result in migration of smooth muscle cells from the media into the intima, where they proliferate. The phenotype of these smooth muscle cells changes from a contractile into a secretory phenotype; these cells synthesize and release large amounts of extracellular matrix, which contributes to the bulk of the lesions. These changes generally occur within 2 to 9 months after balloon dilatation.

Atherosclerotic plaque without intimal fibrous proliferation occurs in a subgroup of previously dilated patients and can be explained in at least two ways: (1) stretching of diseased wall (concentric lesions) or disease-free wall (eccentric lesions) during the initial procedure with subsequent elastic recoil (restenosis) and (2) progression of atherosclerotic disease (accelerated atherosclerosis). Although acute elastic recoil

Table 1 Late Incidence of Amputation, Severe Ischemia, and/or Operation in Patients with Lower Extremity Claudication

Series	Year	No.	Follow-up (yr)	Severe Ischemia and/or Operation No.	%	Amputation No.	%
Juergens et al	1960	336	5	NA*	—	10	3
Humphries et al	1963	1,552†	4 (mean)	356	23	105	7
Stable claudication		661†		171	26	53	8
Progressive claudication		891†		185	21	52	6
McDaniel and Cronenwett	1989‡						
History and physical examination		2,469	7	NA	19	NA	7
Vascular laboratory and/or angiography		1,624	5	NA	27	NA	4

*Not available.
†Limbs.
‡Collected series (weighted means).

shortly after balloon angioplasty is generally a well-recognized mechanism of abrupt narrowing, chronic elastic recoil, as a mechanism of late luminal narrowing, is not well understood.

The absence of morphologic signs of previous balloon angioplasty in necropsied patients with restenosis may be interpreted as indicating progression of underlying atherosclerotic plaque. Two histologic features indicate this type of progression. First, the atherosclerotic plaque is densely fibrotic, with focal calcific deposits, indicating a very mature atherosclerotic lesion. Second, the inner layers of the atherosclerotic plaque are histologically similar to its outer layers. It is also conceivable that many months or years after balloon angioplasty, fibrocellular intimal proliferation may come to resemble more typical atherosclerotic plaque as its cellular components incorporate lipid.

The Simpson directional atherectomy catheter has been used to remove obstructing material from sites of restenosis. Tissue removed by this catheter falls into three histologic categories: (1) intimal proliferation, (2) atherosclerotic plaque with or without thrombus, and (3) thrombus only (Table 2). Usually, restenosis at the site of previous angioplasty or atherectomy is due to intimal proliferation, but occasionally it may represent acceleration or progression of atherosclerosis.

BALLOON CATHETERS AND OTHER INTERVENTIONAL DEVICES

Several generations of interventional catheters have evolved primarily by reducing the catheter diameter, reducing the compliance of the balloon, and increasing the trackability, or axial characteristics. In addition, the development of atherectomy catheters and the immense evolution of research related to laser-assisted treatment have influenced the treatment of percutaneous catheter–directed therapies.

Better results have been obtained with newer balloon catheters that avoid overstretching of the balloon and maldistribution of dilating forces. Balloon rupture rarely occurs with the current technology of balloon catheters. The smaller balloon catheter shafts allow their use in smaller vessels with less trauma to the surrounding normal portions of the artery.

The introduction of atherectomy devices for tissue extraction have also improved our understanding and ability to treat lower extremity atherosclerotic lesions. Directional atherectomy catheters (i.e., the Simpson ather ectomy catheter), allows accurate focal removal of the atherosclerotic plaque by slicing the atheroma and collecting it in a distal collection chamber for removal. Rotational atherectomy devices for the most part rely on pulverization, with or without aspiration of the pulverized material.

Laser methods remove tissue by means of thermal or acoustic energy. Histologic studies of vascular tissue after laser therapy show craters surrounded by concentric zones of protein denaturation and tissue vacuolation. These areas vary with the type of laser energy delivered.

RESULTS OF PERCUTANEOUS INTERVENTION

The reported results of angioplasty in the iliac and femoropopliteal arteries frequently have not adhered to uniform reporting standards. This, and the relative lack of long-term objective follow-up, have made it difficult to evaluate these modalities in most studies.

By adopting precise definitions of essential terms, developing objective criteria by which the various measures of success or failures can be judged, and establishing a standardized scheme by which severity of disease, degrees of improvement or deterioration, and risk factors that affect outcome can be graded, the quality of reports of revascularization of lower extremity ischemia can be greatly improved. In the interim, a careful review of the literature allows some generalizations to be made, as discussed below.

Percutaneous Transluminal Angioplasty (PTA) of the Aorta

Johnston and colleagues at the University of Toronto reported 17 patients with aortic PTA. Sixteen of these were women with an average age of 50.5 years, and in all cases the indication was claudication. The initial success rate was 94 percent, and the long-term success rates were 80 and 70 percent at 1 and 5 years, respectively. Only one major complication occurred

Table 2 Pathologic Findings in 218 Lesions Excised by Means of Peripheral Atherectomy in 100 Patients

Pathologic Findings	Primary Stenosis (n = 170)	After PTA (n = 15)	Restenosis After ATH (n = 29)	After PTA and ATH (n = 4)
Atherosclerotic plaque	150	1	10	1
Fibrous intimal thickening	15	0	0	0
Thrombus	5	0	0	0
Intimal hyperplasia	0	14	19	3

Data from Johnson DE. JACC 1990; 15:419.

after the PTA, resulting in limb ischemia that required treatment with an elective aortobifemoral bypass. Other case reports of angioplasty involving the aorta are similar to Johnston's. Thus, PTA of the infrarenal abdominal aorta for occlusive atherosclerotic lesions is feasible, is associated with reasonably good long-term patency, and carries a low incidence of complications.

PTA of the Iliac Arteries

Table 3 lists the results of angioplasty of the iliac arteries. Two studies are of particular interest. Tegtmeyer and colleagues reported 295 consecutive iliac angioplasties in 200 patients with a 7.5-year mean follow-up on 176 patients. Initial success rates were 99 percent for arterial lesions and 93 percent for patients. Success was determined by the completion angiogram, reduction of pressure gradients, and the clinical results. The primary patency rate was 85 percent at 5 years, although relatively few patients were available for follow-up. Complications occurred in 10.5 percent, but most were minor.

In contrast to Tegtmeyer and colleagues' data, Johnston and colleagues reported 667 iliac angioplasties with an initial success rate of 90 percent and a 5-year success rate of 53 percent. In Johnston and colleagues' study, analysis by the Cox proportional hazards model identified four variables that were a significant predictor of long-term success: (1) site of PTA (the common iliac was better than the external iliac), (2) indication for PTA (patients undergoing PTA for relief of claudication fared better than those requiring PTA for limb salvage), (3) lesion severity (stenosis was better than occlusion), and (4) runoff (the presence of more runoff vessels yielded better results). Using these factors for subsequent analysis, the 5-year success rate was 63 percent in the "best" group and only 6 percent in the "worst" group.

Of Johnston and colleagues' patients, 207 had normal distal vessels, and of these 79 percent were asymptomatic after PTA, but 21 percent had persistent mild claudication. The ratio of ankle:brachial systolic blood pressure increased significantly in all patients; it normalized in 43 percent but remained abnormal in 57 percent. Also in this series, 7.9 percent of patients had complications of which most were minor. One patient died from a myocardial infarction and one from bleeding due to arterial rupture after PTA, yielding a total mortality rate of 0.3 percent. In 1.1 percent of the patients, surgery was required because of severe limb ischemia or false aneurysm. In 2.8 percent, hospital discharge was delayed because of a large hematoma or ischemia.

The differences between Tegtmeyer and colleagues' results and those of Johnston and colleagues can be explained by differences in the patient population and the method of analysis. In the Tegtmeyer series, only six of 340 lesions were occlusions and 58 of 200 patients underwent additional surgical procedures after the PTA. Rest pain or limb salvage was the indication in 40 percent; during follow-up, a surprising 12 of 37 patients with rest pain became asymptomatic. In both series, the life table analysis method was used; however, Tegtmeyer and colleagues excluded patients who were initial failures from the subsequent analysis. In the Tegtmeyer study, only 10 of 186 patients were lost to follow-up; however, many patients received follow-up for only 3 years, suggesting a recent increase in volume of procedures.

Nonetheless, it appears that iliac angioplasty is a durable and safe procedure for patients with localized iliac disease. The ideal patient is the claudicator with focal common iliac disease and satisfactory distal vessels (Fig. 1). The risk:benefit ratio of PTA in the iliac region is favorable compared with surgery.

Table 3 Long-Term Results of Aortoiliac Percutaneous Transluminal Angioplasty (PTA)

Series	Year	No. of Patients	% Mortality	% Patency			All Complications %
				Early	2 yr*	Long-term*	
Gruntzig and Kumpe	1977	186	0	92	83	87†	–
Katzen et al	1979	33	0	95	80	80†	5.4
Spence et al	1981	131	–	92.5	87	79‡	1.9
O'Mara et al	1981	17	0	94.1	–	56.3§	0
Johnston et al	1987	667	0	90	–	53‖	8
Gallino et al	1982	45	–	96	95	87¶	10
Kumpe and Jones	1982	–	–	–	–	82**	–
Kadir et al	1983	112	0	95.7	89	89**	10
Van Andel et al	1985	154	0	96.4	98	82††	2
Tegtmeyer et al	1991	200	0	99	94	85‖	10.5

*Includes only initially successful percutaneous transluminal angioplasty procedures.
†Patency at 2 yr.
‡Patency at 2.5 yr.
§Patency at 1 yr.
‖Patency at 5 yr.
¶Patency at 4 yr.
**Patency at 3 yr.
+ +Patency at 10 yr.

PTA for Femoropopliteal Disease

Pooled data from studies reporting initial or technical results in patients with femoropopliteal PTA show a mean 2- and 4-year patency of 89 and 67 percent, respectively (Table 4). In combined series, 2-year patency for 622 patients with stenotic lesions is 84 percent, whereas for 191 patients with occluded femoropopliteal arteries, it is only 57 percent.

Prospective and randomized trials have been conducted comparing PTA with surgery, although these studies contain serious flaws. For example, all patients randomized to surgery must have lesions that are also amenable to angioplasty. This excludes the less severely diseased patients in either group and probably improves patency rates for bypass graft patients. Nonetheless, data from a study by Martin and colleagues indicate that the initial and 2-year patency rates in this randomized study were equivalent for both bypass grafting and PTA.

Blair and associates conducted a retrospective study comparing the results of PTA with those of infrainguinal bypass in patients with critical limb-threatening ischemia. Thirty-nine of 54 patients (72 percent) initially improved after PTA, but only 18 percent showed improvement on Doppler studies at 2 years. Despite these poor results, limb salvage was 78 percent. In the surgical group, 2-year patency was 68 percent and limb salvage 90 percent. When patency rates were compared, surgery fared better than PTA, but no statistically significant difference was noted for limb salvage.

The rate of nonfatal complications associated with PTA in the femoropopliteal region is believed to be less than 5 percent and of serious complications less than 1 percent. Mortality has been reported to be less than 0.4 percent. This low mortality rate compares favorably with surgical mortalities of 2 to 4 percent for femoropopliteal or femorotibial bypass grafting.

Table 4 Pooled Data on Results of Femoropopliteal Angioplasty

Total number of patients:	1,426
Success rate:	89%
2-year patency:	72%
4-year patency:	67%

PTA of Infrapopliteal Arteries

Table 5 shows combined results of studies of infrapopliteal PTA. Recently, improved results have been achieved with the low-profile balloon catheters now available. In the study by Schwarten and colleagues the primary anatomic success rate was 84 percent, the complication rate 4 percent, and the acute thrombosis rate 16 percent.

Atherectomy

Table 6 shows the published results of atherectomy in femoropopliteal arteries. In summary, it can be stated that atherectomy, although a new procedure with various types of devices, can achieve a good initial mechanical result. The most recent data reveal favorable long-term patency with the Simpson directional atherectomy catheter compared with PTA (Table 6, Fig. 2).

Laser Angioplasty

The results of laser angioplasty have not been encouraging. Table 7 lists the results of selected studies using various types of laser-assisted devices for recanalization of peripheral arteries. A significant effort is currently under way to develop better laser products. At present, we would not recommend laser angioplasty as a primary form of treatment.

ANGIOSCOPY AND INTRA-ARTERIAL ULTRASONOGRAPHY

New and useful information can be obtained from these new imaging devices. Angioscopic images of the luminal morphology add information not seen on arteriograms. The ultrasound instruments generate highly accurate cross-sectional images of the arterial wall and can depict the layers of the wall and the composition of these layers. Features such as plaque localization (concentric versus eccentric), discrimination between plaque characteristics (the presence of calcium, fatty versus fibrous composition), and evaluation of the integrity of luminal surfaces can be determined with this

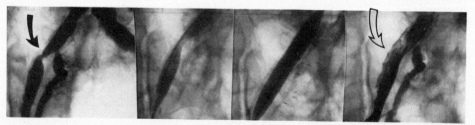

A, B **C, D**

Figure 1 *A,* Arteriogram of the right iliac artery. The arrow highlights a tight stenosis at the proximal portion of the right external iliac artery. *B,* An 8-mm-diameter balloon was inflated across the stenosis. Note the defect in the balloon upon inflation, which resolved with full inflation *(C). D,* Arteriogram after angioplasty reveals a dissection flap (open arrow) in the area of balloon inflation that did not limit flow.

technique. Intra-arterial ultrasound imaging will likely play a role in guidance of percutaneous intervention.

INDICATIONS FOR INTERVENTION

The practice of percutaneous intervention for lower extremity revascularization has grown as a result of the

Table 5 Reported Results of Infrapopliteal PTA

Author	No. of Patients	Initial Success Rate	2-Yr Patency
Schwarten et al	96	94%	83%
Brown et al	57	86%	NA*

*Not available.

Table 6 Results of Directional Atherectomy in Femoropopliteal Arteries

Author	No. Patients	Initial Success	2-Year Patency
Schwarten	41	91.2	83
Simpson et al	30	92	
Graor and Whitlow	214	98	81

spirit of collaboration among vascular surgeons and interventionalists over the past few years. Better data are now available indicating that safe and effective therapy can be applied to certain subgroups of patients. For example, angioplasty of an iliac artery lesion that is focal and in the proximal portion of the arterial segment can provide durable results that compare favorably with those of iliac endarterectomy or bypass grafting.

In the femoropopliteal segment, short-segmental lesions respond favorably to balloon angioplasty or directional atherectomy. In this group of patients, it may be preferable initially to pursue a percutaneous intervention rather than femoropopliteal or femorotibial bypass grafting. In patients with severe limb-threatening ischemia, surgical repair is probably preferable.

Although an in-depth discussion is beyond the scope of this chapter, combined thrombolysis and interventional percutaneous treatment have produced gratifying results (Fig. 3). Dissolving of thrombus within the artery can frequently convert long occlusions into short stenotic lesions that are more ideal for atherectomy or PTA.

For nondisabling claudication, interventional procedures or surgery are probably not appropriate. Patients who have socially or economically disabling claudication without limb-threatening ischemia are very suitable candidates for intervention. If one pursues a

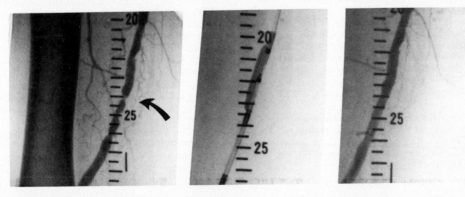

A **B, C**

Figure 2 *A,* Arteriogram of the right superficial femoral artery with the arrow pointing out the tight atherosclerotic stenosis at Hunter's canal. *B,* Directional atherectomy carriage at the site of stenosis. *C,* Arteriogram after atherectomy showing resolution of stenosis with a much smoother-appearing luminal outline.

Table 7 Reported Results of Laser Angioplasty in Femoropopliteal Disease

Author	Type of Laser	No. of Patients	Initial Success (%)	6- to 12-Month Patency (%)
Sanborn	LABA*	124	93	72
Katzen	Excimer	22	90	NA†
Nordstrom	Argon	34	90	68
Leon	Pulsed dye	35	72	NA
Dietrich	LABA	555	90	74
Asela	LABA	49	82	50

*Laser-assisted balloon angioplasty.
†Not available.

A, B   **C, D**

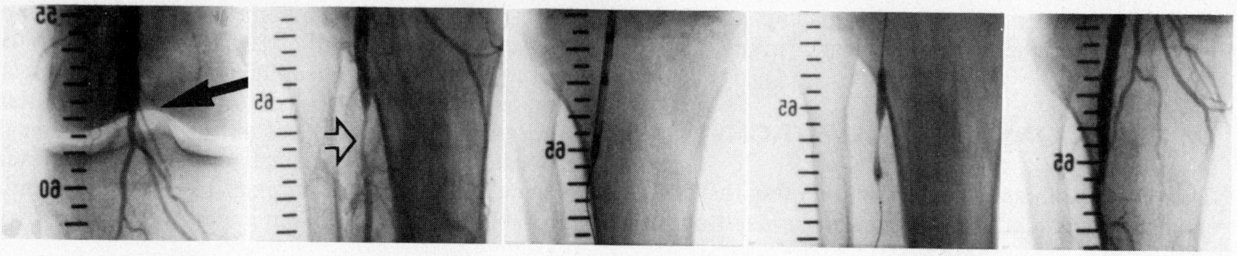

Figure 3 *A,* Arteriogram demonstrating occlusion of the right popliteal artery with collateral vessel flow below the knee. A catheter was placed in the popliteal occlusion, and thrombolytic therapy was administered for 16 hours. *B,* Arteriogram after thrombolytic therapy shows a patent popliteal and peroneal artery. *C,* Atherectomy was performed on the residual popliteal stenosis followed by balloon (2.5 mm in diameter) angioplasty of the tibioperoneal trunk *(D). E,* Arteriogram after the intervention reveals a widely patent popliteal artery with peroneal runoff.

percutaneous intervention to treat lower extremity ischemia, it suggests that appropriate follow-up be provided to these patients in terms of objective assessments by specialists involved in the care of patients with vascular disorders. With these objectives in mind, percutaneous catheter therapies for peripheral arterial disease can be highly successful.

SUGGESTED READING

Blair JM, Gewertz BL, Moosa H, et al. Percutaneous transluminal angioplasty versus surgery for limb-threatening ischemia. J Vasc Surg 1989; 9:698–703.

Brown KT, Schoenbert NY, Moore ED, Saddekni S. Percutaneous transluminal angioplasty of infrapopliteal vessels: preliminary results and technical considerations. Radiology 1988; 169:75–78.

Graor RA, Whitlow PL. Transluminal atherectomy for occlusive peripheral vascular disease. J Am Coll Cardiol 1990; 6:1551–1558.

Johnston KW, et al. Five-year results of a prospective study of percutaneous transluminal angioplasty. Ann Surg 1987; 206:403–413.

Juergens JL, Barker NW, Hines EA Jr. Arteriosclerosis obliterans: review of 520 cases with special reference to pathogenic and prognostic factors. Circulation 1960; 21:118–195.

Kannel WB, McGee DL. Diabetes and cardiovascular disease: the Framingham Study. JAMA 1979; 241:2035–2038.

Liu MW, Roubin GS, King SB. Restenosis after coronary angioplasty: potential biologic determinants and role of intima hyperplasia. Point of view. Circulation 1989; 79:1374–1387.

Mannick JA, Whittemore AD, Donaldson MC. Clinical and anatomic considerations for surgery in tibial disease and the results of surgery. Circulation 1991; 83(Suppl I):I-81–I-85.

McDaniel MD, Cronenwett JL. Basic data related to the natural history of intermittent claudication. Ann Vasc Surg 1989; 3:273–277.

McNamara TO, Bomberger RA, Merchant RF. Intra-arterial urokinase as the initial therapy for acutely ischemic lower limbs. Circulation (Suppl I) 1991; 83:I-106–I-119.

Schwarten DE, Cutcliff WB. Arterial occlusive disease below the knee: treatment with percutaneous angioplasty performed with low-profile catheters and steerable guidewires. Radiology 1988; 169:71–74.

Schwarten DE, Katzen BT, Simpson JB, Cutcliff WB. Simpson catheter for percutaneous transluminal removal of atheroma. AJR 1988; 150:799–801.

Simpson JB, Selmon JR, Robertson GC, et al. Transluminal atherectomy for occlusive peripheral vascular disease. Am J Cardiol 1988; 61:965–1016.

Sullivan KL, Gardiner GA Jr, Kandarpa K, et al. Efficacy of thrombolysis in infrainguinal bypass grafts. Circulation (Suppl I) 1991; 83:I-99–I-105.

Tegtmeyer CJ, Hartwell GD, Selby JB, et al. Results and complications of angioplasty in aortoiliac disease. Circulation 1991; 83(Suppl I):I-53–I-60.

Waller BF. "Crackers, breakers, stretchers, drillers, scrapers, shavers, burners, welders, melters"—the future treatment of atherosclerotic coronary artery disease? A clinical-morphologic assessment. J Am Coll Cardiol 1989; 13:969–987.

CHRONIC ARTERIAL OCCLUSIVE DISEASE: PREOPERATIVE EVALUATION

WILLIAM K. FREEMAN, M.D., F.A.C.C.
BERNARD J. GERSH, M.B., Ch.B. D.Phil, F.A.C.C.

Although cardiac disease, primarily coronary artery disease, is a leading cause of perioperative morbidity and mortality during general noncardiac surgical procedures, it is of particular concern in patients undergoing vascular surgery. Moreoever, the impact of coronary artery disease upon late prognosis is substantial, emphasizing the need for a conscientious cardiac evaluation of the vascular surgical patient both pre- and postoperatively.

Guided by a thorough cardiovascular history and physical examination, supplemented by judicious preoperative laboratory testing, potential cardiac risk can be effectively assessed in the patient with surgical vascular disease. Identification of the high-risk patient in need of further cardiac intervention before vascular surgery and careful perioperative cardiac surveillance are the most important immediate goals and should be pursued in an individualized and cost-effective manner.

ASSOCIATION OF CORONARY ARTERY DISEASE AND PERIPHERAL VASCULAR DISEASE

The prevalence of associated coronary artery disease in patients with surgical vascular disease has been extensively studied by investigators at the Cleveland Clinic and others. In patients having routine coronary angiography before vascular surgery, significant coronary disease (70 percent or more luminal stenosis) involving one or more major epicardial arteries has been found in approximately 80 percent of patients with clinically suspected ischemic heart disease and even in about one-third of all patients without clinical evidence of coronary disease. The spectrum of associated coronary disease is broad, with multivessel disease generally occurring in approximately one-half of all patients. Resultant ischemic segmental or diffuse left ventricular dysfunction can coexist in up to one-third of patients.

In general, approximately one-half of all patients presenting with surgical vascular disease have clinically evident ischemic heart disease, based on a history of myocardial infarction, symptoms of angina, or electrocardiographic evidence of previous infarction or resting repolarization abnormalities consistent with ischemia. In patients with clinically overt coronary artery disease, the highest incidence of severe coronary disease is in those operated on for aneurysmal disease (over 90 percent), being less, but still significant (50 to 80 percent), in patients with occlusive aortoiliac disease or carotid occlusive disease.

IMPACT OF CORONARY ARTERY DISEASE ON EARLY AND LATE POSTOPERATIVE OUTCOME

Over the past two decades, it has become clear that ischemic heart disease accounts for most perioperative morbidity and mortality associated with vascular surgical procedures. This is consistent with the previously documented high prevalence of associated coronary artery disease in this surgical population.

Multiple clinical studies have demonstrated that 40 to 60 percent of all perioperative deaths were cardiac in etiology, the vast majority related to complications of ischemic heart disease, in particular perioperative myocardial infarction. In patients without clinically suspected coronary artery disease, elective vascular surgical procedures have been associated with about 1 to 3 percent risk of cardiac perioperative death. The attendant cardiac mortality generally increases three- to fourfold (usually 3 to 10 percent) in patients with clinically apparent coronary disease, and approaches 20 to 30 percent in emergent operations such as for ruptured abdominal aortic aneurysm.

The magnitude of the vascular surgical procedure itself appears to influence perioperative outcome. Abdominal aortic aneurysm repair is associated with the highest degree of intraoperative cardiovascular hemodynamic and physiologic stress, which may be further complicated by major extra- and intravascular volume shifts and multifactorial respiratory insufficiency in the early postoperative period. Surgery for carotid occlusive disease may be associated with major fluctuations in blood pressure (usually hypertension), but as is the case with peripheral vascular surgery in the lower extremity, is relatively well tolerated, with a low (less than 1 to 2 percent) cardiac mortality even in patients with stable symptomatic coronary disease.

Late survival after surgery for peripheral vascular disease is also primarily influenced by coronary artery disease, and in general at least one-half of all deaths at follow-up have cardiac causes. Multiple studies, including several from the Mayo Clinic, have delineated the late outcome after repair of abdominal aortic aneurysms. In patients without clinically suspected coronary disease preoperatively, late survival was not significantly different from control populations, especially for patients 70 years of age and older. However, in patients having suspected or overt ischemic heart disease at the time of abdominal aortic aneurysm repair, late survival was nearly one-half that of controls, the risk of cardiac death being twice as great as in patients without apparent coronary disease. Of note, one Mayo Clinic population-based study documented a very high (61 percent) cardiac event rate (cardiac death, myocardial infarction, and/or coronary revascularization) in patients with suspected coronary disease during follow-up after abdominal aortic aneurysm repair; this was four times as great as in patients operated on without suspected coronary disease. Patients in the fifth and sixth decades of life with nonrevascularized symptomatic coronary disease at initial presentation have been shown to have the poorest relative long-term survival (in comparison with a control population) after abdominal aortic aneurysm repair. This suggests that vascular disease of this nature presenting at middle age may be a marker for a very aggressive and generalized atherosclerotic process. There is some evidence to suggest a similar but less striking influence of ischemic heart disease on the late survival of patients after surgery for carotid occlusive disease.

CLINICAL EVALUATION PRIOR TO PERIPHERAL VASCULAR SURGERY

Given the high prevalence of coronary artery disease in patients presenting with surgical vascular disease, a careful clinical history focusing on the presence, pattern, and severity of symptoms consistent with ischemic heart disease is an essential component of the preoperative evaluation. The history should provide information regarding the degree of functional limitation due to angina pectoris, details of previous coronary events such as myocardial infarction, and any symptoms of congestive heart failure or arrhythmias. However, owing to the nature of this surgical population, an accurate assessment of functional limitation due to ischemic heart disease may be difficult to obtain, for a variety of reasons. The physical activity of the patient with vascular disease may be severely limited by symptoms of peripheral arterial insufficiency, advanced age, general infirmity, or cardiovascular deconditioning. Long-standing diabetes mellitus, which is very strongly associated with both peripheral vascular and coronary heart disease, may mask or totally conceal the typical symptoms of angina and even myocardial infarction in 20 to 30 percent of patients. As discussed below, further stress testing is often necessary for preoperative risk stratification in such patients. Again, careful attention to the patient's functional limitation from the standpoint of both cardiovascular and noncardiovascular disease is an essential aspect of the decision to pursue either physiologic (exercise) or nonphysiologic stress testing.

The cardiovascular physical examination is the initial step in the identification of hemodynamically significant valvular heart disease. It is most important to recognize severe aortic or mitral stenosis. Severe aortic stenosis constrains cardiac output, markedly increases left ventricular afterload, and in conjunction with increased oxygen demand can cause significant myocardial ischemia. Both severe aortic and mitral stenosis may predispose the patient to precipitous perioperative hypotension due to fixed afterload and preload, respectively. Careful observation of changes in intravascular volume status, best guided by invasive hemodynamic monitoring, is indicated to prevent the development of acute pulmonary edema in such patients. Physical examination may also detect significant left ventricular dysfunction, although the correlation between clinical signs of left ventricular failure and quantitative assessment of left ventricular ejection fraction is far from ideal.

On the basis of the clinical evaluation, a multifactorial cardiac risk index was developed by Goldman and colleagues in an attempt to quantitate the potential cardiac risk of general noncardiac surgery. In descending order of importance, variables independently predictive of perioperative outcome were the following: evidence of congestive heart failure on examination (S_3 gallop, elevated jugular venous pressure), preoperative myocardial infarction within 6 months, arrhythmia other than sinus with atrial ectopy or more than five ventricular premature contractions per minute, age over 70 years, emergency operation, significant aortic stenosis by examination, poor general medical status, and type of operation (intraperitoneal, intrathoracic, or aortoiliac). Although the Goldman cardiac risk index has been validated prospectively for general surgical procedures, it should be emphasized that it was derived from a general surgical population with a low prevalence (less than 10 percent) of symptomatic coronary disease with a minority of patients (16 percent) undergoing vascular procedures.

Applying the Goldman cardiac risk index to patients undergoing aortoiliac vascular surgery (in whom the prevalence of coronary disease is high) has been found by other investigators to underestimate substantially the risk of a perioperative cardiac event. Other clinical cardiac risk indices derived from populations with a higher prevalence of ischemic and other cardiac disorders await prospective validation. Although useful in developing a systematic approach to the preoperative evaluation of the patient, currently available clinical cardiac risk indices are of limited value in risk stratification of the vascular surgical population.

LABORATORY EVALUATION PRIOR TO PERIPHERAL VASCULAR SURGERY

In the contemporary practice of medicine, the cost-effective use of laboratory testing is receiving increasing emphasis. Selective and judicious testing of patients should likewise be employed in an attempt to identify potentially high-cardiac-risk patients before vascular surgery.

Resting Electrocardiography

Although the cost effectiveness of routine 12-lead electrocardiography (ECG) before general noncardiac surgery has been appropriately questioned, it is still useful and indicated before vascular surgery. Resting ECG abnormalities such as left ventricular hypertrophy, ischemic repolarization changes, and particularly Q-wave myocardial infarction have been shown by some investigators to be predictive of perioperative cardiac events. More important, the ECG finding of Q-wave myocardial infarction may direct the identification of significant occult left ventricular dysfunction by noninvasive imaging or the need for stress testing, especially in patients with diabetes mellitus. A baseline preoperative ECG is particularly helpful for future comparison with tracings obtained in the early postoperative state, which may provide the first clue to ongoing (and often otherwise clinically silent) myocardial ischemia.

Echocardiography

Two-dimensional and Doppler echocardiography is indicated to assess patients suspected of having hemodynamically significant mitral and especially aortic stenosis. The detection of such valvular lesions does not automatically imply a need for cardiac surgery or balloon valvuloplasty; this decision depends on the severity of the lesion, presence of symptoms, degree of functional limitation, age, and overall "viability" of the individual patient. However, such findings should at least indicate the need for perioperative hemodynamic monitoring for optimization of left ventricular filling pressures, for guiding fluid balance, and for preload and afterload reduction therapy. The identification of severe mitral or aortic regurgitation in the preoperative setting has variable implications, but is important when associated with significant left ventricular dysfunction and especially clinical congestive heart failure.

The value of assessing resting left ventricular function by two-dimensional echocardiography in the setting of coronary artery disease is not well defined. This technique generally clearly demonstrates the severity of segmental left ventricular dysfunction and offers an estimation of global systolic performance by determination of ejection fraction, but has not been studied systematically for preoperative risk stratification. Some investigators have suggested that the resting left ventricular ejection fraction by radionuclide angiography is predictive of perioperative cardiac events complicating vascular surgery. As discussed below, however, other studies have shown that the degree of functional cardiovascular limitation on exercise radionuclide angiography is a much better predictor of "hard" perioperative events (myocardial infarction or death) and is independent of resting left ventricular ejection fraction.

Exercise Stress Testing

The degree of functional cardiovascular limitation can often be estimated from a thorough clinical history in patients who are not limited by the symptoms and sequelae of cerebrovascular or peripheral vascular disease. If feasible, exercise stress testing is indicated if the patient's functional capacity is unclear by clinical history, particularly in the presence of diabetes mellitus, which may obscure symptoms of ischemia. Patients with overt coronary disease manifested by symptoms of stable angina, previous myocardial infarction, and/or symptoms of ischemic left ventricular dysfunction likewise usually warrant further investigation with exercise stress testing.

Several studies employing exercise ECG have demonstrated that if the patient can exercise to an adequate workload, generally 5 METS or more or achievement of over 75 percent of maximal predicted heart rate, the risk of a significant perioperative cardiac event is reasonably low (approximately 2 to 5 percent), even if the test is positive for ischemia.

Using the more sophisticated technique of exercise radionuclide angiography, other investigators have similarly shown that the exercise workload is the most important independent predictor of perioperative cardiac outcome during vascular surgery. In one Mayo Clinic study, all significant perioperative cardiac events (myocardial infarction, cardiac arrest, or death) occurred in patients unable to exercise to 400 kg-m per minute (4.5 METs for a 70-kg patient). Multiple variables of resting and peak exercise global and segmental left ventricular function, even when positive for ischemia, failed to independently predict perioperative outcome.

The consensus of available studies suggests that the achievement of an adequate functional aerobic capacity on exercise stress testing, in general 5 METs or more, is associated with an acceptably low risk of cardiac mortality and morbidity during vascular surgery. Selected active and nondiabetic patients routinely exceeding physical exertion at this level without cardiovascular symptoms in their daily activity may not require preoperative stress testing to achieve clearance for surgery. If any doubt remains after the initial clinical assessment, the clinician should consider objective functional assessment with stress testing in patients preoperatively, and certainly at some time for long-term prognostication.

Nonphysiologic Stress Testing

In a significant proportion of patients presenting for vascular surgery, physical activity is limited by the symptoms or complications of peripheral arterial insufficiency, or by a variety of neurologic, orthopedic, and other medical factors. In this group of patients, exercise stress testing usually is not possible, and if attempted, leads to inadequate and inconclusive results.

Dipyridamole thallium scintigraphy has been the most thoroughly investigated nonphysiologic stress test before vascular surgery. With this technique, intravenous dipyridamole induces coronary artery vasodilatation, resulting in increased perfusion to myocardium in the distribution of nonstenotic vessels but reduced perfusion in myocardium supplied by stenotic vessels with limited flow reserve. The resultant heterogeneity in coronary blood flow is reflected by differences in segmental myocardial thallium uptake, which result in reversible "redistribution" defects immediately after dipyridamole infusion, with subsequent resolution on delayed imaging 4 to 6 hours later. Such thallium redistribution defects are consistent with myocardial ischemia secondary to dipyridamole-induced hypoperfusion. Thallium defects that are unchanged on delayed imaging are termed "fixed," and imply myocardial infarction, although a significant minority may demonstrate a partial redistribution upon imaging 24 to 72 hours after dipyridamole infusion with repeat thallium injection after initial imaging.

Preoperative risk stratification analysis by multiple investigators has generally shown that dipyridamole thallium scintigraphy demonstrating no redistribution or even "fixed" perfusion defects (consistent with previous infarction but not ischemia) essentially ensures a low perioperative cardiac risk with a high negative predictive value of approximately 95 to 98 percent. However, the positive predictive value of redistribution on dipyridamole thallium scintigraphy for a perioperative ischemic event is low, consistently in the range of only 30 percent. Since at least two-thirds of patients who are positive for redistribution have an uncomplicated perioperative course, attention has been focused on the potential to further stratify these patients by level of risk.

Quantitative analysis of the severity and extent of thallium redistribution, the development of ischemic ECG changes, and angina with dipyridamole infusion all may be useful in identifying the patient at potentially high risk for ischemic events. Eagle and colleagues showed that the predictive value of dipyridamole thallium scintigraphy is improved if used in conjunction with several clinical variables before vascular surgery. On multivariate analysis, these investigators found the following preoperative clinical parameters to be predictive of an adverse postoperative cardiac event (unstable angina, ischemic pulmonary congestion, myocardial infarction, or death): Q-wave myocardial infarction on ECG, a history of angina pectoris, history of ventricular ectopy requiring medical therapy, diabetes mellitus, and age over 70 years; congestive heart failure was a univariate predictor of outcome. Patients with none of the above clinical variables had an acceptably low incidence (3 percent) of perioperative events compared with a high incidence (50 percent) in the small group of patients having three or more variables, regardless of the results of dipyridamole thallium imaging. Further preoperative risk stratification was most effective in patients at intermediate risk (one or two clinical variables) in that patients without dipyridamole-induced thallium redistribution had low risk (3 percent) compared with a tenfold higher risk (30 percent) with thallium redistribution. Nonetheless, other investigators have suggested that thallium scintigraphic parameters remain the strongest predictors of subsequent ischemic events in the analysis of study populations as a whole.

Dipyridamole thallium scintigraphy is not widely available, and although it is generally safe, there is an approximately 5 percent incidence of hypotension during dipyridamole infusion, which may increase the risk of the procedure in patients with symptomatic cerebrovascular disease. An alternative noninvasive assessment before vascular surgery using 24- to 48-hour ambulatory ECG monitoring has been described. Raby and colleagues found that the absence of preoperative myocardial ischemia, defined as 1 mm or more ST-segment depression persisting for 60 seconds or more, had a very high negative predictive value (over 99 percent) for absence of perioperative cardiac complications. However, as in the case with dipyridamole thallium scintig-raphy, ischemia or ambulatory ECG had a relatively low positive predictive value (38 percent). Although ischemia was the most significant predictor of postoperative cardiac events in this study, the relatively low positive predictive value raises the unresolved issues of how to further evaluate and manage patients with a positive test effectively. Moreover, baseline ST-T abnormalities such as those associated with bundle branch block, left ventricular hypertrophy, or digitalis therapy exclude approximately 10 percent of patients from accurate analysis by this technique.

Employing continuous two-dimensional echocardiography for analysis of segmental left ventricular contraction during incremental infusion of dobutamine, dobutamine echocardiography offers another alternative for nonphysiologic stress testing. Preliminary studies suggest promise for this technique as a predictor of perioperative cardiac outcome. This method may be limited by adequacy of endocardial definition for regional wall motion analysis, and rarely by arrhythmias induced by high dobutamine infusion rates. Other potential techniques for nonphysiologic stress testing include atrial pacing with either two-dimensional echocardiographic or nuclear imaging, and intravenous adenosine thallium scintigraphy. These methods are currently under various phases of investigation and await validation as a means of risk stratification before vascular surgery.

STRATEGIES FOR EVALUATION AND MANAGEMENT

Preoperative evaluation of the patient before vascular surgery can be difficult. Owing to the multitude of potential complicating factors that may be encountered in any given patient, algorithms outlining specific approaches can serve only as guidelines, and for the individual patient flexibility should be the watchword. The best approach to evaluation and subsequent management must take into account many factors, including the age and life style of the patient, the comorbidity of associated medical conditions and the magnitude and urgency of the intended vascular surgical procedure itself. Subjective clinical judgment is important and inescapable, but must be individualized to the patient.

There is a complex interplay of impact between coronary and peripheral vascular disease. Patients with both symptomatic coronary and peripheral vascular disease are at significant long-term cardiac risk with medical therapy alone, and the greater the ischemic compromise from coronary disease, the more are the potential benefits of coronary bypass surgery. Nonetheless, with advanced age and peripheral vascular disease, the morbidity and mortality rates associated with coronary bypass surgery are increased and the long-term results are less favorable. Peripheral vascular surgery is not in itself an indication for coronary artery bypass; the decision for coronary revascularization should be made on its own merits, particularly regarding its potential impact on long-term prognosis. However, the timing of coronary artery bypass surgery remains dependent on the severity and stability of the concomitant vascular disease and the magnitude of the intended vascular surgical intervention.

In view of the current availability and utility of exercise and nonphysiologic stress testing, routine coronary angiography before vascular surgery is no longer necessary or indicated as the sole means of identifying potentially high-risk cardiac patients. This approach has been advocated in the past to guide preoperative "prophylactic" coronary bypass surgery, which has been suggested as a way to minimize cardiac risk for vascular as well as general noncardiac surgical procedures. Although this may be the case, it has become increasingly evident that coronary bypass surgery in patients with severe vascular disease carries a significant mortality and morbidity rate in itself that, although justified in some patients, has the potential to outweigh the risks of vascular surgery alone in others. Moreoover, there have been no controlled, randomized studies to investigate this issue. Even in tertiary care centers, the current mortality for coronary bypass surgery in patients 65 years of age or more may range from 1 to 5 percent, which probably exceeds the mortality rate of even abdominal aortic aneurysm repair in active asymptomatic patients. Percutaneous transluminal coronary angioplasty (PTCA) may be an attractive alternative to surgical revascularization but is not without risk, particularly when severe vascular disease impedes intravascular access to the coronary circulation. In the setting of multivessel coronary disease, PTCA is associated with approximately a 0.5 to 4 percent risk of nonfatal myocardial infarction, need for emergent coronary bypass surgery, or even death. The widespread applicability of PTCA in patients with diffuse vascular and coronary disease remains to be determined.

A careful clinical evaluation, based on history and physical examination, is an essential initial step in the preoperative cardiac evaluation. Information thus gained is used to direct the need and nature of further noninvasive testing, particularly stress testing, or need for coronary angiography. On the basis of the clinical evaluation, the patient can be preliminarily estimated to be at low, intermediate, or high risk from ischemic heart disease (Table 1).

High-Clinical-Risk Patients

Patients with significant symptoms of ischemic heart disease, e.g., angina with only mild activity or unstable coronary syndromes such as crescendo or postinfarction angina, are at significant risk for an adverse cardiac event even without antecedent noncardiac surgery. Provided that patients are potential candidates for coronary revascularization, proceeding directly to coronary angiography is indicated in anticipation of coronary artery bypass surgery or PTCA before consideration of any elective vascular surgical procedure. Patients with multiple clinical risk factors (Table 1) and significant cardiovascular functional limitation should also be considered for coronary angiography. Despite advanced age (70 years or more) being a clinical risk factor, this more aggressive approach should be aimed particularly at the "younger" middle-aged vascular patient who may derive the greatest long-term benefit. Patients with ischemic left ventricular dysfunction, even with only mild ongoing angina, also usually warrant coronary angiography with the intent of coronary revascularization in those with multivessel disease. The results of randomized trials of coronary artery bypass surgery versus medical therapy substantiate this approach.

If unstable coronary disease complicates unstable peripheral vascular (especially cerebrovascular) disease, a combined surgical procedure is most often indicated and can be performed in most experienced centers without prohibitive risk. In selected patients with relatively localized coronary disease, coronary revascularization with PTCA or other intravascular modalities may be possible, followed in short sequence by vascular surgery at an acceptable cardiac risk.

In patients who are not candidates for coronary angiography (often because of severe multifactorial

Table 1 Preoperative Cardiac Evaluation

Low Clinical Risk	Intermediate Clinical Risk	High Clinical Risk
Active and asymptomatic No clinical cardiac risk factors*	Variably active Cardiac functional limitation unclear by history Some cardiac risk factors* with clinically evident coronary disease	Unstable coronary syndromes Severe CHF Multiple clinical risk factors*
	Perioperative risk increased with Urgent operation Magnitude of operation (aortic aneurysm repair) Complicating medical disease(s)	

*Age > 70, angina pectoris, history of myocardial infarction, congestive heart failure (CHF), diabetes mellitus, ventricular ectopy requiring medical therapy.
Eagle KA et al. Combining clinical and thallium data optimizes preoperative assessment of cardiac risk before major vascular surgery. Ann Intern Med 1989; 110:859–866.

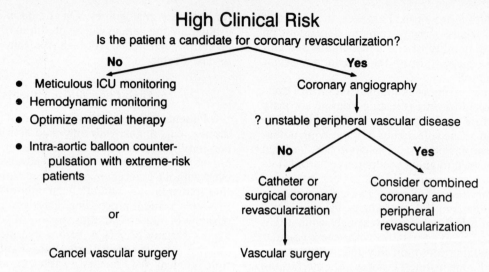

Figure 1 Preoperative cardiac evaluation before vascular surgery for the high-risk patient.

illness combined with extreme age) or who are found to have diffuse coronary disease not amenable to revascularization by either surgery or intravascular techniques, it may be decided to cancel elective vascular surgery altogether. If vascular surgery is to be pursued, intensive medical management will help minimize the otherwise high potential cardiac morbidity and mortality (Fig. 1).

Although the role of perioperative hemodynamic monitoring has not yet been investigated in a controlled, randomized fashion, the overwhelming impression is that such monitoring in conjunction with meticulous intensive care unit observation may significantly reduce the incidence of perioperative myocardial infarction and death. This technique permits optimization of left ventricular filling pressure and systolic performance with medical therapy in the setting of left ventricular dysfunction with or without significant valvular heart disease. Intravenous infusion of nitroglycerin or a beta-antagonist (e.g., esmolol) may be required for control of symptoms of myocardial ischemia or to maximize myocardial protection on an empiric basis. Combinations of intravenous inotropic, vasodilator, and diuretic therapy are effective for the preoperative treatment of refractory left ventricular failure and should be guided by invasive hemodynamic monitoring. Hemodynamic monitoring is indicated in patients with high-risk ischemic heart disease, clinically significant left ventricular failure, severe asymptomatic aortic or mitral stenosis, or emergency surgery. The threshold for hemodynamic monitoring should be lower in patients undergoing vascular surgery with anticipated major intra- and postoperative physiologic derangements, e.g., abdominal or thoracoabdominal aneurysm repair. Intraaortic balloon counterpulsation initiated preoperatively has been reported to be effective in patients at extreme cardiac risk undergoing abdominal aortic aneurysm repair, but clearly carries an increased risk of multiple complications in patients with diffuse atherosclerotic vascular disease. Transesophageal two-

dimensional echocardiographic monitoring of segmental left ventricular dysfunction may also be sensitive for early detection of intraoperative myocardial ischemia and identification of patients at risk for adverse perioperative cardiac events.

Oral medical therapy for ischemic heart disease with long-acting nitrates, beta-antagonists, or calcium channel blockers should be titrated incrementally as the patient tolerates to optimize parameters of myocardial oxygen expenditure. Therapy for left ventricular failure with diuretics and afterload-reducing agents, i.e., angiotensin converting enzyme (ACE) inhibitors, should be aggressive but with the avoidance of hypovolemia and hypotension. Medical therapy not only for ischemic heart disease, but also for hypertension, congestive heart failure, and arrhythmia, should be maintained as continuously as possible before and after surgery. Even temporary discontinuation of therapy may lead to rebound myocardial ischemia, severe hypertension, or exacerbation of arrhythmias.

In the high-risk cardiac patient, invasive hemodynamic monitoring must be accompanied by close and conscientious postoperative observation in the intensive care unit. The symptoms of perioperative myocardial infarction are frequently obscured by postoperative pain and the effects of sedative and analgesic drugs; hence, most perioperative myocardial infarctions are clinically unrecognized until complicated by congestive heart failure, arrhythmia, or even death. Myocardial ischemia can be further exacerbated by high sympathetic autonomic output in the setting of postoperative pain, anemia, multifactorial respiratory insufficiency, and significant extra- to intravascular volume redistribution. Correspondingly, most perioperative myocardial infarctions occur within the first 72 hours postoperatively and usually by the sixth postoperative day.

The mortality rate of perioperative myocardial infarction is high (30 to 50 percent) and delayed diagnosis is probably a contributory factor. Serial ECG

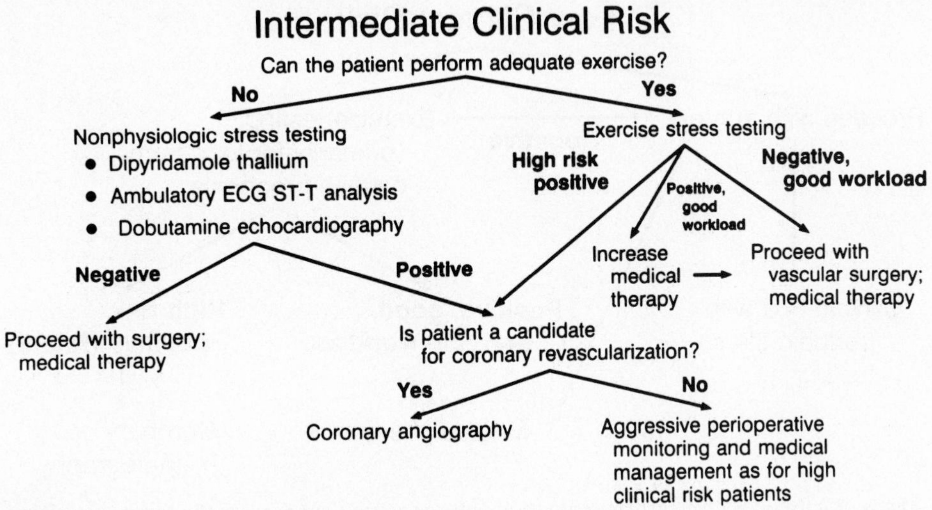

Intermediate Clinical Risk

Figure 2 Preoperative cardiac evaluation before vascular surgery for the intermediate-risk patient.

and creatine kinase enzyme determinations with MB isoenzyme analysis are recommended during the first 3 postoperative days in patients with potentially high-risk ischemic heart disease. Any symptoms suggestive of myocardial ischemia should be promptly evaluated. If perioperative myocardial ischemia or infarction is suspected, analysis of regional left ventricular dysfunction by bedside two-dimensional echocardiography or radionuclide angiography is useful to assess myocardium at risk. In the setting of significant segmental myocardial dysfunction with ongoing myocardial ischemia, acute intervention with coronary angiography and PTCA of the infarct-related artery is often the best approach. Thrombolytic therapy for acute myocardial infarction is not an option in the early postoperative period. Irrespective of any acute invasive intervention, standard therapy for acute myocardial ischemia or infarction should be instituted with aspirin, intravenous heparin (if permitted by the surgeon), intravenous nitroglycerin, and beta-antagonist therapy. Continuous ECG monitoring should be maintained with suppressive antidysrhythmic therapy given for complex ventricular ectopy.

Intermediate-Clinical-Risk Patients

Patients at intermediate cardiac risk (Table 1) for vascular surgery generally have clinically evident ischemic heart disease, but with stable symptoms and little functional disability. Patients with unclear functional cardiovascular limitation by history owing to sedentary life style or limitation by vascular or other noncardiac disease may also be at intermediate risk. The presence of some clinical risk factors such as advanced age, a history of stable angina or congestive heart failure, and especially long-standing diabetes mellitus furthermore necessitates further risk stratification by stress testing, as for all patients clinically assessed to be at intermediate cardiac risk (Fig. 2).

In patients able to perform adequate exercise, symptom-limited exercise stress testing should be undertaken. If the study is negative or even mildly positive at an adequate work load (5 to 6 METs or more), vascular surgery can be pursued with an acceptably low risk (5 percent or less) provided that medical therapy is continued or augmented as indicated. Patients with a high-risk positive exercise test (early onset or prolonged ischemic symptoms or ECG changes, exercise-induced hypotension, or extensive ischemia on noninvasive imaging) should proceed to coronary angiography if deemed appropriate candidates for potential coronary revascularization. If this is not an option, cancellation of elective vascular surgery should be considered rather than proceeding with vascular surgery employing the management and precautions outlined for high-risk patients.

If the patient is unable to exercise, nonphysiologic stress testing using dipyridamole thallium scintigraphy, ambulatory ECG ST-T analysis, or dobutamine echocardiography should be pursued.

Low-Clinical-Risk Patients

Physically active, nondiabetic, and relatively young (65 years of age or less) patients with no clinical history of cardiac disease have an acceptably low (3 percent or less) risk of a significant perioperative cardiac event with vascular surgery (Table 1). It is unlikely that routine screening with exercise or nonphysiologic stress testing solely to ascertain perioperative risk is justified in this low-risk population. Even if stress testing is mildly positive for ischemia, the vast majority of these active and asymptomatic patients can proceed without further investigation to vascular surgery without prohibitive risk, with medical therapy only and careful postoperative clinical monitoring (Fig. 3).

Associated coronary disease is highly prevalent in

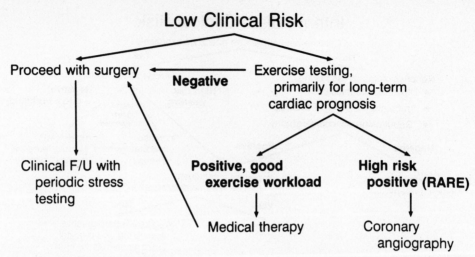

Figure 3 Preoperative cardiac evaluation before vascular surgery for the low-risk patient.

patients presenting with vascular disease and has a major impact on survival, especially that of middle-aged patients after vascular surgery. Thus, although routine stress testing is not mandatory for preoperative clearance of this subset of clinically low-risk patients, it is indicated at some time postoperatively and periodically during follow-up for assessment of long-term cardiac prognosis.

DISCUSSION

Continued advances in the practice of contemporary anesthesiology and vascular surgery, in addition to those in cardiovascular therapeutics and postoperative care, have contributed to the apparent decline in cardiac morbidity and mortality associated with vascular surgery.

A careful clinical cardiovascular evaluation with a high index of suspicion for associated coronary artery disease provides the foundation for effective risk stratification of the patient before vascular surgery. From this, judicious laboratory testing can further identify those patients in need of further preoperative cardiac intervention or intensive perioperative monitoring and medical management.

Through the concerted efforts of the medical consultant, anesthesiologist, and surgeon, cardiac morbidity and mortality rates can be minimized in patients undergoing vascular surgery.

SUGGESTED READING

Culter BS, Sheeler HB, Paraskos JA, Cardullo PA. Applicability and interpretation of electrocardiographic stress testing in patients with peripheral vascular disease. Am J Surg 1981; 141:501–506.

Eagle KA, Boucher CA. Cardiac risk of noncardiac surgery (editorial). N Engl J Med 1989; 321:1330–1332.

Eagle KA, Coley CM, Newell JB, et al. Combining clinical and thallium data optimizes preoperative assessment of cardiac risk before major vascular surgery. Ann Intern Med 1989; 110:859–866.

Foster ED, Davis KB, Carpenter JA, et al. Risk of noncardiac operation in patients with defined coronary disease: the Coronary Artery Surgery Study (CASS) Registry experience. Ann Thorac Surg 1986; 41:42–49.

Freeman WK, Gersh BJ, Gloviczki P. Abdominal aortic aneurysm and coronary artery disease: frequent companions but an uneasy relationship (editorial). J Vasc Surg 1990; 12:73–77.

Freeman WK, Gibbons RJ, Shub C. Preoperative assessment of cardiac patients undergoing noncardiac surgical procedures. Mayo Clin Proc 1989; 64:1105–1117.

Gersh BJ, Rihal CS, Rooke TW, Ballard DJ. Evaluation and management of patients with both peripheral vascular and coronary artery disease. J Am Coll Cardiol 1991 (in press).

Goldman L, Caldera DL, Nussbaum SR, et al. Multifactorial index of cardiac risk in noncardiac surgical procedures. N Engl J Med 1977; 297:845–850.

Hertzer NR. Basic data concerning associated coronary disease in peripheral vascular patients. Ann Vasc Surg 1987; 1:616–620.

Hertzer NR, Beven EG, Young JR, et al. Coronary artery disease in peripheral vascular patients. A classification of 1000 coronary angiograms and results of surgical management. Ann Surg 1984; 199:223–233.

Mangano DT. Perioperative cardiac morbidity. Anesthesiology 1990; 72:153–184.

Raby KE, Goldman L, Creager MA, et al. Correlation between preoperative ischemia and major cardiac events after peripheral vascular surgery. N Engl J Med 1989; 321:1296–1300.

Rao TLK, Jacobs KH, El-Etr AA. Reinfarction following anesthesia in patients with myocardial infarction. Anesthesiology 1983; 59: 499–505.

Reigel MM, Hollier LH, Kazmier FJ, et al. Late survival in abdominal aortic aneurysm patients: the role of selective myocardial revascularization on the basis of clinical symptoms. J Vasc Surg 1987; 5:222–227.

Roger VL, Ballard DJ, Hallett JW Jr, et al. Influence of coronary artery disease on morbidity and mortality after abdominal aortic aneurysmectomy: a population-based study, 1971–1987. J Am Coll Cardiol 1989; 14:1245–1252.

Young JR, Hertzer NR, Beven EG, et al. Coronary artery disease in patients with aortic aneurysm: a classification of 302 coronary angiograms and results of surgical management. Ann Vasc Surg 1986; 1:36–42.

CHRONIC ARTERIAL OCCLUSIVE DISEASE: SURGERY

THOMAS C. NASLUND, M.D.
WILLIAM M. MOORE Jr., M.D.
LARRY H. HOLLIER, M.D., F.A.C.S.

Chronic arterial occlusive disease of the lower extremities most commonly results from progressive atherosclerosis, as described in previous chapters. Treatment is generally directed toward modification of atherosclerotic risk factors, and efforts to increase blood flow to the distal extremity. As previously described, cessation of tobacco use and control of hypertension, diabetes, and hyperlipidemia can all be accomplished by a combination of dietary modification, pharmacologic intervention, and life style changes. These modifications can frequently retard the progression of atherosclerotic occlusive disease of the lower extremities. Increased collateral blood flow and/or physiologic adaptation can be induced by an exercise program for the patient with intermittent claudication (see the chapter *Chronic Arterial Occlusive Disease: Exercise Rehabilitation*). Patients with cardiac dysfunction may also benefit from optimization of cardiac performance, which enhances distal perfusion. However, when such efforts fail to achieve the desired clinical effect, operative intervention must be considered.

INDICATIONS FOR OPERATIVE TREATMENT

Claudication is the most common symptom of chronic peripheral arterial occlusive disease, but by no means should claudication alone be considered an indication for either arteriography or operative intervention. Claudication is exercise-induced pain within a muscle group that is completely relieved with rest and has therefore been referred to by some authors as "functional ischemia." Claudication is frequently associated with occlusion of an isolated arterial segment, such as the iliac or superficial femoral artery (SFA); less commonly, multiple, hemodynamically significant stenoses can produce identical symptoms. Noninvasive evaluation of the arterial supply to the lower extremities frequently locates the level of such occlusions or stenoses. Nonoperative measures with intermittent follow-up is frequently sufficient treatment, since claudication seldom impairs the patient's life style. However, if the previously described nonoperative therapeutic measures fail and claudication continues to interfere with gainful employment or quality of life, angiographic evaluation should be undertaken and operative treatment considered.

The development of ischemic rest pain is indicative of more severe ischemia and is usually associated with arterial occlusion at two or more levels. In contrast to claudication, ischemic rest pain is an indication for angiographic evaluation and consideration of surgery. Ischemic rest pain is frequently improved by placing the limb in a dependent position.

Ischemic rest pain indicates that distal perfusion is inadequate to meet the metabolic demands of the extremity and requires prompt evaluation and treatment. Further impairment of perfusion in these patients may result in tissue or limb loss if untreated. Untreated patients presenting with claudication have an eventual amputation rate of approximately 5 percent, whereas those presenting with rest pain have amputation rates of 20 percent or higher if untreated. This high risk of tissue loss requires timely intervention for patients with ischemic rest pain.

Occasionally, patients with known claudication progress rapidly to limb-threatening ischemia if the distal extremity is compromised by infection or trauma, which can render the arterial supply inadequate to meet the increased metabolic demands required by these circumstances. In these patients, healing is impaired and necrosis frequently occurs unless additional perfusion is provided.

A nonhealing ulcer on an ischemic extremity may lead to amputation if infection supervenes. Vascular bypass to facilitate healing of an ulcer may prevent amputation, provided that the extremity is protected from further injury. Meticulous foot care must be a lifelong commitment for such patients, because subsequent injury to the foot, with or without a patent graft, can result in another nonhealing wound and the potential risk of limb loss.

Patients with diabetes mellitus and chronic occlusive arterial disease represent a challenging problem for the vascular surgeon. The term "small vessel disease" has frequently been used to describe the pathology observed in patients with diabetic vasculopathy. Unfortunately, some physicians have been taught that this type of vasculopathy is not amenable to operative treatment and therefore do not refer such patients to vascular surgeons. In reality, diabetics develop atherosclerotic changes in both large and small vessels. Also, medial calcinosis occurs quite often in diabetic patients and impairs the ability to assess distal blood flow accurately on the basis of pulse volume recordings or ankle-brachial indices (ABIs). The distribution of disease affects the profunda, popliteal, and tibial arteries, all of which can be approached with standard vascular surgical procedures. Diabetic patients with ongoing ischemia and nonhealing ulcers or distal infections must be treated aggressively if limb salvage is to be expected. Such treatment frequently includes balloon angioplasty or vascular bypass.

PREOPERATIVE EVALUATION AND PREPARATION

Preoperative cardiac assessment is imperative for patients with atherosclerotic occlusive disease of the lower extremities, owing to the high prevalence of significant coronary artery disease in these patients (see the chapter *Chronic Arterial Occlusive Disease: Preoperative Evaluation*). Uncompensated congestive heart failure is a relative contraindication to operations for occlusive disease both because of cardiac risk and because of the effect heart failure may have on inflow to a bypass graft. Heart failure should be treated before elective surgery for ischemia is considered, and in fact cardiac optimization occasionally obviates the need for an operation by improving collateral blood flow.

Examination of the saphenous veins is mandatory for patients undergoing lower extremity vascular operations. When veins cannot be seen or palpated, duplex mapping can be of great benefit in order to assess the size of the vein preoperatively. Lesser saphenous and arm veins can likewise be mapped.

All our patients undergoing lower extremity procedures for occlusive disease receive a minimal noninvasive evaluation of ankle-brachial pressure ratio and Doppler waveforms. These measures document the preoperative condition and are useful in assessing graft patency after reconstruction. In diabetics, we also obtain a magnetic resonance flowmeter assessment (Metriflow) of extremity blood flow since, as mentioned, ankle pressure measurements are frequently invalid in diabetics. Angiography provides a visual record of the vascular anatomy and also the opportunity to perform simultaneous angioplasty for a short segment occlusion (see the chapter *Chronic Arterial Occlusive Disease: Percutaneous Interventional Treatment*). Percutaneous transluminal angioplasty is particularly successful in the common iliac arteries. Angioplasty can occasionally provide sufficient increase in blood flow to make immediate surgery unnecessary, or can satisfactorily improve inflow to allow a lower extremity bypass procedure without the need for concomitant iliac reconstruction. The hemodynamic significance of a lesion is occasionally difficult to identify with certainty on the angiogram, even with multiple views. This can be assessed at the time of angiography by measuring arterial blood pressure via the angiography catheter above and below the stenosis. A gradient more than 15 mm Hg is considered hemodynamically significant, and correction with angioplasty or bypass would be expected to improve distal blood flow. However, a stenosis that seems significant on inspection, but has a resting gradient of less than 15 mm Hg, may become significant at the higher flow rates induced by exercise. The physiologic significance of such lesions can be identified by measuring pressure gradients after intra-arterial injection of papaverine hydrochloride, which relaxes smooth muscle and dilates peripheral arteries, thereby increasing blood flow and unmasking hemodynamically significant stenoses.

Whereas the indication for intervention is made on the basis of clinical history, physical examination, and noninvasive vascular assessment, the type of intervention is determined by imaging studies. Collateral flow will fill patent distal vasculature, but it must be appreciated that delayed images are necessary, since flow through collaterals is slower than through native vessels. Using appropriate delayed films and digital subtraction techniques, we have rarely needed to resort to operative exploration and intraoperative angiography to define distal vasculature.

CHOICE OF PROCEDURE

Before distal revascularization is undertaken, it is imperative that satisfactory inflow be established. This is accomplished by optimizing cardiac function and confirming or re-establishing adequate aortoiliac flow.

Femoropopliteal Bypass

The anatomy demonstrated on the angiogram enables the appropriate procedure to be chosen. Short segment occlusions or stenoses may be treated with angioplasty techniques. Long stenoses or occlusions of the superficial femoral artery can be treated with femoropopliteal bypass. The proximal popliteal artery is frequently patent, filling by collateral flow from the profunda by way of the superior geniculate artery, and can be used as a site for the distal anastomosis. When the proximal popliteal artery is heavily calcified or stenotic, it is wise to perform the distal anastomosis below the knee. Careful examination of the angiogram for irregularities in the above-knee popliteal artery will alert the surgeon that atherosclerotic plaque exists, and unnecessary operative exposure of the above-knee popliteal artery can be avoided.

Femoropopliteal bypass can best be performed with saphenous vein or polytetrafluoroethylene (PTFE) grafts. Patency rates of vein and PTFE grafts appear relatively equal in the above-knee position. In below-knee femoropopliteal grafts, vein and PTFE have equal patency for the first 2 years, but thereafter PTFE carries an increased incidence of thrombosis. When vein grafts are used for femoropopliteal bypass, reversed or nonreversed grafts have similar patency; our preference, however, is for use of the nonreversed in situ vein graft for below-knee grafts.

Femorotibial Bypass

Femorotibial bypass is needed by patients with popliteal artery occlusion or stenosis. The tibioperoneal trunk is the preferred site of distal anastomosis when both posterior tibial and peroneal arteries are patent. Alternatively, the posterior tibial, anterior tibial, or peroneal artery can be used as the site of distal anastomosis.

Patients needing distal bypass may have no usable greater saphenous veins because of previous vein stripping, coronary bypass, or simply unsuitable vein quality. Such problems should always be suspected preoperatively either by physical examination or by duplex mapping. When greater saphenous veins are not available, vein can be obtained for more distal bypasses by bilateral lesser saphenous vein harvesting. Alternatively, the upper extremity can be used to harvest the cephalic or basilic veins. When the upper extremities may be needed for vein harvesting, it is prudent to establish central venous access preoperatively.

Segments of vein harvested from various sites can be combined as a composite and used for distal bypass. The use of PTFE and vein composites has been reported, but we have not been impressed with their long-term results. Certainly, if usable vein cannot be located, PTFE graft may be used for limb salvage, but long-term patency rates are reduced. Likewise, human umbilical vein and cryopreserved veins can be used but do not seem superior to PTFE. In any case, the use of umbilical vein grafts is discouraged because of a tendency to develop aneurysms. Occasionally, when autogenous vein is unavailable, a patient can be better served with amputation rather than bypass with a graft that has little chance of success.

Profundoplasty

The profunda femoris artery provides blood to the thigh, and when the superficial femoral artery is occluded, this artery also provides collateral flow to the popliteal and tibial vessels via the geniculate arteries and other unnamed collateral vessels. Atherosclerotic plaque at the origin of the profunda can compromise distal blood flow. Endarterectomy and/or patch angioplasty of this stenosis is generally considered during inflow operations for aortoiliac occlusive disease when there is coexistent superficial femoral artery occlusion. Occasionally, however, a hemodynamically significant stenosis of the proximal profunda treated by primary profundoplasty may avoid the need for a lower extremity bypass operation. The documentation of profunda to popliteal and tibial collaterals should be established preoperatively by angiography and noninvasive assessment with a profundopopliteal collateral index. The profundopopliteal collateral index can be calculated by the difference in above-knee and below-knee systolic pressure divided by the above-knee pressure. An index of less than 0.5 is suggestive of a favorable outcome from isolated profundoplasty.

Isolated profundoplasty is approached through a vertical groin incision, as for an aortofemoral graft but extended distally 5 to 10 cm. The common and superficial femoral arteries are dissected and the profunda is exposed by dividing the lateral circumflex femoral vein that crosses the profunda anteriorly. A length of profunda is exposed so that the distal extent of the plaque can be identified and later removed. Each branch of the exposed profunda is encircled with a vessel loop and the patient systemically heparinized. We frequently use an endarterectomized segment of the superficial femoral artery as a patch for the profunda arteriotomy. This can be accomplished by excision and endarterectomy of a segment of superficial femoral artery, or by endarterectomy of the proximal superficial femoral and incorporation onto the profunda without division of the

superficial femoral origin. The plaque within the profunda is endarterectomized under direct vision and gently teased from the orifices of the branches. Patch closure with endarterectomized superficial femoral artery completes the procedure (Fig. 1).

OPERATIVE TECHNIQUE

The patient is shaved from the umbilicus to the foot and prophylactic antibiotics are administered. In the supine position, general or regional anesthesia is administered and invasive monitoring devices are established based on the patient's overall cardiovascular status. The lower abdomen, groin, and entire lower extremity are scrubbed and painted with povidone-iodine (Betadine).

The incision is started in the groin, and the saphenous vein is identified at its junction with the femoral vein and followed distally by sequentially lengthening the incision. By first identifying the saphenofemoral junction, misidentification of the vein and a misplaced distal incision are avoided. After a vein suitable in both quality and length has been identified,

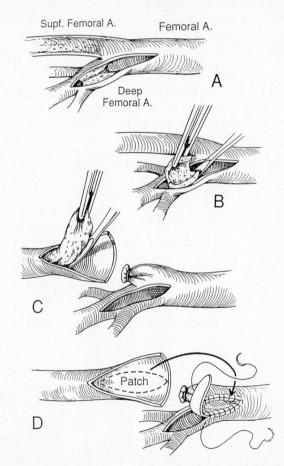

Figure 1 Sequential steps in performing profundoplasty. *A*, Arteriotomy extending throughout the length of diseased profunda. *B*, Endarterectomy. *C*, Resection and endarterectomy of the superficial femoral artery for a patch. *D*, Patch closure.

the points of arterial anastomosis are exposed. The common femoral is usually the point of the proximal anastomosis, and requires cephalad extension of the groin incision several centimeters above the inguinal ligament for adequate exposure and proximal control.

The site of the distal anastomosis is exposed via a medial approach for the above-knee or below-knee popliteal, tibioperoneal trunk, peroneal, and posterior tibial arteries. Approach to the anterior tibial artery is obtained laterally through the anterior compartment.

After exposure of the appropriate arteries, the vein is excised if a reversed or nonreversed-translocated graft is planned. Side branches of the saphenous vein are ligated with fine silk ties. The vein is hydrostatically dilated and placed in a subsartorial tunnel above or below the knee. If a translocated vein is used for an anterior tibial bypass, the tunnel is made subcutaneously across the thigh into the lateral leg incision used to expose the anterior tibial artery. After the development of the tunnel, the patient is heparinized with 100 units of sodium heparin per kilogram of body weight, administered intravenously.

When the in situ technique is used, the saphenous vein is transected at the level of the femoral vein and the latter is repaired with polypropylene suture. The first few vein side branches are ligated and divided so as to mobilize enough saphenous vein to permit anastomosis to the common femoral artery without tension. The transected end of the saphenous vein is everted, allowing direct excision of the first value cusp. Next, an end-to-side anastomosis is constructed with the common femoral artery, using a continuous polypropylene suture. This allows arterial pressure to be delivered to the vein graft while a side branch is entered distally with a valvulotome, and anterior and posterior leaflets of each

valve are destroyed by drawing the valvulotome distally (Fig. 2). The position of each valve is noted with a marking pen, since side branches are frequently adjacent to each valve. After destruction of all valves, pulsatile flow should be observed at the distal end of the graft and a pressure measurement may be obtained at this point. The distal segment of graft is mobilized (in the same manner as was the proximal segment) and a long end-to-side anastomosis created with the recipient native artery. Side branches can be identified and ligated by local dissection at the points of valve cusps, at any point where there is a palpable thrill, and by localization of a fistula with a hand-held Doppler while the distal graft is partially occluded. Every effort is made to locate all side branches. A completion arteriogram is performed in search of fistulas, retained valve cusps, and technical problems with the distal anastomosis and to verify outflow. The wounds are closed in layers with polyglycolic acid suture. Drains are not routinely used unless persistent diffuse bleeding is noted; if so, a soft, large-bore, closed suction drain can be utilized.

OTHER CAUSES OF LOWER EXTREMITY OCCLUSIVE DISEASE

Adventitial cystic disease of the popliteal artery is an uncommon but treatable cause of lower extremity ischemia, presenting most frequently in young men without other evidence of atherosclerotic disease. Calf claudication is the usual presenting symptom. The patient generally has normal distal pulses when the knee is extended, but an obvious pulse decrement appears with flexion of the knee. The diagnosis is frequently

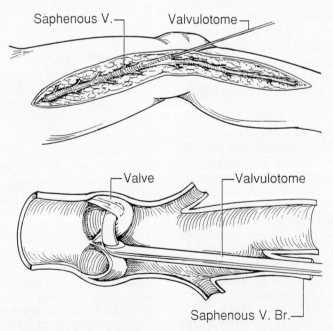

Figure 2 Destruction of venous valves with a valvulotome.

difficult to make preoperatively and may be discovered by ultrasonography or by noting a scimitar sign on angiography (Fig. 3). The exact cause of the cyst is unknown, but the cyst contents are very similar to synovial fluid or the contents of a ganglion cyst. The subadventitial cysts may occur in other arterial segments. Although some authors have reported successful treatment by cyst aspiration, the treatment of choice is cyst wall incision and drainage via a posterior approach (Fig. 4). Chronic compression of the popliteal artery, particularly during knee flexion, may result in thrombosis and occlusion, which requires bypass or interposition grafting. Percutaneous transluminal balloon angioplasty is not an effective mode of treatment and should be discouraged, since intimal rupture occurs with balloon inflation. In order for simple cyst incision and drainage (treatment of choice) to be performed, the intima must remain intact to ensure vascular integrity. Treatment after intimal disruption would therefore require bypass or interposition grafting (Fig. 5).

Popliteal artery entrapment by the medial head of the gastrocnemius muscle can produce claudication in a young patient that may be clinically similar to adventitial cystic disease of the popliteal artery (see the chapter *Other Vascular Compression and Entrapment Syndromes*). The popliteal artery can be trapped medial to the gastrocnemius or popliteus muscles, and this generally presents as claudication in a young patient. Suspicious signs are either absent pedal pulses or pedal pulses that diminish with forced dorsiflexion or plantar flexion of the foot in a patient with otherwise normal vascular examination. Color flow Doppler ultrasonography may show a thrombosed midpopliteal artery or changes in velocity of flow with plantar flexion and dorsiflexion of the foot.

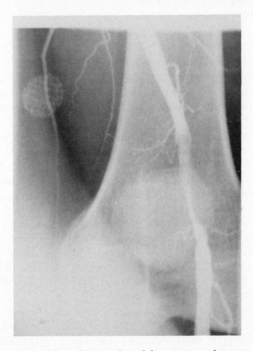

Figure 3 Scimitar sign produced from external compression of the arterial lumen.

Angiography may demonstrate an occlusion of the popliteal artery, medial deviation, or post-stenotic dilatation. Angiography with the feet dorsi- and plantar-flexed may demonstrate entrapment that is not apparent on routine views. Bilateral examination with angiography is needed because a contralateral lesion may be asymptomatic.

Treatment of popliteal entrapment consists of operative release of the muscular origin of the medial head of the gastrocnemius or popliteus muscles. This is easily accomplished by a posterior popliteal approach. If the popliteal artery contains an acute thrombus, it can be removed through a transverse arteriotomy with an embolectomy catheter. Vein graft bypass is the procedure of choice if the popliteal artery is chronically occluded.

POSTOPERATIVE CARE

Postoperative care is generally supportive; however, attention must be directed toward the cardiac and pulmonary status, because these systems are usually compromised in populations of patients with atherosclerotic arterial occlusive disease. We monitor all postoperative patients overnight in the recovery room to facilitate close observation and hourly neurovascular assessment. Pulses must be checked and the ABI recorded frequently in the recovery room and daily thereafter. Any deterioration of pulses or ABI raises the suspicion of graft thrombosis. Sheepskin boots are applied to the feet to cause vasodilation and enhance graft blood flow. Prophylactic antibiotics are continued for 24 hours after surgery. Patients are usually ambulating on the second postoperative day, and discharge from the hospital is generally determined by the patient's mobility and a satisfactory appearance of the wound.

COMPLICATIONS

Wound complications should be uncommon. Use of a vertical groin incision, ligation of lymphatics, and attention to good skin approximation will avoid many wound complications. Lymphatic leaks or lymphoceles are caused by disruption of lymphatics in the incision and can usually be successfully treated with bed rest, aspiration, and pressure dressings. Immediate reaccumulation of lymph is usually indicative of substantial lymphatic injury and should be treated by ligation under direct vision. Minor lymph leaks and lymphoceles usually respond to nonoperative measures. Wound infections require open drainage. If the graft is not exposed, healing should be expected. However, when prosthetic graft is exposed in a wound infection, reoperation with remote vascular reconstruction is indicated. The exception to this rule is when there is a limited length of PTFE graft exposed in an adequately drained wound remote from the anastomoses. These wounds frequently heal with systemic antibiotics and local wound care. However,

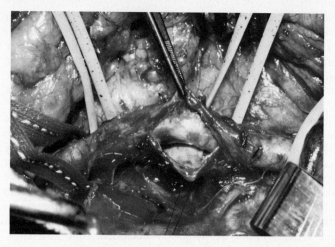

Figure 4 Incision and drainage of cyst contents.

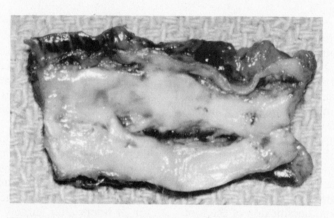

Figure 5 An intimal tear in the popliteal artery caused by balloon angioplasty. Repair required bypass grafting.

if the anastomosis is involved, expeditious intervention is indicated, with remote bypass through noninfected tissues. Exposed vein graft is a less severe problem. When the infection is caused by gram-positive cocci, exposed vein grafts should be treated with open wound care in anticipation of healing. Gram-negative wound infections with exposed vein grafts, however, seem to do poorly, with a high rate of anastomotic disruption.

Graft thrombosis can be diagnosed when there is loss of a peripheral pulse and reduction in the ABI. Graft thrombosis is treated by immediate thrombectomy, restoration of graft flow, and intraoperative angiography to identify any technical errors. Any such errors are corrected, but if none are found the wound is closed over a drain and the patient systemically heparinized for 3 days. Late graft thrombosis (at least 2 weeks postoperatively) can frequently be treated with intra-arterial urokinase, with lysis of the thrombus and diagnostic angiography to identify any technical errors or restenoses.

Wound hematomas may form from unrecognized bleeding postoperatively. They should be treated by operative evacuation, control of bleeding, and closed drainage. Nonoperative treatment of significant hematomas should be avoided, since graft compression and thrombosis, as well as hematoma infection, can occur.

Arteriovenous fistulas and retained valve cusps can occur when the in situ bypass technique is employed. Small asymptomatic fistulas identified postoperatively can be observed, because many thrombose spontaneously and others have no hemodynamic significance. However, when skin changes develop or progressive enlargement occurs, the fistulas can be localized with color flow Doppler and ligated. Retained valve cusps are usually brought to attention by graft thrombosis or reduction in the ABI. All retained valve cusps need reoperation with excision and patch repair of the vein graft, because leaving such an error untreated will contribute to later graft failure.

Swelling in the bypassed extremity is common and usually is due to division of lymphatics. However, the possibility of deep venous thrombosis must not be overlooked and venous duplex imaging should be obtained when this is suspected.

GRAFT FAILURE

Clinical outpatient follow-up is key in identifying significant intimal hyperplasia and progression of disease, the most common causes of late graft failure. By identifying a decrease in the ABI or changes in the velocity profile of the graft, suspicion of a stenosis is raised, and angiography can locate its site. Balloon angioplasty or operative vein patch angioplasty can alleviate localized graft stenosis and avoid later graft occlusion. All patients are counseled on the need to return immediately if ischemic symptoms return, since thrombosed grafts frequently can be opened with intra-arterial urokinase in the first 2 weeks after thrombosis.

Chronic graft thrombosis is not responsive to intra-arterial urokinase and requires re-evaluation prior to a second bypass operation. The possibility of inadequate inflow, cardiac function, or outflow must be considered as possible reasons for graft failure. In addition, complete coagulation studies are warranted in these patients, including measurement of levels of anti-thrombin III, protein C, and protein S.

SUGGESTED READING

Berguer R, Cotton LT, Sabri S. Extended deep femoral angioplasty. Br Med J 1973; 1:469–471.

Flanigan DP, Burnham SJ, Goodreau JJ, Bergan JJ. Summary of cases of adventitial cystic disease of the popliteal artery. Ann Surg 1979; 189:165–175.

Flinn WR, Rohrer MJ, Yao JST, et al. Long-term patency of infragenicular polytetrafluoroethylene grafts. J Vasc Surg 1984; 54:283–287.

Leather RP, Shah DM, Karmody AM. Infrapopliteal arterial bypass for limb salvage: increased patency and utilization of the saphenous vein used "in-situ." Surgery 1981; 90:1000–1008.

Rich NM, Collins GJ, McDonald PT, et al. Popliteal vascular entrapment. Arch Surg 1979; 114:1377.

Sottiurai VS, Yao JST, Flinn WR, et al. Intimal hyperplasia and neointima: an ultrastructural analysis of thrombosed grafts in humans. Surgery 1983; 93:28–38.

Taylor LM, Edwards JM, Porter JM. Present status of reversed vein bypass: five-year results of a modern series. J Vasc Surg 1990; 11:193–205.

ACUTE ARTERIAL OCCLUSION OF THE EXTREMITIES

ROGER F. J. SHEPHERD, M.D.

Acute arterial occlusion is a medical emergency if tissue viability is in jeopardy. The clinical presentation may be dramatic, with sudden onset of leg or arm pain and a cold, pulseless, and pale extremity, or more subtle, characterized by the onset of intermittent claudication. If there is adequate collateral circulation, symptoms may be minimal; however, critical ischemia results if this is inadequate to maintain the metabolic requirements of the tissues under resting conditions. Critical ischemia is manifested by severe pain at rest, loss of cutaneous sensation, and motor weakness. Within hours, irreversible tissue damage occurs, with resultant gangrene if adequate blood flow cannot be re-established. In these circumstances, it is imperative to determine as rapidly as possible the site and cause of arterial occlusion, in order to expeditiously restore circulation to the extremity.

Even when reperfusion is accomplished quickly, these patients may suffer sequelae such as reperfusion injury, postischemic neuropathies, and tissue loss.

CAUSES OF ACUTE ARTERIAL OCCLUSION

Origins of acute arterial occlusion are listed in Table 1.

Thrombosis In Situ

Thrombosis in situ occurs frequently in patients with atherosclerosis obliterans. From studies of the epicardial coronary arteries, it is likely that rupture of an atherosclerotic plaque is often the precipitating factor. The normal arterial endothelium produces relaxing factors, including prostacyclin and endothelium-derived relaxing factor (EDRF), which has been shown to be nitric oxide. These substances, in addition to relaxing the underlying vascular smooth muscle, inhibit platelet adhesion and aggregation. This protective mechanism is absent at sites of atherosclerosis and endothelial damage, allowing platelets to aggregate and to release the vasoconstrictors serotonin and thromboxane A_2. Thrombin is formed and clotting is initiated.

A history of intermittent claudication or the presence of an arterial bypass graft suggest the diagnosis of thrombosis in situ.

Popliteal aneurysms are unique in that they rarely rupture but frequently thrombose. As these aneurysms are often asymptomatic, they may be unnoticed until the onset of sudden leg ischemia.

Embolic

Macroemboli

Approximately 85 to 90 percent of peripheral arterial emboli originate from the heart. These cardiac emboli are likely to obstruct major peripheral leg arteries, including the common femoral, iliac, popliteal, and superficial femoral arteries. The emboli may be multiple or may fragment, often lodging at more than

Table 1 Causes of Acute Arterial Occlusion

Thrombosis in situ
  Pre-existing atherosclerosis obliterans
  Popliteal aneurysm
Embolic
  Macroemboli
    Left atrium: atrial fibrillation, mitral stenosis, atrial myxoma
    Left ventricle: myocardial infarction, dilated cardiomyopathy,
      prosthetic heart valve
    Paradoxical
  Microemboli
    Ulcerated atheromatous plaque
    "Coral reef" plaque
    Aneurysm of thoracic or abdominal aorta
Other causes
  Arteritis, including Takayasu's and giant cell arteritis
  Aortic dissection
  Trauma
  Drugs, ergot
  Hypercoagulable states

one site. Sudden bilateral lower extremity ischemia may result from a saddle embolus at the aortic bifurcation. Emboli may also lodge in the arm arteries, at sites from the subclavian to the ulnar and radial arteries. Other arterial beds may also be involved, including the intracranial vessels, causing a stroke; and the renal arteries, causing renal insufficiency and mesenteric vessels, with resultant ischemia of the bowel.

The most common origin of a cardiac thrombus is the left atrium, owing to stasis of blood flow as a consequence of atrial fibrillation. The risk is increased greatly by the presence of mitral stenosis. It is estimated that up to 20 percent of patients with untreated mitral stenosis have an episode of thromboembolism. Atrial myxoma, a rare tumor, is often associated with systemic embolization.

A mural thrombus overlying the inner surface of the left ventricle is a common occurrence soon after myocardial infarction. If aneurysmal dilatation of the infarcted wall occurs, the thrombus persists. Patients with dilated cardiomyopathy and low ventricular ejection fraction also are prone to intracardiac thrombi. A mural thrombus in an abdominal or thoracic aortic aneurysm may also be a focus of peripheral embolization.

Paradoxical Embolus. An embolus originating from a deep vein may pass through an atrial or ventricular septal defect to the arterial circulation. The most common cause is a patent foramen ovale. With the advent of transesophageal color flow Doppler echocardiography, a patent foramen ovale has been demonstrated in as many as one-third of adults. In this group, shunting of blood from the right to the left atrium may occur due to elevated right-sided pressures (e.g., after pulmonary artery embolization). Right-to-left shunting at the atrial level also occurs transiently in normal subjects, such as when performing a Valsalva maneuver during defecation.

Microemboli

An atheromatous ulcerated plaque anywhere in the arterial tree may cause atheroemboli to the extremities.

Owing to their size, they obstruct small arteries and in particular the digital vessels. These patients present with symptoms of acute digital ischemia; in the legs, this has been labeled the blue-toe syndrome. Similar lesions can be found in the fingers. The pulses are palpable as major vessels remain patent. Livedo reticularis from cutaneous involvement and asymmetric digital ischemia suggests the diagnosis. Atheroemboli may be spontaneous, e.g., associated with a "coral reef" plaque in the thoracic aorta, or may occur during an invasive procedure such as cardiac catheterization.

Other Causes

Vasculitis

Takayasu's disease is an inflammatory arteritis involving large arteries, particularly the aorta and proximal branch vessels. It most commonly affects women in the second and third decades of life. In contrast, giant cell arteritis (temporal arteritis) not only affects the temporal arteries but also may involve extracranial arteries such as the brachial or superficial femoral artery. Systemic symptoms frequently predominate, with polymyalgia rheumatica, headache, fever, jaw claudication, and visual loss. Laboratory abnormalities include an elevated erythrocyte sedimentation rate, mild normocytic anemia, and abnormal liver function tests.

Aortic Dissection

This may result from a defect in the media; however, dissection begins at the site of a transverse intimal tear, creating a false lumen between layers of the aortic wall. As the dissection extends, it frequently involves branch vessels either by dissection or by external compression. Approximately two-thirds of aortic dissections involve the ascending aorta, and usually the greater curvature of the arch. If the dissection extends to the aortic root, it causes aortic incompetence and may also involve the ostium of the right coronary artery, precipitating an acute inferior myocardial infarction. Occlusion of a carotid artery may cause a left or right hemispheric stroke; involvement of the subclavian arteries may result in arm ischemia. Dissection of the descending thoracic aorta may cause visceral ischemia from mesenteric vessel obstruction or the abrupt onset of hypertension from renal artery involvement and renal insufficiency. The iliac arteries are frequently involved in a type III aortic dissection extending distally past the bifurcation of the aorta. A history of severe chest or back pain in a patient with hypertension and nicotine dependence, with widening of the mediastinum on chest x-ray and evidence of pulse deficits, should arouse suspicion of acute aortic dissection. The diagnosis can be confirmed by computed tomography, transesophageal echo, and aortography.

Ergotism

This is a rare but important cause of arterial insufficiency that may also present as an acute arterial occlusion. A retrospective study at the Mayo Clinic identified 38 patients with ergotism. In the majority, Cafergot had been prescribed for migraine headaches. Although intermittent claudication was the most common presentation, lower limb symptoms in 14 patients ranged from cold extremities to rest pain. Unusual presentations included mesenteric insufficiency with intestinal angina and small bowel infarction, isolated upper extremity ischemia, visual disturbances, and angina. Findings on arteriography ranged from localized arterial spasm and occlusion to diffuse narrowing of major vessels and their branches, usually bilateral but at times asymmetric. The mechanism by which ergot derivatives cause vasoconstriction is complex and involves activation of adrenergic and serotinergic receptors. In most patients, discontinuation of ergot is curative. In acute arterial insufficiency from ergot, sodium nitroprusside remains the treatment of choice. Less severe cases may respond to calcium antagonists.

Hypercoagulable States

A number of hematologic disorders, including myeloproliferative disease with thrombocytosis, are associated with venous and arterial thrombosis. Deficiencies of endogenous coagulation inhibitors, including protein C, protein S, and antithrombin III, also increase predisposition to clotting. Recently, the antiphospholipid antibody syndromes have been identified (see the chapter *Lupus Anticoagulant, Anticardiolipin Antibodies, and the Antiphospholipid Syndromes*). These are acquired autoantibodies found in patients with or without autoimmune disorders such as systemic lupus erythematosus. The presence of an anticardiolipin antibody or lupus anticoagulant is associated with up to a 30 percent incidence of thrombosis.

EVALUATION

A focused history and physical examination is necessary. The clinical assessment of the degree of ischemia is important, as this will dictate the time available for evaluation before a definitive procedure to restore blood flow to the extremity. Clinical signs to look for include the level of skin coolness; the color of the skin, which may be pale, mottled, or cyanotic; motor function (especially ability to move the digits); and skin sensation. Documentation of pulse deficit may help determine the level of arterial occlusion. The presence of significant elevation pallor and collapsed veins with prolonged venous filling time (greater than 45 seconds with leg dependent) is an indication of severe occlusive disease. Ankle systolic blood pressure should be obtained using a hand-held Doppler. A ratio of ankle-to-arm blood pressure of less than 0.5 signifies severe occlusive disease. Other noninvasive vascular laboratory assessment may include transcutaneous oximetry, which is helpful in determining the severity of ischemia. A PO_2 value of less than 20 to 40 mm Hg, or severe reduction in the regional perfusion index (PO_2 of the foot divided by reference PO_2 of the chest wall), is indicative of severe ischemia. If the skin is cold with a mottled or cyanotic appearance with loss of sensation, and if there is motor deficit, attempts at revascularization should be made emergently.

If, however, motor and sensory function are intact, more time is available for assessment. Baseline laboratory evaluation should include a chest x-ray; an electrocardiogram; blood tests including creatinine, electrolytes, fasting blood sugar, sedimentation rate, and complete blood count; and urinalysis. Patients with acute arterial occlusion often have significant coexisting cardiac, cerebrovascular, renal, and pulmonary disease. It may therefore be important to assess the operative risk from occult coronary artery disease in patients with silent myocardial ischemia; the risk of intraoperative stroke from associated carotid artery disease; and potential postoperative hypertension with associated renal vascular disease.

After initial evaluation, arteriography is usually necessary to define accurately the arterial anatomy. Angiography may also provide insight into the cause of arterial occlusion: for example, showing evidence of multiple emboli with a meniscus sign, or of thrombosis in situ associated with an atherosclerotic plaque or a smooth-tapered stenosis due to vasculitis.

MEDICAL MANAGEMENT

Heparin anticoagulation should be started immediately if there is no significant contraindication. A bolus of 5,000 to 10,000 units of heparin is given intravenously followed by a continuous infusion, generally beginning at 700 to 1,000 units per hour and titrated to achieve prolongation of the activated partial thromboplastin time to 2.0 to 2.5 times baseline. Patients with a severely ischemic limb should be placed at bed rest. Local care of the extremities is important. Lamb's wool should be placed between the toes. A vascular boot is used to maintain the temperature of the extremity and to protect it from injury.

Embolectomy

Fogarty balloon embolectomy remains a mainstay of therapy for embolic arterial occlusion. A preoperative arteriogram may not be necessary when clinical findings are indicative of embolization. Distal emboli often cannot be retrieved completely, and local thrombolytic therapy can be effective in dissolving these emboli. Other embolectomy techniques are being developed, including percutaneous aspiration with a large-bore catheter.

Surgical Bypass

Thrombectomy usually is not possible for acute thrombosis in an atherosclerotic artery. In these cases, either surgical endarterectomy or a bypass graft with anastomosis distal to the area of thrombosis may be necessary to restore pulsatile blood flow to an extremity. Percutaneous endovascular techniques may open a short segmental occlusion. This may be accomplished at the time of angiography by passing a wire through the occluded segment, followed by laser, atherectomy, or balloon angioplasty.

Thrombolytic Therapy

Recently there has been much interest in the use of thrombolytic agents to treat both thrombotic and embolic arterial occlusion. Thrombolytic agents dissolve fresh clots less than 1 week old. Currently the most widely used agents are streptokinase, urokinase, and tissue plasminogen activator. A number of other thrombolytic agents are currently under investigation, including pro-urokinase (SCU-PA) and acetylated plasminogen:streptokinase complex (APSAC). These thrombolytic agents are all plasminogen activators converting the inactive plasma enzyme plasminogen to plasmin, which acts to degrade fibrin. Tissue plasminogen activator and SCU-PA are fibrin-selective agents, as they act on fibrin-bound plasminogen. Urokinase and streptokinase activate circulating plasminogen as well as that bound to fibrin, leading to a systemic lytic state that has been postulated to increase hemorrhagic complications; however, in clinical use all agents cause a systemic lytic state. Therefore, the incidence of hemorrhagic complications is similar for all thrombolytic agents. Such agents have been used successfully to open arterial bypass grafts and native arteries with fresh thrombus, and to lyse peripheral artery emboli.

Intravenous administration of thrombolytic agents often produces inadequate lysis, which in part is due to shunting of the thrombolytic agent away from the thrombus via collateral vessels. However, encouraging results have been obtained by delivering the thrombolytic agent directly into the occluded artery, with a catheter lodged in the thrombus. This is referred to as regional thrombolysis and is conducted as described below.

Regional Thrombolysis

1. An angiogram confirms the site of the acute arterial occlusion.
2. The angiographic catheter is advanced into the thrombus for local infusion of the lytic agent.
3. Baseline coagulation studies are drawn, including partial thromboplastin time, prothrombin time, thrombin time, fibrinogen level, fibrinogen split products, and fibrinogen monomer. These are repeated at regular intervals during thrombolysis.
4. Repeat angiography is performed at 3- to 6-hour intervals to assess the effect of lytic therapy.

- If there is no significant thrombolysis, the infusion is discontinued.
- If there is significant thrombolysis, the infusion may be continued for up to 48 hours.
- If the fibrinogen level falls to less than 100 mg per deciliter, the lytic agent should be reduced.

In the protocol described by McNamara and Fisher (1985), a bolus of 250,000 units of urokinase is initially infused, followed by 4,000 units per minute over 2 hours and then 1,000 units per minute. It is imperative that a continuous infusion of heparin at approximately 800 units per hour be given to prevent pericatheter thrombosis.

Local infusion of lytic agents is also useful in patients who have residual tibial peroneal thrombosis after undergoing embolectomy. In most patients with a thrombus in situ, the initial thrombotic episode occurs at a site of high-grade stenosis, which may require angioplasty following lytic therapy. Lytic therapy in the case of a thrombosed popliteal aneurysm is controversial and has potential for further embolic occlusion of distal vessels, but in some cases in which no infrapopliteal vessels are visible, thrombolytic therapy may open a distal vessel and allow for surgical revascularization and limb salvage. There is also a risk of precipitating embolization in a patient with cardiac thrombus during thrombolytic therapy, but this complication is unusual. Even when thrombolytic agents are infused directly into the occluded artery, there remains an increased risk of hemorrhage, the most catastrophic of which is cerebral hemorrhage; however, this should be reduced to approximately 1 percent or less by appropriate patient screening. Depletion of fibrinogen may be a major factor in bleeding.

Thrombolytic agents all have systemic actions and will dissolve fibrin clots anywhere in the body. The same contraindications exist for intra-arterial thrombolysis of limb vessels as for other forms of lytic therapy. Specifically, absolute contraindications include aortic dissection, acute pericarditis, and active bleeding. Relative contraindications include a previous cerebral hemorrhage, a stroke within the previous 6 months, gastrointestinal and urinary hemorrhage, surgery, organ biopsy, trauma within the previous 2 to 4 weeks, prolonged cardiopulmonary resuscitation, severe hypertension (greater than 200/110), pregnancy, and malignancy.

FURTHER MANAGEMENT

Reperfusion Injury

Cell necrosis with acute ischemia may lead to loss of potassium and myoglobin from necrotic muscle cells. After reperfusion, these products may rapidly enter the systemic circulation, causing hyperkalemia, further aggravated by acidosis and also the risk of renal tubular obstruction by myoglobin. Pink discoloration of the urine should prompt further assessment for myoglobinuria, which should be aggressively treated with intravenous bicarbonate and maintenance of high urine output with intravenous fluids and loop diuretics. Electrolytes and acid-base balance should be monitored closely.

Another complication of reperfusion is local swelling in the previously ischemic area, which in severe cases can precipitate compartment syndrome. The latter (swelling in a confined fascial space) may cause severe pain, edema, motor weakness, and necrosis of tissues, unless identified early. Postischemic neuropathies (as a complication of prolonged ischemia and/or compartment syndrome) are difficult to manage, but may be helped by tricyclic antidepressant medication.

After angiography or surgery, high-risk patients need close monitoring of cardiac, pulmonary, and renal function. Long-term anticoagulant therapy may be indicated to prevent recurrent emboli. Those with pre-existing atherosclerosis obliterans need strict attention to modification of cardiovascular risk factors, including smoking, hyperlipidemia, and diabetes. These patients also benefit from a supervised exercise program (see the chapter *Chronic Arterial Occlusive Disease: Exercise Rehabilitation*). Mortality in these patients is chiefly due to associated cardiac and cerebrovascular disease. One therefore should not miss the opportunity to complete the evaluation for cardiac and cerebral vascular disease in these complex patients.

SUGGESTED READING

Cranley JJ. Acute embolic occlusion of major arteries. In: Bergan JJ, Yao JT, eds. Vascular surgical emergencies. New York: Grune & Stratton, 1987:487–498.
Deyo WA. Acute peripheral arterial ischemia. In: Dale WA, ed. Management of vascular surgical problems. New York: McGraw-Hill, 1985:54–72.
Fairbairn JF, Joyce JW, Pairolero PC. Acute arterial occlusion of the extremities. In: Juergens JL, Spittell JA, Fairbairn JF, eds. Peripheral vascular disease. Philadelphia: WB Saunders, 1980: 381–401.
Hollier LH. Acute arterial occlusion. In: Spittell JA, ed. Clinical vascular disease. Philadelphia: FA Davis, 1983:49–57.
McNamara TO, Fischer JR. Thrombolysis of peripheral arterial and graft occlusions; improved results using high dose urokinase. Am J Radiol 1985; 144:769–775.
Wells KE, Steed DL, Zajko AB, Webster MW. Recognition and treatment of arterial insufficiency from Cafergot. J Vasc Surg 1986; 4:8–15.

PERIPHERAL ARTERIAL ANEURYSMS

K. CRAIG KENT, M.D.

Aneurysms most frequently involve the aorta and iliac arteries and the potential morbidity and mortality associated wth these lesions is well understood. Peripheral arterial aneurysms are less common and less well understood, but experience has shown that these lesions can also produce a significant threat to "life and limb."

Approximately 70 percent of peripheral aneurysms are found in the popliteal artery and less frequently in the femoral, subclavian, and axillary arteries. The cause is usually atherosclerosis, and in many patients multiple aneurysms coexist. Bilateral incidence and multiplicity is so common that when a peripheral aneurysm is recognized, there must be a thorough search for aneurysms in other locations.

Because the incidence of peripheral aneurysms is low, it has been difficult to determine their natural history. Reports from several large series have described aneurysms in each location, but the majority of patients included in these series were treated surgically at the time their aneurysms were first recognized. Still, peripheral aneurysms frequently develop complications, and the morbidity associated with these complications is significant. Early surgical treatment of most peripheral aneurysms is therefore indicated.

POPLITEAL ANEURYSMS

In 1953, Gifford described the popliteal aneurysm as "a sinister harbinger of sudden catastrophe." Several subsequent reports have drawn attention to the high rate of amputation associated with complications that have arisen as a result of these lesions.

In the 1800s, a popliteal aneurysm might have arisen from syphilis or developed as a consequence of trauma to the popliteal artery. Today, atherosclerosis is the usual cause, and only rarely is trauma or infection involved.

An unusual cause of a popliteal aneurysm is entrapment of the popliteal artery. Lateral deviation and stenosis of the artery results from inappropriate insertion of the medial head of the gastrocnemius muscle. Poststenotic dilatation can develop and may progress to aneurysm formation. With the increased frequency of peripheral bypass surgery, pseudoaneurysms may occasionally develop at an anastomosis between an infrainguinal bypass graft and the popliteal artery.

True atherosclerotic popliteal aneurysms are found almost exclusively in men. Diffuse arteriomegaly is often a coincidental finding. Aneurysms occur bilaterally in 60 to 70 percent of patients, and in 50 percent of patients, aneurysms can be discovered in arteries other than the popliteal. Most often, the aorta is affected, followed in descending frequency by the femoral and the iliac arteries. These statistics underscore the necessity to examine thoroughly all patients in whom a popliteal aneurysm is found. A complete physical examination is necessary, but ultrasonographic evaluation of the opposite popliteal artery, as well as the aorta, iliac, and femoral arteries, should be considered.

Symptoms produced by aneurysms are the result of expansion, rupture, thrombosis, or embolization. In the popliteal artery, thrombosis and distal embolization are the most common complications and rupture is rare.

Thrombosis is the most frequent event associated with this aneurysm (60 to 70 percent of symptomatic cases; Fig 1). The result may be acute or chronic ischemia in the affected limb. Occasionally a patient will remain asymptomatic. Before surgical repair was possible, an asymptomatic thrombosis of a popliteal aneurysm was regarded as a spontaneous cure. Unfortunately, popliteal occlusion usually produces symptoms of claudication or a limb-threatening state with rest pain, ulceration, or gangrene. Acute limb-threatening ischemia is the most serious consequence of thrombosis of the popliteal artery, and despite urgent intervention, amputation is often unavoidable.

Laminar clot, which lines the wall of the aneurysm, may embolize to the distal circulation. This process is responsible for approximately 20 to 30 percent of complications. Necrosis or ulceration of a toe or a portion of the foot may result. The diagnosis of popliteal aneurysm should be considered in a patient who has an acutely painful and ischemic toe despite the presence of palpable pedal pulses.

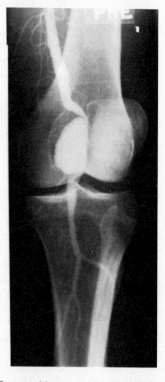

Figure 1 Angiogram in a 65-year-old man with an acutely ischemic right lower leg shows thrombosis of a right popliteal aneurysm (*arrow*). Vascular reconstruction was urgently performed. Note the luminal narrowing produced by the asymptomatic left popliteal aneurysm. This aneurysm was repaired 3 weeks later.

As a popliteal aneurysm expands, it can exert pressure on adjacent structures. Impingement on the popliteal vein may result in lower extremity edema or venous thrombosis. Pressure on adjacent nerves may produce neuralgia, paresthesia, or paralysis. The posterior tibial nerve is most commonly affected.

Rarely, a popliteal aneurysm will rupture (4 percent of cases). In contrast to an aortic aneurysm, rupture of a popliteal aneurysm is almost always contained and exsanguination is not likely. However, severe pain may develop in the popliteal fossa, and a compartment syndrome may ensue. Limb salvage is rare in cases in which rupture has occurred.

Each of the complications may produce a variety of symptoms. Table 1 outlines the symptoms and signs that can be associated with a popliteal aneurysm and gives their relative incidence as well.

The diagnosis of a popliteal aneurysm can usually be made by physical examination. It is easiest to examine the popliteal artery with the patient in a supine position and the knee flexed at 40 degrees. If the aneurysm has formed a thrombus, a pulse will be absent, but usually a mass can be palpated. Plain films of the knee will often suggest the presence of a soft tissue mass and, in 30 percent of cases, will reveal calcification that is associated with the aneurysm. Ultrasonography is the diagnostic test of choice and will allow determination of the diameter of the aneurysm and identification of the intraluminal thrombus. Complications are usually the result of either thrombosis or embolization, and the presence of a clot implies a potentially more severe course. Although computed tomography (CT) scan and magnetic resonance imaging (MRI) can accurately identify a popliteal aneurysm, both procedures rarely provide useful clinical information that cannot be obtained with an ultrasound examination. Angiograms are inaccurate when used to diagnose a popliteal aneurysm (the presence of intraluminal clot makes the lumen of the aneurysm appear smaller than its actual size). Angiographic examination is necessary preoperatively to evaluate the distal circulation so that an appropriate plan of reconstruction can be chosen.

The natural history of symptomatic and asymptomatic popliteal aneurysms should be considered before treatment recommendations are made. The morbidity of an untreated popliteal aneurysm must be compared with

Table 1 Symptoms and Signs Produced by Popliteal Aneurysms*

Claudication	67%
Rest pain	46%
Ulceration or gangrene	9%
Venous obstruction	11%
Neurologic	12%

*More than one symptom or sign may affect each patient. Derived from a series of 98 popliteal aneurysms reported by Vermilion, et al. A review of one hundred forty-seven popliteal aneurysms with long-term follow-up. Surgery 1981; 90:1009–1014.

the risk involved with the only available treatment, which is surgical repair. The majority of patients whose cases were reported in the literature had surgical repair at the time of discovery of their popliteal aneurysm. There are cohorts of patients in several of the series who did not undergo surgery because of coexisting medical disability or patient refusal. It is from these patients that the natural history of the lesion is derived.

Gifford and co-workers followed 45 patients who did not have surgery and whose popliteal aneurysms were uncomplicated at the time of presentation. In an average follow-up of 44 months, complications developed in 13 patients (29 percent), and 5 patients required amputation (11 percent). This experience is similar to that reported by other groups (Table 2).

The prognosis is significantly worse for patients who present with symptoms and do not undergo surgical correction. In Gifford et al's series, 11 patients with complications were followed without intervention. Further complications developed in 8 (73 percent) and 5 required subsequent amputation (45 percent). Patients who present with a thrombosed aneurysm that has not immediately produced a limb-threatening state are exceptions. Of 15 such patients followed by Gifford and co-workers, only 2 subsequently developed gangrene. The authors did not comment on how many of these patients were disabled by claudication.

This high frequency of complications has led to the current recommendation of surgical repair for the treatment of both symptomatic and asymptomatic popliteal aneurysms. Unfortunately, when complications occur, urgent repair is often required, and morbidity and mortality are high. Even with urgent intervention, salvage of the extremity is not always possible, and above-the-knee amputation may be necessary.

The surgical therapy for popliteal aneurysms has undergone an interesting evolution. Originally, an above-knee amputation was performed when complications of the aneurysm led to a threatened limb. In 1785, Hunter described ligation of the superficial femoral artery as a method of treatment. In some cases, this treatment would lead to limb-threatening ischemia. Unfortunately, the aneurysm did not always form a thrombus and additional complications would develop. This therapy was superseded in the next era by resection of the aneurysm, accompanied by lumbar sympathectomy. The popliteal arterial occlusion that resulted from aneurysm resection continued to produce limb-threatening ischemia in many patients despite the peripheral vasodilation produced by the sympathectomy.

Currently, the preferred method for repair of an asymptomatic popliteal aneurysm is exclusion of the aneurysm with saphenous vein bypass (Fig. 2). Through medial incisions in the thigh and calf, the nondiseased popliteal artery above and below the aneurysm is identified. A bypass around the aneurysm is constructed, preferably with saphenous vein. The placement of ligatures above and below the aneurysm allows its exclusion from the circulation. With this approach, it is unnecessary to expose the aneurysm in the popliteal fossa (which can be associated with significant morbidity). It is rare with this technique for the aneurysm not to thrombose.

If thromboembolism has already occurred, the distal popliteal and tibial arteries may be partially obstructed. It may then be necessary for a bypass to be constructed to the tibial or pedal circulation beyond the obstructed vessels. Occasionally, an angiogram will fail to show reconstitution of an open distal vessel. Usually this circumstance occurs when thrombosis or embolization has occurred acutely. If urgent revascularization is required, surgical thrombectomy of the distal vessels can be attempted to create runoff for a surgical reconstruction. If there is time, intra-arterial thrombolytic therapy may enable removal of the clot from the tibial circulation so that a reconstruction can be performed.

Bypass with aneurysm exclusion is effective in preventing and treating the complications of popliteal aneurysm. The rate of limb salvage and the long-term patency of bypass grafts are greatest when aneurysms are repaired before complications develop. This fact has led to our policy of repairing asymptomatic popliteal aneurysms that measure greater than 2 cm in diameter. The 5-year patency of reconstructions with the use of saphenous vein can be greater than 90 percent. When saphenous vein is unavailable, autogenous alternatives such as arm or lesser saphenous vein should be used. Bypass with prosthetic graft to the infrageniculate position has yielded consistently poor results (<50 percent patency at 5 years for femoral to below-knee popliteal bypass) and should be reserved for situations where no autogenous conduit is available.

Coexisting medical disease is common in elderly patients with popliteal aneurysms. Modern anesthetic techniques have allowed elective surgical intervention to be performed with minimal morbidity and mortality. A mortality of less than 2 percent and a morbidity of less than 4 percent should be expected for patients undergoing repair of asymptomatic popliteal aneuryms.

Table 2 Outcome of Asymptomatic Popliteal Aneurysms Followed Without Surgical Intervention

Series	Average Follow-up (mos)	No. of Aneurysms	Complications n (%)	Amputations n (%)
Gifford et al	44	45	13(29)	5(11)
Wychulis et al	36	94	27(29)	3 (3)
Vermilion et al	36	26	8(31)	2 (8)

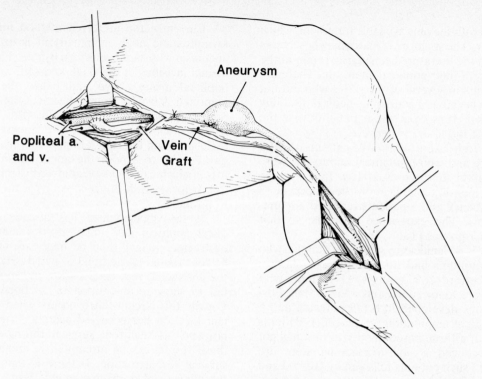

Figure 2 Medial incisions expose the popliteal artery above and below the knee. Saphenous vein is used to construct a bypass around the popliteal aneurysm. Ligatures are placed on the popliteal artery above and below the aneurysm so that it is excluded from the circulation.

FEMORAL ANEURYSMS

True Femoral Aneurysms

Approximately 30 percent of all peripheral aneurysms are located in the femoral artery, but the overall incidence of these aneurysms is low. Patients with femoral and popliteal aneurysms have similar characteristics. The average age is approximately 65 years, and the overwhelming majority of patients are male. Coexisting diseases include hypertension (70 percent) and ischemic coronary artery disease (50 percent). Diabetes is an infrequent occurrence, in contrast to coexisting diseases in patients who have atherosclerotic occlusive disease.

A systemic process with diffuse arterial dilation affects many patients found to have femoral and popliteal aneurysms (Fig. 3). In 40 to 50 percent of patients with femoral aneurysms, the process is bilateral. Seventy to eighty percent of patients have aneurysms in multiple sites, and 50 percent of patients have 3 or more aneurysms. If bilateral femoral aneurysms are present, there is a greater than 75 percent chance that the distal aorta is abnormally dilated. Once a femoral aneurysm is identified, it is important for the clinician to search avidly for the presence of aneurysms in other sites.

Presenting symptoms are the result of thrombosis, embolization, expansion, or rupture. Cutler and Darling found that symptoms developed in 40 percent of femoral aneurysms as a result of thrombosis. In one-half of these aneurysms the thrombosis was chronic, with claudication being the most frequent symptom. In the remaining 50 percent, the process was acute, and limb-threatening ischemia was present. Several of the patients were found to have a cold, pulseless extremity, and urgent surgical intervention was necessary. Evidence of local expansion developed in 20 percent of symptomatic patients. Symptoms and signs include pain and tenderness over the aneurysm, thrombophlebitis, peripheral edema from femoral vein compression, and femoral neuralgia.

Twenty percent of patients in the same series presented with rupture of the aneurysm. With the addition of groin ecchymosis, the symptoms of rupture are the same as those produced by local expansion. Sixteen percent of the patients had occlusion of the distal vessels. Although embolization may have been the cause for this distal disease in some patients, other possibilities include thrombosis of an associated popliteal aneurysm or atherosclerotic occlusion.

Because of the rarity of the condition, the natural history of femoral arterial aneurysms has not been well defined. A group of 44 patients with femoral aneurysms were treated nonsurgically by Pappas and others from the Mayo Clinic. These patients either refused surgery or were thought to be unsuitable candidates. Sixteen percent of these patients eventually underwent amputation of the affected extremity. Unfortunately, the study did not indicate the duration of follow-up or whether the patients were symptomatic or asymptomatic at the time of their initial presentation. Tolstedt and co-workers observed seven patients with asymptomatic aneurysms

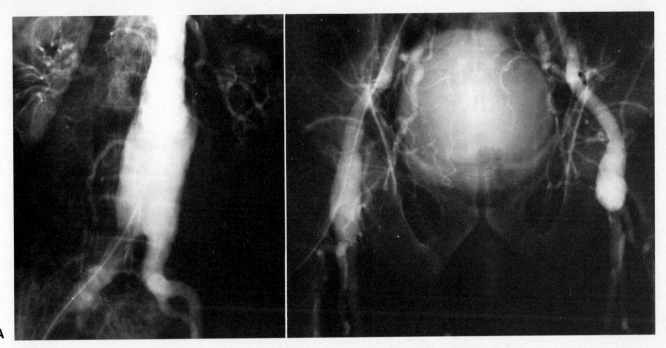

A

B

Figure 3 *A,* This 5.5 cm abdominal aortic aneurysm was discovered during a routine physical examination in a 55-year-old man. *B,* A more thorough examination revealed widening of both femoral pulses. Angiogram confirms the presence of bilateral common femoral artery aneurysms. All three aneurysms were repaired during one operation.

over a 10-year period. Complications that required above-knee amputation eventually developed in five of these seven patients. Although all of the aneurysms studied by Cutler and Darling were treated surgically, 71 percent of the aneurysms in their series were symptomatic at the time of initial presentation and 47 percent of limbs had suffered a major complication. The existing data suggest that a femoral aneurysm carries significant morbidity if left untreated.

The diagnosis of femoral aneurysm can usually be made by physical examination, but size and the presence of intraluminal thrombus can be more accurately assessed by ultrasound examination. An angiogram is usually obtained to evaluate the distal circulation but is not absolutely necessary when distal pulses are intact. The majority of femoral artery aneurysms begin below the level of the inguinal ligament. Two anatomic types can be discerned. In 44 percent of cases, the aneurysm terminates proximal to the bifurcation of the common into the superficial femoral and profunda femoris arteries (type 1). In the second subtype, aneurysmal degeneration extends into the superficial femoral and profunda femoris arteries (type 2). Rarely, an aneurysm will involve only the profunda femoris or superficial femoral arteries. Differences in anatomy affect the surgical approach and the prognosis after surgical repair.

Surgical repair consists of replacement of the aneurysm with a prosthetic graft or saphenous vein. The patency of both conduits is equal as long as the saphenous vein is of appropriate size. I prefer the use of a prosthetic bypass because this approach allows pres-

Table 3 Symptoms Produced by Aneurysmal Degeneration of the Proximal or Mid-Subclavian Artery

Symptoms	Cause
Pain in the neck, chest or shoulder	Expansion or rupture
Upper extremity ischemia, "blue finger" syndrome	Thrombosis or embolization
Upper extremity neurologic dysfunction	Brachial plexus compression
Hemoptysis	Erosion into the lung
Hoarseness	Compression of the recurrent laryngeal nerve
Transient ischemic attack	Retrograde embolization of the carotid or vertebral circulation
Respiratory insufficiency	Tracheal compression

ervation of the saphenous vein for a simultaneous or subsequent distal bypass.

For type 1 aneurysms, proximal and distal control are obtained with minimal dissection of the outer wall of the aneurysm. The aneurysm is then entered and branches are internally ligated. The graft is then sewn end to end proximally and distally. The approach is similar with type 2 aneurysms, but the distal anastomosis is to the superficial femoral artery and a side graft is extended to the profunda femoris artery.

Five-year patencies of greater than 80 percent should be expected as a result of these approaches. With proper preoperative evaluation, perioperative morbidity and mortality should be minimal. If superficial femoral artery occlusion is present, simultaneous femo-

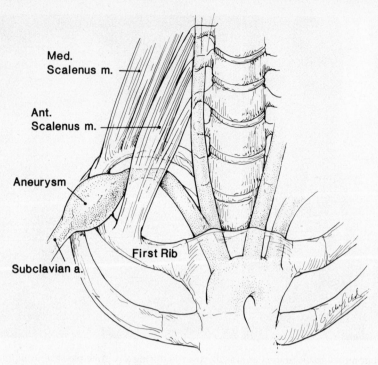

Figure 4 With thoracic outlet syndrome, external compression may narrow the subclavian artery as it passes beneath the scalenus anterior muscle. Poststenotic dilatation leads to aneurysm formation. Distal embolization from intraluminal clot is a frequent complication.

ropopliteal bypass should be performed only if warranted by the preoperative symptoms. When multiple aneurysms are present, the timing of the repairs may be important. In Cutler and Darling's series, three patients had thrombosis of their femoral aneurysms develop soon after repair of an abdominal aortic aneurysm. In many cases, repair of both aneurysms can be performed simultaneously (see Fig. 3).

Femoral False Aneurysms

Pseudoaneurysms (false aneurysms) of the femoral artery resulting from cardiac catheterization or previous bypass grafting have become increasingly common. False aneurysms are described as such because the wall of the aneurysm is composed of a pseudocapsule of periarterial tissue as opposed to being a true vessel wall.

In the case of cardiac catheterization, removal of the femoral sheath leaves a laceration in the femoral artery that rapidly seals under usual circumstances. If the laceration remains patent, blood may circulate outside the femoral vessel, thereby forming a pseudoaneurysm. Pseudoaneurysm formation increases as the size of the sheath used for catheterization increases when patients receive anticoagulation therapy following the procedure and when the arterial puncture is low (through the superficial femoral artery). Occasionally a small pseudoaneurysm will spontaneously form a thrombus, but surgical repair is usually indicated. This requires open-

ing of the aneurysm cavity and direct suture repair of the femoral artery laceration. The procedure can almost always be performed under local anesthesia.

Two to five percent of aortofemoral reconstructions eventually develop pseudoaneurysms at the femoral anastomosis. The cause is a dehiscence of the prosthetic graft from the femoral vessel. Predisposing factors include hypertension, type of suture material used, graft infection, and endarterectomy of the femoral vessel at the time of original bypass. Repair consists of revision of the femoral anastomosis and usually requires insertion of a new bridging prosthetic graft.

SUBCLAVIAN ARTERY ANEURYSMS

Subclavian aneurysms involving the proximal and mid-portion of the artery occur rarely, with atherosclerosis being the usual cause. These aneurysms too can be part of a diffuse aneurysmal process; 30 to 50 percent of patients with these aneurysms will be found to have aneurysms in other sites. Because of their strategic location, symptoms can vary greatly (Table 3).

A subclavian aneurysm may be identified by palpation of a pulsatile supraclavicular mass, or a chest radiograph may reveal a superior mediastinal mass. Frequently, a supraclavicular pulsatile mass can be palpated in thin, elderly patients, particularly in those with chronic obstructive pulmonary disease or in elderly

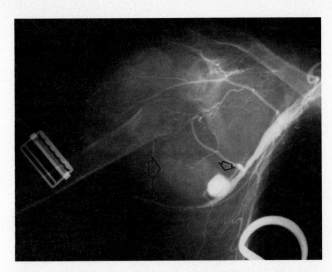

Figure 5 Angiogram in a 55-year-old woman who fractured her proximal humerus and 6 weeks later presented with an insensate and paralyzed right arm. During examination a pulsatile mass was noted in her axilla. Angiogram demonstrates a traumatic pseudoaneurysm of the axillary artery *(small arrow)* that has ruptured and formed a second pseudoaneurysm *(large arrow)*. The patient underwent emergency decompression of the axillary sheath and repair of the pseudoaneurysm; she eventually regained the majority of neurologic function in that arm.

women with hypertension. Most often, this sign occurs as a result of a tortuous, innominate, subclavian, or carotid artery, although aneurysmal disease must be excluded. An ultrasound examination can usually distinguish between these two conditions, and only occasionally is angiography necessary.

An angiogram should be obtained in all cases of subclavian aneurysm in which surgical therapy is anticipated. Surgical correction requires resection of the aneurysm with end-to-end anastomosis or replacement of the aneurysm with an interposition arterial conduit. Ligation without replacement of the aneurysm has been performed but has been shown to lead to ischemic symptoms in 25 percent of patients with these aneurysms. The surgical approach to the proximal portion of the right subclavian artery is through a median sternotomy. A left thoracotomy is often required for exposure of the proximal left subclavian artery. The mid- and distal subclavian arteries can be approached through a supraclavicular incision.

A second cause of subclavian aneurysms is narrowing of the thoracic outlet (thoracic outlet syndrome). Compression of the subclavian artery by a cervical rib, the scalenus anticus muscle, or a fibrous band can produce stenosis of the artery (Fig. 4). Turbulence resulting from this stenosis can lead to poststenotic dilatation and subsequent aneurysm formation. These aneurysms have a significant predominance in women, and the right subclavian artery is more often affected than is the left subclavian artery. Clots form within the aneurysm and embolic complications are common. If the

aneurysm is left unattended, loss of digits and eventually the entire hand may result.

These aneurysms are isolated to the mid- and distal portions of the subclavian artery, and a supraclavicular incision is usually sufficient for repair. Occasionally, the aneurysm can be resected and an end-to-end anastomosis can be performed. Usually, interposition of a prosthetic conduit is required. An embolic event may require simultaneous thrombectomy of the distal circulation through a brachial incision.

If thoracic outlet syndrome or a cervical rib is identified and an asymptomatic dilation of the subclavian artery is present, correction of the anatomic abnormality producing the thoracic outlet syndrome may prevent aneurysm formation. If significant aneurysmal degeneration is already present (greater than two times the normal diameter of the artery) or if ultraluminal clot or intimal disruption has developed, reconstruction of the artery should accompany repair of the thoracic outlet.

AXILLARY ARTERIAL ANEURYSMS

Axillary arterial aneurysms are usually traumatic in origin. Crutch-induced dilation of the axillary artery was first described by Robb in 1956. Repetitive injury leads to dilation of the artery, and a thickened wrinkled intima forms. Complications most frequently arise as a result of thrombosis or embolization. The diagnosis is often made in the patient who has been using crutches for a prolonged period and who presents with signs and symptoms of upper extremity ischemia.

Humeral fractures or anterior dislocation of the shoulder can lead to the formation of a false aneurysm of the axillary artery (Fig. 5). Because of excellent collateral circulation in this area, normal distal pulses may be present despite extensive injury to the artery. Hemorrhage into the axillary sheath may lead to compression of the brachial plexus and neurologic dysfunction. Unless the axillary sheath is rapidly decompressed and the aneurysm repaired, an irreversible neurologic deficit may result.

Surgical treatment of axillary arterial aneurysms involves resection of the aneurysm and either direct anastomosis or interposition of a segment of large-diameter saphenous vein. Traumatic pseudoaneurysms require suture or patching of the artery.

SUGGESTED READING

Abbott WM, Darling RC. Axillary artery aneurysms secondary to crutch trauma. Am J Surg 1973; 125:515.
Anton GE, Hertzer NR, Beven EG, et al. Surgical management of popliteal aneurysms: trends in presentation, treatment, and results from 1952 to 1984. J Vasc Surg 1986; 3:125–134.
Bergan JJ, Yao JST, eds. Aneurysms: Diagnosis and treatment, New York: Grune & Stratton, 1982.
Cutler BS, Darling RC. Surgical management of arteriosclerotic femoral aneurysms. Surgery 1973; 74:764–773.

Gifford RW, Hines EA, Janes JM. An analysis and follow-up study of one hundred popliteal aneurysms. Surgery 1953; 33:284–293.

Hobson RWW, Sarkaria J, O'Donnell J, Neville W. Atherosclerotic aneurysms of the subclavian artery. Surgery 1979; 85:506.

Reilly MK, Abbott WM, Darling RC. Aggressive surgical management of popliteal artery aneurysms. Am J Surg 1983; 145:498–502.

Rutherford RB, ed. Vascular surgery, 3rd ed, vol 2. Philadelphia: WB Saunders, 1989.

Vermilion BD, Kimmins SA, Pace WG, Evans WE. A review of one hundred forty-seven popliteal aneurysms with long-term follow-up. Surgery 1981; 90:1009–1014.

RAYNAUD'S PHENOMENON

JAY D. COFFMAN, M.D.
RICHARD A. COHEN, M.D.

CLINICAL PROBLEM

Primary Raynaud's Phenomenon

Primary Raynaud's phenomenon (Raynaud's disease, idiopathic Raynaud's phenomenon) is a common and usually benign condition that occurs primarily in young women 15 to 40 years of age. The clinical presentation is episodic attacks of well-demarcated white or blue discoloration of the digits; during rewarming the digits may become bright red. Some patients have all three color changes, but most have one of the ischemic manifestations and may have the redness of reactive hyperemia. During the ischemic phase, numbness is present; pain is a more common accompaniment of the reactive hyperemia phase. At first only one or two fingers may be involved, but later all fingers of both hands manifest the color changes. The toes are affected in about 40 percent of patients and rarely the nose tip, earlobes, and tongue tip. The thumbs are often spared. Approximately 13 percent of patients develop trophic changes or sclerodactyly of the digits, but gangrene and ulcers are extremely rare.

The etiology of primary Raynaud's phenomenon is unknown. The strongest evidence points to a local sensitivity of the digital arteries to cold with an intensification of this abnormality by normal sympathetic stimulation. The abnormality may involve the alpha-adrenoceptors.

The diagnosis of Raynaud's phenomenon must often be made on the basis of a history of well-demarcated color changes of the digits on exposure to cold. The hands and feet are not involved. The history is of paramount importance, because vasospastic attacks are often difficult to induce in the office or laboratory. In primary Raynaud's phenomenon the physical examination is normal; radial and ulnar pulses are present and strong. Laboratory study results are also normal. The only test of some diagnostic value is not readily available: this involves the measurement of finger systolic blood pressure after a period of digital ischemia at progressively cooler local temperatures. Body cooling increases the sensitivity of the test. In most patients with Raynaud's phenomenon, digital systolic pressure is abolished at a higher temperature than in normal subjects. Unfortunately, the test does not distinguish between primary and secondary Raynaud's phenomenon. Nailfold capillaroscopy is normal in primary Raynaud's phenomenon and in many of the secondary etiologies. Dilated, elongated capillaries; avascular areas; or "bushy" capillaries help diagnose the connective tissue diseases and eliminate the diagnosis of the primary phenomenon.

Diagnosis of primary Raynaud's phenomenon must still rely on the criteria proposed by Allen and Brown: (1) vasospastic attacks precipitated by exposure to cold or emotional stimuli; (2) bilateral involvement of the extremities; (3) gangrene absent or, if present, limited to the skin of the fingertips; (4) no evidence of an underlying disease associated with vasospastic attacks; and (5) a history of symptoms lasting at least 2 years. The fourth criteria should now include a normal sedimentation rate, antinuclear antibody determination, and nailfold capillaroscopy examination if available. If all criteria are not met, the patient should be classified as having secondary Raynaud's phenomenon.

Secondary Raynaud's Phenomenon

Secondary Raynaud's phenomenon may have a variety of underlying causes (Table 1), the most common being connective tissue disease, drug therapy, traumatic vasospastic disease, and carpal tunnel syndrome. Pain, digital ulcers, and gangrene occur in many of these. Patients with secondary Raynaud's phenomenon usually have systemic symptoms, positive physical findings, or laboratory test results that indicate an underlying disease. Determination of a secondary cause can be very important in planning treatment.

Most of the secondary causes of Raynaud's phenomenon are associated with decreased blood flow or blood pressure in the digits. Low digital artery blood pressure, thickened vessel walls, increased blood viscosity, persistent vasoconstriction, and vasoconstrictor products from platelet breakdown or the endothelium could (alone or in combination) lead to closure of digital arteries during a sympathetic stimulus, with or without an increase in extravascular pressure.

Table 1 Etiologies of Secondary Raynaud's Phenomenon

Connective tissue diseases
  Scleroderma
  Systemic lupus erythematosus
  Mixed connective tissue disease
  Polymyositis and dermatomyositis
  Rheumatoid arthritis
  Sjögren's syndrome
Drugs
  Beta-adrenoceptor blocking agents
  Ergot preparations
  Methysergide
  Vinblastine and bleomycin
  Bromocryptine
  Clonidine
  Cyclosporine
  Amphetamines
  Imipramine

Traumatic vasospastic disease
  Carpal tunnel syndrome
  Thoracic outlet syndrome
  Hypothenar hammer syndrome
Blood dyscrasias
  Cryoproteinemia
  Cold agglutinins
  Polycythemia
Reflex sympathetic dystrophy
Obstructive arterial disease
  Arteriosclerosis obliterans
  Thromboangiitis obliterans
  Arterial emboli
Vinyl chloride disease
Hypothyroidism
Vasculitis and hepatitis B antigenemia
Arteriovenous fistula

THERAPEUTIC ALTERNATIVES

Since all therapy for Raynaud's phenomenon is nonspecific and symptomatic, conservative measures are most important. Pavlovian conditioning or biofeedback training may be suitable for mild to moderate cases. Drug therapy is indicated when the condition interferes with normal daily functioning or when ulcers or gangrene are present. Several classes of drugs have been used, including calcium channel entry blockers, sympatholytic agents, direct-acting vasodilators, eicosanoid agents, serotonin antagonists, and angiotensin converting enzyme (ACE) inhibitors (Tables 2 and 3). In the two most commonly used classes, one or two agents have proved more beneficial than others (Table 2).

Among the calcium channel entry blockers, nifedipine has proved of more benefit than diltiazem, verapamil, nicardipine, and nisoldipine. Guanethidine and reserpine are the most beneficial of the sympatholytic agents. Ketanserin, a selective 5-HT$_2$-receptor antagonist with some alpha$_1$-adrenoceptor inhibitory activity, has been shown to decrease the frequency but not the duration or intensity of vasospastic attacks; it is not available in the United States. Prostaglandins must be used parenterally and need more study. The ACE inhibitors are probably not of value. Upper extremity surgical sympathectomy should not be performed for treatment of primary Raynaud's phenomenon; results are variable and benefits of short duration. Lower extremity sympathectomy has been very useful for vasospastic attacks of the toes, but only in primary Raynaud's phenomenon. Plasmapheresis should be considered only for patients with severe ulcerations or gangrene who have not responded to other therapy.

PREFERRED APPROACH

Conservative Therapy

In primary or secondary Raynaud's phenomenon, all patients except those with constant pain, ecchymoses of the digits, ulcers, or gangrene should receive a trial of conservative therapy. Patients are told that mittens will keep the fingers warmer than gloves. Hands and feet must also be kept dry in cool weather. Avoidance of cold objects is imperative. Pressure on the digits plus cold, as in handling cold drinks and frozen foods, induces attacks more easily than just cold exposure. The fact that cold applications to the neck or most parts of the body cause reflex sympathetic vasoconstriction is explained to patients. Therefore, as much of the body as possible should be covered with warm, loose-fitting clothes in cool weather. A good illustration is the induction of attacks while handling frozen foods during the reflex sympathetic stimulation of the cold environment of the frozen foods section of a supermarket; this has been experienced by most patients. Some patients find battery-operated hand or foot warmers or chemical heat bags of help. Patients should refrain from tobacco smoking, because nicotine causes vasoconstriction of digital vessels via the sympathetic nervous system. Moving to a warm climate may make some patients more comfortable. However, exposure to air conditioning or cool mornings and evenings still induces attacks in most individuals.

Conditioning

Patients with mild to moderate primary Raynaud's phenomenon are offered a trial of Pavlovian conditioning. However, they must be willing to spend the time involved. In daily sessions they must immerse the hands in warm water (43°C) while exposing the body to 0°C temperatures for three 10-minute periods. Patients can do this on the porch or in the backyard in the cold months of the year, but should wear only indoor clothing. Three weeks of this regimen may produce subjective benefit for several months in many patients and can then be repeated.

Drug Therapy

Patients whose symptoms interfere with daily functions despite conservative measures, and patients with ulcers or gangrene, warrant a trial of drug therapy. In our experience, only about 50 percent of patients respond to pharmacologic interventions. Some of these failures are due to the intolerable side effects of the medications. None of the agents affects the underlying disease.

Primary Raynaud's Phenomenon

Nifedipine is the preferred agent for primary Raynaud's phenomenon. It is a calcium blocker that causes arteriolar dilatation and counteracts vasospasm. There is evidence of alpha-adrenoceptor blocking activ-

Table 2 Preferred Drug Therapy for Raynaud's Phenomenon

Agents	Action	Dosage	Limiting Side Effects
Nifedipine	Calcium entry blocker	10–30 mg t.i.d. or XL tablets 30–90 mg daily	Headache, dizziness, palpitations, anxiety
Guanethidine	Inhibits neural release of norepinephrine	10–50 mg daily	Postural hypotension, diarrhea, impotence
Reserpine	Depletes vascular norepinephrine	0.125–0.75 mg daily	Postural hypotension, lethargy, depression
Prazosin	Alpha$_1$-adrenoceptor antagonist	1–3 mg t.i.d.	Nausea, headache, palpitations, dizziness, fatigue, dyspnea, rash, diarrhea
Phenoxybenzamine	Alpha-adrenoceptor blocker	10–30 mg q.i.d.	Postural hypotension, palpitations, impotence, constipation

Table 3 Alternative Drug Therapy for Raynaud's Phenomenon

Agents	Action	Dose	Limiting Side Effects
Diltiazem	Calcium entry blocker	30–90 mg t.i.d.	Headache, dizziness, nausea
Methyldopa	Central alpha-adrenoceptor agonist	0.5–2.0 g daily	Lethargy, headache, diarrhea, postural hypotension
Nitroglycerin ointment (1 or 2%)	Direct-acting vasodilator	1 cm applied t.i.d.	Headache, postural hypotension
Captopril	Angiotensin converting enzyme inhibition	25 mg t.i.d.	Rash, cough, hypotension
Ketanserin*	5-HT$_2$-receptor antagonist	40 mg t.i.d.	Dizziness, sedation, anxiety, prolonged Q-T interval
Thymoxamine*	Alpha$_1$-adrenoceptor antagonist	40 mg daily to 40 mg q.i.d.	Nausea, headache, insomnia

*Not available in the United States.

ity, a beneficial effect on red cell deformability, an antiaggregating action on platelets, and an ability to inhibit thromboxane A_2 synthesis by platelets for some of the calcium entry blockers. They have proved to be effective inhibitors of vascular responses evoked by alpha$_2$-adrenoceptor activity. In several well-controlled studies and in our experience, nifedipine decreases the frequency, duration, and severity of vasospastic attacks in patients with primary or secondary Raynaud's phenomenon. Patients should be started on 10 mg three times a day. Barring side effects, the dosage can be increased to 30 mg three times a day if maximal benefit is not obtained with lower doses. Frequent side effects not interfering with the use of the drug are transient headache, flushing, and edema. The headache often disappears if the drug is taken continuously for 3 days. Side effects that cause discontinuation of the drug are dizziness or lightheadedness due to low blood pressure, anxiety, persistent headache, and palpitations. Less frequent side effects are dyspepsia and pruritus. The new long-acting preparation of nifedipine has been beneficial to our patients and there has been a marked decrease in side effects. It should be started at 30 mg daily but can be increased to 60 or 90 mg daily if needed.

More patients have to discontinue the drug because of side effects than because of a lack of improvement in vasospastic attacks.

In patients who cannot tolerate the side effects of nifedipine, guanethidine or reserpine can be tried. Guanethidine is our current preference. It interferes with the release of norepinephrine at the sympathetic neuroeffector junction and has been shown to increase capillary blood flow in patients with scleroderma during finger cooling. It should be started at a dosage of 10 mg daily and increased by 10 mg weekly until relief of symptoms or side effects occur. Relief of symptoms is defined as a clinically important decrease in the frequency and duration of vasospastic attacks. Patients should be monitored frequently for hypotension in the standing position. Side effects limiting use of the drug include lightheadedness or dizziness due to the postural hypotension, diarrhea, and lethargy. Impotence may also occur. An alternative to guanethidine is reserpine. Reserpine depletes norepinephrine in arterial walls and has been shown to increase the capillary blood flow in the fingertips in warm and cool environments in patients with Raynaud's phenomenon. It also decreases the vasoconstrictor response in the hand to intra-arterial tyramine and to ice applied to the forehead. Reserpine should be started at a dosage of 0.125 mg daily and increased by 0.125 weekly until there is relief of symptoms or induction of side effects. Bradycardia and nasal stuffiness indicate that a therapeutic dosage has been reached that should not be increased. Reserpine may cause depression, and if so should be discontinued immediately; it should not be given to patients with a history of depression. Other side effects limiting use of this drug are postural hypotension and lethargy. Dyspepsia and fluid retention may also occur.

Failing tolerance of the above drugs, prazosin can be administered. This is a specific alpha$_1$-adrenoceptor antagonist that may be of moderate benefit to patients with Raynaud's phenomenon. The first 1 mg of the drug should be given at bedtime, because syncope has been reported with the first dose. Patients should be started on 1 mg three times a day; the dosage may be increased to as much as 3 mg three times a day if side effects do not occur. Intolerable side effects are frequent, including dizziness, nausea, headache, palpitations, fatigue, dyspnea, and rash. Edema and diarrhea may also occur.

The final drug we may try is phenoxybenzamine. It is a potent alpha-adrenoceptor blocking agent whose side effects severely limit its use. We use small doses of 10 to 20 mg twice a day, although as much as 30 mg four times a day has been used. Side effects of postural hypotension, palpitations, blurry vision, and gastrointestinal symptoms limit the dosage. Nasal congestion and impotence are not uncommon.

In the choice of drugs, we start with nifedipine, preferably the long-acting preparation. If this is not tolerated, guanethidine or reserpine is preferred. We have not had much success with prazosin, but have noted some beneficial responses with phenoxybenzamine. In fairness, the latter two drugs may have produced better responses if used first instead of third and fourth. We also have not had success with drug combinations. Methyldopa, nitroglycerin preparations, niacin derivatives, papaverine, isoxsuprine, cyclandelate, nylidrin, and thyroid hormone have not been of value.

Secondary Raynaud's Phenomenon

The treatment of many of the secondary causes of Raynaud's phenomenon has been the subject of few controlled studies. Patients with scleroderma or vinblastine-bleomycin–induced vasospastic attacks often respond to drug therapy as well as patients with the primary phenomenon. In these patients we follow the drug therapy outlined previously. Raynaud's phenomenon in patients with lupus erythematosus or mixed connective tissue diseases may improve with corticosteroid therapy. However, corticosteroids should be used only if there are other manifestations of these diseases. Vasospastic attacks due to beta-adrenoceptor blocking agents may cease if the drug can be withdrawn. Specific beta$_1$-adrenoceptor antagonists have not been shown to benefit the vasospastic attacks or prevent their occurrence. Patients who develop severe vasospasm with ergotamine preparations or methysergide often respond within 3 days to withdrawal of the drugs; if the ischemia is severe, intra-arterial or intravenous nitroprusside or oral nifedipine should be administered. These patients should also be anticoagulated with intravenous heparin to prevent thromboses of small vessels.

In patients who develop vasospastic attacks due to vibratory tools, improvement often occurs with cessation of exposure to the vibration, but the phenomenon usually does not disappear. The calcium entry blocking drugs also improve these patients. The primary effort should be directed toward prevention, limiting use of the tools to 2 hours per day and using antivibratory tools. Raynaud's phenomenon due to the carpal tunnel syndrome may or may not be relieved by surgical decompression of the tunnel. The same is true in the thoracic outlet syndrome, although excellent relief may occur when cervical ribs are causing the problem and are removed. In our experience, the vasospastic attacks have been attenuated only by exercises to build up the shoulder muscles or by surgical treatment. Excision of an occluded or aneurysmal portion of the ulnar artery or medical or surgical sympathectomy often produces satisfactory relief in the hammer hand syndrome.

For vasospastic attacks of the digits of the involved limb with arteriosclerosis obliterans, revascularization procedures produce complete relief. However, if there has been tissue damage in these patients or in patients with arterial emboli, Raynaud's phenomenon may persist after restoration of normal large vessel blood flow. In patients with a prominent vasospastic component in thromboangiitis obliterans, sympathectomy may be beneficial but not curative. Patients must cease smoking. We have had no success with drug therapy in these individuals or those in whom vasculitis is the underlying disease.

In reflex sympathetic dystrophy, medical or surgical sympatholysis with an intense physical therapy program may be curative. Alkylating agents plus steroids, but not steroids alone, alleviate vasospasm in the cryoglobulinemias. Plasmapheresis has also been beneficial. Patients with hypothyroidism and Raynaud's phenomenon often respond remarkably well to thyroid replacement. Raynaud's phenomenon or digital ischemia due to hepatitis B antigenemia usually responds to corticosteroid therapy.

SUGGESTED READING

Coffman JD. Raynaud's phenomenon. New York: Oxford University Press, 1989.

Coffman JD, Cohen AS. Total and capillary fingertip blood flow in Raynaud's phenomenon. N Engl J Med 1971; 285:259–263.

Nielsen SL, Vithing K, Rasmussen K. Prazosin treatment of primary Raynaud's phenomenon. Eur J Clin Pharmacol 1983; 24:421–423.

Porter JM, Rivers SP, Anderson CJ, Baur GM. Evaluation and management of patients with Raynaud's syndrome. Am J Surg 1981; 142:183–189.

Smith CD, McKendry RVR. Controlled trial of nifedipine in the treatment of Raynaud's phenomenon. Lancet 1982; 2:1299–1301.

SURGICAL SYMPATHECTOMY FOR ARTERIAL OCCLUSIVE DISEASE AND VASOSPASM OF THE UPPER EXTREMITY

HEATHER J. FURNAS, M.D.
JOSEPH UPTON, M.D.

Ischemia of the hand and digits is commonly the result of embolization, thrombosis, arteriosclerosis, or vasospasm. Embolic episodes usually lead to acute ischemia, which must be diagnosed and treated urgently. Most patients with vascular symptoms in the hand have chronic ischemia manifested by severe cold intolerance, pain, and, rarely, ulceration and gangrene. A careful diagnostic work-up is imperative to determine the proper treatment modality. We discuss some of the approaches to the treatment of ischemia of the hand, although the management of each individual condition is beyond the scope of this chapter.

CAUSE OF UPPER EXTREMITY ISCHEMIA

Discovering the cause of peripheral upper extremity ischemia will frequently require the collaborative efforts of an internist, a vascular surgeon, and a hand surgeon. Clues that elucidate the cause of ischemia can be invariably traced through a careful medical history. A detailed inquiry should include questions concerning the patients' associated diseases, occupation, nicotine and caffeine use, trauma, and factors that may have precipitated ischemic events. For example, atrial fibrillation or a recent myocardial infarction can predispose to cardiogenic embolism; embolic material may lodge at the bifurcation of the brachial artery, leading to acute ischemia of the hand and forearm. The patient will have clinical symptoms of pain, pallor, lack of pulse, paresthesias, and later, paralysis, in the region of ischemia. Microemboli shed from an ulcerated atherosclerotic plaque or a mural thrombus in the subclavian artery lodge more distally (i.e., in the digital arteries), thereby inducing cyanosis and ischemia of the fingers. Although severe ischemia of the fingers and hands will occasionally improve with the establishment of collateral circulation, distal gangrene is often the end result.

Digital necrosis and gangrene may result from thrombosis or embolism following cardiac catheterization via the brachial artery or after placement of radial artery catheters. Occasionally, the accidental intra-arterial infusion of certain drugs (vasopressors) leads to vasoconstriction and thrombosis. Disseminated intravascular coagulopathy, seen in meningococcal septicemia and malignancies, is also associated with thrombosis affecting the vasculature of the hand. Chronic occupational trauma may also result in compromise of circulation in the hand. The hypothenar hammer syndrome (seen in mechanics or other manual laborers) is associated with repetitive trauma to the hypothenar region. Such trauma can cause intimal injury with resultant thrombosis of a segment of the ulnar artery in the hand. Patients with this complication may complain of a dull ache, burning pain, paresthesias, decreased skin temperature, pallor, cyanosis, and cold intolerance (Figs. 1 and 2).

Chronic ischemia of the hand can result from the advanced vascular disease associated with chronic renal failure. Arterial calcification is a common manifestation that affects vessels as distal as in the forearm, hand, and digits. Many patients without widespread calcification may demonstrate angiographic evidence of segmental occlusions ("skip lesions") of the radial and ulnar arteries, the palmar arch, and the common digital vessels. Whether these segmental occlusions result from disorders such as diabetes mellitus and collagen vascular disease, disorders that often occur in association with renal failure, or from a "steal" phenomenon caused by the arteriovenous fistulas placed for dialysis, is unknown. Additional problems can result from thrombosed fistulas that generate emboli. Vascular occlusion can occur when these emboli lodge distally within the palmar arches and digital arteries.

Collagen vascular diseases can lead to small vessel occlusion through intimal thickening, the possible result of deposition of antigen-antibody complexes. Atherosclerosis, Buerger's disease, and renal vascular disease are also associated with similar intimal thickening that can progress to vascular occlusion. These patients may present with digital ulceration, gangrene, and autoamputation.

Raynaud's phenomenon is a particular manifestation of hand ischemia characterized by pallor of the digits and sometimes followed by cyanosis and post-ischemic rubor. The discoloration may be accompanied by paresthesias or hyperesthesias. Intense hyperemia of the digits accompanies the warming that follows an ischemic attack. This phenomenon may be induced by local or systemic factors, such as exposure to cold temperature or emotional stress. Raynaud's phenomenon may be associated with atherosclerosis, Buerger's disease, scleroderma, systemic lupus erythematosus, blood dyscrasias, or any of the previously mentioned disorders that induce luminal narrowing. *Raynaud's disease* is the term reserved for the entity characterized by Raynaud's phenomenon in the absence of an associated disease process. Vasospasm of the digital arteries in Raynaud's disease may be the result of sympathetic overactivity, or a "local fault" (i.e., an increased sensitivity to circulating vasoconstrictors).

DIAGNOSTIC INVESTIGATION

To identify the cause of symptomatic ischemia of the upper limb, the physician should embark on a systematic

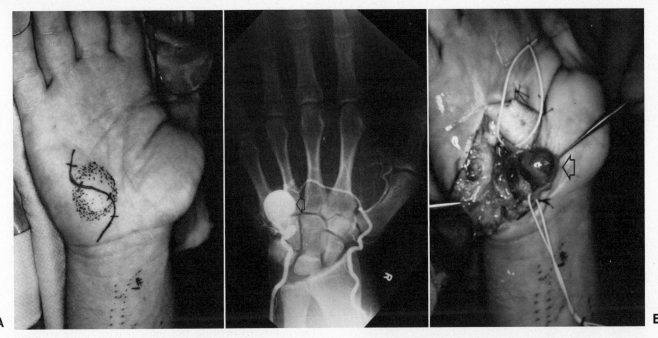

A   B, C

Figure 1 *A,* A large, pulsatile mass *(stippled region)* is seen in a 28-year-old auto mechanic who habitually used the butt of his hand to reinsert wheel hubcaps. He had experienced an episode of transient ischemia of the ulnar three digits. *B,* Retrograde femoral angiogram demonstrating a large aneurysm of the ulnar artery *(arrow). C,* Intraoperative photograph revealing aneurysm of the ulnar artery *(arrow).* Surgical resection with end-to-end reconstitution of the ulnar artery was possible. The location of several donor veins is marked on the distal forearm. Foot veins are generally preferred because their thicker walls (media) resist dilatation following revascularization.

investigation of the vascular system. The hands should be observed for signs of cyanosis, pallor, hyperemia, and masses. The carotid, subclavian, brachial, radial, and ulnar arteries should be palpated and any deficiencies should be documented. An Allen's test can disclose the degree of radial and ulnar arterial inflow. To perform this test, the physician occludes both radial and ulnar arteries at the wrist as the patient makes a tight fist in order to partially exsanguinate the hand (so that the hand appears pale when the fist is released). With the hand relaxed, pressure on one artery is released. The hand should flush immediately. A delayed return of normal coloration of the hand suggests vasospasm or luminal obstruction of the artery under examination. The test is then repeated with occlusion of the other artery.

Blood pressure measurements in both arms can be compared (a difference of more than 20 mmHg is abnormal), and the clavicular area auscultated to check for possible stenosis of the subclavian artery. Segmental blood pressures from the level of the brachial artery to the distal radial and ulnar arteries can be obtained with a Doppler probe to uncover a stenosis or occlusion. A difference of 20 mmHg between segmental pressures suggests a lesion at that level. A plethysmographic evaluation can further identify the extent of vascular abnormalities by providing information for waveform analysis (i.e., reduced pulse wave amplitude suggests luminal narrowing).

Blood flow in the superficial palmar arch, the dorsal branch of the radial artery, and each digital artery can be evaluated with a Doppler probe. Occlusions distal to the superficial palmar arch can be evaluated by performing plethysmography in the fingers.

Cold stress testing of the patient's hands can precipitate the symptoms of vascular insufficiency. During testing the hands are placed in a cooling chamber at a temperature of 6 to 10 degrees Centigrade for 20 minutes. Digital temperatures are recorded every 5 minutes for 20 minutes and then for a further 20 minutes as the temperature is returned to ambient levels. Symptomatic vascular insufficiency is manifested by a lower baseline temperature, a faster rate of cooling, and a slower rate of rewarming. The cold stress test can then be repeated after the administration of a digital block with lidocaine hydrochloride (without epinephrine) for local sympathetic blockade. If an abnormal cold stress reaction normalizes after injection of the local anesthetic, this suggests that sympathetic activity (causing vasoconstriction) is contributing to the vascular insufficiency. The patient who exhibits a beneficial response to blockade of sympathetic vasoconstriction after the administration of local anesthesia is a suitable candidate for a digital sympathectomy (Fig. 3).

An angiogram provides invaluable information about the vascular system of the upper extremity. As an invasive procedure with attendant risks, angiography should be performed judiciously. Indications for this

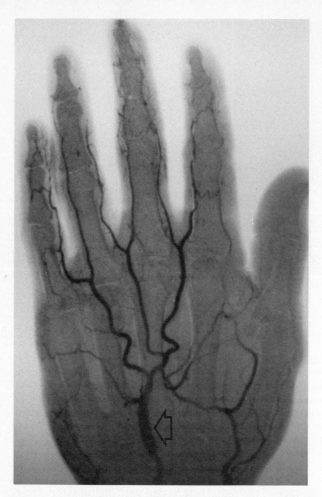

Figure 2 Angiogram revealing dilatation and irregularity of the ulnar artery *(arrow)* in a 34-year-old tree surgeon who had severe distal ischemia of all digits. Microembolization had occluded or obstructed the digital arteries. Reconstitution of flow beyond segmental occlusions is seen in the index and small fingers. Presumably, the ulnar artery abnormality was secondary to chronic occupational trauma (use of hammers and vibrating chain saws).

examination include unilateral Raynaud's phenomenon, recalcitrant or recurrent digital ulceration, and Doppler evidence of a major arterial occlusion.

Patients with diffuse vascular abnormalities of the hands and fingers should be evaluated for a connective tissue disorder. A screening panel initially should include tests for erythrocyte sedimentation rate, serum electrophoresis, antinuclear antibody, and rheumatoid factor.

MEDICAL MANAGEMENT

Treatment of the patient with chronic ischemia of the hand should begin by minimizing the inciting causes of vasoconstriction. Patients should reduce or cease any use of tobacco or other agents known to cause cutaneous vasoconstriction (i.e., cocaine, ergot preparations). They should be instructed in protecting their arms and hands from trauma or exposure to cold temperatures. Patients who have digital ulcerations may benefit from vasodilator therapy with calcium channel antagonists. Because these agents decrease peripheral vascular resistance, blood pressures should be closely monitored.

These agents can also be combined with the hemorrheologic agent, pentoxifylline (Trental), taken in 400 mg doses three times daily. This medication is believed to improve blood flow by decreasing blood viscosity. It is generally well tolerated, but occasionally patients experience gastrointestinal symptoms such as dyspepsia and nausea, dizziness, and tremors. As a methylxanthine derivative, pentoxifylline may potentially lead to angina, hypotension, and arrhythmias, although reported cases are rare. Some patients have experienced bleeding and prolonged prothrombin times.

Some patients with vasospastic ischemia benefit from thermal biofeedback. The goal of biofeedback therapy is to provide the patient with some voluntary control over the autonomic regulation of vasomotor tone. This method can be helpful in some patients who experience cold stress intolerance when vasospasm occurs primarily as a result of anxiety and stress. Biofeedback techniques are frequently offered by outpatient (hand) therapists who work closely with interested vascular medicine physicians and anesthesiologists from pain management clinics.

SURGICAL MANAGEMENT

Microsurgical Reconstruction

Patients with severe symptoms of ischemia, such as rest pain or digital ulcerations, may benefit from medical therapy. Those who do not obtain relief should be considered for surgical revascularization. Those patients who are found to have an occluded arterial segment may benefit from resection of the occluded segment and subsequent arterial reconstruction (see Figs. 1 and 2). The preoperative evaluation in these patients should include angiography to document the presence of segmental occlusions of the radial or ulnar artery, and the superficial palmar arch. Good distal runoff should be present to allow adequate filling of the common digital arteries.

During surgery, the back flow of the common digital arteries should be evaluated directly. If the flow is present and satisfactory, the superficial palmar arch can be reconstructed by using a reversed interposition vein graft. The vein graft, which is commonly taken from the foot, can be anastomosed end to end to the distal ulnar artery and either end to end or end to side to the common digital arteries. Improvement in blood flow may result from increased arterial inflow pressure as well as from the attendant digital sympathectomy that occurs

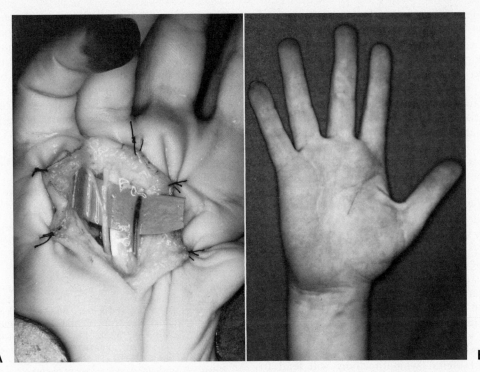

A   B

Figure 3 *A,* Intraoperative photograph displaying the technique of microsurgical sympathectomy. All nerve fibers from the common nerves in the palm to the corresponding arterial
segments are removed. Vessels to both sides of a digit are dissected. Here, the common nerve
to the fourth webspace and the artery to the third webspace are exposed. Note the
gangrenous appearance of the tip of the fifth finger. *B,* Appearance of the same hand 5 years
later following sympathectomy to the index finger. Palmar incisions are well healed. An
additional sympathectomy has been performed at the base of the index and long fingers.
Motion and sensation have been unaffected, and there has been no significant tissue loss.

when dissecting the superficial arch and common digital
arteries at the metacarpal level (see Fig. 3).

The hypothenar hammer syndrome that leads to
ulnar artery thrombosis can be successfully treated by
excising the thrombosed portion of the ulnar artery and
approximating the two ends when the defect is less than
2.0 cm. If the defect is larger, arterial reconstruction is
carried out with a reversed vein graft. In either case,
withdrawal of the causative repetitive trauma is an
essential part of the overall management (see Fig. 2).

Sympathectomy

Revascularization and elimination of the source of
microemboli will *not,* however, completely reverse the
most distal symptoms at the fingertip level, which often
were the symptoms that prompted referral to the
surgeon. These symptoms may be improved by concomitant sympathectomy.

Historically, the cervicothoracic sympathectomy
performed for chronic arterial insufficiency of the upper
arm and hand has had mixed results because the brachial
plexus is supplied, not only by the cervicothoracic
sympathetic trunk, but also by the vertebral nerve
through the sinuvertebral nerve, the carotid plexus, and
the nerve of Kuntz. Intermediary sympathetic ganglia of

the spinal nerve roots or rami communicantes bypass the
sympathetic trunk. Some sympathetic fibers leave the
median and ulnar nerves at the level of the wrist to
innervate the radial and ulnar arteries and superficial
palmar arch, while other sympathetic fibers travel in the
common digital and proper digital nerves to their
corresponding arteries and the superficial palmar arch.
Within the forearm, the distal third of the radial artery
is innervated by a contribution from the superficial
branch of the radial nerve and additional branches from
the lateral cutaneous nerve of the forearm. The deep
palmar arterial arch receives contributions from the
deep branch of the ulnar nerve and one branch from the
medial nerve. Of the patients with distal arterial
problems, most have ischemia in the fingers from the
level of the mid-palm to the tips. Therefore, a very distal
digital sympathectomy results in the best possible
sympathetic blockade of the digital arteries.

Those patients who are good candidates for a digital
sympathectomy demonstrate marked improvement in
cold stress testing after the administration of local
anesthetic block in the distal palm.

The dissection during digital sympathectomy includes isolation and resection of the sympathetic fibers
within the adventitial layer of the common (proper)
digital arteries. The adventitia from the vessel is

visualized through a microscope and then stripped for a length of at least 1.0 to 2.0 cm. All connections between the nerve and vessel are divided sharply before the adventitia is removed from the vessel circumferentially. The media and intima of the artery must be left undisturbed to prevent thrombosis. An increase in the temperature of the fingers is usually apparent within 12 to 24 hours. Initial improvement may be a result of the regional block anesthesia used for the surgical procedure.

In patients with isolated digital ischemia, the sympathectomy can be carried out at the level of the proximal interphalangeal joint to assure that all possible connections between the digital nerve and the digital arteries are divided. Vincular and dorsal arborizations of the digital artery should be preserved under microscopic visualization.

Common digital arteries sometimes appear totally occluded prior to resection of the adventitia. Stripping of the adventitia can result in a pliable and patent vessel. In such cases the patient may benefit from the mechanical release of the external pressure caused by periadventitial fibrosis, which is commonly seen in patients with collagen diseases.

A successful digital sympathectomy will lead to relief from acute digital pain, healing of ulcers, and improvement in the severity of cold intolerance (see Fig. 3). The best results are obtained in those patients who experience symptoms after cold injury and post-traumatic vasospasm, although symptoms in patients suffering from hand ischemia caused by scleroderma, mixed connective tissue disease, and systemic lupus erythematosus may also alleviate. Results are less permanent in those patients with occlusive disease.

SUGGESTED READING

Egloff DV, Mifsud RP, Verdan C. Superselective digital sympathectomy in Raynaud's phenomenon. The Hand 1982; 15:110–114.

Flatt AE. Digital artery sympathectomy. J Hand Surg 1980; 5:550–556.

Given KS, Puskett CL, Kleinert HE. Ulnar artery thrombosis. Plast Reconstr Surg 1978; 61:405–411.

Jones NF. Ischemia of the hand in systemic disease: the potential role of microsurgical revascularization and digital sympathectomy. Clin Plast Surg 1989; 16:547–556.

Morgan RF, Reisman NR, Wilgis EF. Anatomic localization of sympathetic nerves in the hand. J Hand Surg 1983; 8:283–288.

Newmeyer WL. Vascular disorders. In: Green DP, ed. Operative hand surgery 2nd ed. New York: Churchill Livingstone, 1988:2391.

Pin GP, Sicard GA, Weeks PM. Digital ischemia of the upper extremity: a systematic approach for evaluation and treatment. Plast Reconstr Surg 1988; 82:653–657.

Wilgis EF. Evaluation and treatment of chronic digital ischemia. Ann Surg 1981; 193:693–698.

VASCULITIS

VASCULITIC SYNDROMES

GENE G. HUNDER, M.D.

The vasculitides are a group of diverse diseases characterized by the presence of inflammation in blood vessel walls. The inflammation causes narrowing or occlusion of the lumen and ischemia of the tissues supplied by the blood vessel. Alternatively, aneurysms may develop and sometimes rupture. Vessels of different sizes and parts of the body may be involved, giving rise to a broad spectrum of symptoms and signs. The various forms of vasculitis may be transient or chronic, localized or widespread. The inflammatory lesions are usually distributed irregularly in an interrupted fashion, but in some instances longer segments may be involved continuously. Vasculitis may occur as a primary disease or as a secondary manifestation of another illness.

Immunologic processes are generally thought to be involved in the development of most forms of vasculitis, but the exact pathogenetic mechanisms are poorly understood.

Because of the variability of the different types of vasculitis, there is no single or uniform way to study patients suspected of having one of these conditions. Careful history taking is indicated to obtain information about exposure to infectious agents or drugs, as well as a detailed physical examination and appropriate laboratory tests. These measures provide data about the type of onset, course of illness, organ systems involved, and extent of tissue damage. Conditions that might be mistaken for vasculitis must be ruled out, including fibromuscular dysplasia, ergotism, cholesterol embolization, thromboembolic disease, systemic infections, and thrombocytopenia or other processes causing purpura.

Some patients cannot easily be classified diagnostically because of insufficient or atypical findings, or manifestations of more than one type of vasculitis. The physician needs to use experience and judgment about management of such cases. This discussion focuses on well-defined forms of vasculitis.

TAKAYASU'S ARTERITIS

Takayasu's arteritis is a chronic vasculitis that affects the aorta and its primary branches. It begins between the ages of 10 and 30 years and may remain active for years. Most patients are women. The pathology is that of a continuous or patchy granulomatous inflammation with lymphocytes, histiocytes, and multinucleated giant cells infiltrated throughout the segments of larger arteries involved.

Fever, fatigue, and arthralgias may precede vascular symptoms and delay the diagnosis for 1 or more years. Later, symptoms of claudication of the extremities develop. Compromised cranial circulation may result in syncope, blurred vision, and dementia. When the disease is active, the erythrocyte sedimentation rate (ESR) is elevated and a moderate normochromic normocytic anemia is present.

Examination reveals decreased peripheral pulses and bruits over proximal arteries. Diagnosis depends on aortography, which shows focal or lengthy narrowing of affected vessels with smooth-tapered walls and other areas of dilation. Because of the chronicity, collateral circulation is often well developed.

Adrenocorticosteroids effectively and rapidly suppress the systemic symptoms and usually halt the progression of arterial narrowing. The usual starting dose is 40 to 60 mg of prednisone per day or the equivalent of a similar corticosteroid, given as a single morning dose or in divided doses throughout the day. If the patient is treated early, pulses may return. Because the vasculitis has often been present for some time before treatment is started, reversibility is often limited. However, in younger individuals, collateral circulation often develops to provide adequate perfusion of peripheral structures.

After 4 to 6 weeks, when the systemic symptoms have been suppressed and laboratory values have reverted to normal, the prednisone dosage can be reduced by 2.5- to 5-mg decrements every 2 to 4 weeks as tolerated. If severe ischemic symptoms persist after initial treatment, arterial bypass grafting may prove successful. Surgery should not be performed under most circumstances while the disease is still active (i.e., an elevated ESR). In addition, the prednisone dose should be as low as possible or discontinued at the time surgical procedures are performed. Angioplasty may also be useful, but restenosis occurs in a sizable proportion of cases. Cytotoxic drugs can be considered in patients not responding adequately to corticosteroids, but are not needed often.

In most patients the disease tends gradually to become less active with time. However, cases of persistent arteritis for 10 or more years have been reported.

Late in the course of treatment when the prednisone dosage is at a reduced level, it is sometimes difficult to determine whether or not a low degree of inflammation persists. There currently is no perfect way to evaluate and follow such patients. Testing of acute-phase reactants and the ESR is useful but not always reliable. Because of its associated risks, arteriography cannot be performed repeatedly. Careful examination of the pulses and extremity blood pressures should be made periodically. Doppler examination is also useful. Magnetic resonance imaging (MRI) may be helpful, but further refinements are needed.

Current management practices have resulted in a 5-year survival rate of over 90 percent.

GIANT CELL (TEMPORAL) ARTERITIS

Giant cell arteritis most often involves the arteries of the head and neck and spares the intracranial arteries. The disease affects persons over the age of 50, and women more commonly than men. It is one of the more common types of vasculitis in the United States.

Histologically, granulomatous inflammatory infiltrations are found in the vessels that originate from the arch of the aorta. The branches of the external carotid artery are affected most prominently clinically. Microscopic examination of tissue sections shows infiltrations of histiocytes, lymphocytes, and multinucleated giant cells.

Giant cell arteritis may present with a wide range of symptoms or findings, including fatigue, malaise, low-grade or high-spiking fever, aching and stiffness (polymyalgia rheumatica), persistent nonproductive cough, or even hepatic dysfunction. Because these symptoms do not directly suggest vasculitis, the diagnosis may be delayed. The usual symptoms related to vascular involvement include headaches, tender scalp, blindness, and aortic arch syndrome. However, careful history taking and examination reveals evidence of vascular involvement in most cases. Temporal and occipital arteries should be carefully palpated for enlargement, thickening, or tenderness. Tenderness of the scalp away from these vessels is of much less significance. New bruits over the cervical areas or brachial regions are of importance diagnostically. Temporal artery biopsies should be performed to confirm the diagnosis in all patients suspected of having giant cell arteritis. The most abnormal portion of the artery should be selected for biopsy. If the artery is frankly abnormal, only a small section is needed to confirm the clinical diagnosis. However, if the temporal arteries are not obviously involved clinically, a 4- to 6-cm piece should be removed under local anesthesia and cut

into 3- to 5-mm sections, each of which should be examined for giant cell arteritis. If the first biopsy is not positive and the clinical suspicion is high, the opposite temporal artery should be removed and examined in a similar fashion. The occipital artery can be biopsied if it is most clinically abnormal. The scalp has abundant collateral circulation, and removing such long segments of temporal artery does not compromise local circulation. However, an occasional case of active temporal arteritis is associated with ischemia and necrosis of portions of the scalp or tongue as a result of extensive vasculitis.

In some instances when the diagnosis seems apparent, the need for a confirmatory temporal artery biopsy may be questioned. However, later in the course of the disease, after several months of corticosteroid therapy, the original diagnosis may not seem so clear-cut, and a positive biopsy assists decisions regarding treatment at that point. Follow-up studies have shown that if an adequate temporal artery biopsy has been performed, the correct clinical diagnosis is obtained in over 90 percent of cases. Arch aortography should be considered in patients with an aortic arch syndrome.

Initial treatment of giant cell arteritis consists of an initial dose of prednisone, 40 to 60 mg per day; other corticosteroids can be used if desired. The response of the arteritis to corticosteroids is very rapid, and patients are likely to feel improved within 24 hours. If blindness or other complications have occurred or seem imminent, treatment can be started before a biopsy has been obtained. The biopsy can still be done for as long as 3 to 5 days afterward and may still show changes helpful in the diagnosis.

Prednisone can be given as a single morning dose or in divided daily doses. If a vascular complication has occurred recently, the initial doses can be given parenterally, or pulse doses of 500 to 1,000 mg of methylprednisolone can be administered intravenously. Nevertheless, if blindness has developed and has persisted for more than 1 or 2 hours, some permanent visual deficit is likely. With more awareness of this disease in recent years, the frequency of blindness in giant cell arteritis has dropped to approximately 15 percent. Corticosteroids appear to block the development of blindness and other vascular complications in nearly all patients. If blindness or another vascular complication develops after corticosteroids are started, it almost always occurs within the first few days of starting treatment.

The initial dose of corticosteroids should be continued for 2 to 4 weeks, at which time all reversible symptoms and blood tests should be back to normal. The initial dose can be reduced by 5 mg per week to approximately 30 mg per day, and 2.5 mg per week thereafter to 20 mg per day. Subsequently, 2.5 mg decrements every 2 to 4 weeks should be continued unless symptoms return. Below a daily dose of 10 mg, 1-mg decrements per month are recommended. At some point in the reduction schedule, the ESR may rise. At that point, further reductions are interdicted until the clinical situation is assessed. If the ESR elevation was only slight and no other manifestations are present, the steroid withdrawal program may be cautiously resumed. In some patients, moderate doses of corticosteroids may be needed for several months or a year or more; in most patients the prednisone dose can be discontinued after 1 or 2 years. Recurrences develop occasionally, and resumption of low to moderate doses of corticosteroids may be necessary. Follow-up studies indicate that there is no statistically significant increased mortality related to giant cell arteritis. However, occasional patients die from occlusion of large vessels in the neck that cause strokes, rupture of aortic aneurysms, or even coronary artery occlusions.

A variety of steroid-sparing drugs have been tried, including dapsone, azathioprine, cyclophosphamide, and methotrexate, but these have not proved clearly helpful in most patients. They can be tried in patients with persistently active disease who have needed continued high doses of corticosteroids.

POLYARTERITIS NODOSA

Polyarteritis nodosa is defined as an acute necrotizing arteritis involving medium-sized and small muscular arteries. In typical cases it is a toxic, multisystem illness with fever, fatigue, and a variety of other manifestations such as mononeuritis multiplex, muscular and joint pains, glomerulonephritis, mesenteric ischemia, and skin ulcers. It may present as a slowly progressive illness over weeks or months or a sudden overwhelming process associated with early death. There probably are multiple causes of polyarteritis. Hepatitis B virus infection is a well-documented etiology but accounts for only a minority of cases.

Histologically, an acute vasculitis is present with infiltration of the artery wall structures by neutrophils and lesser numbers of other leukocytes. The internal elastic lamina becomes disrupted, resulting in aneurysms and occasional vessel rupture. Fibrinoid necrosis may be prominent. At times only a portion of the artery wall is affected. In the healing phase, mononuclear cells predominate. Acute and healing lesions may be seen in the same biopsy specimen.

Diagnosis is best made by biopsy of a symptomatically involved area. This includes skin ulcers, sural nerve in patients with neuritis, and muscle biopsy in patients with pain and tenderness of other tissues. A percutaneous renal biopsy generally shows glomerulonephritis but does not yield a blood vessel large enough to diagnose vasculitis. If symptoms are not localized but the diagnosis is suspected, a mesenteric angiogram may be appropriate. Typical cases show multiple aneurysms of small and medium-sized vessels, irregularities of the vessel lumen, and occlusions of blood vessels that support a clinical impression. Left atrial myxoma and bacterial endocarditis with embolism may produce a similar picture. Diagnostic findings need to be correlated with the overall clinical picture. The results of biopsy obviously depend on the tissue examined, and the stage of the vessel lesion, i.e., acute or healing vasculitis. If skin or sural nerve is biopsied, any changes are likely to be noted in very small vessels. If a muscle specimen is taken, a larger vessel may be visualized. Angiograms show aneurysmal changes in small and medium-sized conduit vessels. Because other syndromes may be mistaken for polyarteritis, it is important to try to secure a positive histologic diagnosis before embarking on treatment.

Therapy consists of adrenocorticosteroids, often combined with cyclophosphamide. In cases that do not seem urgent and are more limited in organ involvement, adrenocorticosteroids alone may be sufficient. An initial dose of 40 to 60 mg of prednisone may be tried. If the patient's response is not rapid, larger doses can be given. The starting dose should be continued until all reversible signs, symptoms, and laboratory tests have returned to normal, generally in about 1 to 2 months. Subsequently, the dose can be reduced by small decrements of approximately 10 percent of the total daily dose every 2 to 4 weeks as tolerated. Lower doses of corticosteroids may be needed over several months to keep the disease under control.

In patients with rapidly developing symptoms or with widespread involvement, cyclophosphamide should be started with the prednisone. A single dose of 1.5 to 2 mg per kilogram body weight is usually prescribed in the morning. Patients should drink large amounts of water to avoid hemorrhagic cystitis or bladder neoplasms due to toxic metabolic products of this drug. Recently it has been suggested that monthly pulses of cyclophosphamide of approximately 500 to 1,000 mg may be helpful and result in less toxicity because the total dose is reduced.

There is no uniformity of opinion regarding the duration of use of cyclophosphamide, but if the disease is brought under control, the dosage can be reduced and discontinued as tolerated. Subsequently, the corticosteroid dose should be lowered and discontinued. There is no evidence that continuing corticosteroids or cytotoxic drugs for a fixed period, such as 1 year, even though symptoms remit in a month or two, results in a better outcome or "cure." The physician should evaluate the relative toxicities of these drugs in the individual patient, and on that basis decide which of the drugs to lower initially. In chronic cases with relatively stable symptoms in which moderate or larger doses of prednisone are required, azathioprine can be used as a steroid-sparing agent instead of cyclophosphamide. An initial dosage of 1.5 to 2 mg per kilogram body weight can be used. Several weeks are likely to elapse before any beneficial effect is noted. The antiviral drug vidarabine has been used experimentally in a few patients with hepatitis-associated vasculitis, with some apparent success.

Gastrointestinal ischemia and renal insufficiency are causes of early death. Infection and cardiovascular complications are causes of later death. Side effects of therapeutic agents have also been a contributor to later death. The mortality rate is greatest early in the first year of the disease. The 5-year survival rate in patients with polyarteritis nodosa has been greater than 50 percent in recent years.

ALLERGIC ANGIITIS AND GRANULOMATOSIS (CHURG-STRAUSS SYNDROME)

The most common manifestations of this infrequent vasculitis are asthma, eosinophilia, small and medium-sized artery vasculitis, and extravascular eosinophilic granulomas. The clinical spectrum of clinical findings is similar to those of polyarteritis, except that pulmonary involvement is usually present in Churg-Strauss syndrome but exceptional in polyarteritis nodosa.

Histologically, eosinophils are usually the predominant leukocyte infiltrating the vessel walls, but neutrophils and other cells may also be present. Fibrinoid necrosis, disruption of the elastic lamina, thrombosis, or rupture may also occur. Extravascular necrotizing eosinophilic granulomas may be found in a wide variety of tissues such as lung, skin, and prostate.

The diagnosis should be suspected in a patient who has a systemic illness with eosinophilia, asthma, pulmonary infiltrations or progressive interstitial changes, mononeuritis multiplex, palpable purpura, or other vasculitic findings. The diagnosis is confirmed by biopsy of affected tissue.

Initial therapy consists of adrenocorticosteroids in dosages sufficient to control the inflammatory manifestations. As in most other forms of vasculitis, the initial dose is 40 to 60 mg of prednisone per day as a single morning dose or in divided doses. Patients with Churg-Strauss syndrome appear to respond better as a group to corticosteroids than patients with polyarteritis nodosa. Experience with cytotoxic drugs is not extensive, but cyclophosphamide or azathioprine may be used in patients not responding adequately to corticosteroids, or as steroid-sparing agents later in the course of treatment.

The long-term survival has not been studied extensively, but a 5-year survival rate of 62 percent was found in one series. Common causes of death include myocardial infarction, congestive heart failure, and pulmonary complications. As in other forms of vasculitis, deaths also occur as a result of infections related to immunosuppressive drugs.

WEGENER'S GRANULOMATOSIS

Wegener's granulomatosis consists of granulomatous inflammation and vasculitis of the upper and lower respiratory tracts and kidneys. In some instances the involvement may be limited to the nasal structures or respiratory tract, but in others the disease is more generalized and any organ may be involved. Long-term survival without treatment is rare.

Diagnosis is based on the combination of clinical features and typical histopathology. In smaller biopsy specimens the vasculitic component may not be seen, and correlation with the clinical findings is necessary to make the diagnosis. Cultures and stains should be taken to exclude mycobacterial and fungal infections that have similar pathologic changes.

Recently the diagnostic importance of antineutrophil cytoplasmic antibodies (ANCAs) has been recognized. The titer of these antibodies is usually higher in active and generalized disease and may aid in the follow-up of patients. A variety of techniques for testing these antibodies is being developed. The most widely used test at this time is an immunofluorescent method using peripheral blood polymorphonuclear leukocytes as the substrate. A bright granular fluorescence is characteristic of Wegener's granulomatosis; less intense staining is seen in other vasculitides. A perinuclear pattern is seen in glomerulonephritis.

The combination of cyclophosphamide and prednisone is extremely effective for control of the disease. The initial dosage of prednisone is 40 to 60 mg per day or an equivalent dose of a similar corticosteroid. Cyclophosphamide is given at 1.5 to 2 mg per kilogram body weight. The prednisone dosage can usually be reduced and discontinued after 1 to 3 months, but cyclophosphamide is continued longer. Patients generally improve quickly on this regimen, and all reversible signs and symptoms may have resolved within 1 to 2 months. Remission develops in over 90 percent of patients on this regimen. Most rheumatologists empirically continue cyclophosphamide for 1 year after the patient has gone into remission, after which the dose is reduced and then discontinued. However, relapses may occur after 1 or more years. In such instances, cyclophosphamide should be started again and continued for another year. The risk of neoplastic complications increases with the total dosage of cyclophosphamide used. Some attempts have been made to treat Wegener's granulomatosis patients with pulse cyclophosphamide in a dosage of 500 to 1,000 mg at 3- to 4-week intervals intravenously. Although trials have not been extensive, early experience suggests that pulse cyclophosphamide may not control the disease as well as daily oral therapy. Opportunistic infections are a common cause of death with long-term treatment.

Trimethoprim-sulfamethoxazole has been advocated as an adjunctive treatment of Wegener's granulomatosis. It may be tried in milder or limited cases, but is clearly not helpful for all patients.

Follow-up may be aided by measurement of ANCA in serum. Relapses are frequently preceded by a rise in antibody titer. The role of these antibodies in the pathogenesis of Wegener's granulomatosis is not known, however.

VASCULITIS WITH RHEUMATIC DISEASES

Vascular inflammation is central to many rheumatic diseases. In rheumatoid arthritis, perivascular collections of lymphocytes and intimal proliferation commonly occur in the synovium and other tissues. These changes are not referred to as necrotizing vasculitis because the circulation appears to remain unimpaired and there is no evidence of damage to the blood vessels themselves.

In some instances, however, more marked intimal proliferation develops, leading to impaired circulation in the digits or resulting in skin infarctions and leg ulcerations. In a small percentage of patients with severe seropositive nodular rheumatoid arthritis and other rheumatic diseases, a necrotizing vasculitis develops. Small or medium-sized muscular arteries and arterioles may be affected. Microscopically the vascular lesions are indistinguishable from those of polyarteritis nodosa.

For localized or less systemic involvement, observation or more aggressive therapy for the underlying rheumatic disease may suffice. Low or medium doses of corticosteroids may be indicated in other cases if progression develops. When mononeuritis multiplex, mesenteric artery ischemia, or other serious problems develop, large doses of corticosteroids are indicated, 40 to 60 mg of prednisone per day or more. Cytotoxic drugs such as cyclophosphamide and azathioprine may also be considered.

Rheumatoid vasculitis and the necrotizing vasculitis associated with lupus erythematosus tend to be self-limited processes and may regress after weeks or months. The aim of therapy is to prevent irreversible changes during the active phase. The dosage of corticosteroid or cytotoxic agent should be reduced gradually as tolerated.

VASCULITIS OF SMALL BLOOD VESSELS

This group includes a number of diverse conditions with acute necrotizing inflammation of the small blood vessels, especially arterioles, capillaries, and venules of the skin and other organs. Palpable purpura is the most characteristic finding in this group of conditions. These syndromes also are sometimes grouped under the term *hypersensitivity vasculitis* because it is suspected that hypersensitivity mechanisms are important in their pathogenesis. The histopathologic findings are similar in most cases, and these syndromes have also been categorized as *leukocytoclastic vasculitides*. Typically, neutrophils infiltrate the vessel wall and perivascular areas. As the inflammatory process evolves, leukocytes fragment, and cellular and nucleolar remnants are visible. In some instances, however, lymphocytes predominate.

Hypersensitivity Vasculitis

This term is most appropriate for cases that develop after exposure to a sensitizing agent or in which one is strongly suspected. Maculopapular lesions are present over various areas of the body. Careful history taking may help determine the presence of a possible inciting agent. Biopsy of a lesion is recommended to confirm the presence of vasculitis as a cause of the purpura. Any potential inciting agent or drug should be eliminated. Mild cases with a brief episode and limited skin rash may require no specific treatment. If the rash is extensive and internal organs are involved, corticosteroids can be given in doses of 20 to 40 mg per day, reduced as symptoms resolve.

Henoch-Schönlein Purpura

This syndrome usually occurs in childhood and includes palpable purpura, abdominal pain, glomerulonephritis, and arthritis. It is often self-limited but may be worse when it occurs in adults. Corticosteroids can be used if necessary but are required in only a few cases.

MIXED CRYOGLOBULINEMIA

This syndrome includes palpable purpura, arthralgias, glomerulonephritis, hepatic abnormalities, or other symptoms. It tends to be chronic and may be progressive. Small amounts of cryoglobulins are found in plasma that contain IgG and IgM and other proteins. The IgM component usually has rheumatoid factor activity.

Treatment depends on the extent of the disease. Penicillamine has been used in some cases, 1 to 1.5 g per day. Corticosteroids can be used in doses similar to those for polyarteritis nodosa. Cyclophosphamide may be given as a steroid-sparing agent in chronic cases. In addition to these drugs, plasmapheresis may be helpful for acute flares.

SUGGESTED READING

Conn DL, Hunder GG. Necrotizing vasculitis. In: Kelley WN, Harris ED, Ruddy S, Sledge CB, eds. Textbook of rheumatology. 3rd ed. Philadelphia: WB Saunders, 1989:1137.

Devaney KO, Travis WD, Hoffman G, et al. Interpretation of head and neck biopsies in Wegener's granulomatosis. Am J Surg Pathol 1990; 14:555–564.

Hunder GG, Arend WP, Bloch DA, et al. The American College of Rheumatology 1990 criteria for the classification of vasculitis: introduction. Arthritis Rheum 1990; 33:1065–1144.

Jennette JC, Wilkman AS, Falk RJ. Antineutrophil cytoplasmic antibody–associated glomerulonephritis and vasculitis. Am J Pathol 1989; 135:921–930.

Machado EBV, Michet CJ, Ballard DJ, et al. Trends in incidence and clinical presentation of temporal arteritis in Olmsted County, Minnesota, 1950–1985. Arthritis Rheum 1988; 31:745–749.

KAWASAKI DISEASE

ROBERT P. SUNDEL, M.D.
JANE W. NEWBURGER, M.D., M.P.H.

Kawasaki disease (KD) is an idiopathic childhood vasculitis of small- and medium-sized vessels that has become a leading cause of acquired heart disease in American children. The syndrome was first described by a Japanese pediatrician in 1967 and is characterized by fever, conjunctivitis, rash, mucosal inflammation, lymph-adenopathy, and extremity changes. The major morbidity of KD, however, occurs in the heart: coronary artery aneurysms or ectasia develop in approximately 15 to 25 percent of children with the disease and may lead to myocardial infarction, sudden death, or chronic coronary artery insufficiency. Intravenous gamma globulin decreases the incidence of coronary artery aneurysms three- to fivefold if given within 10 days of disease onset. Management of children with suspected KD therefore requires accurate and expeditious diagnosis and close monitoring of the cardiovascular system. This chapter outlines our approach to the KD patient, from initial evaluation to long-term follow-up (Fig. 1).

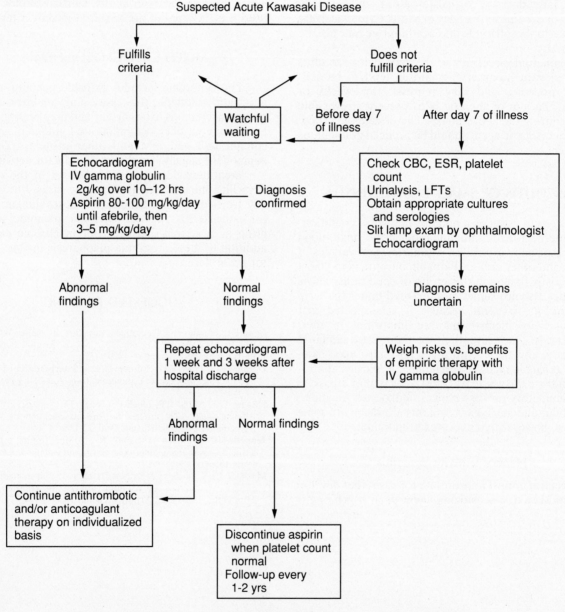

Figure 1 Algorithm for evaluation of patients with suspected Kawasaki disease.

DIAGNOSIS

Clinical Criteria

The diagnosis of KD rests on fulfilling at least five of six clinical criteria of mucocutaneous inflammation (Table 1). These criteria vary considerably in frequency. For example, fever is thought to reflect the underlying inflammation incited by proinflammatory lymphokines, including tumor necrosis factor and interleukin-1. Therefore, even if a child has the remaining five signs of mucocutaneous inflammation, a diagnosis of KD in the absence of fever must be suspect. On the other hand, lymphadenopathy is most likely to be absent at diagnosis: up to one-half of children with KD do not have lymphadenopathy at presentation, and this is especially likely to be the case in younger children.

As with other diseases diagnosed on the basis of clinical manifestations (e.g., acute rheumatic fever, systemic lupus erythematosus), the diagnostic criteria were constructed in an attempt to minimize false-positive diagnoses. Nonetheless, a percentage of children who meet the criteria have other diseases, while some of those subsequently shown to have KD do not fulfill the criteria (so-called partial, incomplete, or atypical KD). The illnesses most likely to mimic KD are viral infections (measles, adenovirus infection), toxin-mediated illnesses (beta-hemolytic streptococcal infection, toxic shock syndrome), and idiopathic immune or autoimmune diseases (drug reactions, juvenile rheumatoid arthritis). While the absence of a diagnostic test prevents absolute distinction in some cases, certain characteristics of the clinical criteria may be helpful:

1. Discrete intraoral lesions are virtually never seen in KD, so Koplik's spots, vesicles, or purulent tonsillitis all strongly suggest alternative diagnoses.
2. The conjunctivitis of KD is rarely exudative. During the first week of illness, mild inflammation of the anterior chamber is observed in approximately 80 percent of patients. Slit-lamp evidence of anterior uveitis may thus be helpful in supporting a diagnosis of KD, whereas ocular discharge makes KD less likely.

Table 1 Diagnostic Criteria for Kawasaki Disease

Fever of at least 5 days' duration not explained by other disease processes, plus at least four of the following five conditions:
1. Bilateral conjunctival injection
2. Changes in the oropharyngeal mucous membranes (including one or more of injected and/or fissured lips, strawberry tongue, injected pharynx)
3. Changes of peripheral extremities, including erythema and/or edema of the hands or feet (acute phase) or periungual desquamation (convalescent phase)
4. Polymorphous rash, primarily truncal; nonvesicular
5. Cervical lymphadenopathy

Modified from Centers for Disease Control. Kawasaki disease—New York. MMWR 1980; 29:61–63.

3. Lymphadenopathy in KD, for unknown reasons, is generally restricted to the anterior cervical region, especially that overlying the sternocleidomastoid muscle. Diffuse lymphadenopathy or splenomegaly therefore should prompt a search for other possibilities.
4. The rash in KD is described as polymorphous and literally may have almost any appearance. However, in two-thirds of patients it begins in the perineal region, followed 48 hours later by desquamation. Bullous or vesicular lesions almost never occur in KD.
5. Extremity involvement includes erythema and an indurative edema. One-third of patients develop arthralgia or arthritis, typically involving the small joints during the acute phase and the large joints during the second and third weeks of illness. During convalescence, periungual desquamation and, later, transverse grooves in the nails (Beau's lines) typify KD.

On the other hand, certain clinical characteristics of KD are not included among the diagnostic criteria, but are frequently noted. Most striking of these is irritability: children with KD, especially infants, are often inconsolable. This is thought to be due to meningeal irritation (as evidenced by abnormalities of the cerebrospinal fluid [CSF]) and possibly encephalitis (with demonstrable electroencephalographic changes). KD occurs most often in males, with a male:female ratio of 1.6:1. Children with KD tend to be young, with a peak incidence in the toddler years; approximately 80 percent of patients are younger than 5 years of age, and the disease is extremely rare over age 15. KD in adolescents therefore must be diagnosed with caution. Finally, recent evidence suggests that KD may frequently be accompanied by transient, mild, sensorineural hearing loss, in addition to the tympanitis previously reported.

The conventional diagnostic criteria are particularly useful in preventing overdiagnosis, but they may result in failure to recognize incomplete forms of the illness. Signs and symptoms of KD are particularly obscure in infants less than 6 to 12 months of age, the subgroup at highest risk for coronary lesions. Fever is probably the only universal symptom. Accordingly, the diagnosis should be considered in all infants with prolonged, unexplained fever; irritability; and laboratory signs of inflammation. If possible, these children should be referred to a regional KD center for further evaluation.

Laboratory Studies

No laboratory values are included in the criteria for KD, but in ambiguous cases certain trends may be helpful. As already noted, KD is characterized by widespread release of inflammatory mediators, and blood test results reflect this. Early in the disease course, acute-phase reactants (e.g., erythrocyte sedimentation rate [ESR], C-reactive protein [CRP], alpha$_1$-antitrypsin) tend to be elevated, and there is usually a leukocytosis and left shift in the white blood cell (WBC) count. By the second week of fever, platelet counts are generally elevated, rising to over 1 million per cubic millimeter in the most severe cases.

For reasons that are poorly understood, children with KD usually have significant anemia. The hematocrit may be more than two standard deviations below normal even early in the disease course, before the effects of decreased reticulocytosis should be clinically evident. Similarly, urethritis, aseptic meningitis, and hepatitis may be part of the illness. Evaluation of urine commonly reveals WBCs on microscopic urinalysis; these cells are monocytes and are not detected by dipstick tests for leukocyte esterase, so macroscopic examination alone is inadequate. Although lumbar punctures are not routinely performed in KD, the CSF characteristically displays a mononuclear pleocytosis without elevated protein or decreased glucose. Measurement of liver enzymes reveals elevated transaminase levels or mild hyperbilirubinemia; in a small percentage of children, obstructive jaundice from hydrops of the gallbladder may complicate the disease course.

Cardiovascular Findings

Cardiac abnormalities dominate the pathology of KD. Clinical examination is often remarkable for tachycardia and gallop rhythms that are more prominent than expected from the degree of fever and anemia. These findings are thought to be secondary to myocarditis, which has been demonstrated in autopsy and myocardial biopsy studies to be a universal feature of early KD. Rarely, myocardial inflammation may progress to frank congestive heart failure. The severity of myocarditis does not appear to be associated with the risk of coronary artery aneurysms, nor does it correlate with the pericardial effusion that may develop during the second week of illness. The effusion rarely progresses to tamponade and resolves spontaneously in most instances. Valvulitis, presenting as either aortic or mitral regurgitation, may be seen in a small percentage of children during the early phases of KD. Late-onset mitral regurgitation, from papillary muscle dysfunction or myocardial infarction, may also complicate the clinical course.

Most characteristic of KD is inflammation of the coronary arteries. This progresses to ectasia or aneurysm formation in 15 to 25 percent of untreated children. Several scoring systems have been developed to identify those children at highest risk for formation of coronary artery abnormalities. Male gender, age under 1 year, duration of fever, and degree of elevation of CRP and absolute band count and depression of albumin level are among the best predictors. However, at the time of early presentation, no algorithm can clearly differentiate those children who will develop aneurysms from those who will remain unaffected.

The electrocardiogram (ECG) in acute KD may show mild abnormalities consistent with myocarditis, most commonly prolonged PR interval and nonspecific ST-segment and T-wave changes. Of greatest utility in evaluating children with suspected or documented KD, however, is the two-dimensional echocardiogram. This may be used both for detecting coronary artery abnormalities (where the sensitivity approaches that of angiography) and pericardial effusions and for quantifying myocardial dysfunction. Echocardiographic evaluation of myocardial function early in the course of the disease frequently reveals reduced left ventricular function and contractility. Dilatation of the coronary arteries may be detected by echocardiography as early as 7 days after the first appearance of fever, and usually peaks 3 or 4 weeks after the onset of illness.

The normal ranges of coronary artery segment diameters measured by two-dimensional echocardiography in children are not well established and show wide variation by body surface area. A baseline two-dimensional echocardiogram before coronary dilatation ordinarily begins (i.e., before the seventh day of illness) provides a baseline for comparison with later studies. Cardiac catheterization need not be performed in patients with normal echocardiograms and ECGs throughout the disease course, as the likelihood of finding unsuspected lesions is negligible.

Echocardiographic examinations should be repeated about 2 weeks and again 1 month after the onset of illness. Additional examinations may be necessary in some patients with persistent fever or abnormalities on their early examinations; uncooperative young patients should be sedated to obtain optimal visualization. Complete studies should include visualization of the left main coronary artery, the left anterior descending branch to a point beyond the level of the pulmonic valve, the left circumflex artery, and the right coronary artery from ostium to posterior crux and posterior descending branch. Doppler interrogation of the mitral and aortic valves, quantitative assessment of left ventricular function, and the presence or absence of pericardial effusion should also be evaluated.

It is often difficult to obtain agreement on the exact configuration and extent of coronary artery lesions as demonstrated by two-dimensional echocardiography, in large part owing to the variability of coronary artery caliber in normal children. To address this issue, the Japanese subcommittee on standardization of diagnostic criteria and reporting of coronary artery lesions in Kawasaki disease has combined ectasia and aneurysm into the single category of "dilated lesions." We prefer to use their definition: a coronary artery whose internal lumen is at least 3 mm in a child under age 5 years, or 4 mm in a child at least age 5 years, is considered abnormal. In addition, if the internal diameter of a segment measures at least 1.5 times that of an adjacent segment, or if its lumen is clearly irregular, then the coronary artery is classified as abnormal even if its greatest internal diameter is less than 3 mm.

Selective coronary arteriography can provide definitive delineation of coronary artery anatomy. This technique is especially useful for visualization of coronary artery lesions that are difficult to define by two-dimensional echocardiography (e.g., the presence of stenoses, distal lesions). Because of the potential morbidity and mortality of invasive studies, we perform angiography only in patients with persistent aneurysms. Using a percutaneous femoral approach, right and left heart studies are performed. Selective coronary angiograms, using specially formed No. 4.5 Fr pediatric coronary artery catheters, are then obtained in at least two projections for each coronary artery. Large-volume injections of nonionic contrast (up to 0.5 ml per kilogram) may be necessary to obtain excellent images of large aneurysms.

Coronary aneurysms in early KD usually occur in the proximal segments of the major coronary vessels; abnormalities that occur distally are almost always associated with proximal coronary dilatations (Fig. 2). Aneurysms may also occur in arteries outside the coronary system, most commonly the subclavian, brachial, axillary, iliac, or femoral vessels and occasionally in the abdominal aorta and renal arteries. For this reason, abdominal aortography and subclavian arteriography are often performed in patients undergoing coronary arteriography for KD. The arterial lesions gradually transform with the passage of time, sometimes with apparent partial or total regression of aneurysms, and sometimes with development of stenoses or occlusion. Coronary angiography is therefore repeated at intervals of 1 to 5 years in some patients with multiple severe coronary lesions, especially in those for whom future surgical management is contemplated.

THERAPY

Aspirin

Aspirin was the first medication to be used for treatment of KD because of its anti-inflammatory and antithrombotic effects. Few prospective studies have examined its efficacy and optimal dosing regimen. Typically, high doses (80 to 100 mg per kilogram per day in divided doses four times a day) are employed during the inflammatory phase of illness; salicylate levels are monitored to avoid toxicity. Once the child has been afebrile for 48 hours (evidence that active vasculitis has subsided), aspirin is decreased to antithrombotic doses of 3 to 5 mg per kilogram per day. Finally, when platelet counts normalize, aspirin is discontinued. All elements of this recommendation are empiric; although retrospective studies have suggested that aneurysms may be less common among children treated early with high-dose aspirin, selection bias renders these data uninterpretable. Further, many clinicians have the impression that high-dose aspirin makes children less uncomfortable and benefits the associated arthritis seen in up to one-third of cases of KD. Following the acute inflammatory stage of KD, platelet counts may remain elevated for weeks, and coronary artery endothelium is thought to have diminished antiaggretory potential. Accordingly, low-dose aspirin is conventionally continued to provide some antithrombotic effects.

There is considerable variability in actual salicylate dosing because of the lack of objective data and because of various theoretical and potential risks. Of greatest concern is the risk of Reye's syndrome; there are anecdotal reports of three children being treated for KD with aspirin who developed this complication. Additionally, aspirin binding studies suggest that the hypoalbuminemia of children with KD predisposes them to toxic-free salicylate levels despite measured (bound) values within the therapeutic range. Weighing the absence of objective evidence of benefit from salicylates against these concerns, we accept relatively low serum salicylate levels (i.e., 10 to 15 mg per deciliter). We rapidly discontinue aspirin upon exposure to, or signs of,

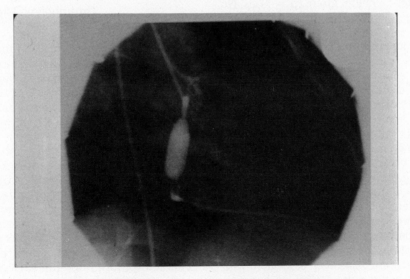

Figure 2 Selective right coronary arteriogram in the right anterior oblique projection demonstrating a fusiform aneurysm of the right coronary artery.

varicella or influenza, and we attempt to limit treatment with high-dose aspirin to periods of fever or severe arthritis. Alternatives to aspirin, especially nonsteroidal anti-inflammatory drugs such as ibuprofen, have not received widespread use in the United States. In Japan, however, these are employed regularly, without obvious differences in outcome compared with salicylates.

Intravenous Gamma Globulin

Intravenous gamma globulin (IVGG) treatment has revolutionized the care of children with KD. Studies in Japan suggested relative protection from coronary artery aneurysms when IVGG was administered in doses analogous to those used in idiopathic thrombocytopenia. Since then, further trials in the United States and Japan have confirmed this finding and documented the safety of high-dose infusions of gamma globulin when administered early in the course of the disease.

In a prospective, randomized, multicenter, controlled trial performed in the United States, investigators compared the efficacy of IVGG plus aspirin with that of aspirin alone in reducing the frequency of coronary artery abnormalities in children with acute KD. Children assigned to the gamma globulin group received IVGG, 400 mg per kilogram per day, for 4 consecutive days; both treatment groups received aspirin, 100 mg per kilogram per day, through the 14th day of illness, then 3 to 5 mg per kilogram per day. Two-dimensional echocardiograms were interpreted blindly and independently by two or more readers. Two weeks after enrollment, coronary artery abnormalities were present in 18 of 78 children (23 percent) treated with aspirin alone, compared with 6 of 75 (8 percent) treated with gamma globulin plus aspirin (p = .01). Seven weeks after enrollment, abnormalities were present in 14 of 79 children (18 percent) in the aspirin group and in 3 of 79 (4 percent) in the gamma globulin group (p = .005). No children had serious adverse effects from receiving gamma globulin.

Therapy with gamma globulin has additional benefits. Treatment results in a reduced prevalence of giant aneurysms, the most serious form of coronary abnormality caused by the disease, and accelerates normalization of abnormalities of left ventricular systolic function and contractility. Finally, high-dose IVGG reduces fever and laboratory indices of inflammation, suggesting a rapid, generalized, anti-inflammatory effect in addition to specific cardioprotective effects. A recently completed U.S. trial compared the four-dose regimen with a single infusion of 2 g per kilogram of IVGG. Single dosing appears to be more effective than the conventional regimen, with a similar safety profile. No studies have compared the relative efficacies of the seven IVGG preparations currently available in the United States. However, none has been associated with a human immunodeficiency virus (HIV) or hepatitis infection, and all are thought to be free of transmissible agents.

Antithrombotic Therapy

The risk of coronary artery thrombosis is greatest after the acute inflammation has subsided. At that point, beginning approximately 2 to 3 weeks after disease onset, smoldering coronary vasculitis coincides with marked thrombocytosis and hypercoagulability due to both endothelial and fluid-phase abnormalities. Low-dose aspirin (3 to 5 mg per kilogram per day given as a single dose) is the mainstay of antithrombotic therapy in KD. Dipyridamole (3 to 6 mg per kilogram per day in three divided doses) may be substituted for aspirin when salicylates are contraindicated. For children without evidence of coronary artery ectasia or aneurysms, antiplatelet therapy is usually discontinued approximately 2 months after the onset of illness.

Children with coronary artery abnormalities require long-term antithrombotic therapy, usually with low-dose aspirin. Dipyridamole is sometimes added to aspirin therapy, although its value in this setting is controversial. The risk of coronary thrombosis and myocardial infarction is especially great in children with rapidly increasing coronary dimension or with giant aneurysms (internal diameter greater than 8 mm). Blood flow in these cavernous vascular segments is turbulent and sluggish, so some investigators advocate treatment with systemic heparin together with an antiplatelet agent during the subacute phase. For chronic antithrombotic therapy, options include aspirin with or without dipyridamole, anticoagulation using warfarin, or a combination of antiplatelet and anticoagulant therapy, usually dipyridamole or sulfinpyrazone with warfarin. No prospective data exist to guide the clinician in choosing an optimal regimen, and anecdotal reports suggest cases of thrombosis despite treatment with each of these drug combinations. Currently, aspirin plus dipyridamole is the most popular regimen because of its safety and ease of administration.

Thrombolytic Therapy

Despite the use of antithrombotic agents, myocardial infarction secondary to thrombotic occlusion of coronary aneurysms may develop in some children, especially those with giant aneurysms. In others, the presence of a coronary artery thrombus may be detected on serial two-dimensional echocardiography. Treatment with thrombolytic agents in adults with myocardial infarction has been conclusively demonstrated to decrease mortality and improve function. In children with KD and coronary artery thrombosis, thrombolytic agents—mainly urokinase and streptokinase, either intravenous or intracoronary—have been used with variable success. Thrombolytic therapy for coronary artery thrombosis is most effective if begun within 3 to 4 hours of symptom onset. Immediately following clot lysis, systemic heparin is begun in combination with aspirin. Maintenance of reperfusion then requires chronic oral antithrombotic therapy (e.g., warfarin with dipyridamole), although the ideal regimen has not been established.

Surgical Management

Surgical management in KD is composed primarily of coronary artery bypass grafts for obstructive lesions, although mitral valve replacement is occasionally necessary in children with papillary muscle dysfunction or valvulitis. The decision to recommend coronary artery bypass grafting in children with KD must take into account the technical complexity of anastomosis of grafts to very small coronary arteries, the absence of symptoms or evidence of heart failure in the majority of cases with coronary artery occlusion, and the remarkable capacity of children to form collaterals. The indications for coronary bypass graft procedures in children have not been established, but such surgery should be considered when stenosis is demonstrated to be progressive, the myocardium to be perfused through the graft is still viable, and no appreciable lesions are present in the artery peripheral to the planned graft site. When these conditions are satisfied, surgery is an option if arteriography demonstrates critical stenosis of the left main coronary artery, or occlusions or progressive critical stenosis in two or more of the other coronary vessels. Isolated stenotic lesions in the proximal left anterior descending artery or the right coronary artery are probably not an indication for bypass grafting.

The earliest coronary artery bypass surgery in children with KD was performed using autologous saphenous veins, or veins obtained from a parent. Results with this approach, however, were unsatisfactory, with late occlusion rates of 32 to 87 percent due to marked myointimal proliferation and graft shortening. Recently, Japanese groups have reported improved results with the use of internal mammary artery grafts. These grafts increase in both diameter and length as the children grow, and late patency rates of up to 100 percent have been achieved. After surgery, patients show improvement of abnormalities on exercise ECG, of thallium-20 myocardial scintigraphy during exercise, and of the response of stroke volume to the increase in end-diastolic pressure during exercise. Greater patient accrual and further follow-up are necessary to assess the long-term results of coronary artery bypass surgery for obstructive lesions in KD.

Miscellaneous

Patients who fail to respond completely to IVGG pose the greatest therapeutic dilemma. Prolonged fever itself correlates with increased risk of developing coronary artery abnormalities; males under 1 year of age are of special concern, because their risk of developing aneurysms is approximately 20 percent despite treatment. Although this is a significant improvement over their risk without IVGG, it obviously represents an unsatisfactory failure rate. Approaches to this problem vary; our preference, based on experience with a handful of patients as well as on data that indicate a correlation between defervescence and postinfusion serum IgG levels, is to treat nonresponders with a second dose of gamma globulin, 1 g per kilogram over 5 hours. The risk appears to be minimal: no patient given a second dose has had adverse effects from the additional IVGG, and many seem to improve. Specific second-line therapy for gamma globulin failures would be ideal, but this is currently in the experimental stages. Finally, children who have had KD, particularly those with active or regressed coronary lesions, should be monitored and treated aggressively for other risk factors for adult atherosclerotic vascular disease, such as hyperlipidemia or hypertension. The parents, caretakers, and teachers of children with coronary artery lesions, especially giant aneurysms, should be instructed in cardiopulmonary resuscitation.

MONITORING

Coronary artery lesions resulting from KD change dynamically over time. Angiographic resolution 1 to 2 years after disease onset has been observed in approximately one-half to two-thirds of vessels with coronary aneurysms. The likelihood of resolution appears to be determined largely by the initial size of the aneurysm, with smaller lesions having a greater tendency to regress. Other factors that have been reported to correlate with regression of aneurysms include age less than 1 year, saccular rather than fusiform morphology, and location within a distal coronary segment. Vessels that do not undergo apparent resolution of abnormalities may show persistence of aneurysmal morphology, development of stenosis or occlusion, or abnormal tortuosity. Whereas aneurysm size tends to diminish over time, stenotic lesions secondary to marked myointimal proliferation are frequently progressive.

Even those aneurysms that undergo angiographic resolution do so by myointimal proliferation or organization of thrombus, resulting in fibrous narrowing of the vessel lumen despite normal external artery diameter. Regressed axillary aneurysms have been noted to exhibit histologic characteristics similar to those seen in early atherosclerosis. These findings have raised concerns that sites of coronary artery abnormalities may be predisposed to accelerated atherosclerosis. Conversely, it is possible that some cases of early atherosclerosis in patients without known risk factors may be attributable to unrecognized KD.

Coronary artery segments in which aneurysms have regressed also show abnormalities of function. Vascular distensibility in such segments has been studied by examining the variation in artery size between systole and diastole, as well as by examining vascular reactivity during pharmacologic vasodilation. In each of these systems, previously affected arteries display markedly reduced vascular reactivity. The diminished distensibility of arteries that have undergone spontaneous regression of aneurysms may affect their ability to accommodate to increased myocardial metabolic demands during exercise and stress. Such clinical effects have not been documented to date, however.

Myocardial infarction caused by thrombotic occlusion of an aneurysmal and/or stenotic coronary artery is the principal cause of death in KD. A Japanese registry of 195 children with myocardial infarction revealed that almost 40 percent had a myocardial infarction within 3 months of disease onset, and 73 percent had their infarctions during the first year after KD. About two-thirds of myocardial infarctions were associated with symptoms (shock, crying, chest pain, abdominal pain, vomiting, dyspnea, or arrhythmia), but only three patients had a history of antecedent angina. Myocardial infarction occurred during sleep or at rest in 63 percent of patients, whereas only 14 percent experienced myocardial infarction while playing, walking, or exercising.

The clinical course after myocardial infarction is variable and depends on the extent of damage to the myocardium. Mortality from the first infarction was 22 percent; most fatal attacks were associated with obstruction either in the left main coronary artery or in both the right main and left anterior descending coronary arteries. In survivors, obstruction was frequently present in a single vessel, most commonly in the right coronary artery. Almost half of these survivors did well, without cardiac symptoms; in general, children seem to have a greater capacity for recovery of myocardial function following infarction than do adults. However, follow-up is thus far inadequate to allow delineation of the natural history of children with coronary artery abnormalities and/or myocardial infarctions. As these children are followed prospectively over a longer period, it is possible that progressive myocardial ischemia will further increase the cardiac morbidity and mortality resulting from KD.

Data concerning the long-term status of the coronary arteries in children who never had demonstrable abnormalities are inadequate to enable conclusions to be drawn. Although coronary artery aneurysms are the most serious sequelae of KD, vascular inflammation during the acute stage is diffuse. Abnormalities in prostaglandin and lipid metabolism may persist for weeks or months after clinical resolution of the disease, suggesting long-term endothelial cell dysfunction. Further research is needed to elucidate these abnormalities and to prospectively assess their long-term course. From the purely clinical perspective, however, children without known cardiac sequelae during the first month of KD appear to return to their previous, usually excellent, state of health without signs or symptoms of cardiac impairment. We evaluate such children every 3 to 5 years after recovery from the acute illness. Meaningful knowledge about long-term myocardial function, late-onset valvular regurgitation, and coronary artery status in this population must await their careful surveillance over the coming decades.

OUTLOOK

KD was first noted less than three decades ago, although echocardiographic and autopsy evidence of coronary artery aneurysms long before this time suggest that it is not a new disease. IVGG treatment has significantly improved the outlook in acute KD, decreasing the incidence of permanent coronary artery abnormalities from 20 to 3 percent. Nonetheless, the more than 100,000 documented cases worldwide to date are a cause for concern. A significant percentage of these have had coronary artery abnormalities demonstrable on the echocardiogram. As a group they are at increased risk for future coronary artery disease, with the most acute risks occurring among those with persistent coronary artery lesions. Since the criteria for diagnosis of KD are imperfect, it is likely that additional patients develop incomplete KD in whom the disease is never recognized but who present with late coronary artery disease. Also, even those without demonstrable coronary artery abnormalities may have subtle perturbations of endothelial cell architecture and function. A sensitive test for the disease is urgently needed, as is a more specific therapy directed at the mechanism of coronary artery damage apparently unique to KD. Ideally, these will follow closely upon identification of the cause of KD. In any event, continued surveillance of KD patients with or without detected coronary artery abnormalities will be necessary to determine the long-term sequelae of this fascinating disease.

SUGGESTED READING

Fujiwara T, Fujiwara H, Hamashima Y. Frequency and size of coronary arterial aneurysms at necropsy in Kawasaki disease. Am J Cardiol 1987; 59:808–811.

Fujiwara H, Hamashima Y. Pathology of the heart in Kawasaki disease. Pediatrics 1978; 61:100–107.

Kawasaki T, Kosaki F, Okawa S, et al. A new infantile acute febrile mucocutaneous lymph node syndrome (MLNS) prevailing in Japan. Pediatrics 1974; 54:271–276.

Landing BH, Larson EJ. Pathological features of Kawasaki disease (mucocutaneous lymph node syndrome). Am J Cardiovasc Pathol 1987; 1:215–229.

Newburger JW, Sanders SP, Burns JC, et al. Left ventricular contractility and function in Kawasaki syndrome. Circulation 1989; 79:1237–1246.

Newburger JW, Takahashi M, Beiser AS, et al. A single intravenous infusion of gamma globulin as compared with four infusions in the treatment of acute Kawasaki syndrome. N Engl J Med 1991; 324:1633–1639.

Newburger JW, Takahashi M, Burns JC, et al. The treatment of Kawasaki syndrome with intravenous gamma globulin. N Engl J Med 1986; 315:341–347.

Rowley AH, Gonzalez-Crussi F, Shulman ST. Kawasaki syndrome. Rev Infect Dis 1988; 10:1–15.

Shulman ST, ed. Management of Kawasaki syndrome: a consensus statement prepared by North American participants of the Third International Kawasaki Disease Symposium, Tokyo, Japan, December, 1988. Pediatr Infect Dis J 1989; 8:663–667.

Shulman ST, ed. Kawasaki disease. Proceedings of the Second International Kawasaki Disease Symposium. New York: Alan R Liss, 1987.

Suzuki A, Kamiyq T, Ono Y, et al. Aortocoronary bypass surgery for coronary arterial lesions resulting from Kawasaki disease. J Pediatr 1990; 116:567–573.

THROMBOANGIITIS OBLITERANS (BUERGER'S DISEASE)

JEFFREY W. OLIN, D.O.
J. T. LIE, M.D.

Thromboangiitis obliterans (TAO) was first described by von Winiwarter in 1879. Twenty-nine years later, Leo Buerger provided an accurate description of the pathology of TAO in 11 amputated limbs. Since that time, TAO has become known as Buerger's disease.

TAO is a nonatherosclerotic inflammatory disease that most commonly affects the small and medium-sized arteries and veins. It is often classified in the miscellaneous category of vasculitis. In the past, TAO was considered a disease predominantly of male, heavy cigarette smokers, but recently more women have been described with this entity.

The true incidence of TAO is unknown. It has been estimated that in a group of U.S. Army World War II servicemen between the ages of 20 and 44 years, the incidence was 6.8 cases per 100,000 per year. In another study of Israeli Jews over 25 years old, the incidence was one in every 5,000 individuals. The Mayo Clinic has demonstrated a progressive decline in the clinical diagnosis of TAO from 1947 to 1986. In 1947 there were 121 cases per 116,232 registrants (0.1 percent) compared with 28 cases per 221,000 registrants (0.01 percent) in 1986. This represents an almost tenfold decline in incidence. The reason for this is unknown but probably relates to stricter criteria being used to diagnose TAO. In the past some patients with premature atherosclerosis had been misdiagnosed as TAO. Japan and Eastern European countries have not shown a similarly sharp decline in the incidence of TAO. It is clear that the prevalence is greater in Southeastern Asia, Eastern Europe, India, and Israel.

The etiology is unknown. There is an extremely strong association with tobacco use, which suggests that some factor in tobacco either causes TAO or is strongly associated with the development and continuation of symptoms in this disease. It has been suggested that some patients may in fact be allergic or sensitive to tobacco, and that this sensitivity leads to small-vessel occlusive disease. Patients with TAO have higher tobacco consumption and higher levels of carboxyhemoglobin than patients with atherosclerosis or a control group.

Other studies have suggested that TAO is primarily a thrombotic disorder and that patients with this disease actually have blood that is hypercoagulable. This point is disputable. There has been an occasional familial clustering of patients with TAO, and HLA-A9 and HLA-B5 antigens are more common in patients with Buerger's disease than in the general population. Adair demonstrated a higher index of cell-mediated sensitivity to types I and III collagen in patients with TAO. Although patients may have an increased genetic predisposition to TAO or an abnormality in cell-mediated response to collagen, tobacco in some unknown way plays a major role in the initiation and continuation of disease activity in patients with TAO.

Pathologically, small and medium arteries and veins, and at times nerves, are involved in the inflammatory process. The acute phase of the disease is characteristic: a panvasculitis with involvement of the intima, media, and adventitia. There is a highly cellular thrombus with lymphocytes, neutrophils, giant cells, and microabscesses in the thrombus. The presence of microabscesses is characteristic. Segments of normal-appearing artery and vein are interspersed with segments showing an acute inflammatory reaction. There is no disruption of the internal elastic laminae or fibrinoid necrosis as is seen in necrotizing vasculitis. During the subacute phase, the amount of cellularity and microabscess formation is lessened and recanalization of thrombus begins. Late in the course of the disease, there may be only organized and recanalized thrombus with evidence of marked fibrosis around the artery, vein, and nerve. This end-stage lesion is not pathognomonic of Buerger's disease, because it may occur in other vascular diseases.

CLINICAL ASPECTS

The signs and symptoms of TAO are usually distinctive. It generally involves young smokers. The ischemia that occurs in patients with Buerger's disease begins distally and usually involves the small and medium-sized arteries and veins. Occasionally large artery involvement has been reported, but this is distinctly uncommon.

In a series of 112 patients with Buerger's disease evaluated at the Cleveland Clinic, the mean age at diagnosis was 42 years, with a range of 20 to 75 years; 77 percent of patients were male and 23 percent female. In the past, Buerger's disease was considered to be primarily a disease of men, with a male:female ratio of 9:1. A large series by Shionoya and colleagues still reports only a 2 percent incidence of Buerger's disease in women. However, recent reports, including ours, have demonstrated that this disease occurs much more commonly in women than was previously thought; the reason is probably the increase in cigarette smoking among women. Some early reports of patients with Buerger's disease suggested that it was more common in Jews than in other ethnic and religious groups. However, this has not been borne out; in our recent series, there was no religious or ethnic predisposition.

The presenting signs and symptoms of TAO are shown in Table 1.

The intermittent claudication that occurs in patients with TAO usually starts distally. It is not uncommon for patients to present with arch claudication; when this is

265

Table 1 Signs and Symptoms in 112 Patients with Thromboangiitis Obliterans (Buerger's Disease)

Signs and Symptoms	No. (%)
Intermittent claudication	70 (63)
Ischemic rest pain	91 (81)
Ischemic ulcers	85 (76)
Upper extremity ulcers only	24 (28)
Lower extremity ulcers only	39 (46)
Both upper and lower extremity ulcers	22 (26)
Abnormal Allen's test	71 (63)
Superficial thrombophlebitis	43 (38)
Raynaud's phenomenon	49 (44)
Nonspecific sensory findings	77 (69)

Adapted from Olin JW, Young JR, Graor RA, et al. The changing clinical spectrum of thromboangiitis obliterans (Buerger's disease). Circulation 1990; 82 (Suppl IV):IV-1–IV-7; with permission.

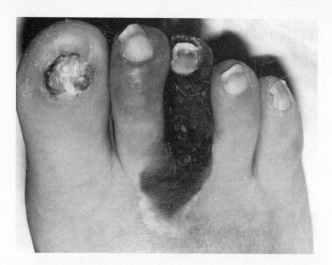

Figure 2 Gangrene of the third toe in a patient with TAO.

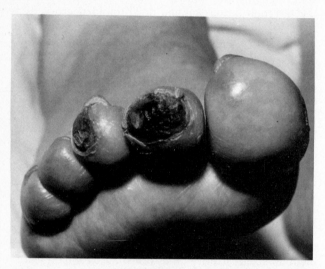

Figure 1 Ischemic ulcers on the first (medial aspect), second, and third toes in a young man with thromboangiitis obliterans (TAO).

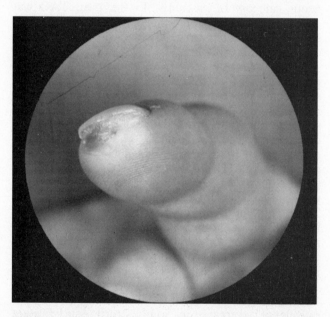

Figure 3 Ischemic ulcer of the index finger in a patient with Buerger's disease.

present in a young smoker, it is highly suggestive of TAO. As the disease progresses more proximally, patients may present with typical calf claudication similar to that of patients with arteriosclerosis obliterans.

Up to 76 percent of patients with Buerger's disease present with ischemic ulcers in the upper and/or lower extremities (Figs. 1 to 3). In patients with lower extremity ulceration in whom Buerger's disease is a consideration, an Allen's test should be performed to assess the circulation in the hands and fingers (Fig. 4). An abnormal Allen's test in a young smoker with lower extremity ulceration is highly suggestive of TAO since it demonstrates small-vessel involvement of *both* the upper and lower extremities.

The inflammatory reaction that occurs in patients with Buerger's disease may cause encasement of the artery, vein, and nerve in densely fibrotic tissue. Approximately 40 percent of patients with Buerger's disease develop superficial thrombophlebitis at some time dur-

ing the course of the disease (Fig. 5), and about 40 percent have associated Raynaud's phenomenon. It is also interesting to note that up to 70 percent of patients may have significant sensory impairment such as numbness or tingling. This may be due to either severe ischemia or ischemic neuropathy secondary to encasement of the nerve fibers.

DIFFERENTIAL DIAGNOSIS

Diseases that may mimic TAO are shown in Table 2.

The most important and common diseases to exclude are premature atherosclerosis or emboli. At times, emboli may be excluded only by arteriographic

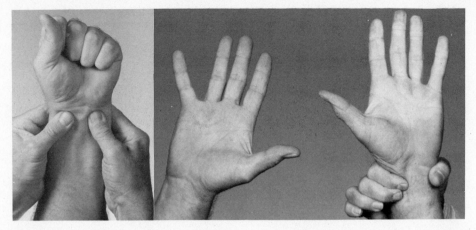

Figure 4 *A,* Allen's test with occlusion of the radial and ulnar pulse by compression. *B,* The pressure on the ulnar pulse is released, while the radial is still compressed. The hand does not fill with blood; note the paleness of the hand on the right compared with the left, indicating occlusion of the ulnar artery.

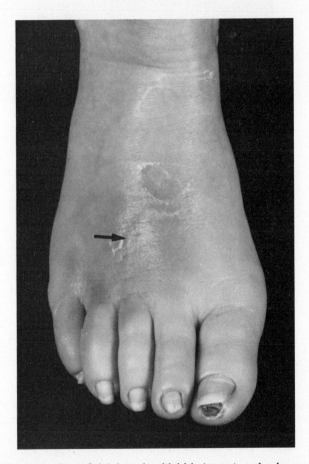

Figure 5 Superficial thrombophlebitis *(arrow)* on the dorsum of the foot in a patient with TAO. There is an area of erythema around the phlebitis. Note the ischemic ulcer on the distal portion of the great toe.

Table 2 Differential Diagnosis of Thromboangiitis Obliterans

Atherosclerosis
Emboli
Connective tissue diseases/vasculitis
   Systemic lupus erythematosus
   Rheumatoid arthritis
   Scleroderma
   Polyarteritis nodosa
   Antiphospholipid antibody syndrome
   Giant cell or Takayasu's arteritis
   Leukocytoclastic vasculitis
Miscellaneous
   Idiopathic arterial thrombosis (i.e., cancer, infection, ulcerative colitis, congestive heart failure)
   Blood dyscrasias (polycythemia vera)
   Ergotamine abuse
   Occupational hazards (vibratory tools, hypothenar hammer syndrome)
   Ehlers-Danlos syndrome
   Pseudoxanthoma elasticum
   Calciphylaxis
   Thrombosis of aneurysms

evaluation. Unless the history is absolutely classical, patients presenting with ischemic ulcers of the hands or feet should undergo echocardiography and Holter monitoring to exclude a cardiac source of emboli. Also, upper extremity or lower extremity arteriography is helpful to rule out a more proximal source of emboli originating in the arteries.

Differentation of TAO from premature atherosclerosis may be difficult. Table 3 illustrates differentiating features of these two entities. However, there are times when arteriography is mandatory in distinguishing between these two diseases, and in rare instances biopsy is necessary.

Abnormal serology is usually present in patients with systemic lupus erythematosus, rheumatoid arthritis, cryoglobulinemia, and other forms of vasculitis. Patients with the antiphospholipid antibody syndrome may present with evidence of both arterial and venous thrombosis. These patients usually have positive titers for circulating lupus anticoagulant and anticardiolipin antibodies. Patients with scleroderma are usually obvious from a clinical examination of the skin and a history of systemic features (e.g., esophageal motility disturbance and pulmonary involvement). It is also important

Table 3 Comparison of Thromboangiitis Obliterans with Arteriosclerosis Obliterans

	Thromboangiitis Obliterans	*Arteriosclerosis Obliterans*
Age	Usually young (< 40 yr)	Usually older (> 55 yr)
Distribution of disease	Distal: toes, feet, hands, fingers	Proximal: hands and fingers rarely involved
Tobacco use	Invariably present	Usually present
Other cardiovascular risk factors (obesity, hypertension, increased lipids, family history, etc.)	Usually absent	Usually present
History of superficial thrombophlebitis	Present in approximately 40%	Absent
Raynaud's phenomenon	Present in approximately 40%	Rare

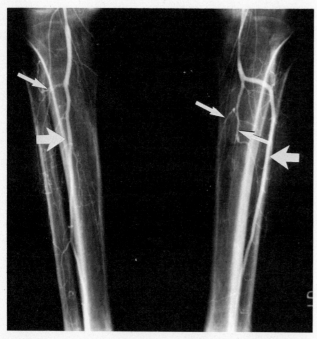

Figure 6 Severe infrapopliteal disease in a patient with TAO. In the right leg the anterior tibial artery *(small arrow)* and the posterior tibial artery are occluded at their origin. The peroneal artery is patent *(large arrow)*. In the left leg the anterior tibial is patent *(large arrow)*, but the posterior tibial and peroneal artery *(small arrow)* are occluded proximally.

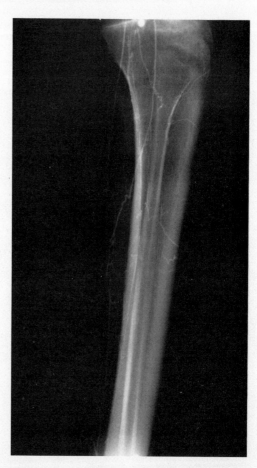

Figure 7 Severe disease of the infrapopliteal vessels in a patient with TAO. No major vessels are seen. This patient subsequently underwent an above-knee amputation.

to recognize that patients with scleroderma rarely, if ever, have involvement of the toes and feet, whereas lower extremity involvement in Buerger's disease is common. Nailfold capillaroscopy may be helpful in differentiating scleroderma from TAO. The ischemic ulcerations of the upper extremity and the arteriographic appearance may be identical in patients with scleroderma and TAO.

Patients with Takayasu's arteritis or giant cell arteritis usually have elevated acute-phase reactants (erythrocyte sedimentation rate and C-reactive protein) as well as evidence of more proximal vascular involvement. However, at times it may be necessary to perform

arteriography to help differentiate TAO from large-vessel vasculitis. It should be noted that as a general rule TAO is a distal disease and Takayasu's arteritis a proximal disease, but there can be some overlap.

A careful history should be taken for the possibility of ergotamine abuse, as this may cause severe ischemia. When this is uncertain, ergotamine blood levels can be obtained. Rarely, Ehlers-Danlos syndrome, pseudoxanthoma elasticum, blood dyscrasias, idiopathic arterial

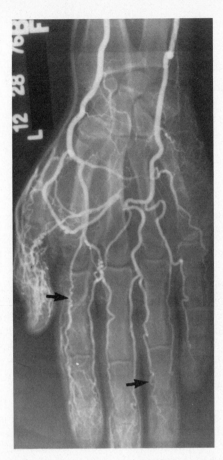

Figure 8 Multiple digital artery occlusions wth evidence of collateralization (corkscrew collaterals) *(arrows)* around areas of occlusion.

thrombosis, calciphylaxis (metastatic and vascular calcification related to an increased calcium-phosphate product), or thrombosed aneurysms may be the cause of distal extremity ischemia.

LABORATORY AND ANGIOGRAPHIC FINDINGS

There are no specific laboratory tests to assist the diagnosis of TAO. As mentioned previously, serologic markers for other connective tissue diseases are usually not present. Occasionally, there may be low titers of antinuclear antibody, but this is not a universal finding.

As Juergens stated,

"The typical patient with thromboangiitis obliterans is a man less than 40 years of age with evidence of occlusive arterial disease distal to one or both popliteal arteries with the presence or a strong history of superficial thrombophlebitis in non-varicose veins, and with evidence of chronic ischemia in one or more fingers of one or both hands. The patient does not have roentgenographically demonstrable calcification of the peripheral arteries, diabetes mellitus, hyperlipidemia, xanthomas, scleroderma, organic heart disease, arterial aneurysms or bruits that can be heard over the abdominal aorta or the iliac or

Table 4 Therapy

1. Stop smoking or using tobacco in any form
2. Treat local ischemic ulcerations:
   a. Foot care
      1. Lubricate skin with lanolin-based cream or lotion
      2. Use lamb's wool between toes to prevent "kissing" ulcers
      3. Avoid trauma with use of a bed cradle and heel protectors
   b. Trial of calcium channel blocking agents such as nifedipine or nicardipine and/or pentoxifylline
   c. Although not currently available, Iloprost may help heal ischemic ulcers
   d. Sympathectomy for ischemic ulcers that fail to heal with conservative therapy
3. Treat cellulitis with antibiotics and superficial phlebitis with nonsteroidal anti-inflammatory agents as needed
4. Amputate when all else fails to control ischemic rest pain and/or pain associated with ischemic ulcerations

femoral arteries. When this clinical picture is present, the clinical diagnosis can be made almost with certainty. When the patient is a woman less than 40 years of age with normal ovarian function and the clinical picture is the same, the diagnosis can be made with almost equal certainty."

Therefore, if the clinical scenario is compatible with Buerger's disease and there are no proximal sources of emboli as demonstrated by echocardiography or arteriography, the diagnosis of TAO can be made without pathologic proof. However, if there are any unusual features (e.g., older age group, unusual distribution of disease) or if there is coexistent atherosclerosis, a pathologic specimen may be necessary to confirm the diagnosis. We are reluctant to biopsy patients with ischemic ulcerations or with ischemic rest pain for fear that the biopsy site will not heal. In fact, most pathologic specimens from patients with Buerger's disease are obtained at the time of amputation.

The classic arteriographic findings of TAO are demonstrated in Figures 6 to 8. Usually, the proximal arteries are normal with no evidence of arteriosclerosis obliterans proximally and no proximal source of emboli. The disease is most severe distally with evidence of occlusion of the infrapopliteal vessels or vessels distal to the elbow. Small and medium-sized vessels are involved, such as the digital arteries in the fingers and toes and palmar and plantar arteries in the hand and foot, as well as the tibial, peroneal, radial, and ulnar arteries. *Isolated* disease below the popliteal artery almost never occurs in arteriosclerosis obliterans even if the patient has coexistent diabetes mellitus.

TAO is a segmental disorder with areas of diseased vessel interspersed with normal segments. There may be multiple sites of vascular occlusion with evidence of collateralization around the obstructions (corkscrew collaterals). Corkscrew collaterals are not pathognomonic of Buerger's disease, because they may be seen in any small-vessel occlusive disease. The arteriographic appearance in scleroderma may be identical to that in patients with TAO.

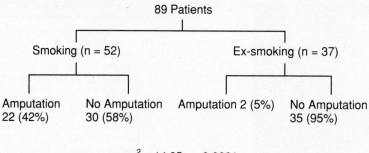

$$x^2 = 14.95, p<0.0001$$

Figure 9 Smoking status related to amputation. (Adapted from Olin JW, Young JR, Graor RA, et al. The changing clinical spectrum of thromboangiitis obliterans [Buerger's disease]. Circulation 1990; 82(Suppl IV):IV-1–IV-7; with permission.)

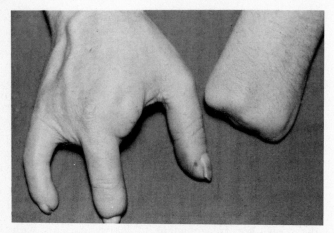

Figure 10 The result of multiple amputations in a patient with TAO who was unable to stop smoking.

THERAPY

The therapies available for patients with TAO are listed in Table 4. The only effective way to halt the progression of the disease is to discontinue smoking and the use of tobacco in any form. Even one or two cigarettes a day are enough to allow the disease to remain active. It has been shown repeatedly that patients who discontinue cigarette smoking rarely have to undergo amputation (Fig. 9). In the 89 patients followed in our series, there was a direct relationship between amputation and persistent tobacco use. If the patient does not have gangrene at the time of smoking cessation, the risk of amputation is extremely small. Figure 10 shows an example of a patient who could not stop cigarette smoking despite multiple amputations. It is imperative that these patients realize the need to stop using tobacco, in any form, in any amount. Whether involuntary smoking (secondary smoke) can cause the disease is unknown. However, patients with active TAO should probably try to avoid involuntary smoking as much as they can until the disease becomes quiescent.

Other than the discontinuation of tobacco, all forms of therapy are palliative. If ischemic ulcers are present, local care is outlined in Table 4. It may be worthwhile to give patients a trial of calcium channel blocking agents such as nifedipine or nicardipine or of pentoxifylline (Trental), although there are no controlled studies to support this approach. Iloprost, a prostacyclin analog, may be effective in healing ischemic ulcerations in some patients with TAO. In one study, 58 of 68 Iloprost-treated patients (85 percent) showed healing of ischemic ulcerations and/or relief of ischemic rest pain compared with 11 of 65 patients (17 percent) treated with aspirin (P = <.05). Although this form of therapy is still experimental, it merits a trial in patients with critical ischemia.

When medical therapy is unsuccessful in healing ischemic ulcers, a sympathectomy (either chemical or surgical) may be of benefit. There are no good studies to assess the efficacy of sympathectomy, but of 23 patients at our institution who underwent sympathectomy, 13 avoided amputation and ten required amputation. Of these ten, eight had continued to smoke.

Surgical revascularization generally is not an option in patients with Buerger's disease, since the disease is distal and there usually is not a good target for bypass. In a few patients who have had arterial bypass, the long-term results are not good.

SUGGESTED READING

Buerger L. Thrombo-angiitis obliterans: a study of the vascular lesion leading to pre-senile spontaneous gangrene. Am J Med Sci 1908; 136:567–580.

Fiessinger JN, Schafer M. Trial of Iloprost vs. aspirin treatment for critical limb ischaemia of thromboangiitis obliterans. Lancet 1990; 335:555–557.

Juergens JL. Thromboangiitis obliterans (Buerger's disease, TAO). In: Juergens JL, Spittell JA Jr, Fairborn JF II, eds. Peripheral vascular diseases. Philadelphia: WB Saunders, 1980:467.

Lambeth JT, Yong NK. Arteriographic findings in thromboangiitis obliterans: with emphasis on femoral popliteal involvement. Am J Roentgen 1970; 109:553–562.

Lie JT. Thromboangiitis obliterans (Buerger's disease) in women. Medicine 1987; 66:65–72.

Lie JT. Thromboangiitis obliterans (Buerger's disease) revisited. Pathol Annu 1988; 23(Part II):257–291.

Mills JL, Taylor LM, Porter JM. Buerger's disease in the modern era. Am J Surg 1987; 154:123–129.

Olin JW, Young JR, Graor RA, et al. The changing clinical spectrum of thromboangiitis obliterans (Buerger's disease). Circulation 1990; 82(Suppl IV):IV-1–IV-7.

Shionoya S, Zan I, Nakata Y, et al. Diagnosis, pathology and treatment in Buerger's disease. Surgery 1974; 75:695–700.

VASCULAR TRAUMA

ACUTE ARTERIAL INJURY

MALCOLM O. PERRY, M.D.

Trauma is the fourth leading cause of death in the United States; it is responsible for over 50 million injuries each year and more than 100,000 deaths. Wounds of major arteries are the sole cause or a major contributing cause in many deaths. Most of these injuries are the result of aggressive acts of violence that cause penetrating trauma, usually from bullets and stabbings. However, as motor vehicle accidents increase in frequency, vascular injuries as a result of blunt trauma have also increased (Table 1). These pose more difficult problems in diagnosis and management than injuries caused by penetrating trauma.

CLINICAL FEATURES

The distribution of major arterial injuries is shown in Table 2. The vessels in the extremities are more

Table 1 Arterial Injuries: Etiology

Etiology	%*
Gunshot	55
Edged instruments	36
Blunt trauma	9

*Expressed as a percentage of total cases (665 cases over a 6-year period).

Table 2 Arterial Injuries: Distribution

Distribution	No. of cases*
Extremity	501
Aorta	31
Visceral	37
Cervical	96
	665

*A total of 665 patients in whom adequate follow-up could be obtained, presenting to Parkland Memorial Hospital over a 6-year period.

vulnerable, being located superficially, and victims may attempt to defend themselves with arms or legs, thus inviting injuries to these arteries.

Injuries of large arteries usually can be readily identified because of severe hemorrhage, but wounds in the trunk and chest may be more difficult to evaluate (Fig. 1). Table 3 lists clinical signs that help establish the diagnosis of a major arterial injury. Weak or absent pulses beyond the arterial wound are a fairly common finding, but distal pulses may be normal in up to 20 percent of patients who have surgically proved arterial injuries. The pulse wave is a pressure wave that attains velocities of up to 13 meters per second, and this pressure wave can be transmitted through limited areas of soft clot, via collateral vessels, or beyond intimal flaps; thus, a palpable pulse may be misleading.

DIAGNOSIS

A detailed history that establishes the mechanism of injury and a careful physical examination form the basis

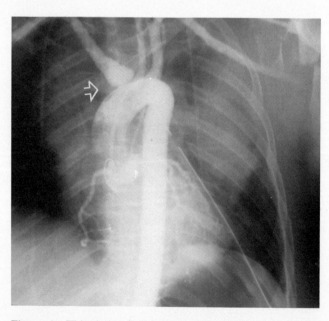

Figure 1 This victim of blunt chest trauma has near-avulsion of the innominate artery. Normal pulses and arm blood pressures were observed.

for the diagnosis, but certain adjunctive procedures may be helpful. The detection of Doppler signals and measurements of distal arterial systolic blood pressure may be useful, but the specificity of these tests is influenced by the same hemodynamic features that govern distal pulses. Although subtle abnormalities in these measurements are common, relatively normal values are also seen.

Injuries of the heart and great vessels present special diagnostic problems because of inaccessibility to direct examination. Table 4 lists the clinical features that suggest injuries to these arteries. In most situations the diagnosis depends on detection of continued bleeding into the chest or abdomen.

ARTERIOGRAPHY

In stable patients, preoperative arteriography can be of value in establishing the diagnosis of an arterial injury. Arteriography is generally performed for one of three reasons: (1) to exclude the need for an operation in patients who have no other indications for surgery, (2) to detect lesions not otherwise discernible by clinical evaluation, and (3) to help plan an operation when complex vascular injuries are suspected. The validity of arteriography in arterial trauma was assessed by Snyder and colleagues in a study of 177 patients with 183 penetrating extremity wounds. All patients had biplane arteriography and all were operated on regardless of the arteriographic findings. Surgical exploration revealed that 36 arteriographic results were true positives and 132 true negatives; there were 14 false-positive results and one false-negative result. From this study it was concluded that arteriography, although not infallible, offers reliable information as to the presence or absence of major arterial injuries (Fig. 2).

In patients who are hemodynamically unstable, immediate surgery is necessary and should not be delayed for arteriography. If further evaluations are required, they can be performed in the operating room while the patient is prepared for surgery. If sudden cardiovascular collapse does occur, an immediate operation can be undertaken and bleeding rapidly controlled. These unstable patients should not be sent to the radiology department nor admitted to an intensive care unit, because an emergency operation may be required at any time.

PREOPERATIVE PREPARATION

The management of trauma requires a rapid and thorough evaluation, and because many of these patients have associated injuries, certain priorities must be set if a successful conclusion is to be gained. As seen in Table 5, there often are other injuries that must be evaluated and treated. Initial attention to control of the airway and of bleeding is the first priority. Next, an overall assessment is completed, baseline studies are recorded, and a rapid physical examination is performed to make certain that all injuries are identified. Fluid and blood requirements in injured patients are often impressive, and adequate intravenous access lines are needed. Large catheters are placed into an uninjured upper and lower extremity, and one line is reserved for fluid replacement. This line is not used

Table 3 Arterial Injuries: Signs

Highly reliable
  Distal circulatory deficit
    Ischemia
    Pulses diminished or absent
  Bruit
  Expanding or pulsatile hematoma
  Arterial bleeding
Less reliable
  Small or moderate-sized stable hematoma
  Adjacent nerve injury
  Shock (unexplained by other injuries)
  Proximity of penetrating wound to a major vascular structure

Table 4 Arterial Injuries: Evidence
of Great-Vessel Involvement

Cardiac arrest
Persistent shock
Cardiac tamponade
Widened mediastinum
Recurring hemothorax

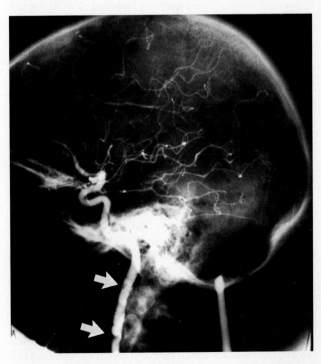

Figure 2 Hyperextension of the internal carotid artery can cause multiple injuries that predispose to thromboembolism.

Table 5 Arterial Injuries: Associated Injuries

Associated Injuries	%*
Significant trauma to	
Vein	34
Major nerve	18
Additional artery	7
Thoracic/abdominal viscera	39
Shock	36

*Expressed as a percentage of total cases (665 cases over a 6-year period).

Table 6 Arterial Injuries: Results of Surgical Repair

Results	%*
Failure of repair	5.2
Bleeding	2.0
Infection	3.1
Amputation	1.8
Death	10.4

*Expressed as a percentage of total cases (665 cases over a 6-year period).

for drug administration or anesthetic manipulations because, if hemorrhage is severe, large volumes of blood must be infused rapidly through it.

OPERATIVE MANAGEMENT

During the preparation for surgery, the selection of anesthetic agents can be important, especially in patients who are already hypotensive. Certain other precautions need to be observed, because in patients with multiple injuries these areas must be protected from further damage during positioning. Trauma patients are usually placed supine in the anatomic position to afford access to the chest, the abdomen, and all four extremities. In most situations, vertical exploratory incisions are best because they can be extended easily in either direction to obtain proximal and distal control of the major arteries. Moreover, vertical incisions parallel the neurovascular structures and thus reduce the risk of injuring superficial veins that may be needed for autograft interposition. Midline abdominal incisions can be extended into the chest as a median sternal splitting incision, and vertical incisions along the border of the anterior sternomastoid muscle to expose the carotid and jugular vessels can easily be enlarged into a median sternal incision if there are injuries in the root of the neck.

Most external bleeding can be controlled with direct arterial pressure, but if the wound is not bleeding it is not disturbed during resuscitation, and no attempt is made to remove foreign bodies or to evacuate clots until surgical control is possible. Penetrating objects still in the wound are left in place, protected, and not removed until the patient is in the operating room. No attempt is made to blindly clamp vessels in the depths of a wound. If fatal hemorrhage appears imminent, the wound can be extended and vascular clamps applied accurately under direct vision.

Surgical Methods

The wounds are approached directly through vertical incisions, and proximal and distal control are gained before the clots are evacuated and direct exposure of the injured area is attempted. Every effort should be made to avoid fragmenting and dislodging clots, or extending damage to the vessel, a problem particularly likely to occur in patients who have arteriosclerosis. Repairs of the arteries are not begun until all hemorrhage is arrested and the extent of associated injuries is assessed. Priorities can then be established as to which vessel should be repaired first. Certain organs, such as the kidney and liver, are more susceptible to hypoxia than others, and repair of major vessels supplying these organs should be undertaken first while less vulnerable tissues are given lower priority.

Vessels are repaired by the usual vascular techniques with continuous over-and-over sutures in larger arteries, but in small vessels, especially in children, interrupted vascular sutures are preferred to ensure adequate patency. Although tangential lacerations of larger vessels can be successfully treated by lateral suture techniques, debridement is as important in these structures as in other areas. If there is widespread vascular damage, it may be necessary to use an interposition graft of autogenous tissue, usually saphenous vein, if it is of an appropriate size. If a direct end-to-end anastomosis without tension cannot be accomplished, interposition grafts are used. Although autogenous tissues are favored, plastic prostheses will be required to repair large arteries in the aortoiliac system and the arch of the aorta. Most surgeons prefer polytetrafluoroethylene grafts to fabric grafts when they must be placed in potentially contaminated fields. If there is soilage, such as might occur from a gunshot wound to the colon, it may be preferable to insert remote bypass grafts through clean tissue planes and avoid direct arterial repairs in a field where heavy contamination exists. In such situations the artery is oversewn with monofilament sutures, and the remote bypass grafts are placed so as not to interfere with the exploratory incisions.

In most patients an arterial repair is followed by the immediate return of pulsatile flow, but in people who remain hypotensive and cold and have vasoconstricted arteries it may be difficult to determine clinically whether the repair is satisfactory. A sterile Doppler probe can help document distal patency of the vessels, but if there is any doubt about the adequacy of the repair, completion arteriography is recommended.

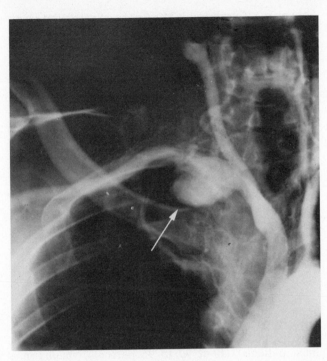

Figure 3 This false aneurysm of the subclavian artery was the result of a steering wheel injury in a motor vehicle accident.

POSTOPERATIVE CARE

Most arterial injuries occur in young people, and a satisfactory vascular reconstruction can be expected to remain patent and free of complications. As mentioned above, heavy bacterial contamination may be present in certain patients, and delayed infection is always a threat, although unusual. Postoperatively, any question about the adequacy of flow is an indication for a repeat arteriogram to examine the repair. The sine qua non for viability of the extremity is continued perception of light touch and intrinsic motor function. Any deterioration in these findings is reason to perform arteriography, regardless of skin color, temperature, presence or absence of pulses, and limb blood pressures.

Evaluation of the vascular reconstruction in other areas may be somewhat more difficult because of the lack of direct accessibility for clinical examination. Repair of arteries to the major viscera can usually be followed by assessment of organ function, such as continued monitoring of urinary output, liver function, and intestinal viability. Repeated examinations by certain adjunctive laboratory evaluations may be needed in these situations. If there is any doubt about continued function, a repeat arteriogram is needed.

COMPLICATIONS

The results of immediate repair of acute arterial injuries are excellent, as shown in Table 6. The direct

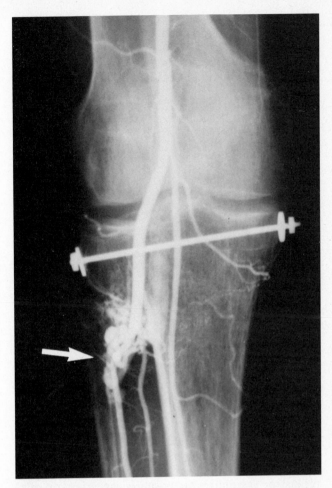

Figure 4 The arteriovenous fistula at the knee was discovered after treatment of the fracture. A difficult vascular reconstruction was successful.

repair of normal arteries is usually followed by continued patency, and few complications occur from the vascular injury itself. Associated injuries are common, and this must be taken into account during the follow-up period because patients often have complications related to the other injuries. Failure to repair injuries of major arteries is likely to lead to the development of false aneurysms or arteriovenous fistulas, or delayed thromboembolism (Fig. 3); these are unusual because now most vascular injuries, once identified, are treated. If false aneurysms and arteriovenous fistulas do occur, they should be repaired. The natural history of these lesions reveals that spontaneous cure is unlikely, occurring in approximately 6 percent of false aneurysms and less than 3 percent of arteriovenous fistulas (Fig. 4). Spontaneous cure can occur only by thrombosis, and this may or may not be tolerated by the organ supplied by the afflicted artery. Once an arteriovenous fistula or false aneurysm is identified, there is little reason for procrastination; early elective repair is recommended.

Delayed bleeding or disruption of the vascular repair is rare in the absence of a coagulopathy or invasive infections. Most of the delayed complications can be prevented by aggressive and appropriate surgical treatment.

SUGGESTED READING

Feliciano DV, Burch JM, Graham JM. Vascular injuries of the chest and abdomen. In: Rutherford RB, ed. Vascular surgery. Philadelphia: WB Saunders, 1989.

Liekweg WG, Greenfield LJ. Management of penetrating carotid arterial injury. Ann Surg 1978; 188:587.
Snyder WH, Thal ER, Bridges RA, et al. The validity of normal arteriography in penetrating trauma. Arch Surg 1978; 113:424.
Snyder WH, Thal ER, Perry MO. Vascular injuries of the extremities. In: Rutherford RB, ed. Vascular surgery. Philadelphia: WB Saunders, 1989.

THORACIC OUTLET SYNDROME

KENNETH J. CHERRY Jr., M.D.

Thoracic outlet syndrome is a constellation of symptoms involving the upper extremity and, to a lesser extent, the head and neck. It is due to nerve (brachial plexus) or vascular (axillary-subclavian artery or vein) compression at or near the thoracic outlet. The thoracic outlet is essentially a triangle, bounded anteriorly by the anterior scalene muscle, posteriorly by the middle scalene muscle, and inferiorly by the first rib. The subclavian artery anteriorly and the brachial plexus traverse this outlet. The subclavian vein is anterior to the anterior scalene muscle (Figs. 1 to 4). The compression may be from bony or soft tissues or a combination thereof and may or may not be traumatic, although careful history taking will reveal a history of trauma in

most patients. Presenting symptoms are neurologic in most patients (about 90 to 95 percent), venous in a smaller group (about 5 to 7 percent), and arterial in a few (about 1 to 5 percent). Differential diagnoses include other vascular, neurologic, and orthopedic problems such as Raynaud's disease, Buerger's disease, collagen vascular diseases, atherosclerotic disease of both the great vessels and extremity vessels as well as the coronary arteries, cervical disc disease, cervical spondylitis, brachial plexus lesions, carpal and cubital tunnel syndromes, and shoulder disorders.

NEUROLOGIC SYMPTOMS (COMPRESSION OF THE BRACHIAL PLEXUS)

Neurologic compression at the thoracic outlet, although the most common manifestation of thoracic outlet syndrome, is the most difficult to diagnose

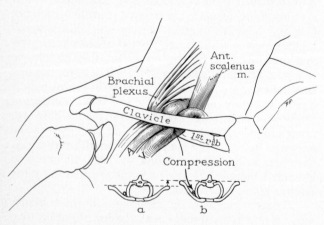

Figure 1 Anatomy of the thoracic outlet.

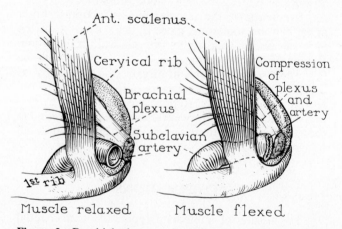

Figure 2 Brachial plexus and subclavian artery overriding the cervical rib.

accurately. Women outnumber men in a ratio of 2 to 3:1, and the symptoms are most often seen in young women from the teenage years through the 40s. Most have a history of trauma to the neck or the extremity, which may include repetitive minor occupational trauma and also torsion or jerking injuries involving the neck, extremities, or upper torso. Often the symptoms do not become apparent until months after the injury. With both traumatic and nontraumatic etiologies, the onset is often insidious and progressive.

Diagnosis

Compression of C5 to C7 is termed "upper cord involvement" of thoracic outlet syndrome. Symptoms include unilateral neck pain, often with one-sided headaches, and radiation into the upper chest or scapular region and down the lateral surface of the arm

and forearm to the radial distribution of the hand. Compression of C8 and T1 is termed "lower cord involvement" and is manifested by pain in the supraclavicular area, the inner aspect of the arm and forearm, and the ulnar aspect of the hands. There are combinations of these two types of involvement. Symptoms include paresthesias as well as pain and weakness, and are classically brought on by exertion with the extremity in an elevated or abducted position, such as brushing the hair, driving with the hands atop the steering wheel, or stacking items. Symptoms are usually intermittent at first, but with progression may become more constant. These are always exacerbated by use. Cervical spine lesions and brachial plexus lesions must be ruled out before making a diagnosis of thoracic outlet syndrome. The history of cervical spine lesions may be one of classical radiculopathy and easily distinguished from thoracic outlet syndrome, but the symptoms of the two may overlap. Careful and detailed neurologic examination is a strict necessity.

Electromyelography and nerve conduction studies should be obtained if indicated. Classical physical examination tests for thoracic outlet syndrome, such as the hyperabduction maneuver and Adson's maneuver, are really examinations of arterial and not neurologic compression. As such, they are perhaps more useful with suspected arterial involvement, but are of limited value in patients with compression of the brachial plexus. The elevated arm stress test (EAST) advocated by Roos, in which the patient's arms are placed in basically a surrender position and the hands opened and closed for several minutes with reproduction of the symptoms, is perhaps the most useful. The supraclavicular space should be inspected, as cervical ribs, bands, and other abnormalities may be palpated. Supraclavicular tenderness should be sought.

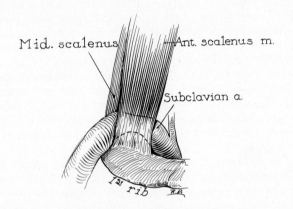

Figure 3 Muscular compression by scalene muscles.

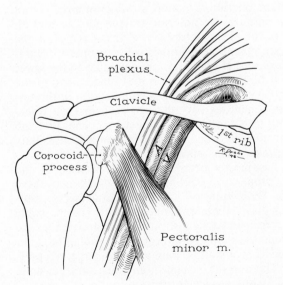 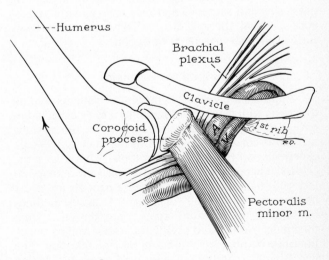

Figure 4 *A* and *B,* Muscular compression by the pectoralis minor muscle.

There is no satisfactory laboratory or roentgenologic test which is pathognomonic of thoracic outlet syndrome, nor are there any that rule in or out the diagnosis. The most helpful x-ray finding in any of the three forms of thoracic outlet syndrome (neurologic, venous, or arterial) is a cervical rib. This is most commonly identified with arterial disorders. Its presence does not guarantee the diagnosis but it makes it more likely. Other bone abnormalities, such as nonunion of the clavicle or hypertrophic union or exostosis, have also been implicated as causes of thoracic outlet syndrome.

Careful history taking is necessary to determine the time of onset, any history of trauma or exacerbating factors, and uni- or bilaterality. It is also important to determine whether there is any evidence of vascular involvement. Physical examination in conjunction with the history taking are the principal elements of diagnosis, because tests, as previously mentioned, add little in the way of confirmatory or definitive diagnosis. Electromyelography, nerve conduction studies, plain x-rays, and electrocardiography are useful in excluding other causes of the upper extremity or neck symptoms. Arteriography and phlebography are neither necessary nor indicated in the evaluation of patients with neurologic symptoms of thoracic outlet syndrome in the absence of clear vascular indications for angiography.

The diagnosis is therefore both a clinical and an exclusionary one. Patients first seen with neurologic symptoms of thoracic outlet syndrome, especially those diagnosed early in the disease process, should be given a trial of physical therapy to strengthen the shoulder girdle and open the thoracic outlet. Thoracic and vascular surgeons probably take a pessimistic view of such physical therapy because they see a select population. However, it has been reported that up to 75 percent of patients respond positively to these conditioning exercises and do not require an operation. If no improvement is made in 4 to 6 weeks, surgery may be considered. Patients with long-standing thoracic outlet syndrome, who have often been seen by a host of physicians and surgeons and may have already undergone physical therapy, are unlikely to benefit from further physical therapy at this point.

Surgical Management

Approximately 80 to 85 percent of patients coming to surgery with neurologic symptoms may be expected to have complete or partial relief. Most of the others show no improvement, and only a very small percentage experience worsening of symptoms. There is some evidence that patients in whom trauma is the etiology do less well than others. Many of these patients are often nervous and emotionally distraught. It may sometimes be difficult to separate appropriate anxieties from functional overlay, and psychiatric testing and consultation may be necessary to aid in patient selection. The necessity for careful diagnosis and patient selection cannot be overemphasized. No surgeon wishes to operate on patients without the correct diagnosis, especially if they are chronic pain patients with a history of multiple operations and a strong emotional component to their symptoms. On the other hand, it is disadvantageous to patients to withhold operation when clearly indicated. If the diagnosis is missed for many years, atrophy of the muscle groups subserved by the brachial plexus may ensue in rare cases. In one patient with a cervical rib and symptoms of thoracic outlet syndrome who presented with marked wasting of the intrinsic muscles of her hand, the diagnosis was missed for over 20 years.

Surgery is performed in patients whose history and physical examination are consistent with thoracic outlet syndrome, who have no other diagnosis to account for the extremity symptoms, and who are good emotional candidates for surgery. Cervical spine and chest films and electrocardiograms should be obtained in all patients. The advisability of other testing has been discussed previously, but essentially other tests such as electromyelography and nerve conduction studies are performed to determine the presence of other lesions that may give rise to the symptoms in the extremity. Negative tests do not preclude the diagnosis of thoracic outlet syndrome but rather enhance it. At my institution, patients are seen by a neurologist and a vascular surgeon, and usually by a vascular internist also. If there is not a clear diagnosis, medical management is instituted or intensified and the patient is re-examined in 6 to 8 weeks.

If no cervical rib or elongated transverse process of C7 is encountered, surgery is limited to first rib resection and/or total anterior scalenectomy. Classically, all patients have undergone first rib resection. As experience has been gained in differentiating upper cord from lower cord symptoms, operations are tailored to each patient. If symptoms are purely related to the upper cord, total anterior scalenectomy alone is performed. The older operation, anterior scalenotomy, is not advised, because the anterior scalene muscle and elements of the plexus interdigitate. If not removed, the muscle scar tissue and fibrosis will continue to aggravate the plexus. If symptoms are referable to the lower cord, first rib resection alone is performed. Most of the patients I see, however, have a combination of the two symptom complexes and undergo both first rib resection and total anterior scalenectomy. The first rib resection may be done through either a transaxillary or a supraclavicular approach. The old posterior approach has mostly been abandoned because of the severe postoperative pain manifested by many of these patients. Both transaxillary and supraclavicular approaches have their proponents and are probably equally effective. At my institution both approaches are used, depending on the presenting complaints, anatomy, and concomitant repair and the surgeon's preference. The anterior scalenectomy, of course, is done through a supraclavicular incision.

The most common complication of first rib resection is pneumothorax, which is of little import. Routine chest tubes may be used, or the pleural space may be aspirated at the conclusion of the procedure, with a small catheter left in the pleural space and withdrawn after skin closure is complete. Inner arm numbness is encountered from traumatic injury to the intercostobrachialis nerve arising from the second intercostal nerve. If the long thoracic nerve is injured, a winged scapula will result. This nerve exists through the belly of the middle scalene muscle. Injury to this is a rare complication, since most surgeons do not resect this muscle but detach it from the first rib at its distal extent. Traumatic injuries to the brachial plexus may occur and are the most feared complication, usually in the form of a neuropraxia due to stretching of the nerve. If the transaxillary approach is used, the extremity should be periodically rested, in the interest both of the patient and of the assistants. If the supraclavicular approach is used, gentle retraction of the plexus is mandatory.

Injury to the subclavian vessels is a potential problem. If this occurs through the transaxillary incision, the wound should be packed and the vessels approached from supraclavicular or infraclavicular incisions to gain control and effect repair. Blood loss may be dramatic but is easily controlled with packing.

The anterior component of the rib should be excised sharply and not avulsed from its sternal attachments. If it is avulsed, a significant chondritis often ensues.

Postoperatively, patients are kept with their heads elevated 15 to 30 degrees, and the extremity is gently elevated anteriorly on pillows. Most patients are discharged in 2 to 3 days, depending on their level of comfort. Analgesics are used liberally at this time to break the cycle of pain that these patients have been experiencing. All are asked to refrain from heavy or repetitive use of the extremities for 6 weeks, at which time they are seen in follow-up. Such restrictions include driving and routine housework. Shoulder mobility exercises are used in the postoperative period to prevent "freezing" of the joint. "Walking the wall" with the fingers and rotating the torso, as well as hooking the hands over the head, two to three times each day is sufficient for this purpose. Patients should return to full work levels gradually to allow return of muscle tone and a sense of health. Some modification of work may be necessary to decrease use of the extremity.

If a bilateral condition exists, the contralateral side may be operated on as early as 4 days after the initial procedure, although I prefer to wait 6 weeks to determine whether there has been improvement sufficient to encourage expectations of similar results on the opposite side. If results are as anticipated, a similar operation is performed on the opposite side. If results are poor and no improvement has been noted, first rib resection for contralateral suspected neurologic involvement is not carried out.

VENOUS SYMPTOMS (COMPRESSION OF AXILLARY-SUBCLAVIAN VEIN)

Unlike patients with neurologic symptoms, patients with venous symptoms from thoracic outlet syndrome have so far been predominantly male. This probably reflects the fact that the injury is usually on the basis of soft tissue, i.e., muscle and ligament compression rather than bony compression. Again, the patients are youthful adults.

Physical examination may reveal an increased venous pattern about the shoulder and upper lateral chest as well as the extremity. Such engorgement may not be seen when the patient is at rest, but may be present with the classic maneuvers for diagnosis of thoracic outlet. Venous compression is a vexing problem. Patients may present with intermittent heaviness and easy fatigability of the extremity, or with venous engorgement. Phlebography should be performed in all patients suspected of having the venous symptoms of thoracic outlet syndrome. If the vein is patent, resection of the rib and appropriate soft tissue structures should be performed. All patients presenting with thrombosis of the subclavian-axillary system should be anticoagulated. Those presenting with occlusion should undergo repeat phlebography in 3 to 6 months. If recanalization has occurred, surgery should be offered. If the vein is still occluded, there is little benefit in removing the first rib unless there are associated nervous or arterial components to the thoracic outlet syndrome. It is most important that patients be alert to the onset of similar problems on the contralateral side. At the first evidence of symptoms, they should consult their physician or surgeon for consideration of operative therapy. If bone abnormalities are seen initially on the contralateral side, operation may be offered prophylactically to prevent the development of contralateral symptoms.

Patients presenting with venous thrombosis within 48 to 72 hours of onset should be treated with venous thrombectomy or thrombolysis. Once patency is reestablished, the underlying cause must be corrected. In addition to rib resection, excision of the subclavius muscle and the costoclavicular ligament is indicated. The subclavian vein lies anterior to the anterior scalene muscle and is not part of that triangular compression between the two scalene muscles and the rib. If tendons such as the pectoralis minor are incriminated, they too should be divided. Intervention past this "golden period" provides little long-lasting relief, and poor maintenance of vessel patency. Supportive medical care (elevation anteriorly on pillows and anticoagulation) is indicated. Approximately 60 percent of patients have swelling of the extremity for life, and half of these have moderate or severe symptoms. Internal jugular-subclavian vein bypass, in which the internal jugular vein is divided, swung laterally, and sewn end to side to the subclavian vein to circumvent a localized obstruction, may offer a viable option for patients with occlusion who heretofore have not been offered operation.

ARTERIAL SYMPTOMS (SUBCLAVIAN-AXILLARY ARTERY INVOLVEMENT)

Patients with arterial symptoms of thoracic outlet syndrome may present with upper extremity claudication, ischemic pain or ulcers, microembolization, or aneurysms. The arteries themselves may be stenotic or occluded, may have localized areas of traumatic ulceration, or may exhibit post-stenotic dilatation or aneurysmal changes. These patients on presentation may be young, or may be members of an older age group when the degeneration of the artery manifests itself. Unilateral hand ischemia in a young woman or man should make the clinician consider thoracic outlet syndrome with arterial involvement. The classical tests for thoracic outlet syndrome are best suited for these patients with arterial symptoms. Bruits may be elicited. "High-riding" subclavian pulses or aneurysms may be palpated as well as cervical ribs. Patients with microembolization exhibit splinter hemorrhages under the nails or areas of painful, bluish discoloration in the fingertips and hands. More severe cases present with severely ischemic hands, with ulcers and pregangrenous changes and perhaps absent pulses at the wrist. In the early stages of microembolization, pulses are usually palpable.

In these patients, cervical ribs are commonly found with the artery draped over them. Abnormal bands running from elongated transverse processes or from shorter cervical ribs may also account for the structural abnormality. Post-stenotic dilatation with thrombus formation in the ectatic portion of the artery, or traumatic ulcerated lesions of the artery, are the two sites that give rise to embolus-producing lesions.

At operation, the first rib should be resected in all cases, including those in which a cervical rib is incriminated. Usually these two are joined, but even if they are not, the rib should be removed. In addition to bony and soft tissue resections, arterial reconstruction is necessary to repair aneurysms and to replace stenotic, ulcerated arteries. Those arteries that are simply dilated beyond the rib and are not embolizing or causing ischemia need not be replaced. Claviculectomy is not necessary, and supraclavicular and infraclavicular incisions can be placed appropriately to allow reconstruction. In severe cases of distal ischemia in which digital and palmar arteries have been filled with embolic debris, upper extremity sympathectomy should be added to the procedure. This may be done through a supraclavicular (cervical) or a transaxillary approach. Reconstruction of the artery may be performed using vein if suitably sized, or Dacron or expanded polytetrafluoroethylene.

Patients undergoing arterial reconstructions need to be followed, as does any patient with an arterial reconstruction, with periodic physical examination and noninvasive laboratory testing. If indicated, conventional or digital arteriograms should be obtained.

SUGGESTED READING

Cormier JM, Amrane M, Ward A, et al. Arterial complications of the thoracic outlet syndrome: fifty-five operative cases. J Vasc Surg 1989; 9:778.

Etheredge S, Wilbur R, Stoney RJ. Thoracic outlet syndrome. Am J Surg 1979; 138:175.

Gloviczki P, Kazmier RJ, Hollier LH. Axillary-subclavian venous occlusion: the morbidity of a non-lethal disease. J Vasc Surg 1986; 4:333.

Pairolero PC, Walls JT, Payne WS, et al. Subclavian axillary artery aneurysms. Surgery 1981; 90:757.

Qvarfordt PG, Ehrenfeld WK, Stoney RJ. Supraclavicular radical scalenectomy and transaxillary first rib resection for the thoracic outlet syndrome—a combined approach. Am J Surg 1984; 148:111.

Reilly LM, Stoney RJ. Supraclavicular approach for thoracic outlet decompression. J Vasc Surg 1988; 8:329.

Roos DB. The place for scalenectomy and first rib resection in thoracic outlet syndrome. Surgery 1982; 92:1077.

Roos DB. New concepts of thoracic outlet syndrome that explain etiology, symptoms, diagnosis and treatment. Vasc Surg 1979; 13:313.

Sanders RJ, Pearce WH. The treatment of thoracic outlet syndrome: a comparison of different operations. J Vasc Surg 1989; 10:626.

Sanders RJ, Raymer S. The supraclavicular approach to scalenectomy and first rib resection; description of technique. J Vasc Surg 1985; 2:751.

OTHER VASCULAR COMPRESSION AND ENTRAPMENT SYNDROMES

DAVID NAIDE, M.D.

Although not common, various forms of vascular compression and entrapment do exist and are seen in clinical practice. Patients with these conditions may present with symptoms of acute arterial occlusion, with a history of episodic ischemia with exertion (intermittent claudication), or with symptoms mimicking vasospastic phenomenon (i.e., Raynaud's phenomenon). Diagnosis is often delayed and management is often suboptimal. This discussion is meant to heighten clinical awareness of the entrapment and compression syndromes.

VASCULAR COMPRESSION SYNDROMES

Vascular structures, particularly veins, may be compressed by a variety of masses. This occurs more commonly in the lower abdomen and pelvis than in the extremities. A common cause of venous compression in the pelvis is the enlarged uterus in pregnancy. Compression of the pelvic and iliac veins leads to increased venous pressure in the lower extremities. If a pregnant woman has incompetent communicating veins, the tendency to develop varicosities will be accentuated. In the postpartum period, the venous pressure markedly diminishes and the varicose veins often recede significantly.

In men, prostatic hypertrophy with outlet obstruction can lead to chronic enlargement of the urinary bladder, occasionally resulting in iliac vein compression, venous insufficiency, and peripheral edema. In this case, pelvic computed tomography (CT) will demonstrate the enlarged urinary bladder and iliac vein compression. This clinical problem can be relieved by transurethral resection of the prostate. Rarely, an intra-abdominal abscess may significantly impede iliac venous outflow; likewise, an abscess in the lower extremity can lead to compression of the deep leg veins. Proper treatment includes administration of intravenous antibiotics and drainage of the abscess. Rarely, fibrous bands may compress portions of the deep venous system (Fig. 1). This may be resolved by surgically cutting the fibrous bands.

Other causes of vascular compression in the abdominal area include retroperitoneal fibrosis, which may be idiopathic or secondary to drugs such as methysergide. When present, retroperitoneal fibrosis can lead to significant vascular compression that may involve the iliac veins and vena cava as well as the abdominal aorta and iliac arteries (Figs. 2 and 3). Cessation of the

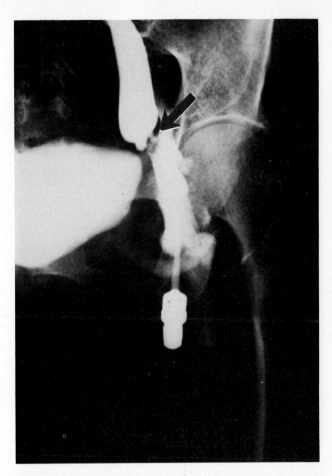

Figure 1 Fibrous band causing external iliac vein compression.

offending drug usually halts the process. Occasionally, when dialysis access is placed in a lower extremity, venous hypertension and insufficiency may become significant. This is especially true in some patients who have pre-existing subclinical venous insufficiency on the basis of proximal (iliac) venous compression. Because of this possibility, some people advocate noninvasive venous studies or radionuclide venography before placement of a vascular access in the lower extremities, although this may not be cost effective since the syndrome is not that common.

Tumors can cause significant vascular compression or invasion in the pelvic and retroperitoneal area. These include adenocarcinoma of the prostate, female pelvic organs, or gastrointestinal tract; various types of lymphoma, including Hodgkin's disease; renal tumors; leiomyosarcomas; and testicular tumors. These tumors may induce leg edema by compressing the iliac vein and/or vena cava; by invading and obstructing the venous lumen; or by infiltrating nodes, producing lymphatic obstruction. It is axiomatic that unilateral edema in a man over the age of 60 should be considered to be caused by prostate cancer until proven otherwise. When any of these entities are suspected, in addition to a good physical and rectal or gynecologic examination, CT of

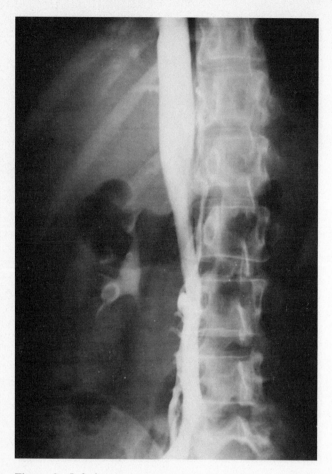

Figure 2 Inferior vena cava compression caused by retroperitoneal fibrosis.

the abdomen and pelvis (with contrast material) or ultrasonography should be performed. Occasionally, however, it may be necessary to resort to venography, arteriography, or lymphoscintigraphy to establish a diagnosis. Management depends on the etiology; palliation can occasionally be achieved by surgery, radiation therapy, or chemotherapy.

Another cause of vascular compression, especially in the extremities, is hematoma secondary to trauma, arterial puncture, or cannulation. Lastly, aneurysms or pseudoaneurysms of the aorta or its branches may compress adjacent vessels. For example, superior vena cava syndrome may be caused by an aneurysm of the ascending aorta. Similarly, the false lumen of an aortic dissection may compress adjacent vascular structures, branches of the aorta, or even the true lumen.

POPLITEAL ENTRAPMENT SYNDROME

The popliteal artery entrapment syndrome is caused by an abnormal anatomic relationship between the popliteal artery and the muscles within the popliteal fossa. Normally, the popliteal artery courses between the two heads of the gastrocnemius muscle. In this disorder, the artery deviates medially around the inner border of the medial head of the gastrocnemius or an accessory muscle or fascial slip arising more laterally than the medial head. The typical patient is a teenager or young adult with typical intermittent claudication of the foot and calf, although on rare occasions patients have reported leg pain at the onset of walking or with walking but not running. The severity of symptoms depends on

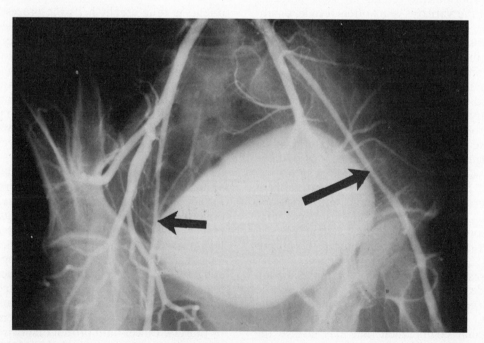

Figure 3 External iliac artery compression caused by retroperitoneal fibrosis (oblique view).

whether the popliteal artery is compressed or thrombosed. On physical examination, patients demonstrate disappearance of pedal pulses with passive dorsiflexion of the foot, or occasionally with active plantar flexion. This syndrome of popliteal entrapment is often bilateral and appears to be significantly underdiagnosed. Noninvasive vascular studies before and after exercise, as well as arteriography, may help establish the diagnosis. Angiographic findings include narrowing of the popliteal artery with post-stenotic dilatation, or popliteal artery occlusion in the absence of generalized atherosclerosis. Differential diagnosis includes adventitial cystic degeneration of the popliteal artery, also usually found in younger patients, which if present, should be surgically corrected to avoid thrombosis and/or distal embolization.

ANTERIOR TIBIAL COMPARTMENT SYNDROME

The usual causes of anterior tibial compartment syndrome (Table 1) include muscular swelling due to blunt trauma, revascularization of a severely ischemic limb, and direct arterial trauma. For example, a patient with severe ischemia due to acute arterial occlusion who undergoes a corrective procedure such as embolectomy, thrombectomy, or thrombolysis to restore blood flow is susceptible to developing this complication. The pathophysiology of this syndrome is not well understood but may represent a tissue response to hypoxemia with ischemic injury to the capillary and venous bed subserving the previously ischemic area. This leads to excessive permeability, permitting transudation of fluid and/or bleeding into the muscle. Once the pressure increases, certain compartments bounded by fascial planes, such as the anterior tibial compartment, are unable to expand. If compartment pressure exceeds capillary pressure, ischemic muscle necrosis may ensue. This is most often an acute process, but rarely may be subacute or chronic. The increased compartment pressure leads to ischemic damage to peripheral nerves and muscles and can result in weakness, anesthesia, and paralysis. If increased pressure is not relieved within 24 hours or less, neurologic deficits may become permanent; even before 24 hours have elapsed, muscle breakdown can occur.

Less common causes of anterior tibial compartment syndrome include segmental spasm of the anterior tibial artery, venous obstruction (e.g., phlegmasia cerulea dolens), and muscle hemorrhage secondary to trauma. The physical signs and symptoms of compression syn-

drome include swelling, tenseness, paresis, pain (with or without passive stretching of the involved muscles), and paresthesias. The pain may be out of proportion to what is expected. Although tissue arterioles are compromised by the increased pressure, peripheral pulses often remain palpable, especially in the early stages.

In order to institute prompt therapy, it is essential to make the diagnosis as early as possible. To expedite this, it is most helpful to take pressure measurements of the compartment involved. The normal compartment pressure is 0 to 10 mm Hg. A tissue pressure greater than 30 mm Hg is usually associated with significant compromise of muscle and nerve perfusion, but even lower pressures may be equally harmful if the patient has concomitant hypotension. Before one proceeds to fasciotomy, the physical findings must be considered along with the compartment pressures.

Sometimes, fasciotomy may be indicated prophylactically, such as with delayed revascularization after acute ischemia; with marked swelling of an ischemic limb postoperatively; with severe crush injuries to the leg; after combined arterial and venous injury, especially in situations in which the damaged vein must be ligated; and, on rare occasions, with phlegmasia cerulea dolens. If the diagnosis of compartment syndrome is entertained but immediate fasciotomy is not warranted by the clinical evidence (physical signs and compartment pressures), careful observation must be maintained, including serial tissue perfusion measurements, until all danger of increased compartment pressure has disappeared.

THIGH OR ARM COMPARTMENT SYNDROME

Thigh compartment syndrome is occasionally observed, usually secondary to femoral fracture. The compartment syndrome in these patients often develops after femoral intramedullary stabilization. Other case reports describe the same syndrome after blunt trauma to the thigh or after prolonged compression by body weight or vascular injury. One of my patients presented after 28 hours of drug-induced coma while in a yogi position with his legs sharply crossed. This was attended by marked swelling of the legs, leading to femoral nerve compression, lower extremity paralysis, and acute renal failure secondary to myoglobinuria. Renal function recovered, but neurologic dysfunction of the lower extremities persisted despite fasciotomy to decompress both thighs shortly after hospitalization. These sequelae are consistent with the available literature that documents a significant incidence (40 to 50 percent) of permanent neurologic deficit after thigh compartment syndrome as well as a moderate incidence of secondary infection.

Compartment syndromes affecting the upper extremities may be observed after crush injuries, supracondylar fractures of the humerus with damage to the brachial artery, or angiography performed via an axillary or brachial artery approach, at which time adjacent nerves may be damaged directly by the cannulation procedure or indirectly by hematoma compressing

Table 1 Anterior Tibial Compartment Syndrome

Closed anatomic compartment: limited expansion
Bounded by bone, interosseous membrane, bone
Ischemia leads to muscle necrosis and to swelling with damage to nerves and blood vessels
Usual cause is either severe ischemia or revascularization after sudden ischemia
Treatment: fasciotomy

nerves. If this is not recognized and treated promptly, irreversible muscle or nerve injury may result in Volkmann's ischemic contracture.

Uncommonly, some athletes may develop chronic compartment syndrome secondary to muscular overuse and overdevelopment. This can lead to neural or arterial compression, and rarely can produce claudication. In addition, if not treated, these athletes may develop neurologic involvement. Diagnosis can be established by noninvasive testing and measurement of compartment pressures, which are often elevated at rest.

SUGGESTED READING

Harris RD. The etiology of inferior vena caval obstruction and compression. CRC Crit Rev Clin Radiol Nucl Med 1976; 8:57–86.

Patman RD. Fasciotomy: indications and techniques. In: Rutherford RB, ed. Vascular surgery. Philadelphia: WB Saunders, 1984.

Rob C, May AG. Neurovascular compression syndromes. Adv Surg 1975; 9:211–239.

Rohrer MJ, et al. Axillary artery compression and thrombosis in throwing athletes. J Vasc Surg 1990; 11:761–769.

Schurmann G, Mattfeldt T, Hofmann W, et al. The popliteal artery entrapment syndrome. Eur J Vasc Surg 1990; 4:223–231.

Schwartz JJ, et al. Acute compartment syndrome of the thigh. J Bone Joint Surg 1989; 71A:392–400.

VENOUS AND LYMPHATIC DISEASE

DEEP VENOUS THROMBOSIS

SAMUEL Z. GOLDHABER, M.D.

Deep venous thrombosis (DVT) is responsible for approximately 200,000 hospitalizations per year in the United States (Fig. 1). It is notoriously difficult to recognize and the number of hospitalizations therefore underestimates the true frequency of this disease. Nevertheless, DVT is diagnosed twice as often as pulmonary embolism (PE) and is the underlying cause of both PE and chronic venous insufficiency (CVI). About one-third of DVTs are recurrent rather than first episodes. Recently, there have been important advances in our understanding of the coagulation disorders implicated as etiologies of DVT. There has also been a revolution in the diagnosis of DVT with high-resolution B-mode ultrasonography and color Doppler imaging. Therapy now focuses with increasing frequency on thrombolysis as an adjunct to heparin. Furthermore, a new generation of inferior vena caval filters has recently received Food and Drug Administration (FDA) approval. Finally, there is augmented emphasis on employing proven preventive mechanical and pharmacologic measures against venous thrombosis.

DVT occurs more often with increasing age and is slightly more common in men than in women. The risk of DVT also increases in any of the following conditions: previous DVT, cancer (especially adenocarcinoma), surgery (especially hip or knee reconstruction, cesarean section, or any operation requiring more than 1 hour of general anesthesia), pregnancy (especially among women confined to bed because of placenta previa, preeclampsia, or eclampsia and particularly among all women during the postpartum period), and use of oral contraceptives. DVT, especially when bilateral, may herald the presence of occult malignancy. This suggests that patients with DVT should be screened and followed carefully for cancer when no cause of the venous thrombosis is clinically apparent.

COAGULATION MARKERS FOR DEEP VENOUS THROMBOSIS

The best marker of a coagulation disorder is a carefully taken family history for venous thrombosis that is positive for DVT or PE. Undoubtedly, most coagulation abnormalities have not yet been elucidated. Those that are implicated include (1) increased plasminogen activator inhibitor (PAI) and (2) deficiencies of antithrombin III, protein C, or protein S. In a study of 88 patients with venous thrombosis, 19 percent with DVT had increased PAI levels (Tabernero et al, 1989). An earlier study of 752 patients with venous thromboembolism demonstrated antithrombin III levels below the normal range in 7 percent (Vikydal et al, 1985). Nevertheless, the best available studies indicate that deficiencies of protein C and protein S are the most commonly identified offenders, accounting for 5 to 9 percent of associated coagulation abnormalities in an unselected population of patients with DVT. An evaluation for hypercoagulopathy as the underlying cause of DVT usually includes antithrombin III, protein C, protein S, and anticardiolipin antibody levels. It is not cost effective to screen all patients for hypercoagulopathy; rather, these tests should be se-

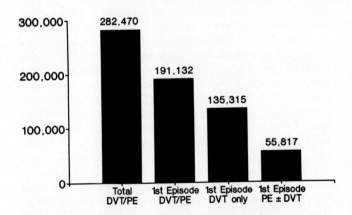

Figure 1 Estimated cases of diagnosed deep venous thrombosis (DVT) and pulmonary embolism (PE) in the United States. (Based on data from Anderson FA Jr, Wheeler HB, Goldberg RJ, et al. A population-based perspective of the incidence and case-fatality rates of venous thrombosis and pulmonary embolism: the Worchester DVT Study. Arch Intern Med 1991, in press.)

lectively applied, particularly in young patients with no obvious risk factor for DVT.

THE DEEP VENOUS THROMBOSIS–PULMONARY EMBOLISM RELATIONSHIP

Among patients with venographically proved proximal leg DVT, approximately half endure concomitant PE that is often clinically silent. As many as 15 to 30 percent of patients with isolated calf vein thrombosis have asymptomatic PE, a much higher frequency than is generally appreciated. With the advent of ultrasonography, the visualization of ominous-appearing, free-floating venous thrombi in the deep leg veins can easily panic the treating physician. Fortunately, most free-floating thrombi do not embolize, but instead are seen on serial noninvasive examinations to become attached to the vein wall or to resolve.

Anatomically large DVT (Fig. 2) can cause fatal PE even when a relatively small portion of the underlying DVT embolizes. When venous thrombi dislodge, they flow through the venous system to the pulmonary arterial circulation and may embolize to the bifurcation of the pulmonary artery, forming a "saddle embolus" or, more commonly, may occlude a major pulmonary vessel. The pathophysiologic response to acute PE depends on (1) the extent to which pulmonary artery blood flow is obstructed, (2) pre-existing cardiopulmonary disease, and (3) the release of vasoactive humoral factors from activated platelets that accumulate at the site of new clot.

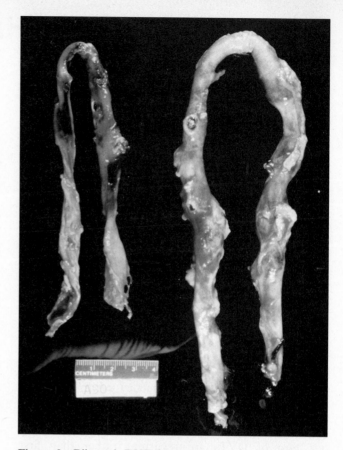

Figure 2 Bilateral DVT involving the external iliac and femoral veins in a 48-year-old woman who died of pulmonary embolism in association with adenocarcinoma of the lung.

CHRONIC VENOUS INSUFFICIENCY

DVT causes permanent damage to the valves of deep leg veins, which in turn causes venous reflux that results in CVI. The cardinal signs of CVI are darkened skin pigmentation due to hemosiderin deposition, varicosities of the veins, and, ultimately, ulceration of the skin. Among a group of DVT patients followed by Strandness and co-workers for an average of 3 years, two-thirds developed leg pain or swelling, the predominant symptoms associated with CVI. Among another group of patients examined on average 7 years after suffering a DVT, Lindner and co-workers found that four-fifths had both clinical and laboratory evidence of CVI. Figure 3 shows a patient with moderate CVI, and Figure 4 demonstrates a patient with severe CVI whose disease has progressed to the extreme of bilateral venous ulceration. Although CVI is almost always clinically apparent, its presence can be confirmed by objective measurements of impairment of the microcirculation. Direct measurement of abnormally elevated ambulatory venous pressure will confirm the superficial venous hypertension that is responsible for the physical findings of CVI. However, direct pressure measurement is almost never used for clinical purposes and is considered to be

a research procedure that has been mostly replaced clinically by noninvasive testing methods.

In patients with CVI, venous refilling time is shortened. For the past decade, photoplethysmography (PPG) has been the most widely used noninvasive method to assess venous refilling time. A recent variation of this technique, light reflection rheography (LRR), has been gaining acceptance. LRR uses a probe that emits infrared light. Light reflected from the cutaneous dermal circulation is detected by a phototransistor receiver built into the probe. The intensity of reflected light is inversely proportional to the blood content of the microvasculature. With venous emptying, blood content decreases; with venous refill, blood content increases. These changes in blood content of the microvasculature are detected by the probe. After the patient is instructed to dorsiflex the foot, an increase in reflected light correlates with venous emptying. The patient is then instructed to stop dorsiflexing, in order to allow venous refill. A refill time greater than 20 to 25 seconds indicates normal venous valvular competence. With CVI, the refill is abnormally rapid because of venous valvular incompetence. Unlike PPG, LRR is not affected by ambient light, the color of a patient's skin, the degree of skin pigmentation, or edema.

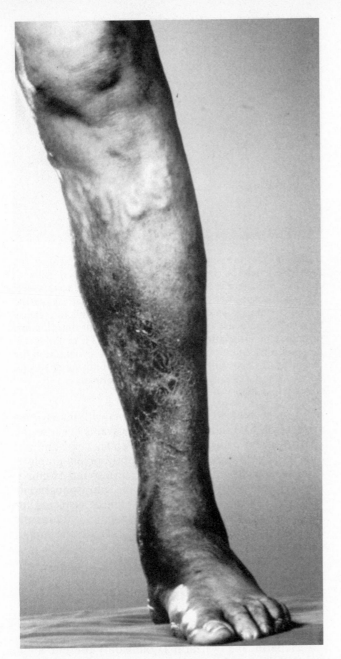

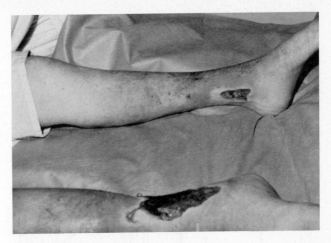

Figure 4 Patient with severe chronic venous insufficiency of the legs manifested by bilateral venous ulcerations that will require surgical repair. Venous ulcers are typically found on the medial malleolus.

Figure 3 Patient with moderately severe chronic venous insufficiency, indicated by abnormal skin pigmentation, varicosities of the veins (particularly below the knee), and ankle edema.

UPPER EXTREMITY THROMBOSIS

Upper extremity DVT is posing an increasingly frequent problem for two reasons: expanded indications for indwelling central venous lines and escalating abuse of intravenous drugs. First, many patients with cancer receive indwelling central venous lines for chemotherapy, routine blood testing, and nutritional supplementation. These lines often stay in place for many months. Thrombus frequently forms at the distal tip of the indwelling catheter and can extend distally to the right atrium. The thrombus can occur commonly despite daily flushing of the line with heparin. Second, intravenous drug abusers, especially those who use cocaine, appear to be particularly susceptible to upper extremity thrombosis. At the University of Texas Medical Branch, upper extremity thrombosis constituted 25 percent of all cases of DVT during a recent 1-year period. Of these upper extremity cases, 42 percent were associated with intravenous cocaine abuse.

DIAGNOSIS OF DEEP VENOUS THROMBOSIS

Clinical Features

DVT often occurs without any symptoms or signs. When present, however, the major symptoms are leg pain, tenderness, and swelling; the major signs are leg edema, discomfort in the calf upon forced dorsiflexion of the foot (Homans' sign), venous distention of subcutaneous vessels, discoloration, and a palpable cord (i.e., thrombus). Unfortunately, these clinical features are not specific for DVT, so that diagnosis based on physical findings is often incorrect. Therefore, clinical suspicion of DVT should prompt definitive radiologic evaluation.

Noninvasive Testing

Impedance plethysmography (IPG) has served as the classic noninvasive test for DVT. IPG measures blood volume changes in the lower leg on the basis of changes in electrical resistance (impedance) during testing. A pneumatic cuff is placed around the patient's thigh and inflated to a low pressure in order to obstruct temporarily the venous outflow. Electrodes are placed on the patient's calf to measure changes in electrical resistance. An imperceptible high-frequency current is then passed through the patient's leg. Under normal circumstances, the conductivity should increase slowly as

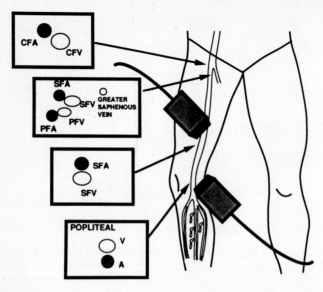

Figure 5 Ultrasound examination of the leg involves compressing the femoral and popliteal veins. The transducer is held transversely to the vein and artery. Manual pressure is applied to the skin, and this in turn is transmitted to the vein and artery. Beginning at the groin, the transducer is moved distally in increments of 2 cm, and the compression maneuver is repeated. At the level of the knee, imaging is performed from the back. CFA, common femoral artery; CFV, common femoral vein; SFA, superficial femoral artery; SFV, superficial femoral vein (which, despite its name, is a deep leg vein); PFA, profunda femoris artery; PFV, profunda femoris vein; V, vein; A, artery. (From Polak JF. Doppler ultrasound of the deep leg veins: a revolution in the diagnosis of deep vein thrombosis and monitoring of thrombolysis. Chest 1991; 99:165S–172S; with permission.)

the veins fill and should decrease rapidly when the cuff pressure is released, because blood is a good conductor of electricity. However, in the presence of DVT, there is little or no change in conductivity as the cuff is inflated and subsequently deflated. A carefully designed prospective study carried out in Amsterdam demonstrated that four normal serial IPG examinations on days 1, 2, 5, and 10 after presentation of ambulatory patients with suspected DVT can exclude DVT in this population almost as accurately as venography.

More recently, the use of high-resolution B-mode ultrasonography with color Doppler flow imaging appears to be supplanting IPG as the most widely used noninvasive test for DVT in the United States. For diagnosing DVT proximal to the calf, B-mode imaging is almost as accurate as venography when inability to compress the popliteal or femoral vein with a hand-held ultrasound probe (Figs. 5 and 6) is used as the major criterion for a positive test. With expensive ultrasound devices, calf vein thrombosis can often be detected.

Contrast Phlebography

Venography is costly, invasive, and occasionally results in complications due to allergy to contrast media

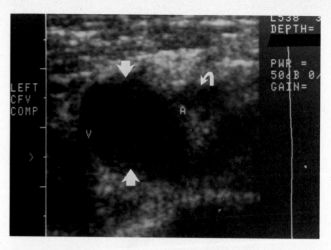

Figure 6 Despite vigorous hand-held pressure against the skin, the common femoral vein (straight arrows) fails to collapse. Sufficient pressure has been transmitted to this level of the soft tissues to cause the common femoral artery (curved arrow) to deform. The common femoral vein fails to collapse because of increased venous pressure and/or intraluminal thrombus in association with acute DVT. (From Polak JF. Doppler ultrasound of the deep leg veins: a revolution in the diagnosis of deep vein thrombosis and monitoring of thrombolysis. Chest 1991; 99:165S–172S; with permission.)

or contrast-induced phlebitis. Patients with massive leg DVT often have nondiagnostic venograms because the contrast agent cannot reach the deep leg veins and fills only the superficial veins. Consequently, phlebography is reserved for patients in whom the ultrasound examination is equivocal, or in whom the ultrasonographic results are normal despite a high clinical suspicion for DVT. We continue to perform venography frequently for patients suspected of thrombosis of the upper extremity and of the calf.

THERAPY

Anticoagulation

Heparin and warfarin (Coumadin) prevent additional thrombus formation and provide the foundation of therapy for DVT. I believe that symptomatic DVT should be treated with anticoagulation unless the patient is actively bleeding. In particular, I do not withhold anticoagulation from patients with symptomatic DVT that is limited to the calf.

An initial heparin bolus of 5,000 to 10,000 units should be administered, followed by a continuous infusion of 1,000 to 1,500 units per hour. For heparin, the target partial thromboplastin time (PTT) is 1.5 to 2.5 times the upper limit of the control value, and the PTT should be checked every 4 hours until the target PTT range is obtained. When the PTT is less than 1.5 times the control, the continuous heparin infusion dose should be increased rapidly, by an increment of at least 25 percent. Conversely, if a PTT level exceeds three times

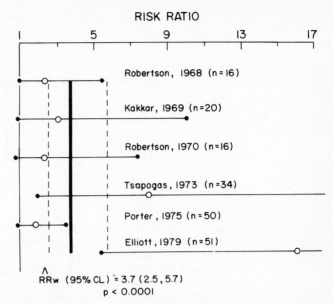

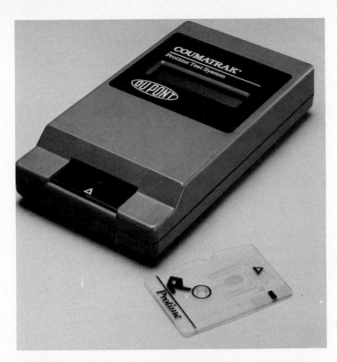

Figure 7 The Coumatrak is a laser photometer. When a drop of whole blood is applied to the disposable plastic reagent cartridge, it is drawn by capillary action into a reagent chamber that contains a dry rabbit brain thromboplastin preparation. Coagulation begins when the blood rehydrates the thromboplastin. The reaction mixture continues flowing in the capillary channel beyond the reagent chamber before a clot develops. The laser photometer detects the cessation of blood flow (clotting) by sensing variation in light scatter caused by the movement of red blood cells.

Figure 8 Overview of six randomized trials of streptokinase (SK) versus heparin for acute DVT indicates an overall 3.7 times superior lysis rate *(heavy vertical line)* for SK compared with heparin. A risk ratio greater than 1 indicates a beneficial effect of SK for clot lysis. The pooled risk ratio is statistically significant (p <.001), with 95 percent confidence limits (CL) *(hatched vertical lines)* of 2.5 to 5.7. In each of the six individual trials, SK achieved superior lysis *(open circles)*, but the lower 95 percent confidence limit *(closed circle, left side of each solid horizontal line)* was greater than 1, indicating statistical significance, in only two of six individual trials. (From Brown WD, Goldhaber SZ. How to select patients with deep vein thrombosis for tPA therapy. Chest 1989; 95:276S–278S; with permission.)

the control value, a reduction rate of no more than 25 percent of the dose should be made.

It is my practice to overlap heparin and warfarin for at least 5 days, except in pregnant women or patients with cancer and DVT in more than one limb (i.e., Trousseau's syndrome), whom I treat with heparin alone. Warfarin is teratogenic, especially during weeks 6 to 12 of pregnancy. Patients with cancer and DVT in more than one limb rarely respond to warfarin therapy. My usual practice for these two groups of patients is to maintain continuous intravenous heparin for 5 to 7 days and then switch to full dose-adjusted subcutaneous heparin.

For most patients, I ordinarily administer heparin for 5 to 7 days and initiate warfarin on the second hospital day. I usually begin with 10 mg of warfarin daily for 3 days and maintain a target prothrombin time (PT) of 15 to 17 seconds for an initial DVT and 16 to 20 seconds for a recurrent DVT. If risk factors are transient, I give warfarin for 6 months. Otherwise, I advise indefinite anticoagulation.

Most warfarin is administered in the outpatient setting. Until recently, I adjusted the dose of warfarin on the basis of plasma PT. After the laboratory telephoned with PT results, patients were contacted either to

reassure them that their dosing regimen was appropriate or to advise dosage adjustments. Unfortunately, it can be difficult to explain changes in anticoagulation dosing by telephone. I therefore now use the Coumatrak (Fig. 7) to make in-office assessments of warfarin dosing regimens. This device provides the PT result in 2 minutes by analyzing a drop of whole blood obtained from a fingertip puncture. A study at Boston City Hospital showed that switching from Coumadin to generic warfarin was associated with increased morbidity and increased expense owing to widely fluctuating PT levels. Therefore, my practice is to prescribe Coumadin.

For pregnant women with DVT, I never use warfarin. Instead, I treat initially with continuous intravenous heparin and then teach self-injection of full-dose subcutaneous heparin for the remainder of the pregnancy. With subcutaneous injections, peak heparin levels are usually obtained at approximately 3 hours, and the effect may last for 12 hours if the heparin dose is adequate. To monitor the heparin, my target is either a mid-interval PTT of approximately 1.5 times control or, more commonly, a trough PTT at least several seconds elevated above the upper limit of normal. It was once thought that women taking warfarin post partum could not breast feed, but it is now evident that breast feeding

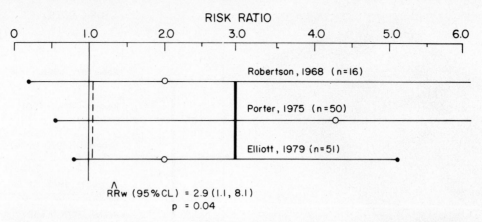

Figure 9 Overview of three trials of SK versus heparin (three of the trials in Figure 8 provided inadequate information on bleeding complications) for acute DVT indicates an overall 2.9 increase in the major bleeding rate *(heavy vertical line)* for SK compared with heparin. A risk ratio greater than 1 indicates more major bleeding complications associated with SK than with heparin. The pooled risk ratio is statistically significant (p = .04), but the 95 percent confidence limits are wide, reflecting the small sample size among the individual trials. (From Brown WD, Goldhaber SZ. How to select patients with deep vein thrombosis for tPA therapy. Chest 1989; 95:276S-278S; with permission.)

is safe. The level of warfarin in breast milk is so low (approximately 25 ng per milliliter) that it cannot be detected in the baby's plasma.

The most important adverse effect of anticoagulation is hemorrhage. Major bleeding during anticoagulation may unmask a previously silent lesion such as bladder or colon cancer. For most cases of moderate bleeding, cessation of heparin therapy will suffice. Resumption of anticoagulation at a lower dose, or an alternative means of therapy such as inferior vena caval interruption, depends on the severity of the bleeding, the risk of recurrent DVT, and the extent to which bleeding may have resulted from excessive anticoagulation (i.e., a PTT or PT greater than three times the baseline value).

Thrombolysis

Thrombolysis for DVT has been advocated as important adjunctive therapy to accelerate clot lysis that would otherwise occur only to a limited extent with endogenous fibronolytic processes. Theoretically, thrombolysis should aid in lysing clot in situ, thereby decreasing the frequency of PE. In addition, thrombolysis should decrease the frequency of chronic venous insufficiency if it minimizes the damage to venous valves caused by residual thrombus. The principal challenge is finding an effective and safe thrombolytic regimen for DVT. Currently, the only FDA-approved thrombolytic treatment of DVT consists of streptokinase (SK) in a dose of 250,000 units as a 30-minute bolus followed by 100,000 units per hour for 24 to 72 hours. Overviews of randomized trials demonstrate that SK followed by heparin is approximately four times more effective than heparin alone in lysing DVT (Fig. 8). However, major bleeding complications occur about three times more often (Fig. 9). In addition, thrombolysis for DVT is often pre-

cluded by the high frequency of patients who are postoperative or who have gastrointestinal or other major bleeding. A survey at our institution showed that only about one in five patients with venographically documented DVT is an acceptable candidate for thrombolysis, even if elderly patients are not excluded from therapy.

A recently completed randomized, controlled study of recombinant human tissue–type plasminogen activator (rt-PA) for DVT versus rt-PA plus heparin versus heparin alone indicated that the addition of heparin to rt-PA does not improve the lysis rate. Surprisingly, heparin did not increase the risk of bleeding from rt-PA therapy. This trial employed a low-dose, 24-hour continuous infusion of rt-PA (Goldhaber et al, 1990). However, future DVT thrombolysis trials should probably investigate more front-loaded and accelerated dosing regimens in order to help improve further the efficacy and safety of thrombolysis.

Thrombolysis Followed by Anticoagulation versus Anticoagulation Alone

Among patients in whom there are no contraindications to thrombolysis, I consider the use of thrombolytic therapy followed by a full course of heparin anticoagulation, and subsequently warfarin. I am currently investigating the use of bolus thrombolytic therapy for DVT.

Inferior Vena Caval Interruption

There are three major indications for IVC filter placement in DVT patients: (1) contraindication to anticoagulation, (2) failure of adequate anticoagulation, and (3) prophylaxis against PE. In most circumstances

Table 1 Percutaneous Insertion of Inferior
Vena Caval Filters

Indications
   Anticoagulation contraindicated in patients with known
     pulmonary emboli
     Bleeding or known risk of bleeding (e.g., gastrointestinal)
     Patients with complications of anticoagulation (e.g., CNS
      hemorrhage, heparin-induced thrombocytopenia)
   Anticoagulation failure despite adequate therapy (e.g., recurrent
     pulmonary embolism)
   Prophylaxis for high-risk patients
     Extensive or progressive deep vein thrombophlebitis
     Following surgical pulmonary embolectomy
     Severe pulmonary hypertension; cor pulmonale

Contraindications (conditions in which surgical venotomy is
* preferred)*
   Severe blood coagulopathy, predisposing to bleeding from
     puncture site
   Anticipated patient noncompliance with postprocedure rest
     orders (especially with No. 24 Fr filter systems)
   Obstructing thrombus along available route(s) of insertion

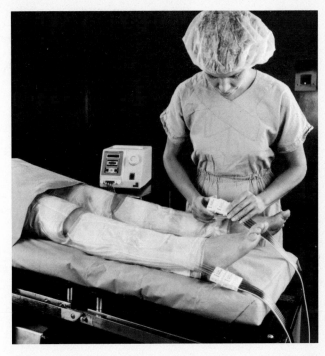

Figure 10 Intermittent pneumatic compression using the Kendall sequential compression device (SCD), which provides separate compression cuffs at the ankle, calf, and thigh.

the filter is placed percutaneously, but occasionally a surgical venotomy is preferred (Table 1). My current preference is percutaneous placement of a Bird's Nest filter, which has the advantage of a small sheath size (No. 12 Frh) that can minimize the risk of bleeding during and after the procedure.

Chronic Venous Insufficiency

As an adjunctive measure, I prescribe thigh-high graduated compression stockings, 30 to 40 mm Hg, to patients with proximal DVT of the leg when they are ready to ambulate (usually after the first 24 hours of hospitalization). The stockings help prevent distension of the vein wall and may mitigate the syndrome of CVI that most DVT patients experience. For patients who do develop the postphlebitic syndrome, preliminary reports indicate potentially dramatic improvement with intermittent pneumatic compression.

PREVENTION

DVT is easier and less expensive to prevent than it is to diagnose and to treat. Virtually all hospitalized patients should undergo mechanical, pharmacologic, or combined mechanical and pharmacologic prevention against venous thromboembolism. The most commonly used mechanical measures are graduated elastic compression stockings (e.g., T.E.D. stockings) or intermittent pneumatic compression (IPC) devices (Fig. 10). IPC boots provide intermittent inflation of air-filled cuffs that prevent venous stasis in the legs and probably stimulate the endogenous fibrinolytic system. For pharmacologic prophylaxis, low-dose subcutaneous heparin is most commonly employed. A typical dose is 5,000 units subcutaneously beginning 2 hours after surgery and continuing every 8 to 12 hours until hospital discharge.

This regimen provides protection against the development of DVT and also minimizes bleeding complications. Adjusted-dose Warfarin is used most often among orthopedic surgery patients. Its use is frequently extended for approximately 1 month after hospital discharge.

Each patient should be assessed individually for the level of risk, and those at highest risk should receive the most aggressive prophylaxis, usually a combination of IPC and low-dose heparin or adjusted-dose warfarin (Table 2). When no incremental blood loss is acceptable (e.g., for neurosurgery), IPC is the best choice. Physicians who consult about preoperative patients for any reason should discuss DVT prophylaxis before surgery with the surgeon who requested the consultation.

THE FUTURE

During the next decade, diagnosis of DVT is expected to be facilitated by ultrasound equipment that will provide greater resolution, increased portability, and decreased cost. Thrombolytic therapy will become a more widely used adjunct if an agent can be found that is both safe and convenient to administer. This undoubtedly will require administering an innovative dosing regimen that employs higher concentrations of drug over shorter periods than has been customary for DVT treatment. Other approaches during the next decade promise to include the development of specific thrombin inhibitors such as hirudin, and refinement of low-

Table 2 Strategy for Risk Stratification and Prophylaxis

Condition	Degree of Risk	Strategy
Orthopedic or gynecologic cancer surgery	Very high	Intermittent pneumatic compression plus adjusted-dose warfarin
General surgery for patients with prior DVT, cancer, or obesity	High	Intermittent pneumatic compression or graded-compression stockings plus low-dose subcutaneous heparin
General or urologic surgery (without prior VTE) or gynecologic surgery for benign condition	Moderate	Graded-compression stockings plus low-dose subcutaneous heparin or intermittent pneumatic compression
Neurosurgery, eye surgery, or other surgery for patients in whom pharmacologic prophylaxis is contraindicated	Moderate to high	Graded-compression stockings or intermittent pneumatic compression
Pregnancy	Moderate to high	*Antepartum*: graded-compression stockings plus daily exercise program plus serial leg examinations ± subcutaneous heparin *Peripartum*: intermittent pneumatic compression plus low-dose subcutaneous heparin *Postpartum*: warfarin for 6 wk if high risk
Medical conditions	Moderate to high	Graded-compression stockings ± low-dose subcutaneous heparin or intermittent pneumatic compression

DVT, deep venous thrombosis; VTE, venous thromboembolism.

molecular-weight heparins for treatment and prevention of DVT. With increased emphasis on cost effectiveness, strategies to prevent DVT will most likely receive increased emphasis and implementation.

SUGGESTED READING

Albada J, Nieuwenhuis HK, Sixma JJ. Treatment of acute venous thromboembolism with low molecular weight heparin (Fragmin). Circulation 1989; 80:935–940.

Anderson AJ, Krasnow SH, Boyer MW, et al. Thrombosis: the major Hickman catheter complication in patients with solid tumor. Chest 1989; 95:71–75.

Anderson AJ, Krasnow, SH, Boyer MW, et al. Hickman catheter clots: a common occurrence despite daily heparin flushing. Cancer Treat Rep 1987; 71:651–653.

Anderson FA Jr, Wheeler HB, Goldberg RJ, et al. A population-based perspective of the incidence and case-fatality rates of venous thrombosis and pulmonary embolism: the Worchester DVT Study. Arch Intern Med 1991; in press.

Baldridge ED, Martin MA, Welling RE. Clinical significance of free-floating venous thrombi. J Vasc Surg 1990; 11:62–69.

Brown WD, Goldhaber SZ. How to select patients with deep vein thrombosis for tPA therapy. Chest 1989; 95:276S–278S.

Collins R, et al. Reduction in fatal pulmonary embolism and venous thrombosis by perioperative administration of subcutaneous heparin: overview of results of randomized trials in general, orthopedic, and urologic surgery. N Engl J Med 1988; 318: 1162–1173.

Dorfman GS. Percutaneous inferior vena cava filters. Radiology 1990; 174:987–992.

Doyle DJ, Turpie, AGG, Hirsh J, et al. Adjusted subcutaneous heparin or continuous intravenous heparin in patients with acute deep vein thrombosis. Ann Intern Med 1987; 107:441–445.

Ginsberg JS, Brill-Edwards P, Kowalchuk G, Hirsh J. Intermittent compression units for the postphlebitic syndrome. A pilot study. Arch Intern Med 1989; 149:1651–1652.

Gladson, CL, Scharrer I, Hach V, et al. The frequency of type I heterozygous protein S and protein C deficiency in 141 unrelated young patients with venous thrombosis. Thromb Haemost 1988; 59:18–22.

Goldberg RJ, Seneff M, Gore, JM, et al. Occult malignancy in patients with deep venous thrombosis. Arch Intern Med 1987; 147:251–253.

Goldhaber SZ. Venous thromboembolism: how to prevent a tragedy. Hosp Pract 1988; 23:164–174.

Goldhaber SZ, Buring JE, Hennekens CH. Cancer and venous thromboembolism. Arch Intern Med 1987; 147:216.

Goldhaber SZ, Buring JE, Lipnick RJ, Hennekens CH. Pooled analysis of randomized trials of streptokinase and heparin in phlebographically documented acute deep venous thrombosis. Am J Med 1984; 76:393–397.

Goldhaber SZ, Meyerovitz MF, Green D, et al. Randomized controlled trial of tissue plasminogen activator in proximal deep venous thrombosis. Am J Med 1990; 88:235–240.

Grassi CJ, Goldhaber SZ. Interruption of the inferior vena cava for prevention of pulmonary embolism: transvenous filter devices. Herz 1989; 14:182–191.

Heijboer H, Brandjes DPM, Büller HR, et al. Deficiencies of coagulation-inhibiting and fibronolytic proteins in outpatients with deep-vein thrombosis. N Engl J Med 1990; 323:1512–1516.

Huisman MV, Büller HR, ten Cate, JW, et al. Unexpected high prevalence of silent pulmonary embolism in patients with deep venous thrombosis. Chest 1989; 95:498–502.

Huisman MV, Büller HR, ten Cate JW, Vreeken J. Serial impedance plethysmography for suspected deep venous thrombosis in outpatients. The Amsterdam General Practitioner Study. N Engl J Med 1986; 314:823–828.

Kakkar VV, Djazaeri B, Fok J, et al. Low-molecular-weight heparin and prevention of postoperative deep vein thrombosis. Br Med J 1982; 284:375–379.

Lagerstedt CI, Olsson C-G, Fagher BO, et al. Need for long-term anticoagulant treatment in symptomatic calf-vein thrombosis. Lancet 1985; 2:515–518.

Lensing AWA, Prandoni P, Brandjes D, et al. Detection of deep-vein thrombosis by real-time B-mode ultrasonography. N Engl J Med 1989; 320:342–345.

Lindner DJ, Edwards JM, Phinney ES, et al. Long-term hemodynamic and clinical sequelae of lower extremity deep vein thrombosis. J Vasc Surg 1986; 4:436–442.

Lisse JR, Davis CP, Thurmond-Anderle ME. Upper extremity deep venous thrombosis: increased prevalence due to cocaine abuse. Am J Med 1989; 87:457–458.

Lucas FV, Duncan A, Jay R, et al. A novel whole blood capillary technic for measuring the prothrombin time. Am J Clin Pathol 1987; 88:442–446.

McEnroe CS, O'Donnell, TF, Mackey WC. Correlation of clinical findings with venous hemodynamics in 386 patients with chronic venous insufficiency. Am J Surg 1988; 156:148–152.

McKenna R, Cole ER, Vasan U. Is warfarin sodium contraindicated in the lactating mother? J Pediatr 1983; 103:325.

NIH Consensus Development Statement. Prevention of venous thrombosis and pulmonary embolism. JAMA 1986; 256:744–749.

Norris CS, Beyrau A, Barnes RW. Quantitative photoplethysmography in chronic venous insufficiency: a new method of noninvasive estimation of ambulatory venous pressure. Surgery 1983; 94: 758–764.

Orme ML'E, Lewis PJ, de Swiet M, et al. May mothers given warfarin breast-feed their infants? Br Med J 1977; 1:1564–1565.

Pearce WH, Ricco J-B, Queral LA, et al. Hemodynamic assessment of venous problems. Surgery 1983; 93:715–721.

Polak JF. Doppler ultrasound of the deep leg veins: a revolution in the diagnosis of deep vein thrombosis and monitoring of thrombolysis. Chest 1991; 99:165S–172S.

Polak JF, Culter SS, O'Leary DH. Deep veins of the calf: assessment with color Doppler flow imaging. Radiology 1989; 171:481–485.

Reis SE, Hirsh DR, Wilson MG, et al. A program for the prevention of venous thromboembolism in high risk orthopedic patients. J Arthroplasty 1991; in press.

Richton-Hewett S, Foster E, Apstein CS. Medical and economic consequences of a blinded oral anticoagulant brand change at a municipal hospital. Arch Intern Med 1988; 148:806–808.

Rogers LQ, Lutcher CL. Streptokinase therapy for deep vein thrombosis: a comprehensive review of the English literature. Am J Med 1990; 88:389–395.

Strandness, DE, Langlois Y, Cramer M, et al. Long-term sequelae of acute venous thrombosis. JAMA 1983; 250:1289–1292.

Tabernero MD, Estellés A, Vicente V, et al. Incidence of increased plasminogen activator inhibitor in patients with deep venous thrombosis and/or pulmonary embolism. Thromb Res 1989; 56: 565–570.

Vikydal R, Korninger C, Kyrle PA, et al. The prevalence of hereditary antithrombin-III deficiency in patients with a history of venous thromboembolism. Thromb Haemost 1985; 54:744–745.

Weitz JI, Hudoba M, Massel D, et al. Clot-bound thrombin is protected from inhibition by heparin–antithrombin but is susceptible to inactivation by antithrombin III–independent inhibitors. J Clin Invest 1990; 86:385–391.

VENOUS THROMBOSIS IN OTHER CIRCULATIONS

JOHN A. HEIT, M.D.

Although infrequent, thrombosis involving venous circulations other than the lower limb can be devastating. The introduction of new imaging techniques has expanded the clinical spectrum of these syndromes and changed our concepts regarding their pathophysiology. Many of these syndromes previously described as "idiopathic" are now recognized as an imbalance in hemostasis promoting abnormal thrombosis (thrombophilia). However, our knowledge regarding their natural history remains incomplete. Furthermore, there are virtually no randomized clinical trials regarding treatment, making rational management recommendations tenuous at best.

SUBCLAVIAN/AXILLARY VEIN THROMBOSIS

The incidence of subclavian/axillary vein thrombosis is increasing owing to the use of large-bore multilumen intravenous catheters. These thromboses are frequently asymptomatic but may be associated with clinically significant pulmonary embolism. Other secondary causes include trauma, compression due to tumor or other soft tissue mass, thrombophilia (polycythemia vera, thrombocythemia, or in association with neoplasm), and conditions causing stasis or elevated venous pressure of the upper extremity (right heart failure). Primary or "effort" thrombosis (Paget-Schroetter syndrome) represents a unique entity affecting healthy young patients with a recent history of upper extremity exertion. In these patients, venographic studies usually demonstrate compression of the subclavian vein by musculoskeletal structures of the thoracic inlet during upper extremity hyperabduction (clavicle, subclavius muscle, and costocoracoid ligament anteriorly and the first rib posteriorly). Up to 80 percent of patients may have a history of intermittent venous compression causing chronic vessel wall injury and stricture. Often this anatomic predisposition is bilateral and associated with bilateral thromboses or other symptoms of the thoracic outlet syndrome.

Common symptoms of subclavian/axillary vein thrombosis include upper extremity heaviness, fatigue, swelling, and pain. The edema is nonpitting and associated with cyanosis; prominent superficial veins over the arm, shoulder, or anterior chest; and occasionally a palpable cord. Shoulder motion may be limited and patients may complain of arm paresthesias. Upper extremity venous hypertension is manifested by failure of distended superficial arm veins to collapse with arm elevation. Arm edema usually resolves within 2 days to 3 weeks, although upper extremity exercise may exacerbate these symptoms. Collateral veins become apparent with resolution of the acute swelling.

Older noninvasive diagnostic tests such as phleborrheography and Doppler ultrasound flow studies are inaccurate for initial diagnosis but may be useful for serial monitoring during acute therapy. Duplex ultrasonography allows direct imaging from the basilic vein proximally to the distal innominate vein. Thrombosis is indicated by absence of a Doppler signal within the vein lumen, inability to compress the lumen with gentle pressure, or luminal narrowing by nonocclusive thrombus. The superior vena cava and proximal innominate vein cannot be imaged with this technique. In addition, the clavicle may obscure a short segment of the subclavian vein. Concomitant computed tomography (CT) or magnetic resonance imaging (MRI) provides complementary noninvasive information. However, accurate anatomic detail for either thrombolytic therapy or surgical intervention requires venography (Fig. 1), often with simultaneous bilateral arm injections to visualize the superior vena cava. Venographic evaluation may be especially important in planning appropriate management for "effort" thrombosis.

Conservative management with arm elevation and local heat rarely leads to vein recanalization; the vast majority proceed to thrombus organization with formation of extensive venous collaterals. Acutely, arm viability is seldom in question. Therefore, treatment is directed toward prevention of associated complications: acute pulmonary embolism and chronic postphlebitic syndrome. On the basis of a reported pulmonary embolism incidence of 12 to 36 percent, most authors recommend acute heparin anticoagulation followed by oral anticoagulation for 3 months. Acute anticoagulation does not promote vein recanalization. However, most patients develop adequate venous collaterals and remain asymptomatic or develop minor arm symptoms with exercise. Patients with an intravenous catheter–associated thrombosis do well with anticoagulation and removal of the indwelling catheter. Percutaneous transluminal balloon venoplasty has relieved chronic axillary/subclavian vein stenosis associated with permanent transvenous pacemaker electrodes and the high-flow state associated with hemodialysis access fistulas. However, recurrent stenosis may require repeated dilations.

Patients with "effort" thrombosis have a higher incidence of residual symptoms and recurrent thrombosis. Aggressive therapeutic intervention may have a role to play in this patient group. Acute surgical thrombectomy is uniformly unsuccessful owing to recurrent thrombosis. Although there are no randomized trials, several case series have reported successful vein recanalization with thrombolytic therapy given either

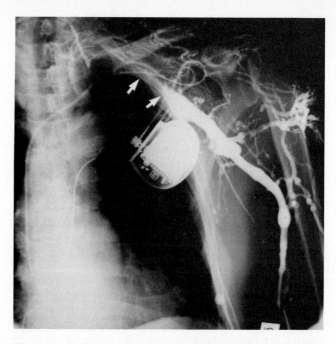

Figure 1 Left upper extremity venogram. A 75-year-old man with left subclavian vein thrombosis due to transvenous pacemaker leads 11 years after pacemaker placement.

systemically or via local infusion. Insufficient data exist to recommend a specific thrombolytic agent, dosing regimen, or mode of delivery. Local low-dose infusion may cause a systemic lytic state and is unlikely to be associated with fewer hemorrhagic complications. Venography immediately after thrombolysis frequently demonstrates underlying vein stenosis. Attempts at immediate balloon venoplasty have usually been unsuccessful; systemic heparin anticoagulation followed by oral anticoagulation for 3 months is preferable. Despite efforts at acute restoration of vein patency, up to 70 percent of patients with "effort" thrombosis continue to develop symptoms with minimal arm exertion. Surgical decompression with first rib resection, partial clavicle resection, patch or balloon venoplasty, or a combination thereof may offer further symptomatic improvement.

SUPERIOR VENA CAVA THROMBOSIS

Malignancy is the most common cause of the superior vena cava syndrome, but up to 20 percent have benign causes, especially thrombosis associated with intravenous catheters. Seven percent of patients with chronic indwelling catheters placed for hyperalimentation develop caval thrombosis. Hickman or Broviac catheters placed for chemotherapy may have associated thrombosis in an even higher proportion. In a prospective study of catheters placed via the internal jugular vein for hemodynamic monitoring, 66 percent of patients developed asymptomatic jugular vein thrombosis. These clots may propagate to the superior vena cava, especially in patients with prolonged low-flow states, and eventually embolize to the pulmonary arteries. Up to 38 percent of malignant superior vena cava obstruction may have associated caval thrombosis. Less commonly, transvenous pacemaker electrodes may be associated with superior vena cava thrombosis, especially in patients requiring multiple pacing interventions or who have infected pacemaker leads.

The hallmarks of superior vena cava thrombosis include facial swelling and cyanosis, dyspnea, and prominant superficial veins of the face, neck, and arms. With rapid onset, symptoms of cerebral edema may rarely occur (headache, visual disturbance, altered consciousness). In patients with known malignancy, these symptoms have been considered sufficiently characteristic to prompt initiation of treatment (usually radiotherapy) without further investigation. This practice originated from the belief that acute superior vena cava obstruction represents a rapidly fatal emergency in the absence of urgent intervention. However, an extensive review of reported cases suggests that the superior vena cava syndrome is seldom fatal. Mortality correlates best with the underlying etiology, especially the tumor cell type in cases due to malignancy. Clinical improvement occurs despite persistent caval obstruction, probably because of the development of venous collateral circulation. Therefore, therapeutic intervention can be safely delayed while appropriate diagnostic testing is made.

CT after intravenous contrast injection readily identifies the mediastinal structures contiguous with the superior vena cava. Compared with venography and bilateral simultaneous arm injections (Fig. 2), CT was superior in visualizing mediastinal vessels and central collaterals. Venography better demonstrated extension of thrombi peripherally into the jugular, basilic, or cephalic veins, and determined the degree of superior vena cava obstruction. Venography appears to be safe despite venous hypertension. In general, MRI currently offers little advantage over CT, with the possible exception of improved discrimination between recurrent tumor and radiation fibrosis.

Patients with intravenous catheter–associated superior vena cava thrombosis improve with systemic anticoagulation and catheter removal. For other causes of caval thrombosis, it is unclear whether anticoagulation contributes significantly to restoration or maintenance of caval patency. However, the risk of pulmonary embolism is sufficient for systemic anticoagulation to be recommended in the absence of other contraindications. There are several reports of pulmonary embolism in association with superior vena cava obstruction from malignancy. Although no concomitant studies of the lower extremity venous system have been reported, these emboli may arise from asymptomatic leg or pelvic deep vein thrombosis, a common complication in patients with malignancy.

Approximately 50 percent of patients with permanent transvenous pacemaker–associated caval thrombosis treated with anticoagulants improve and remain

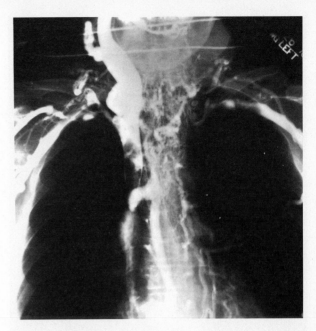

Figure 2 Bilateral simultaneous upper extremity venogram. A 66-year-old woman with thrombosis of the superior vena cava and innominate veins due to extrinsic compression from chronic fibrosing mediastinitis and a thoracic aortic aneurysm. There are extensive mediastinal and neck collaterals with filling of the inferior vena cava via retrograde flow through the azygous and hemiazygous veins.

relatively asymptomatic. Despite improvement, post-treatment venography seldom shows caval recanalization. Unless there is infection, removal of pacemaker leads is usually unnecessary. There are several case reports of clinical improvement after thrombolytic therapy, but the risk of intracerebral hemorrhage may be increased owing to venous hypertension. Patients remaining symptomatic despite anticoagulation or thrombolytic therapy should be considered for percutaneous transluminal venoplasty or surgery. Composite spiral autologous saphenous vein graft anastomosis of the left innominate or jugular vein to the right atrial appendage has been employed successfully for patients with intractable symptoms of superior vena cava obstruction, usually those from benign causes.

HEPATIC VEIN THROMBOSIS

Hepatic vein thrombosis (Budd-Chiari syndrome) is a rare disorder causing obstruction of hepatic venous outflow (Fig. 3). In addition to thrombosis, obstruction may be caused by venous webs, tumor, or hepatic veno-occlusive disease. The obstructive process may be further characterized as involving either the small hepatic veins (veins not clearly seen on hepatic venography or ultrasonography), large hepatic veins (intrahepatic veins visible on hepatic venography), hepatic inferior vena cava, or suprahepatic inferior vena cava. Thrombotic obstruction affects primarily the large he-

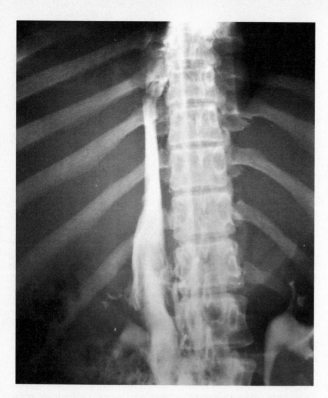

Figure 3 Hepatic vein venogram and inferior vena cavagram. A 20-year-old woman on oral contraceptives with hepatic vein thrombosis complicated by massive pulmonary embolism and cardiac arrest requiring emergency pulmonary embolectomy. There is marked caudate lobe hypertrophy causing compression and elevated pressure within the infrahepatic inferior vena cava.

patic veins and may extend to the inferior vena cava and small hepatic veins. Venous outflow from the caudate lobe of the liver may be spared owing to its separate venous drainage into the inferior vena cava. Hepatic caudate lobe hypertrophy often compresses the infrahepatic inferior vena cava, an important factor to note when planning surgical decompression. Nonthrombotic obstruction predominantly involves the inferior vena cava.

The pathologic picture of hepatic venous outflow obstruction consists of centrilobular congestion followed by cell atrophy and impaired hepatocyte regeneration. With chronic obstruction, fibrosis and cirrhosis eventually occur, although this process requires several months to evolve. After successful surgical decompression, the histologic picture may change rapidly with repopulation of areas of cell loss.

Hepatic vein thrombosis is most commonly seen in conditions known to cause thrombophilia, including polycythemia vera, paroxysmal nocturnal hemoglobinuria, thrombocythemia, oral contraceptive use, lupus-like anticoagulants, antithrombin III deficiency, pregnancy, and the puerperium. Hepatoma, adrenal and renal cell carcinoma, and trauma have also been noted as potential causes. However, in reported series, up to 30 percent of cases have no recognized etiology.

Most patients present clinically with acute right upper quadrant abdominal pain, hepatomegaly, and rapidly developing ascites. Splenomegaly occurs less frequently and jaundice is rare. Alternatively, the presentation may be an insidious wasting disease with slowly progressive ascites formation. Gastrointestinal bleeding and portosystemic encephalopathy are rare and represent late complications of advanced cirrhosis. Routine liver enzyme tests and blood chemistries are either normal or nondiagnostic.

Duplex ultrasonography has replaced the liver scan as the preferred initial diagnostic procedure. The large hepatic veins and inferior vena cava can be imaged for echogenic thrombus, and obstruction can be detected by Doppler. Compression of the infrahepatic inferior vena cava by caudate lobe hypertrophy is easily identified, and the status of the portal and splenic veins can be determined. Up to 30 percent of patients have inferior vena cava stenosis and 20 percent develop portal vein thrombosis. Duplex scanning also provides information regarding the direction of portal vein flow (hepatopetal versus hepatofugal). CT with contrast enhancement and MRI provide valuable information regarding the status of the retrohepatic inferior vena cava, an area not easily visualized by ultrasonography. However, infrahepatic inferior vena cava pressure measurements are necessary to plan appropriate surgical shunting procedures, and inferior vena cavography may be necessary to exclude webs or membranes.

Attempts at medical management with sodium restriction and diuretic therapy may improve symptoms due to ascites. However, thrombosed hepatic veins seldom recanalize, and the natural history is an inexorable progression to cirrhosis and death due to hepatic failure. Anticoagulant therapy is of no benefit. Peritoneovenous (LeVeen) shunting may improve control of ascites but will not alter the natural history. Although there are isolated case reports of successful thrombolytic therapy, too little information is available for any firm recommendations to be made.

Surgical shunting procedures decompress the hepatic venous outflow system by converting the portal vein to a venous outflow tract. As mentioned, successful shunts can provide dramatic improvement in liver histology and restore liver function to normal in the absence of cirrhosis. Therefore, periodic liver biopsy is imperative in the timing of surgical shunting. Portocaval shunts are preferable if the inferior vena cava is patent and the portal vein pressure exceeds that of the cava. Mesocaval shunts may be necessary when the portal vein is impossible to approach surgically owing to hepatomegaly. Stenosis of the inferior vena cava with caval pressures exceeding portal pressures dictates mesoatrial shunting for effective decompression. However, the risk of shunt thrombosis or kinking increases with the length and complexity of the shunt. Some authors have advocated a two-stage procedure for patients with inferior vena cava obstruction due to caudate lobe hypertrophy. An initial mesoatrial shunt provides hepatic venous decompression, which may resolve caudate lobe hypertrophy and relieve inferior vena cava compression. A subsequent mesocaval shunt can be performed when the inferior venal cava pressure is appropriately reduced. Liver transplantation should be considered when portal vein thrombosis precludes surgical shunting.

PORTAL VEIN THROMBOSIS

Portal vein thrombosis can be divided into two pathophysiologic entities depending on the presence or absence of pre-existent portal hypertension. Extrahepatic portal vein thrombosis associated with pre-existent portal hypertension primarily occurs in hepatic cirrhosis, affecting up to 10 percent of cirrhotic patients. Other causes of portal hypertension leading to portal vein thrombosis include conditions associated with elevated right heart pressure (constrictive pericarditis, right-sided heart failure, right atrial tumors), hepatic vein occlusion (Budd-Chiari syndrome, hepatic veno-occlusive disease), and portal vein compression (hepatoma, liver metastases, porta hepatis adenopathy, pancreatic carcinoma, pancreatitis/pancreatic pseudocyst).

Portal vein thrombosis in the absence of pre-existent portal hypertension occurs in conditions associated with pylephlebitis or thrombophilia syndromes. Umbilical sepsis during the neonatal period accounts for a substantial portion of childhood portal vein thrombosis. Intra-abdominal infection or septicemia may lead to pylephlebitis and thrombosis. Conditions commonly associated with thrombophilia and portal vein thrombosis include polycythemia vera, thrombocythemia, sickle cell anemia, paroxysmal nocturnal hemoglobinuria, and pregnancy. Splenectomy often leads to splenic vein thrombosis, which may propagate to involve the portal vein.

Acute massive portal vein thrombosis presents a catastrophic picture with severe abdominal pain and ascites. Portal vein clot propagation to the superior mesenteric vein with associated intestinal ischemia or infarction may account for some patients presenting in this fashion, but fortunately this presentation is rare. More commonly, portal vein thrombosis presents with the manifestations of chronic portal venous hypertension, usually bleeding esophageal or gastric varices. Other manifestations include splenomegaly (especially in children), hypersplenism, and mesenteric vein thrombosis. Portosystemic encephalopathy may occur in up to one-third of patients and is most commonly precipitated by hemorrhage, infection, or anesthesia. Ascites may occur at some time in 35 percent of patients.

The normal portal vein is readily imaged with real-time ultrasonography. In a series of normal patients, the portal vein could be seen in 97 percent of patients as it entered the porta hepatis. Therefore, failure to visualize the portal vein in the absence of technical limitations should encourage a further search for possible portal vein thrombosis. Other sonographic features include echogenic thrombus within the portal vein, portal vein collateral circulation, and enlargement of the thrombosed segment of vein. Venous collaterals may

appear as multiple wormlike vascular channels (cavernomatous transformation) in the region of the portal vein, a finding indicative of chronic thrombosis. Normal portal vein size and respiratory variation in caliber are strong supportive evidence of portal vein patency. Portal vein imaging by CT is limited by inability to scan in the vessel's axis. MRI is capable of providing views in multiple axes and provides complementary information to that obtained by ultrasonography.

Management recommendations for portal vein thrombosis depend on the clinical presentation and the presence or absence of associated hepatic parenchymal disease. Acute portal vein thrombosis is best managed with systemic anticoagulation and a search for associated mesenteric vein thrombosis and bowel ischemia. In most patients with acute portal vein thrombosis in the absence of mesenteric ischemia, symptoms are resolved by simple anticoagulation. In the absence of contraindications, thrombolytic therapy may be a viable option for patients who fail to improve despite anticoagulation.

Esophageal variceal bleeding in patients with portal vein thrombosis associated with cirrhosis is probably best managed with endoscopic variceal sclerotherapy. Gastric variceal bleeding is especially common in this group and may be difficult to manage with sclerotherapy. Portocaval shunting procedures in these patients are technically difficult owing to portal vein thrombosis.

Management of patients with variceal bleeding due to isolated portal vein thrombosis is controversial. Many of these patients are children who seem better able to tolerate bleeding episodes, possibly because their liver function is normal. In addition, there is a common perception that the frequency of bleeding episodes decreases as these patients grow older. Endoscopic variceal sclerotherapy may be a viable option for these patients. Splenectomy for hypersplenism is rarely indicated and should be avoided.

The reported incidence of portosystemic encephalopathy after central (portocaval, mesocaval, proximal splenorenal) shunting is variable. If surgical shunting is deemed necessary, distal splenorenal shunting may provide the best results, although extensive preoperative evaluation is necessary to ensure an appropriate anatomy and patency of the splenic and mesenteric veins.

MESENTERIC VEIN THROMBOSIS

Superior mesenteric vein thrombosis accounts for 15 percent of all cases of small bowel infarction. The incidence of superior mesenteric vein thrombosis may be much higher, since its clinical presentation is nonspecific and spontaneous recovery is possible. Because of extensive collateral circulation, less than 50 percent of superior mesenteric vein thromboses progress to bowel infarction. In this regard, mesenteric vein thrombosis is a more benign disease than mesenteric artery thrombosis. Inferior mesenteric vein thrombosis primarily affects the distal colon and rarely leads to infarction.

Idiopathic or primary superior mesenteric vein

thrombosis accounts for 25 to 50 percent of all cases of mesenteric vein thrombosis; up to one-third have a history of lower limb deep vein thrombosis. A significant percentage of these "idiopathic" cases represent manifestations of a thrombophilic state. Superior mesenteric vein thrombosis has been described in patients with reduced anti-thrombin III, protein C or S, and vascular plasminogen activator, and in women using oral contraceptives. Frequent secondary causes include portal hypertension, pylephlebitis, myeloproliferative disease, abdominal neoplasm (especially pancreatic and colon cancer), trauma, and postsplenectomy (with or without thrombocytosis). Often the thrombosis originates in the portal vein and spreads to the superior mesenteric vein.

Patients may be symptomatic for up to 3 weeks with vague abdominal discomfort that eventually progresses to colicky abdominal pain. Typically, patients continue to eat until late in their course when vomiting, abdominal distention, and rectal bleeding may occur. Abdominal pain is usually out of proportion to the physical findings. Hypotension, abdominal distention without tympany, and hemoconcentration may occur owing to fluid sequestration in the abdomen.

The plain abdominal x-ray view may be abnormal in 50 to 75 percent of cases. Classic findings include small bowel dilatation with separation of loops due to bowel-wall thickening, thumbprinting of the bowel wall due to mucosal hemorrhage, ascites, ileus, and air in the bowel and portal system late in the clinical course. Similar findings may be noted in barium studies of the small bowel. Selective superior mesenteric artery angiography with venous phase images has been the traditional definitive method of diagnosis. Typical findings include reflux of contrast medium into the aorta, mesenteric artery spasm, prolongation of the arterial phase, intense opacification of the thickened bowel wall, and failure to opacify the mesenteric venous-portal system. Duplex ultrasonography and CT after intravenous contrast injection have largely replaced angiography as initial diagnostic procedures. With ultrasonography, thrombosed portal, superior mesenteric, or splenic veins appear as dilated tubular structures filled with intraluminal echogenic material, and have an aberrant or absent Doppler flow signal. In addition, ultrasonography may demonstrate abnormal thickening of the bowel wall (more than 5 mm) and loss of peristalsis. Contrast-enhanced CT demonstrates a sharply defined vein wall with a rim of increased density and a central area of low attenuation. The sharply defined vascular wall is thought to represent contrast enhancement by vein wall vasa vasorum. In addition, ischemic segments of small bowel have persistent contrast enhancement.

Initial management includes volume replacement, nasogastric decompression, and systemic anticoagulation. The use of broad-spectrum antibiotics is of unproved benefit. Death is directly related to the presence of bowel infarction. Thrombi usually originate in the venous arcades and propagate to the arcuate channels. Hemorrhagic infarction occurs when the vasa recta and intramural vessels are occluded. Systemic anticoagulation aims to prevent thrombus propagation, and thereby bowel infarction. Any suspicion of bowel infarction should prompt emergent surgical exploration. At surgery, the intestine is thick-walled and full of blood. Thrombi extrude from the cut surface of mesenteric veins, and arteries are patent but in spasm. Most authors recommend early resection of affected small bowel and mesentery to include the entire thrombotic process. In early surgical series, recurrent thrombosis at the anastomotic margins occurred in up to 60 percent of patients, with associated anastomosis breakdown and mortality approaching 80 percent. This experience has prompted the use of wide surgical resection margins to include at least 10 cm of viable small bowel, and postoperative anticoagulation. Intraoperative examination of the bowel under a Wood's lamp immediately after intravenous fluorescein infusion may improve identification of nonviable bowel and guide the placement of resection margins. Because of the high rate of recurrent thrombosis and further bowel infarction, some authors have advocated an arbitrary "second look" abdominal exploration 24 hours after the initial surgical intervention. Using management recommendations as outlined, a more selective re-exploration policy seems reasonable, especially for patients with lack of a clear demarcation zone at the first operation, extensive small intestinal ischemia without evidence of necrosis, or questionable viability of resection margins. With these guidelines, current series suggest a mortality rate of 25 percent. Some authors have advocated surgical thrombectomy in the absence of bowel infarction. At present, there are insufficient data to recommend this procedure. Isolated case reports of successful restoration of mesenteric vein patency suggest that thrombolytic therapy might be considered in patients without evidence of bowel infarction.

RENAL VEIN THROMBOSIS

In recent years, it has become clear that renal vein thrombosis is a consequence rather than a cause of the nephrotic syndrome (Fig 4). The incidence of renal vein thrombosis in patients with nephrotic syndrome is approximately 20 percent. It is especially common in nephrosis due to membranous glomerulopathy, affecting up to 35 percent of patients. In addition to renal vein thrombosis, lower limb deep vein thrombosis occurs in 20 percent of nephrotic patients, with an associated 8 percent incidence of pulmonary embolism. Up to 50 percent of renal vein thrombi extend into the inferior vena cava, and in older case series pulmonary embolism was the most common cause of death. Arterial thromboses of the femoral, coronary, and mesenteric arteries have also been described. This epidemiologic evidence, together with a number of coagulation anomalies, strongly suggests a nephrosis-associated thrombophilia.

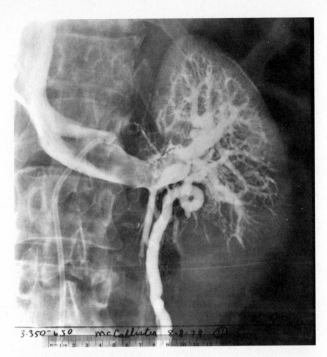

3-350-450   McCollister   8-8-79

Figure 4   Left renal venogram. A 70-year-old woman with left renal vein thrombosis due to nephrotic syndrome associated with chronic membranous glomerulopathy.

These anomalies include urinary loss of the physiologic anticoagulants antithrombin III and protein C and S; relative intravascular volume loss and hemoconcentration; elevated plasma levels of the procoagulant factors I (fibrinogen), V, and VIII; thrombocytosis with increased platelet aggregability; and possibly altered fibrinolysis.

In addition to membranous glomerulopathy, renal vein thrombosis occurs in nephrosis associated with membranoproliferative glomerulonephritis, lipoid nephrosis, focal sclerosis, rapidly progressive glomerulonephritis, amyloidosis, lupus nephritis, diabetic nephropathy, and renal sarcoidosis. Renal vein thrombosis may rarely occur in the absence of the nephrotic syndrome, such as with sickle cell anemia, trauma or surgery involving the retroperitoneum, acute pancreatitis, and syndromes associated with local compression (retroperitoneal fibrosis, abscess, or tumor).

In nephrotic patients, the clinical presentation of renal vein thrombosis is dependent on the rapidity of onset and the extent of renal vein obstruction. Nephrotic patients with acute renal vein thrombosis typically are younger and present with acute flank pain, flank tenderness to percussion, macroscopic hematuria, and deterioration of renal function. The affected kidney is acutely swollen owing to either complete renal vein obstruction or partial obstruction with inadequate collateral circulation. Chronic renal vein thrombosis commonly affects older nephrotic patients and usually is asymptomatic. In prospective studies of nephrotic patients, the presence or absence of chronic renal vein thrombosis had no effect on initial renal function,

24-hour urinary protein excretion, serum albumin, or serum cholesterol. Furthermore, blinded histologic interpretation of renal biopsy specimens failed to detect any of the common pathologic findings associated with acute renal vein thrombosis such as dilatation of peritubular blood vessels or interstitial edema and fibrosis. For unknown reasons, patients with chronic renal vein thrombosis either maintain adequate renal vein flow despite partial obstruction, or develop thrombotic obstruction at a rate or location that allows adequate collateral circulation. Asymptomatic renal vein thrombosis causing complete venous outflow obstruction is probably rare.

Several findings characteristic of acute renal vein thrombosis have been described on intravenous pyelography, including renal enlargement and pelvicaliceal irregularity due to interstitial edema and congestion. The nephrogram is reduced commensurate with renal function, a finding common to both acute and chronic renal vein thrombosis. Ureteral notching due to enlargement of the ureteral veins is most commonly seen in chronic renal vein thrombosis. However, the intravenous pyelogram in chronic renal vein thrombosis is usually normal. Previously, selective renal artery angiography with venous phase images and retrograde venography were required for diagnosis. In addition to intraluminal thrombus, this technique may demonstrate venous collaterals in a substantial percentage of patients with chronic renal vein thrombosis. Complications of retrograde venography include acute pulmonary embolism, inferior vena cava perforation, and contrast-induced acute renal failure. Digital subtraction venography avoids the risks of catheter-associated complications but still requires a substantial dye load with its attendant risk of contrast-induced nephropathy and anaphylaxis. These procedures are indicated in patients symptomatic with an acute renal vein thrombosis, but are unsuitable for screening of asymptomatic nephrotic patients at high risk for renal vein thrombosis. Currently, contrast-enhanced CT is the preferred diagnostic modality in such cases. MRI may offer similar accuracy without the need for contrast injection. Duplex ultrasonography can usually image an acutely thrombosed renal vein with absent flow. However, its accuracy is limited in chronic renal vein thrombosis by difficulty in imaging the affected veins and mistaken identification of a venous collateral as a patent renal vein.

Traditional treatment for acute renal vein thrombosis has consisted of rapid systemic heparin anticoagulation followed by prolonged oral anticoagulation. Available information indicates that such patients have a definite, albeit slow, improvement in renal function associated with at least partial renal vein recanalization or development of collateral circulation. Several case reports of successful thrombolytic therapy indicate that this form of therapy restores vein patency and improves renal function more rapidly than standard anticoagulation. Neither treatment affects the underlying glomerulopathy. Given the increased risk of hemorrhage, thrombolytic therapy should be reserved for symptomatic patients with acute renal vein thrombosis whose clinical course or renal function continues to deteriorate despite therapeutic heparin anticoagulation.

For chronic renal vein thrombosis, the goal of therapy is to prevent additional thrombotic complications. Oral anticoagulation for at least 1 year clearly reduces the incidence of subsequent thrombotic complications, including fatal pulmonary embolism. For patients whose nephrosis enters remission, the associated thrombophilia also resolves, negating the need for continued anticoagulation. The duration of anticoagulation for patients who remain nephrotic is not well defined, although one may reasonably continue anticoagulation as long as the patient remains nephrotic. Because of the high risk of fatal pulmonary embolism in asymptomatic nephrotic patients with renal vein thrombosis, it is reasonable to screen nephrotic patients at initial presentation and anticoagulate those found to have thrombosis. There is insufficient evidence to enable recommendations to be made regarding periodic screening of nephrotic patients not found to have renal vein thrombosis on presentation. Nephrotic patients at especially high risk of thrombosis (i.e., membranous or membranoproliferative glomerulopathy, particularly in the presence of any additional risk factor for venous thromboembolism) should be considered for prophylactic anticoagulation.

SUGGESTED READING

Adelstein DJ, Hines JD, Carter SG, Sacco D. Thromboembolic events in patients with malignant superior vena cava syndrome and the role of anticoagulation. Cancer 1988; 62:2258–2262.
Ahmann FR. A reassessment of the clinical implications of the superior vena cava syndrome. J Clin Oncol 1984; 2:961–969.
Clavien P-A, Durig M, Harder F. Venous mesenteric infarction: a particular entity. Br J Surg 1988; 75:252–255.
Donayre CE, White GH, Mehringer SM, Wilson SE. Pathogenesis determines late morbidity of axillosubclavian vein thrombosis. Am J Surg 1986; 152:179–184.
Harward TRS, Green D, Bergan JJ, et al. Mesenteric venous thrombosis. J Vasc Surg 1989; 2:328–333.
Kunkel JM, Machleder HI. Treatment of Paget-Schroetter syndrome: a staged, multidisciplinary approach. Arch Surg 1989; 124:1153–1158.
Laville M, Aguilera D, Maillet PJ, et al. The prognosis of renal vein thrombosis: a re-evaluation of 27 cases. Nephrol Dial Transplant 1988; 3:247–256.
Llach F. Hypercoagulability, renal vein thrombosis, and other thrombotic complications of nephrotic syndrome. Kidney Int 1985; 28:429–439.
Ludwig J, Hashimoto E, McGill DB, van Heerden JA. Classification of hepatic venous outflow obstruction: ambiguous terminology of the Budd-Chiari syndrome. Mayo Clin Proc 1990; 65:51–55.
Millikan WJ Jr, Henderson JM, Sewell CW, et al. Approach to the spectrum of Budd-Chiari syndrome: which patients require portal decompression? Am J Surg 1985; 149:167–175.
Warren WD, Millikan WJ Jr, Smith RB III, et al. Noncirrhotic portal vein thrombosis: physiology before and after shunts. Ann Surg 1980; 192:341–349.

PULMONARY EMBOLISM

JACK HIRSH, M.D.

Pulmonary embolism (PE), a long-recognized complication of hospitalized patients, is now being recognized in patients who present to the emergency departments of hospitals with nonspecific clinical manifestations. It has been estimated that PE is responsible for approximately 250,000 deaths per year in the United States. Most of these deaths occur in hospitalized patients in whom PE is the most common preventable cause of death. PE usually complicates the venous thrombosis that forms in proximal leg veins. Therefore, the treatment of venous thrombosis and PE are closely linked. PE may also originate from thrombi that form around central venous catheters, in the vena cava, in pelvic veins, or on the right side of the heart.

DIAGNOSIS

Despite an increasing awareness among physicians of the importance of PE, the reports of its high prevalence in medical publications, and the anxiety provoked by the medicolegal implications of its misdiagnosis, fewer than one-third of patients who die with clinically important PE are diagnosed before death. Fewer than 10 percent of patients over the age of 70 with fatal PE had the correct diagnosis established in life. The main reasons for the high frequency of missed diagnoses of clinically important PE are that its clinical manifestations are nonspecific, the diagnostic process can be difficult and complex, and physicians have been slow to accept results of studies demonstrating that some of the time-honored approaches to the diagnosis of PE are inaccurate.

Approach to Diagnosis

In most circumstances the diagnostic process can be approached in an orderly manner, although usually with some sense of urgency. The diagnosis of PE is suspected initially on clinical grounds. Although the clinical manifestations are nonspecific, the setting in which they occur and the associated clinical features allow the clinician to classify patients as "highly likely," "possible," or "unlikely" on clinical grounds. With this approach, patients classified as "highly likely" for PE on clinical grounds have a 60 to 70 percent probability of having PE diagnosed by pulmonary angiography, and those classified as "unlikely" have an 85 percent probability of not having PE. Those classified as "possible" on clinical grounds have a 50 percent probability of having PE. The classification of patients into "highly likely" (high previous probability) and "unlikely" (low previous probability) influences decision making in the subsequent diagnostic work-up.

A diagnosis of PE is considered highly likely on clinical grounds if the clinical features are compatible with such a diagnosis, the patient has one or a number of risk factors, and there are no other obvious causes for the clinical manifestations. The main risk factors for PE are recent trauma or surgery to the leg or pelvis; recent major general surgery; recent bed rest for a medical illness; malignancy (especially if treated with chemotherapy); recent or previous proved venous thrombosis or PE; chronic heart failure; leg paralysis; congenital deficiencies of antithrombin III, protein C, or protein S; anticardiolipin antibody; and the presence of a central line catheter. Patients with PE frequently have a history over the past 6 months of admission to the hospital for a major medical or surgical illness, or a history of enforced bed rest, chronic illness, or leg trauma.

A diagnosis of PE would be considered unlikely on clinical grounds if there is an obvious alternative explanation for the clinical manifestations, if the latter are highly atypical, and if the patient has none of the recognized risk factors for venous thromboembolism. For example, chest pain or dyspnea in association with features of a viral illness or pneumonia provide an obvious alternative explanation for the respiratory symptoms. Transient, sharp chest pain lasting for seconds or 1 to 2 minutes, chronic dull chest pain, sighing respirations, and episodic difficulty in taking a breath are atypical features of PE and are most unlikely to be caused by acute PE. In a recent report 10 to 41 percent of patients were considered on clinical grounds to be likely for PE, 14 to 26 percent unlikely, and the remaining 44 to 64 percent possible.

The likelihood that PE is present in symptomatic patients is increased by demonstration of deep vein thrombosis on objective testing. Approximately 70 percent of patients with angiographically proved PE have deep vein thrombosis at venography, and 50 to 60 percent have a positive impedance plethysmograph (IPG) or B-mode imaging test. Patients with negative findings on venography but with PE shown by angiography may have had their source of embolism in the deep pelvic veins, renal veins, inferior vena cava, or right atrium. Alternatively, the pulmonary emboli may have been derived from the deep veins in the legs, which

embolized in toto, leaving no residual thrombi. Thus, although a positive venogram, B-mode imaging test, or IPG can be used to make a therapeutic decision, a negative result for venous thrombosis cannot be used to exclude venous thromboembolism.

Diagnostic Accuracy Using Clinical Probabilities and Simple Diagnostic Tests in Combination with Ventilation-Perfusion Lung Scanning

Reliable information from two large prospective studies provides the clinician with practical guidelines for the diagnosis of PE. Participating clinicians were asked to rate their clinical suspicion of PE into three categories: "highly likely," "uncertain (probable)," and "unlikely." These previous probabilities were based on clinical findings (history and physical examination), chest x-ray, electrocardiogram (ECG), and either IPG (in one study) or blood gases (in the second study). As assessed by comparison with pulmonary angiography, these clinical probabilities provided clinically useful estimates (see below) for patients in the "highly likely" and "unlikely categories" (Table 1).

The perfusion and ventilation scans were interpreted independently of knowledge of the clinical previous probabilities and results of pulmonary angiography. The lung scans were classified as "high probability" or "non–high probability" in one study and as "high probability," "intermediate probability," "low probability," or "normal or near-normal" in the other study. The predictive values of the different combinations of categories of clinical suspicion and lung scan probabilities were assessed by comparison with pulmonary angiography (Table 2). In both studies the combination of a high clinical suspicion and a high probability scan was highly predictive of PE (96 percent). Similarly, the

Table 1 Comparison of Clinical Estimates of Pulmonary Embolism with Diagnosis by Pulmonary Angiography

Hull et al 1985 (175 Patients)		
Clinical Estimates of PE*	*No. in Category*	*PE by Angiography*
Highly likely (>85%)	76 (42%)	60 (79%)
Possible (10–85%)	81 (44%)	31 (38%)
Unlikely (<10%)	26 (14%)	4 (15%)

PIOPED 1990 (887 Patients)		
Clinical estimates of PE†	*No. in Category*	*PE by Angiography*
Highly likely (80–100%)	90 (10%)	61 (68%)
Uncertain (20–79%)	569 (64%)	–
Unlikely (0–20%)	228 (26%)	21 (9%)

*Clinical estimates based on clinical impression plus ECG, chest x-ray, and IPG.

†Clinical estimates based on clinical impression plus ECG, chest x-ray, and blood gases.

Table 2 Diagnostic Approach Based on Combination of Clinical Impression and Lung Scan Findings

Clinical suspicion	High	Uncertain	Low	Low	High	Low or uncertain	Uncertain
Lung scan	High	High	Low	High	Intermediate or low	Intermediate	Low
Management	Diagnosis of PE		PE excluded*	Pulmonary angiogram		Pulmonary angiogram or serial testing for DVT for 10–14 days‡	
Likelihood of PE*	96%	80–88%	2–6%	53–56%		10–50%†	
Frequency of combination		12–32%	9–17%			59–71%	

*Data from Hull RD et al. Ann Intern Med 1983; 98:891 and PIOPED Study. JAMA 1990; 263:2753.
†Estimated likelihood
‡Serial testing for DVT for 10–14 days would reduce risk of false–negative result.

combination of a low clinical suspicion and a low (or non–high probability scan) was associated with a low frequency of PE (2 to 6 percent). When the clinical suspicion was intermediate and the lung scan pattern "high probability," the frequency of PE was between 80 and 88 percent. All other combinations of categories of clinical suspicion and lung scanning were associated with frequencies of PE that were either too low to rule in or too high to rule out PE. It is interesting that a high probability scan in combination with low clinical suspicion was associated with PE in only 53 and 56 percent of patients, respectively, in the two studies. It should be noted, however, that only a few patients (less than 2 percent) had this combination of findings. On the basis of these observations, and provided that an error rate of 12 to 20 percent for false-positive diagnosis and an error rate of 2 to 6 percent for false-negative diagnosis are accepted, clinical suspicion and lung scan findings can be used to rule in or rule out PE without further testing in between 29 and 41 percent of patients. The rate for false-positive diagnoses can be reduced to less than 5 percent if a diagnosis of PE is accepted only when a high clinical suspicion is combined with a high probability scan. The rate for false-negative diagnoses can be reduced further by performing tests to exclude venous thrombosis (both at presentation and follow-up) and by making a diagnosis of venous thromboembolism if the test for venous thrombosis is positive.

Practical Approach to Diagnosis

A diagnostic algorithm for the management of clinically suspected PE is shown in Figure 1. If a diagnosis of PE is considered possible after history taking and physical examination, ECG, and chest x-ray, all patients should undergo perfusion lung scanning. For practical purposes, the finding of a negative perfusion scan rules out clinically significant PE.

If the perfusion scan results are abnormal, a ventilation scan should be performed. Testing for venous thrombosis with IPG, B-mode imaging, or venography can also be performed, since if tests for deep vein thrombosis are abnormal, the likelihood of PE is very high and in most circumstances the patient can be treated for venous thromboembolism. If these tests for venous thrombosis are negative, subsequent manage-

ment decisions are based on the combination of clinical suspicion and the ventilation-perfusion scan patterns.

An approach to the diagnosis of PE in patients with an abnormal perfusion scan (and negative tests for venous thrombosis) is presented in Figure 2. Patients who have a high probability scan with high or uncertain (possible) clinical probabilities can usually be treated for PE. The exception may be patients with uncertain clinical probabilities and a lung scan that shows a single unmatched segmental defect (classified as "high probability" in one study but not in the other). In the latter circumstance the likelihood of PE is only 80 percent, so a decision could be made to perform pulmonary angiography. Less than 35 percent of patients with abnormal perfusion scan results fall into the category of a greater than 90 percent probability of PE based on clinical features and lung scanning.

In patients who have a low probability scan pattern (particularly subsegmental perfusion defects), with a low clinical probability, the diagnosis of PE can usually be excluded. However, if the perfusion defect is large (a matched segmental defect or an indeterminate scan), pulmonary angiography should be performed. It should also be performed in patients with high probability lung scans who are in the "unlikely" category, because their risk of PE is approximately 50 percent. Similarly, pulmonary angiography should be performed in patients with high clinical probabilities and either low or indeterminate lung scan patterns, and in those with low or uncertain clinical probabilities and an intermediate lung scan pattern, since in these individuals the risk of PE is likely to be up to 50 percent.

There is preliminary evidence that it is safe to follow certain patients who have non–high probability scans by screening for 14 days with noninvasive tests sensitive to proximal vein thrombosis. In patients with low or uncertain clinical probabilities, serial testing with IPG or B-mode imaging could be used to replace pulmonary angiography if they (1) are clinically stable, (2) do not have proximal vein thrombosis at presentation, and (3) have relatively small perfusion defects.

TREATMENT

The objectives of treating patients with PE are to prevent death from either the initial or recurrent PE, to

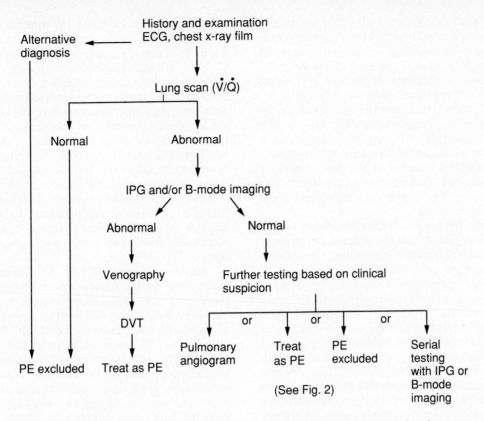

Figure 1 Diagnostic approach to the management of clinically suspected pulmonary embolism.

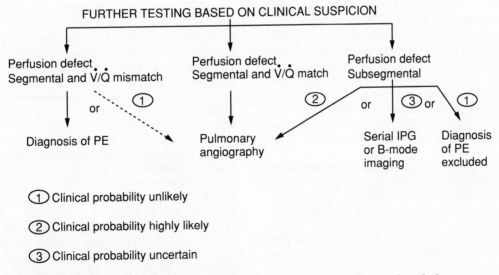

Figure 2 Diagnosis of pulmonary embolism in patients with an abnormal perfusion scan.

prevent recurrent PE arising from the associated venous thrombosis, to reduce morbidity from the acute event, and to prevent thromboembolic pulmonary hypertension.

Untreated, patients with PE have a mortality rate of more than 25 percent, which can be reduced markedly by appropriate treatment. The therapeutic approaches available for patients with PE are anticoagulants, thrombolytic agents, vena caval interruption, and pulmonary embolectomy. Anticoagulants prevent the growth of the associated venous thrombosis, and by so doing prevent recurrent PE; they also prevent thrombotic extension of the existing PE. Anticoagulants also are effective in preventing death and recurrent embolism in patients with PE. The mortality rate in patients with PE who are treated with heparin in adequate doses, and who are hemodynamically stable at the time of presentation, is less than 5 percent. However, the mortality rate is approximately 20 percent in patients who have persistent hypotension due to major PE.

Vena caval interruption prevents recurrent PE by intercepting emboli that arise in the deep veins of the legs or pelvis. Vena caval interruption, usually with a Greenfield filter, is indicated when anticoagulant therapy is contraindicated because of the risk of serious hemorrhage, and in the small percentage of patients who experience recurrent PE despite an adequate anticoagulant dosage and response.

Thrombolytic therapy accelerates the dissolution of pulmonary emboli, and so has the potential to prevent death in the hemodynamically compromised patient who would otherwise have not survived the many hours or days required for spontaneous thrombolysis. Thrombolytic therapy with streptokinase, urokinase, or tissue plasminogen activator (tPA) is more effective than heparin alone in correcting the angiographic or perfusion scan defects produced by pulmonary emboli, and may be more effective than heparin in preventing death in patients with shock due to massive PE. Thrombolytic therapy is recommended for hemodynamically compromised patients with massive PE or for patients who have submassive embolism with underlying cardiac or pulmonary disease in whom even a small or moderate-sized embolus may be life-threatening.

Surgical removal of the embolus by pulmonary embolectomy has the potential to rapidly restore the obstructed pulmonary circulation, but this procedure requires open heart surgery, carries considerable risk, and may be difficult to organize on an emergency basis. For these reasons, urgent pulmonary embolectomy is usually restricted to patients with a saddle embolism lodged in the main pulmonary artery, or patients with massive embolism whose blood pressure cannot be maintained despite thrombolytic therapy and vasopressor agents. An algorithm for treating acute PE is shown in Figure 3.

Pulmonary thromboendarterectomy has been shown to relieve chronic thromboembolic obstruction in patients with thromboembolic pulmonary hypertension who have proximal pulmonary arterial obstruction. In recent years, this procedure has been performed in over 200 patients and has been highly effective in carefully selected patients with chronic thromboembolic pulmonary hypertension.

Anticoagulation Therapy

Anticoagulant therapy with heparin followed by warfarin (Coumadin) for 3 to 6 months is the mainstay of treatment for most patients with PE. Most information on the effectiveness of anticoagulants has come from clinical trials in patients with venous thrombosis, but the results of these studies are applicable to most patients with PE.

Heparin can be given by continuous intravenous infusion, intermittent intravenous injection, or subcutaneous injection. Heparin is equally safe and effective whether administered by continuous infusion or by high-dose subcutaneous injection. In one study, thrombosis recurrence was more common in the group treated with subcutaneous heparin, but the initial dose of subcutaneous heparin was subtherapeutic in most patients randomized to this group. When heparin is administered by the intravenous route, less bleeding occurs with continuous intravenous infusion than with intermittent intravenous injection. The incidence of clinically important recurrence is less than 5 percent and that of clinically important bleeding 5 to 10 percent when heparin is administered in adequate doses by either continuous intraveous infusion or subcutaneous injection.

Heparin has a half-life that varies considerably among individuals. After a single intravenous injection, there is an initial rapid disappearance due to a saturable clearance mechanism, followed by a more gradual linear clearance with a mean heparin half-life of approximately 60 minutes. Intravenous heparin has an immediate anticoagulant effect, and when it is administered as a single bolus this effect lasts for 3 to 5 hours, depending on the dose. High-dose subcutaneous heparin injections produce a measurable heparin effect in 1 to 2 hours, and peak heparin levels are usually obtained at approximately 3 hours; the effect of subcutaneous heparin injections may last for 12 hours or more, depending on the dose.

The anticoagulant response to heparin varies considerably from patient to patient. Therefore, in order to achieve an adequate effect, the amount of heparin administered must be monitored by an appropriate laboratory test. Such tests include global tests of blood coagulation such as the activated clotting time and the activated partial thromboplastin time (aPTT), and heparin assays that measure the interaction of heparin with either thrombin or activated factor X. The responsiveness of aPTT reagents to heparin varies from reagent to reagent, but for many reagents in present use the therapeutic range for the aPTT is a ratio of 1.5 to 2 times the mean laboratory control value. The mean dose of heparin administered by intravenous infusion that is required to produce a heparin effect in the therapeutic range is approximately 33,000 U per 24 hours. The mean dose is about 10 percent higher if heparin is administered by high-dose subcutaneous injection. There is good evidence that the risk of recurrent thromboembolism is influenced by the patient's anticoagulant response, and that clinically important recurrence is less than 3 percent if the aPTT is maintained in the therapeutic range.

Patients treated with heparin by continuous intravenous infusion are given a bolus of 5,000 to 10,000 U followed by continuous infusion of 32,000 U per 24 hours. The aPTT test should be performed approximately 6 hours after the bolus injection, at which time the heparin response reflects the effect of the continuous

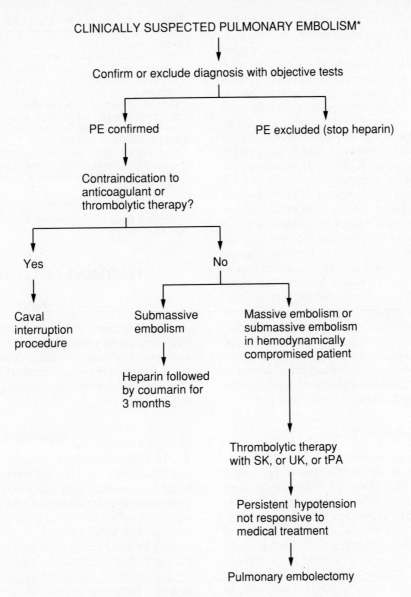

CLINICALLY SUSPECTED PULMONARY EMBOLISM*

Confirm or exclude diagnosis with objective tests

PE confirmed

PE excluded (stop heparin)

Contraindication to anticoagulant or thrombolytic therapy?

Yes

No

Caval interruption procedure

Submassive embolism

Massive embolism or submassive embolism in hemodynamically compromised patient

Heparin followed by coumarin for 3 months

Thrombolytic therapy with SK, or UK, or tPA

Persistent hypotension not responsive to medical treatment

Pulmonary embolectomy

Figure 3   Treatment of acute pulmonary embolism.

intravenous infusion. The test used to monitor heparin therapy should then be repeated once more in the first 24 hours, and then twice daily until an appropriate heparin dose is determined; thereafter, it can be performed once daily.

If heparin is administered by subcutaneous injection, it should be given twice daily and the dose adjusted according to the result of the monitoring test, which is performed 6 hours after each injection. The dose should be adjusted to produce a heparin response in the middle of a therapeutic range 6 hours after each injection. Monitoring should be performed twice daily until the appropriate dose is determined, and then once daily.

It has been common practice to administer heparin for 7 to 10 days, to start oral anticoagulants after 4 to 5 days, and to overlap heparin with oral anticoagulants for 4 to 5 days. This approach has recently been challenged by two studies (one in patients with venous thrombosis and submassive PE and the other in patients with proximal vein thrombosis), which demonstrated that a regimen of 9 to 10 days of heparin with a 4-day warfarin overlap was not superior to one of 4 to 5 days of heparin with 4 days of overlapping warfarin. The rationale for a period of overlap between heparin treatment and oral anticoagulants is based on experimental studies demonstrating a delay before the antithrombotic effects of oral anticoagulants are expressed, and on the short circulating half-life of protein C, a natural vitamin K–dependent anticoagulant. This rapid reduction in protein C levels means that the early anticoagulant effect of warfarin is potentially counteracted by the prothrombotic effect of low levels of protein C. Thus, by overlapping heparin and warfarin for 4 days, the early prothrombotic state is neutralized by the anticoagulant effect of heparin.

Patients with proximal vein thrombosis and with PE require continuing anticoagulant therapy after hospital discharge to prevent recurrent episodes. There is good evidence that 3 months of treatment with either oral anticoagulants or adjusted-dose subcutaneous heparin is effective in preventing recurrent thromboembolism in patients with proximal vein thrombosis, and since most patients with PE have proximal vein thrombosis, it seems reasonable to treat them for at least 3 months. Oral anticoagulants are more convenient and less expensive than subcutaneous heparin. If oral anticoagulants are used, the dose should be adjusted to maintain the PT ratio of 1.3 to 1.5, using a North American Thromboplastin International Normalized Ratio (INR) of 2.0 to 3.0.

An alternative approach to oral anticoagulants is the use of adjusted-dose subcutaneous heparin on an outpatient basis. With this regimen, heparin is given twice daily with subcutaneous injection, and the dose is adjusted to maintain the PTT at 6 hours at the lower therapeutic range (PTT 1.5 times control, heparin level 0.2 U per ml). The heparin regimen is particularly convenient if there is difficulty in laboratory monitoring because of geographic inaccessibility, since the dose can be adjusted in the hospital and the patient sent home without further monitoring. Subcutaneous heparin is also the treatment of choice for pregnant patients who require out-of-hospital anticoagulant therapy.

Thrombolytic Therapy

Thrombolytic therapy with streptokinase, urokinase, and tPA has been shown to be effective in producing early lysis of acute PE. None of the studies using thrombolytic therapy have been large enough to be able to demonstrate clinically important differences in mortality rates when the thrombolytic agent was compared with heparin. Thrombolytic therapy should not be used for all patients with acute PE, because most recover uneventfully if treated with anticoagulants. However, on the basis of available evidence it would be reasonable to use thrombolytic therapy for patients in whom there are no contraindications if they have massive embolism or submassive embolism with evidence of circulatory collapse, syncope, or acute cor pulmonale. The dosage regimens for the three thrombolytic agents are shown in Table 3.

Thrombolytic therapy with streptokinase and urokinase is administered for 12 to 24 hours; thrombolytic therapy with tPA can be administered either in a dose of 40 mg over 10 minutes or in a dose of 80 to 100 mg over 2 hours. Thrombolytic therapy should be followed by heparin for 5 to 10 days and then oral anticoagulants for at least 3 months.

Bleeding occurs more frequently with thrombolytic therapy than with heparin. The risk of hemorrhage increases with the duration of thrombolytic infusion and usually occurs at a site of previous surgery or trauma. Intracranial hemorrhage occurs in approximately 1 percent of patients given thrombolytic therapy, about twice as often as with heparin treatment.

Table 3 Recommended Doses for Thrombolytic Therapy*

Streptokinase
The standard regimen for streptokinase therapy is 250,000 U as a loading dose over 20–30 min followed by a continuous infusion of 100,000 U/hr for 24 h
Urokinase
Different dosing schedules of urokinase have been used; one approach is to give 4,400 U/kg/h as a bolus followed by a continuous infusion of 4,400 U/kg/h for 12 h
Tissue plasminogen activator (tPA)
Experience with this agent in treatment of pulmonary embolism is limited—optimal dosage regimens are under investigation; one effective approach is 100 mg of tPA as a continuous infusion over 2h

*Heparin should be started without a bolus after the PTT falls below twice the control value.

TREATMENT OF COMPLICATIONS

Pain

Pleuritic chest pain can be severe in patients with PE. Pain can be controlled with regular analgesia, using acetaminophen with codeine given every 4 hours. Pain control improves patient comfort and improves oxygenation by facilitating deep breathing, thus reducing the risk of atelectasis.

Hypoxemia

Hypoxemia occurs commonly in patients with large pulmonary emboli. Hypoxic patients may become confused and agitated. Hypoxia also leads to an increase in pulmonary hypertension and may produce arrhythmias, especially when there is underlying cardiopulmonary disease. For these reasons, continuous oxygen therapy should be used for hypoxic patients with acute pulmonary emboli. Oxygen can be administered intranasally or by a facemask; the latter is more effective but less comfortable for the patient. Oxygen saturation should be measured regularly by ear or finger oximetry, and the role of oxygen delivery adjusted to ensure an arterial oxygen saturation of at least 90 percent.

Hypotension

Hypotension may occur with massive PE or in patients with submassive pulmonary emboli who have serious underlying cardiorespiratory disease. Patients should be treated with intravenous fluids initially to counteract hypovolemia. If rehydration does not improve the blood pressure, vasopressor agents are indicated. Emergency embolectomy should be considered only in patients who fail aggressive medical management, including thrombolytic therapy.

PREVENTION OF LATE EFFECTS

It is unknown whether thrombolytic therapy for acute pulmonary emboli prevents the development of thromboembolic pulmonary hypertension. In the randomized trials comparing heparin with either streptokinase or urokinase in patients with acute PE, follow-up serial lung scanning performed 2 weeks, 3 months, and 1 year after treatment demonstrated no apparent difference in the rate of lysis between heparin and thrombolytic agents after the first week of treatment. A subsequent study in a subgroup of these patients reported that pulmonary capillary blood volume and pulmonary diffusion lung capacity were significantly better at 2 weeks and at 1 year in patients treated with thrombolytic therapy than in those given heparin. A recent follow-up study of this same group suggests that patients given thrombolytic therapy performed at a higher functional level than those treated with heparin.

Most patients who survive the initial episode of acute PE make a full recovery, but a few develop thromboembolic pulmonary hypertension. The latter may be more common in patients with underlying chronic heart or lung disease or in patients who sustain recurrent PE, but in most instances pulmonary hypertension is insidious in onset and there are no obvious predisposing factors. When a diagnosis of thromboembolic pulmonary hypertension is made, long-term anticoagulant therapy should be instituted. Most patients show a steady deterioration once their mean pulmonary arterial pressure exceeds 30 mm Hg and will die unless the obstruction is relieved by surgical intervention.

There has been a renewed interest in performing pulmonary thromboendarterectomy in patients with chronic thromboembolic hypertension. Patient selection has been improved by the preoperative use of pulmonary artery angioscopy, and postoperative complications due to reperfusion noncardiac pulmonary edema have been markedly reduced by the use of high-dose preoperative corticosteroids. The results of pulmonary thromboendarterectomy in a fairly large series of patients with thromboembolic pulmonary hypertension have been encouraging, although potential candidates should be carefully screened to ensure that they have an operative lesion (e.g., that the obstruction is proximal), and even with improved perioperative care the mortality rate from the procedure is still high.

PRACTICAL CONSIDERATIONS: USE OF ANTICOAGULANTS (Table 4)

Commencing Heparin

The starting dose of heparin is 5,000 U as an intravenous bolus followed by 32,000 U over 24 hours by continuous intravenous infusion, or heparin, 5,000 U as an intravenous bolus followed by 20,000 U by subcutaneous administration every 12 hours. The starting dose should be lowered to an intravenous bolus of 3,000 U followed by 30,000 U every 24 hours in elderly patients or those at high risk for bleeding according to the nomogram (Table 5). PTT monitoring should be repeated daily.

Table 4 Guidelines for Use of Anticoagulants

1. Bolus dose of heparin	5,000 U IV
2. Initial maintenance dose of heparin	32,000 U IV per 24 h by continuous infusion or 20,000 U SC to be repeated after adjustment at 12 h

3. Adjust dose of heparin at 6 h according to nomogram; maintain aPTT at 1.5–2.0 times control
4. Repeat aPTT q6h until in therapeutic range and then daily (see Table 5)
5. Start warfarin 10 mg at 24–72 h and then at 5–10 mg on next day
6. Overlap heparin and warfarin for 4 days
7. Perform PT at 48 h and adjust warfarin dose to maintain INR at 2.0–3.0 (PT 1.3–1.5 times control)
8. Stop heparin after 5–7 days provided PT is in therapeutic range
9. Continue warfarin for 3 mo and monitor PT daily until in therapeutic range, then 3 times in first wk, then twice weekly for 2 wk or until dose response is stable, and then weekly

aPTT, activated partial thromboplastin time; INR, International Normalized Ratio.

Continuing Therapy

Administer warfarin at 5 to 10 mg daily, starting 24 hours after heparin is begun. Perform PT testing at 48 hours and then daily. Adjust the dose of warfarin to obtain an INR of 2.0 to 3.0 (PT ratio of 1.3 to 1.5 using thromboplastin with ISI of 2.0 to 2.4). Stop heparin after 5 to 7 days provided that the PT ratio is in the therapeutic range. Continue warfarin therapy for 3 months. The effect of warfarin should be monitored by the PT three times in the first week, then twice weekly for 2 weeks or until the dose response is stable, and then weekly.

RECURRENT VENOUS THROMBOEMBOLISM

During Anticoagulant Therapy

Recurrent venous thromboembolism during adequate anticoagulant therapy is uncommon. If recurrence is noted in patients whose anticoagulant effect is subtherapeutic, the dose of anticoagulant should be increased and the coagulation test (PTT or PT) monitored frequently. If there is recurrence in patients whose anticoagulant effect is therapeutic, either the anticoagulant dose should be increased or a caval filter inserted while the patients are maintained at a slightly higher therapeutic range. It is important to confirm the clinical suspicion of recurrence with appropriate objective tests before concluding that the new symptoms have been caused by recurrent venous thromboembolism. Some patients who develop recurrence during warfarin therapy at an INR of 2.0 to 3.0 (PT 1.3 to 1.5 times control) respond to a higher dose of warfarin (PT 1.5 to 2.0 times control; INR 3.0 to 4.5), while others respond only to subcutaneous heparin every 12 hours adjusted to maintain the PTT at 6 hours at 1.5 to 2.0 times control. Since long-term heparin therapy may be complicated by osteoporosis, any trial of heparin treatment should be

Table 5 Intravenous Heparin Dose-Titration Nomogram

Start dose		5,000 IV bolus then 32,000 U/24 h			
aPTT sec	Bolus dose	Stop infusion min	Rate change ml/h*	(U/24 h)	Repeat aPTT
<50	5,000 U	0	+3	(2,880)	6 h
50–59	0	0	+3	(2,880)	6 h
60–85	0	0	0	(0)	Next AM
86–95	0	0	−2	(1,920)	Next AM
96–120	0	30	−2	(1,920)	6 h
>120	0	60	−4	(3,840)	6 h

*1 ml/h = 40 U/h.

limited to 2 or 3 months, at which time warfarin treatment should be restarted. Patients who develop recurrent venous thromboembolism while being treated with anticoagulants should probably be given anticoagulants indefinitely unless a specific cause of recurrence can be identified and reversed.

When Anticoagulant Therapy is Stopped

Patients who develop recurrent venous thrombosis without provocation after a 3-month course of adequate anticoagulant therapy carry a high risk of further recurrence unless their recurrent episode is treated with long-term warfarin. My approach has been to treat the first recurrence with a 12-month course of anticoagulants, and subsequent recurrences with anticoagulants for an indefinite period.

SUGGESTED READING

Barritt DW, Jordon SC. Anticoagulant drugs in the treatment of pulmonary embolism: a controlled trial. Lancet 1960; 1:1309–1312.

Basu D, Gallus A, Hirsh J, Cade JF. A prospective study of the value of monitoring heparin treatment with the activated partial thromboplastin time. N Engl J Med 1972; 287:324–327.

de Swart CAM, Nijmeyer B, Roelofs JMM, Sixma JJ. Kinetics of intravenously administered heparin in normal humans. Blood 1982; 60:1251–1258.

Goldhaber SZ, Hennekens CH, Evans DA, et al. Factors associated with correct antemortem diagnosis of major pulmonary embolism. Am J Med 1982; 73:822–826.

Hull RD, Hirsh J, Carter CJ, et al. Diagnostic value of ventilation-perfusion lung scanning in patients with suspected pulmonary embolism. Chest 1985; 88:819–828.

Hull RD, Raskob GE, Carter CJ, et al. Pulmonary embolism in outpatients with pleuritic chest pain. Arch Intern Med 1988; 148:838–844.

Hull RD, Raskob GE, Rosenbloom D, et al. Heparin for 5 days as compared with 10 days in the initial treatment of proximal vein thrombosis. N Engl J Med 1990; 322:1260–1264.

Moser KM, Auger WR, Fedullo PF. Chronic major-vessel thromboembolic pulmonary hypertension. Circulation 1990; 81:1735–1743.

The PIOPED Investigators. Value of the ventilation/perfusion scan in acute pulmonary embolism: results of the prospective investigation of pulmonary embolism diagnosis (PIOPED). JAMA 1990; 263: 2753–2759.

VENOUS DISEASE: SURGICAL TREATMENT

MAGRUDER C. DONALDSON, M.D.

Chronic venous disorders are most frequently treated by surgeons, not because surgery is invariably indicated, but because surgeons have traditionally been heavily exposed through their training to patients with all forms of peripheral vascular disease. In fact, facility with recognition, early conservative management, and indications for surgical measures are important to all physicians.

DISORDERS OF THE SUPERFICIAL VEINS

Varicose veins are abnormally enlarged subcutaneous venous channels that involve the greater and lesser saphenous systems and their tributaries. An estimated 12 percent of the adult population harbor significant varicose veins for which symptomatic relief might be sought from time to time. In *primary* varicose veins, the problem originates within the superficial system, with no involvement of the deep subfascial veins. In the case of *secondary* varicose veins, superficial veins become enlarged as a result of disease that originates in the deep system and communicating veins. About 75 percent of patients who seek therapy have primary varicose veins and 25 percent have secondary veins. The greater saphenous system is involved about five times more often than is the lesser saphenous system.

Clinical Features

The most common complaint patients have concerning varicose veins is unsightly appearance of the legs. Most patients with involvement of a long segment of vein that extends across the knee or ankle joint also have some discomfort. The typical syndrome involves a dull ache or heavy sensation in the area of the vein, particularly after a period of standing, that is relieved when the leg is elevated. Superficial phlebitis may become an episodic problem. A small percentage of patients with extensive primary varicose veins develop eczema and ulceration at the ankle level. Finally, some varicose veins become extremely thin walled and superficial, so that trauma to the skin causes rupture of the vein with a startling amount of bleeding.

Simple examination of the legs allows visualization of most varicose veins, which are more easily seen over the calf and ankle than over the thigh. The dependent position with oblique lighting enhances visibility. Palpation is very helpful because ballottement of the enlarged veins can generally be done with the leg dependent. Percussion of a distal portion of a vein transmits a fluid wave proximally, proving continuity. When valvular competence is in question, percussion of a vein proximally transmits a strong fluid wave distally when the valves are not functional; the wave is dampened by a competent valve.

Primary and secondary varicose veins can be differentiated by a simplified Brodie-Trendelenberg test. The leg is raised and a tourniquet or compressing hand is placed above the knee to obstruct the flow of blood through the superficial veins. The leg is then lowered to a dependent position while watching for filling of the varicose veins over the calf and ankle. If the veins fill promptly, there must be reflux of blood through incompetent communicators from an incompetent deep venous system, thus rendering the varicose veins *secondary*. On the other hand, if prompt filling occurs only after the removal of the venous obstruction, the source of reflux is the superficial system and the varicose veins are *primary*. In some patients, both deep-communicator and superficial incompetence are identified by the Brodie-Trendelenberg test.

Laboratory study of varicose veins is rarely necessary to perform, but certain techniques may be helpful to supplement the physical examination when there is a question about the status of the deep venous system (Table 1). Most importantly, if significant deep vein obstruction is present superficial varicose veins may be acting as collateral channels and must not be removed. The presence of venous occlusions in the deep system can be determined with either the continuous wave Doppler probe or, preferably, duplex ultrasound examination to image the veins and to assess flow velocity.

Table 1 Laboratory Evaluation Before Vein Surgery

Varicose veins
    Venous ultrasound examination to confirm status of deep veins
        if varicose veins are suspected to be *secondary*

Deep venous insufficiency
    Venous ultrasound examination
    Ascending venography for obstruction or communicators
    Descending venography for proximal valvular reflux

Management

Conservative Measures (Table 2)

An important aspect in the management of varicose veins is patient education about the natural history of this disorder and the minor potential for major impact on the patients' health. A differentiation between venous disease and more ominous arterial disease and between superficial and deep venous disease should be made. With some understanding of the pathophysiologic mechanisms that lead to varicose veins, patients will be more likely to avoid activities such as prolonged standing, which might enhance progression of vein enlargement. Control of symptoms and the natural progression of varicose veins are improved by wearing proper elastic support hose. To be effective, stockings must fit firmly with diminishing compression as the garment ascends the leg to avoid a proximal constricting band. The most precise physiologic control is afforded by prescription stockings measured to fit properly, although many less expensive nonprescription brands are usually satisfactory. Compression at the ankle of 20 to 30 mm Hg is sufficient for most patients with primary varicose veins. A knee-length garment is adequate, although thigh-length or leotard style are usually preferred by women; special maternity brands are advisable during the last trimester of pregnancy.

Ablative Measures

Occasionally varicose veins cause discomfort to such a degree that they interfere with productive activity; at this point ablative therapy should be considered. Although cosmetic concerns alone are usually insufficient grounds for direct intervention, large venous systems can present a major impediment to normal social function.

Sclerotherapy has the major advantage of eliminating hospital costs because the procedure can be performed easily in an office setting. The principle of treatment is to inject a material into the varicose veins that induces inflammation and scarring sufficient to seal

Table 2 Conservative Measures for the Treatment of Chronic Venous Disease

Varicose veins
    Moderate elastic support (20–30 mm Hg)
    Slight changes in activity

Deep venous insufficiency
    Strong elastic support (30–40 mm Hg)
    Moderate changes in activity
    Skin protection

the lumen. After the involved veins are carefully mapped, a 25-gauge needle on a 3 cc syringe containing 1% sodium tetradecyl sulfate (Sotradecol) is inserted into the vein with the leg in the dependent position. The syringe is taped to the leg while two or three other veins are similarly punctured. The leg is then elevated to empty the veins and about 0.5 cc of the sclerosing agent is slowly injected into the vein at each site. Compression with a gauze pad and tape is provided over the vein as the needle is withdrawn. At the completion of the injections, with the leg still elevated, a firm elastic bandage is wrapped carefully from the foot to 6 inches above the most proximal injection site.

Patients are instructed to maintain necessary activities, to avoid prolonged sitting or standing, and to leave the bandage in place for several days. Some physicians recommend continuous compression for as long as 6 weeks but this inconvenience is probably unnecessary because similar results may be obtained with periods of as short as 8 hours. The patient returns to the office for removal of the bandages and inspection of the early results. Further injections can be performed at this visit, and the cycle repeated until all troublesome veins have been removed. The occluded veins are palpable as sclerotic cords and may be faintly visible after sclerosis.

Severe complications from sclerotherapy occur in about 0.1 percent of patients, with mild local reactions occurring in up to 10 percent. Occasionally, extravasation of the sclerosing agent from the injection site takes place, which can cause subcutaneous inflammation or even slough of a small disc of skin. Very rarely, a systemic reaction occurs as a result of the injection, although only small amounts of the drug should reach the systemic veins if small volumes are used. Extension of the sclerotic process to the deep veins also rarely occurs. There is minimal discomfort, but the need for prolonged compression and repeat visits to the office are relative inconveniences.

Early results for the first 1 to 3 years are generally excellent in over 80 percent of patients. In smaller superficial veins the recurrence rate at 5 years was 19 percent in a controlled study by Hobbs that compared sclerotherapy and surgery. The 5-year recurrence rate in the large main venous trunks was 69 percent, however, presumably because the causative valvular defect in the main saphenous or communicating vein continued to exist. Most investigators would agree that such large saphenous varicose veins are treated most effectively with surgery.

Surgical therapy is directed at ligating the varicose system at its origin and removing the varicose veins to prevent recanalization by collateral routes. The procedure requires the administration of at least a spinal or epidural anesthetic agent, but can usually be performed without overnight hospitalization. After the veins have been carefully mapped with an indelible marker, small incisions are placed at both ends of the involved vein — at the saphenofemoral junction and the medial malleolus in the case of the greater saphenous system. An internal stripper is advanced proximally from the distal end of the vein and secured at the saphenofemoral junction. The ends of the vein are ligated and divided, which leaves it flush with the common femoral vein. The vein is then pulled out downward toward the foot, because the incidence of traumatic saphenous neurologic abnormality is less than that when the vein is pulled upwards. Side branches and perforators are avulsed during this process, and hemorrhage is controlled by a few minutes of leg elevation and compression. Any significant residual branches can be stripped separately or simply ligated through a series of several small incisions. The leg is wrapped with an elastic bandage and elevated for 12 hours to minimize the risk for hemorrhage. Ambulation with elastic support stockings is encouraged the day following surgery.

There is some postoperative pain for a few days and ecchymosis and edema over the track of the vein, both of which resolve within 2 to 3 weeks. A return to many activities is possible within several days of surgery while using compression for comfort. Occasional hemorrhage, infection, and local neurologic disorder occur, but deep vein thrombosis and other significant morbidity are rare. With a thorough surgical approach to the treatment of saphenous varicose veins, at least 85 percent of patients remain free of recurrences at 5 years. Hobbs found a 12 percent incidence of recurrence at 5 years among patients treated surgically for large saphenous system veins. The 5-year recurrence rate of communicating veins and superficial small veins in the lower leg treated surgically was 56 percent, however, which suggests that these smaller veins are probably best treated by primary sclerotherapy. The optimal therapy for varicose veins combines both surgery and sclerotherapy, depending on the presenting pathology.

DISORDERS OF THE DEEP VEINS

The general term *venous insufficiency* refers to the physiologic consequence of either deep vein obstruction, valvular incompetence, or a combination of both lesions. The terms *postphlebitic* or *post-thrombotic* are commonly used to describe the pathologic and clinical features of venous insufficiency that result from deep vein thrombosis, a common cause of deep venous insufficiency. Within 5 years after the diagnosis of deep vein thrombosis, up to 80 percent of patients have signs, symptoms, or laboratory findings of venous insufficiency. The prevalence of severe venous insufficiency, including chronic eczema and ulceration, has been estimated at about 0.5 percent of the population.

Clinical Features

Symptoms of deep venous insufficiency consist of dull, bursting aching in the lower leg when in a dependent position, which is often associated after more prolonged periods with edema of the foot and ankle. These symptoms are relieved when the leg is elevated. Secondary superficial varicose veins may appear, usually over the medial aspect of the leg and ankle where communicating veins emerging from the deep system are most plentiful. Pain, itching, and dermatitis focus over these areas, and hyperpigmentation is often visible in the subcutaneous tissues. Weeping of serum or overt skin ulceration occur spontaneously with chronic conditions or after trivial injury. Subcutaneous inflammation becomes prominent, with varying degrees of cellulitis. If significant venous obstruction is present, symptoms may be relatively mild at rest when collateral channels more easily decompress the lower leg. Exercise will elicit the most important symptoms of obstruction, with intense pressure in the distal leg relieved after rest and elevation.

Physical examination may show the leg circumference to be increased, and cyanosis and plethora of the feet are often evident when the leg is in a dependent position. Secondary varicose veins are often present, and hyperpigmentation (hemosiderin deposition) is obvious in areas of healed skin ulcers and other sites of healed trauma or inflammation. Most of these lesions are distributed medially over the ankle and lower leg, with the majority being located just above the medial malleolus. Untreated ulcerations are edematous and porky, with copious drainage from the ulcer. There may be signs of surrounding cellulitis, occasionally ascending up the leg with lymphangitic involvement. Chronicity results in stiffening of the ankle joint and loss of proximal muscle bulk and strength.

Laboratory evaluation in patients with suspected deep vein disease is useful to document valvular insufficiency or chronic obstruction. It is particularly helpful to know if there is an element of venous obstruction (usually a result of fibrotic organization of old thrombus). Symptoms of venous insufficiency can mimic those of acute deep vein thrombosis and can be acutely exacerbated by warm weather and by having the leg maintained in a dependent position for a prolonged period. In this setting, pre-existing fibrotic lesions could be mistaken for fresh thrombus. In addition, any patient with venous insufficiency severe enough to warrant surgical intervention should be examined to understand the anatomic and physiologic disorder. Duplex ultrasound imaging is the mainstay of current laboratory investigation, showing blood flow and obstruction as well as actual valve structure in some instances. Plethysmography and ambulatory venous pressure studies are generally used only as research tools. Venography, on the other hand, should precede any venous reconstruction. Valvular reflux through incompetent communicating veins is evident on ascending venograms when the superficial system is visualized above the level of an occluding tourniquet. Properly performed ascending venography also accurately outlines occluded veins and often necessitates direct puncture of the femoral vein to demonstrate clearly the iliocaval system. Descending venography dramatically demonstrates valvular function, allowing dye to cascade down the leg after the fluoroscopy table has been tilted.

Management

Conservative Measures

Therapy for venous insufficiency is directed at countering the damaging effects of peripheral venous hypertension (see Table 2). The patient should be thoroughly educated as to the underlying problem and its pathophysiologic mechanisms; counseling as to beneficial changes in lifestyle is also important. Prolonged standing or sitting should be avoided because these positions promote stasis and sustained venous hypertension in the lower leg. Prescription graduated knee-length compression stockings (with 30 to 40 mm Hg pressure at the ankle) should be worn during the day. Exercise and habitual ambulatory activities are recommended as ways to enlarge and maintain venous collateral channels, provided adequate stocking support is used. Jogging or other types of exercise that involve forceful pounding of the legs on a hard surface should be substituted by gentler sports like bicycling or swimming. Moderate tipping of the bed into a head-down position promotes mobilization of edema and relief of muscle compartment tension at night.

When eczema and skin ulceration supervene, efforts to reduce venous hypertension must be increased and other measures must be directed at the skin itself. Enforced temporary bedrest combined with careful hygiene and gentle protective dressings of nonadherent gauze are the most important aspects to the control of eczema. If cellulitis or lymphangitis are suspected, antibiotic regimens should be directed initially against staphylococcal and streptococcal skin colonizers and modified later if culture samples yield a wider variety of

Table 3 Surgery for Deep Venous Insufficiency

Communicating vein incompetence
  Subfascial ligation of communicating veins

Deep vein valvular incompetence
  Direct valvuloplasty
  Saphenofemoral or profundafemoral transposition
  Segmental vein interposition

Deep vein obstruction
  Femorofemoral bypass
  Popliteal-femoral bypass

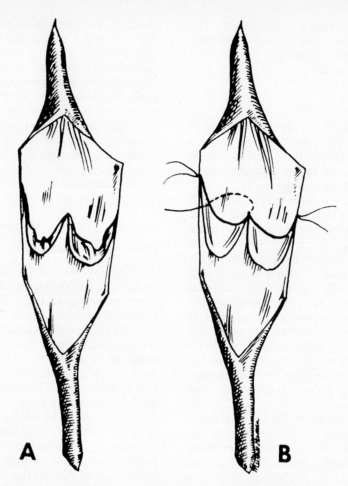

Figure 1 Valvuloplasty to repair floppy valve causing reflux. *A,* Vein opened through valve commissure during surgery, which shows redundant leaky valve leaflets. *B,* Fine sutures placed at valve corners to correct redundancy by reefing leaflets. (From Kistner RL. Transvenous repair of the incompetent femoral vein valve. In: Bergan JJ, Yao JST, eds. Venous problems. Chicago: Year Book, 1978:503; with permission.)

organisms. Open ulcers should be treated with a gentle debriding regimen of dressing changes two to four times a day using wet to dry normal saline or a dilute antibiotic solution (bacitracin, neomycin) on coarse mesh cloth gauze. Once the ulcer is clean and cellulitis appears to have been controlled, less frequent dressing changes combined with continued compression with stockings or Ace bandages are appropriate. Perhaps most practical and effective is Unna's paste boot, which is a mixture of zinc oxide, calamine, and gelatin that gently medicates the open ulcer. Essentially no care is required of the patient, with changes of the boot every 1 to 4 weeks. Because cellulitis may be exacerbated if the ulcer is infected, the boot should only be used on clean ulcers. Gradual healing frequently occurs under the boot even as the patient maintains most normal activities. If the ulcer is large or persistent, split-thickness skin grafts should be applied to ulcers after sufficient preparation.

Surgical Measures

Previous ulceration or a prolonged history of venous insufficiency will make durable success with conservative measures unlikely. In these instances surgical measures directed at the underlying causes of venous hypertension are indicated (Table 3).

The interruption of incompetent communicating veins reduces barotrauma to the subcutaneous tissues. Optimally, any ulcer should be either healed or small and free of cellulitis prior to surgery, and preoperative venography or duplex ultrasonography are helpful procedures for demonstration of communicator anatomy. Surgery should be directed at all communicating veins in the region of the ulcer, not only at the single vein that may appear to be at the base of the ulcer, because collateral channels connected to adjacent communicators from a severely diseased deep system predispose to

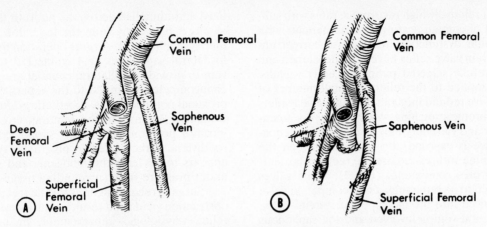

Figure 2 Vein transposition. *A,* Anatomy of proximal femoral region, with incompetent valves in superficial femoral vein. *B,* Restoration of superficial femoral competence by transposition below normal valve in saphenous vein. (From Queral LA, Whitehouse WM, Flinn WR, et al. Surgical correction of chronic deep venous insufficiency by valvular transposition. Surgery 1980; 87:688–695, St. Louis: CV Mosby Company; with permission.)

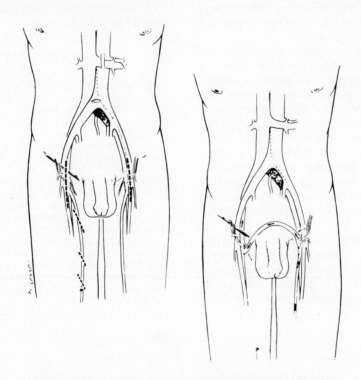

Figure 3 Palma-Dale cross-pubic bypass, using mobilized saphenous vein *(left)* to drain contralateral femoral system through a subcutaneous tunnel *(right)* to relieve symptoms from iliac vein obstruction. (From Bergan JJ, Yao JST, Flinn WR, et al. Surgical treatment of venous obstruction and insufficiency. J Vasc Surg 1986; 3:174–181, St. Louis: CV Mosby Company; with permission.)

recurrent ulceration. The most definitive surgery involves an incision from the ankle to the proximal calf, with subfascial ligation of all communicating veins. Although the reported ulcer recurrence at 5 years varies from 2 to 55 percent after subfascial ligation, results appear to be best when the extent of underlying deep venous disease is limited and when long-term postoperative use is made of support stockings. Slough of the skin edge, infection, deep vein thrombosis, hemorrhage, inadvertent nerve injury, and delayed contracture of the ankle joint all occur with varying degrees of combined morbidity (4 to 30 percent in published series).

Because of relatively high recurrence rates with subfascial ligation of communicating veins in patients with extensive valvular dysfunction, methods to correct underlying deep vein valve reflux have been developed and applied in carefully selected patients. Direct valvuloplasty can be applied to the relatively small number of patients who have redundancy and laxity of valve leaflets as a result of chronic stretching. After careful documentation of reflux and valve anatomy by descending venography, the valve is exposed and opened between the valve leaflets. Fine sutures are used to reef the lax leaflets, which restores competency (Fig. 1). When valves are too damaged to be reparable, a new competent valve may be juxtaposed into the incompetent system. If the superficial femoral vein is involved and the saphenous vein is normal, end-to-end transposition of the competent proximal saphenous vein into the distal femoral vein introduces a valve into the system (Fig. 2). Alternatively, the profunda femoris vein can be transposed into the superficial femoral vein. When no normal valve is available nearby, a segment of the axillary or brachial vein containing a competent valve may be transplanted into the femoral or popliteal vein.

All of these valvular reconstructive procedures are applicable only in patients who have been found by careful evaluation to have appropriate pathophysiologic features and a favorable anatomic situation. Experience is still limited, but it appears that about 80 percent of selected patients clinically improve for varying lengths of time after surgery. Evidence suggests that restoration of a single competent valve in an extensively diseased femoral vein may not be sufficient for the long-term control of venous ulceration, and it appears that subfascial communicator interruption may have the most important impact in patients with extensive valvular reflux.

Surgical bypass of venous occlusions is appropriate in selected instances. Most commonly, a cross-femoral bypass is used to relieve symptoms of iliac vein occlusion; this method is often used in patients with pelvic malignancy. The contralateral saphenous vein is mobilized and tunnelled across the pubis to the femoral vein to direct flow away from the leg below the obstructed iliac system (Fig. 3). A rarer operation makes use of the ipsilateral saphenous vein connected to the popliteal vein to provide a collateral channel around obstruction or incompetence limited to the superficial femoral and proximal popliteal veins. Prosthetic grafts are applicable from time to time in the femoral, cross-femoral, and iliocaval positions. Externally supported polytetrafluoroethylene is the preferred prosthetic agent because it appears to be least thrombogenic and resists collapse under pressure from surrounding tissues.

Surgical reconstructions for the treatment of venous obstruction yield good results when assessed by symptom relief, physiologic improvement, or bypass patency. Clinical improvement occurs in about 80 percent of patients at 1- to 3-year postoperative intervals. A period of anticoagulation with coumadin is recommended after surgery, although there are no data clearly indicating that bypass patency improves. Overall, surgical morbidity is acceptably low, particularly with regard to thromboembolic complications.

SUGGESTED READING

Bergan JJ, Yao JST, Flinn WR, McCarthy WJ. Surgical treatment of venous obstruction and insufficiency. J Vasc Surg 1986; 3:174–181.

Ferris EB, Kistner RL. Femoral vein reconstruction in the management of chronic venous insufficiency. Arch Surg 1982; 117: 1571–1579.

Hobbs JT. Surgery and sclerotherapy in the treatment of varicose veins: a random trial. Arch Surg 1974; 109:793–796.

Johnson WC, O'Hara ET, Corey C, et al. Venous stasis ulceration: effectiveness of subfascial ligation. Arch Surg 1985; 120:797–800.

Lofgren EP. Treatment of long saphenous varicosities and their recurrence: a long-term follow-up. In: Bergan JJ, Yao JST, eds. Surgery of the veins. New York: Grune & Stratton, 1985:285.

O'Donnell TF, Mackey WC, Shepard AD, Callow AD. Clinical, hemodynamic and anatomic follow-up of direct venous reconstruction. Arch Surg 1987; 122:474–482.

Raju S, Fredericks R. Valve reconstruction procedures for nonobstructive venous insufficiency: rationale, techniques, and results in 107 procedures with two- to eight-year followup. J Vasc Surg 1988; 7:301–310.

LYMPHEDEMA

SASKIA R. J. THIADENS, R.N.
THOM W. ROOKE, M.D.
JOHN P. COOKE, M.D., Ph.D., F.A.C.C.

Although lymphedema has long afflicted untold numbers of people, the condition has been sadly neglected until recently. Even today, neither the disease nor the lymphatic system itself is widely understood. The result is that too many patients are untreated or undertreated. Many patients and many health care professionals as well are unaware of the treatments now available and the preventive measures that can be taken for patients at risk of developing lymphedema.

Lymphedema is the result of hypoplasia, dysfunction, or obstruction of the lymphatic vessels. This reduces lymphatic drainage so that interstitial and lymphatic fluid accumulates and the extremity becomes swollen. Pitting edema is a prominent feature of the early stage, and proper treatment can significantly reduce the diameter of the extremity. With chronicity of the disease, subcutaneous fibrosis and hyperplasia of connective tissue occurs and "nonpitting" edema is observed. At this stage, the condition is less responsive to conservative measures to reduce the girth of the limb.

Lymphedema may be primary (an inborn defect) or secondary (acquired loss of lymphatic patency due to trauma, infection, or other disorders). *Primary lymphedema* may be manifested in the neonatal period (congenital lymphedema), in adolescence (lymphedema praecox), or in patients over age 35 (lymphedema tarda). In about 15 percent of cases, there is a family history of the disease.

In about one-third of patients with primary lymphedema, the lymphatic channels in the *distal* part of the extremity are hypoplastic, absent, or obstructed. Most of these patients are female, and the disorder is bilateral and relatively mild. However, the girth of the affected portion may continue to increase, in the absence of proper treatment.

In about half of patients with the primary form, the *proximal* lymphatics are involved. Surgical biopsy of lymph nodes reveals an intranodal fibrotic process occurring in the absence of a history of cellulitis. This form of the disease is often unilateral, is more likely to progress, and leads to disabling symptoms requiring surgery. It is slightly more common in women.

In the remaining patients with primary lymphedema, the lymphatic tributaries are hyperplastic or tortuous and dilated (megalymphatics). In these less common forms, there is a slight male predominance. Patients with megalymphatics carry a worse prognosis for progression.

Secondary lymphedema is an acquired loss of lymphatic patency. According to the World Health Organization, approximately 250 million people annually acquire lymphedema, primarily from filarial infection in tropical third-world regions. The microfilaria are transmitted by a mosquito vector and lead to recurrent lymphangitis and fibrosis of the lymphatics. Ivermectin is now replacing diethylcarbamazine as the treatment of choice for this disease.

In Western industrialized countries, the most common cause is tumor. Prostate cancer in men (causing leg lymphedema) and breast cancer in women (causing lymphedema of the arm) are the most common malignancies involved. Late onset of lymphedema must be assumed to be secondary to malignancy until proved otherwise. The incidence of lymphedema after surgery for breast cancer was as high as 40 percent of patients who had Halsted-type radical mastectomies. Although with more conservative procedures the incidence has decreased, the rate of lymphedema after mastectomy is still high. Adjunctive radiation therapy contributes to the likelihood of developing lymphedema after these surgeries, with as many as 52 percent of these patients developing lymphedema, compared with 25 percent of patients not treated with radiation. Radiation induces fibrosis of the remaining lymph nodes and channels, thus worsening an already distressed lymphatic system. Radiodermatitis is another complication that can initiate skin trauma and streptococcal infection that will predispose to lymphedema. Although rare, lymphangiosarcoma may be associated with chronic lymphedema after mastectomy.

Other causes of secondary lymphedema include trauma, tuberculosis, and iatrogenic injury. Chronic subcutaneous injections of drugs (such as pentazocine [Talwin]) may also injure the lymphatics sufficiently to induce this disorder.

At present, there is no cure, but a variety of effective treatment methods are available. Treatment is especially effective when the diagnosis is made early after onset.

HISTORY AND PHYSICAL EXAMINATION

The diagnosis of lymphedema can usually be made after a thorough clinical history and complete physical examination. However, because clinicians are faced with a lack of uniform diagnostic criteria, much variation exists in the reported incidence of lymphedema. A diagnosis can be based subjectively on the appearance, size, heaviness, and function of the limb. Circumferential (i.e., tape measure) or volumetric (i.e., water displacement) measurements are useful to gauge the severity of the condition and to assess the response to therapy. Computed tomographic (CT) scanning or magnetic resonance imaging (MRI) of the abdomen and pelvis are prudent measures to rule out lymphatic obstruction due to tumor. Of course, these do not replace a careful examination for prostatic, pelvic, or breast malignancy.

Delineation of the lymphatic anatomy is not always necessary, particularly when a diagnosis of primary lymphedema is clear. However, if an acquired form of lymphedema is suspected and there is a possibility of a discrete obstruction of major lymphatic conduits, surgical correction is possible. In such a case, lymphoscintigraphy or lymphangiography will provide useful information.

DIAGNOSTIC TESTS

Lymphoscintigraphy

For 35 years, isotopic lymphoscintigraphy has had the potential to evaluate lymph movement. However, during the past 10 to 15 years improvements in radiopharmaceuticals and in imaging have increased interest in the use of lymphoscintigraphy to assess the location of and damage to lymphatics in patients with lymphedema. The principle of lymphoscintigraphy is that lymphatic vessels and nodes are viewed sequentially, using a radionuclide tracer and a gamma camera. This process detects movement of fluid in the lymphatics and collateral pathways, and allows interpretation of morphologic and functional alterations. Currently, the colloids used are rhenium sulfide and antimony sulfide labeled with technetium. This diagnostic test has been used to determine the location and amount of obstruction in primary and secondary lymphedema.

Lymphangiography

Lymphangiography, an invasive diagnostic study, involves injecting a water-soluble contrast agent into the lymphatic system. The dye is followed radiographically and can define the location of the lymphatic obstruction. This test, however, is not without risks and unwanted complications. It is frequently performed under general anesthesia because of patient discomfort and must be done only by a highly skilled individual. Complications include allergic reactions to the dye and potential further damage to the lymphatic system, which can lead to lymphangitis. Lymphangiography provides much better anatomic detail than lymphoscintigraphy, but this advantage is outweighed in most instances by the discomfort and risks to the patient.

THERAPY

The course of the disease can be modified by aggressive treatment at an early stage. Conversely, if the edema is left untreated, there are serious pathophysiologic and clinical consequences. The protein-rich lymphatic fluid appears to have potent growth properties and its presence is associated with cellular proliferation and generation of connective tissue. This process inexorably leads to the final stage of elephantiasis, which not only is extremely debilitating and disfiguring but is associated with the life-threatening entity of lymphangiosarcoma.

Most patients can be satisfactorily treated with conservative, nonsurgical therapy that includes mechanical and pharmacologic measures. This approach limits further damage to the lymphatics by reducing stasis of lymphatic fluid and preventing infection or inflammation of the remaining lymphatic tributaries. A skilled therapist and physician, working with a willing and compliant patient, can successfully achieve these goals.

Hygiene, Nutrition, and Prevention

Hygiene must be scrupulously maintained so as to keep the skin clean and dry. Emollients (such as Eucerin) should be applied twice daily (after a bath or shower) to keep the skin soft and supple, thereby avoiding potential sources of cellulitis as with neurodermatitis and cutaneous fissuring. Fungal infections should be vigorously treated. Protective clothing (e.g., gloves for patients with upper extremity lymphedema) should be used when performing tasks that can result in even minor injuries. Patients must be warned about exposing the affected extremity to needless trauma. Any injury to the affected limb, no matter how insignificant, can be a source of cellulitis in these patients.

Isotonic exercises such as bike riding and walking (in conjunction with the use of proper compressive support) should be encouraged so that the patient does not feel disabled by the disease. Swimming or walking in thigh-high water at the beach is particularly good therapy, since the hydrostatic pressure of the water provides excellent compression and, together with the movement of large muscle groups, increases lymphatic transport. The patient should maintain a low sodium diet and reduce alcohol intake.

Elevation

In the very early stages of lymphedema, swelling can be decreased somewhat by elevating the limb for periods during the day. As the condition progresses, however, elevation alone does not decrease the swelling, because the transport capacity of the lymphatics is severely limited. At this stage, more dynamic treatment is indicated.

Manual Lymph Drainage

Manual lymph drainage (MLD) is a method of massage aimed at moving the stagnant interstitial lymph out of the affected limb. The lymphatic tributaries include not only the limb but also the quadrant in which the lymphatic plexus resides. That is, the territory governed by the axillary lymph nodes includes the arm and the ipsilateral quadrant of the trunk; the plexus of the inguinal lymph nodes includes the leg, the genitalia, and the ipsilateral lower quadrant of the trunk. According to Foldi, these quadrants are separated by "lymphatic watersheds," over which there is some bridging that allows lymph drainage into the contralateral quadrant and the adjacent quadrant on the ipsilateral side.

MLD differs from other massage therapies in that it focuses on connective tissue rather than muscle tissue. The first step in MLD treatment is to stimulate the lymphokinetic activity on the normal lymphatics in the contralateral quadrant to begin drainage across the lymphatic watershed. The second step is to massage gently the edema fluid from the affected quadrant to the normal, contralateral quadrant.

Sequential Compression Pumps

In Europe, Australia, and Asia, massage has long been known to reduce the swelling and to promote circulation of lymph fluid through existing, undamaged vessels. With this in mind, clinicians and researchers have developed multicell compression pumps that mechanically and sequentially push the edematous fluid through the affected limb, past the damaged lymph vessels, and into viable lymph tissue and vessels.

The earliest compression machine was the Jobst single-cell, single-pressure compression pump. Although this machine has been used on patients for more than 40 years, it has had only limited success. High pressure (80 mm Hg) is applied at intermittent intervals through a special sleeve to the entire limb. However, when pressure is applied equally and simultaneously to the entire limb, the fluid is likely to move in a distal direction because of increased tissue resistance proximally. Moreover, applying the same static high pressure throughout the limb can cause more damage to already diseased tissues and the existing fragile lymphatic system.

The multicell sequential compression pumps represent an improvement over this technique. Air is pumped into a sleeve fitted over the extremity, but this sleeve has multiple overlapping compartments that are inflated sequentially, ensuring that the pressure is applied in a distal-to-proximal direction. These machines have demonstrated good success in promoting the flow of lymph through existing channels by exerting pressure on the interstitial tissue and thus increasing transcapillary exchange of extravascular protein and water. Currently, in the United States, there are three models available: the Lympha press, developed in Israel; the Sequential Circulator; and the Wright Linear Pump.

The high-pressure (80 to 100 mm Hg) Lympha press pumps air into a sleeve containing 10 to 12 overlapping cells. Each cell is inflated separately, beginning with the first distal cell. The successive inflation creates a centripetal distal-to-proximal "milking" mechanism. This intermittent pressure, promoting a distal-to-proximal flow, is able to mobilize large volumes of edema rapidly through the lymphatic system and has effectively reduced edema in many patients, especially those who receive treatment in the early stages before the subcutaneous tissues become fibrotic.

The Sequential Circulator pumps air into a sleeve with five compartments and provides a sequential distal-to-proximal pressure. Unlike other pumps, the Sequential Circulator provides two complete full-length, distal-to-proximal compressions per cycle. The rate of inflation and the time between cycles are adjustable.

Like the Lympha press, the Wright Linear Pump was developed to overcome the inherent reverse flow of single-cell pressure devices. This pump operates on the principle of a distal-to-proximal pressure gradient through a multicell sleeve (in this case, three cells). The pump operates at lower average pressures that can be programmed to counterbalance the hydrostatic pressure gradients to which the extremity is usually exposed; i.e., the distal lower extremity is exposed to the greatest hydrostatic pressure, whereas the proximal part is generally exposed to a lower pressure. The advantages of this sequential pump are that the pressure gradients between the cells (1) promote lymph flow proximally and (2) prevent overpressurization in the upper limb that might cause damage to the underlying tissue.

Pressure Sleeves or Stockings

Specially fitted compression sleeves or stockings control the accumulation of residual fluid after massage or compression pump therapy. These garments increase tissue pressure, thereby enhancing entry of interstitial fluid into the lymphatics, and increase the velocity of transport of lymph fluid. A few reliable manufacturers of compression garments in Europe and the United States will custom-make garments according to the patient's measurements. The best sleeves and stockings are seamless, thus avoiding any potential skin irritation that could lead to infection. The patient should be instructed to wear the garment immediately after therapy and at all other times except at night. The patient must wear only clean stockings or sleeves. The extremity should be measured and refitted every few months to maintain adequate pressure.

Pharmacologic Therapy

The mainstay of pharmacologic therapy is antibiotics, to prevent or treat episodes of cellulitis. Infection and inflammation lead to further fibrosis and obliteration of the remaining lymphatics and must be avoided. Generally the patient is given a prescription for a 7-day course of oral penicillin, to be initiated at the first signs of cellulitis (i.e., rigor and fever followed by erythema of the affected part). In patients who have sustained three or more episodes of cellulitis, we generally initiate chronic use of antibiotics as a prophylactic measure. Usually the patient is given a course of antibiotics the first week of each month. We alternate a course of penicillin with one of erythromycin, to avoid selecting out a resistant strain of bacteria. Alternatively, a first-generation cephalosporin or penicillinase-resistant agent (e.g., dicloxacillin) may be used.

In patients with lymphedema affecting the lower extremity, vigilance should be maintained for fungal infections. For these, we use a topical antifungal agent such as miconazole cream. Diuretics should be used judiciously and only as an adjunct to more effective measures, such as sequential compression.

Agents designed to reduce generation of connective tissue associated with lymphedema are under investigation. Benzopyrones are being used in Europe, Canada, and Australia to promote proteolysis of the lymphatic protein, thus hastening its resorption into the systemic circulation.

Heat Therapy

In Asia, researchers are reporting on the development and use of microwave-generated heat to reduce the swelling in the limb. The reports state that microwaves can penetrate to a considerable depth, where they are absorbed by the interstitial fluid, which is warmed. They note a marked reduction of edema after microwave heating plus bandaging. They also claim a 35 percent reduction in acute inflammations among the patients studied, and they report no skin burns or other side effects. The mechanism of these beneficial effects remains to be determined. This treatment has not yet been adopted in the United States.

Surgery

Surgery for lymphedema is of two types: (1) reduction surgery designed to reduce the mass of the extremity and (2) drainage procedures to surgically restore lymphatic flow. Reduction surgery should be reserved for patients whose lymphedema has progressed to the point that the increased girth and weight of the extremity disables them. This surgery involves extensive removal of subcutaneous tissue, often combined with skin grafting. This surgery is not cosmetic (the patient is left with long surgical scars), does not restore lymphatic flow, and does not obviate the need for compressive support and mechanical lymphatic drainage. However, it does allow disabled patients to return to the activities of daily life.

Surgical restoration of lymphatic flow may be considered in patients with lymphedema secondary to a proximal obstruction, with dilated but otherwise normal lymphatics distally. In the upper extremity, myocutaneous flaps using the latissimus dorsi muscle have been attempted with mixed results. The rationale behind this approach is that the normal lymphatics in the transposed myocutaneous flap will anastomose with lymphatics in the affected arm that are distal to the obstruction, thus providing an alternative route for lymphatic flow. The same principle is behind the use of omentum to bridge lymphatics in the lower extremity with mesenteric channels. Experience with lymphatico-venous and lymphatico-lymphatic bypass grafts is being gained in a few patients at selected centers. Currently, successful drainage is initially achieved in less than half of patients. In sum, surgical therapy is only appropriate for a minority of patients, and success rates are only modest. Medical therapy (skin hygiene, compressive therapy, prevention, and treatment of infection) is the mainstay of treatment for lymphedema.

With the refinement of microsurgical techniques, some centers have been gaining experience with lymphatic bypass operations. Direct anastomoses between dilated distal lymphatics and small veins allow lymphatic drainage into the venous system. Lymphatic-lymphatic anastomoses have been made using autogenous lymph vessels as bypass grafts. All these techniques require dilated but otherwise normal lymphatic channels that are distal to a proximal obstruction. Therefore, these techniques cannot be applied to patients with primary lymphedema, or patients with long-standing secondary lymphedema whose distal lymphatic channels have been damaged by prolonged lymph stasis and/or recurrent bouts of cellulitis.

COMPLICATIONS

Infection

Lymphedema is often complicated by infection. This may be manifested by frank cellulitis or lymphangitis, heralded by the onset of rigors and fever, and followed by development of a diffuse erythema (or, alternatively, discrete lymphangitic streaks), pain, and warmth. Sometimes the infection presents in a chronic and less flagrant form with only slight tenderness and elevation of local temperature. Stasis of lymphatic fluid predisposes to bacterial infection. The protein-rich fluid is an excellent medium for bacterial growth. In addition, a local immunodeficiency has been proposed. Studies show that

lymphoid cell composition of stagnant lymph in patients with lymphedema is quite different from that of normal lymph.

In the Western hemisphere the most common cause of recurrent lymphangitis is streptococcal infection. Fungal infection of the feet predisposes to this infectious process and should be aggressively treated.

For all lymphedema patients, infection is a constant possibility that too often becomes a reality. In a retrospective study of 304 lymphedema patients by the author (SRJT), over 25 percent of patients had incurred an episode of cellulitis over a period of 3 years.

Malignancy

Chronic lymphedema carries not only the constant risk of infection but also the rare but virulent complication of lymphangiosarcoma. The precise cause of this disease is unknown, but it seems to be associated with chronic lymphedema and most often involves the upper extremity after mastectomy with or without radiation therapy; it has also been reported in the lower extremity.

The symptoms appear on the edematous limb as slightly raised, purplish, bruiselike nodules, followed by satellite tumors. Amputation is the usual approach to this aggressively metastatic malignancy. Vigilance must be maintained by the physician and patient for any cutaneous manifestations of this malignancy.

PREVENTION

In breast cancer, the modified radical mastectomy, lumpectomy, or segmental resection have almost totally replaced the Halsted radical mastectomy. The incidence of lymphedema has declined with the preferential use of these procedures, but still represents a significant cause of postsurgical morbidity, particularly when followed by radiation of the affected area or when complicated by postsurgical infection.

The patient must be told of the possibility of lymphedema and instructed in preventive measures. Meticulous skin hygiene must be incorporated into the patient's daily life to prevent infection, and the patient must avoid injections, venipunctures, or other trauma to the affected limb.

SUGGESTED READING

Casley-Smith JR, Casley-Smith Judith R. High protein edemas and the benzopyrones. Philadelphia: JB Lippincott, 1986.

Foldi E, Foldi M, Clodius L. The lymphedema chaos: a lancet. Ann Plast Surg 1989; 33:505–515.

Foldi E, Foldi M, Weisleder H. Conservative treatment of lymphedema of the limbs. Angiology 1985; 36:171–180.

Gloviczki P. Microsurgical treatment for chronic lymphedema: an unfulfilled promise? In: Bergen JJ, Yao JST, eds. Venous disorders. Philadelphia: WB Saunders, 1991.

Hammond SL, Gomez JAC, Lauer CG, et al. Involvement of the

lymphatic system in chronic insufficiency. In: Bergen JJ, Yao JST, eds. Venous disorders. Philadelphia: WB Saunders, 1991.

Horsley JS III, Styblo T. Lymphedema in the postmastectomy patient. In: Bland KI, Copeland EM III, eds. The breast. Philadelphia: WB Saunders, 1991.

Olszewski WL, Engeset A, Romaniuk A, et al. Immune cells in peripheral lymphedema and skin of patients with obstructive lymphedema. Lymphology 1990; 3:23–33.

Thiadens SRJ. Advances in the management of lymphedema. Perspect Plast Surg 1990; 4:181–197.

Wolfe JHN. The prognosis and possible cure of severe primary lymphedema. Ann R Coll Surg Eng 1984; 66:251.

MISCELLANEOUS VASCULAR DISORDERS

ARTERIAL FIBROMUSCULAR DYSPLASIA

THOMAS F. LÜSCHER, M.D.
J. T. LIE, M.D.
SHELDON G. SHEPS, M.D.

Fibromuscular dysplasia (FMD) is a nonatherosclerotic and noninflammatory vascular disease that primarily involves medium-sized and small arteries (Fig. 1; Lüscher and co-workers, 1987, 1990). The most commonly involved are the renal and carotid arteries. Although FMD is an arterial disease, the involvement of renal veins has also been documented.

PREVALENCE

Fibromuscular dysplasia is diagnosed in 3.8 percent of potential kidney donors at angiography. In an autopsy study involving 819 consecutive examinations, 9 cases of renovascular FMD were found, which suggests an incidence of about 1 percent. FMD was found in 1 percent or less of patients undergoing carotid angiography. In the hypertensive population, renovascular FMD represents the underlying cause in less than 2 percent. In patients with renovascular hypertension, FMD is the underlying arterial lesion in 20 to 50 percent.

ANATOMIC DISTRIBUTION

The majority of patients with FMD (i.e., 60 to 75 percent) have renovascular disease, whereas in about 25 to 30 percent of patients with FMD, the cerebral circulation is involved (Fig. 1). Multivessel involvement is very common, particularly in patients with bilateral FMD lesions. Less frequent manifestations of FMD involve the mesenteric, subclavian, and iliac arteries (see Fig. 1).

PATHOLOGIC CLASSIFICATION AND RADIOLOGIC ASPECTS

The pathologic classification of FMD was introduced by Harrison and McCormack in 1971. The classification is based on the site of involvement within the arterial wall; i.e., intima, media, or adventitia (Fig. 2). Thus, three main forms of FMD have been delineated: intimal fibroplasia, medial fibromuscular dysplasia, and periarterial fibroplasia. Lesions involving the medial layer of the blood vessel wall have been further subclassified into medial fibroplasia, perimedial fibroplasia, and medial hyperplasia. Medial dissection, which originally was considered a fourth subtype of medial fibromuscular dysplasia, is a complication of FMD rather than a separate or distinct disorder (Fig. 3). This classification of FMD has the advantage of showing an excellent correlation between the angiographic appearance and the pathologic findings.

Medial fibromuscular dysplasia and in particular its subtype, *medial fibroplasia,* are the most common forms of FMD, accounting for 70 to 95 percent of all fibromuscular lesions (Fig. 4). Angiographically, medial fibroplasia appears as the classical "string of beads" stenosis (Fig. 5A). The "beads" exceed the diameter of the proximal unaffected part of the artery. Thickened fibromuscular ridges alternating with areas of thinning and widening of the arterial wall are the pathologic basis of the radiologic aspects (Fig. 6). In the renal artery the distal two-thirds (often extending into the branch arteries) are typically involved (Fig. 5A and 7). In the cerebrovascular circulation, medial fibroplasia typically is located in the distal internal carotid artery at the level of the C1 and C2 vertebrae (Fig. 8A). Less frequently, this classical form of FMD may be found in the iliac, axillary, and coronary arteries.

In *perimedial fibroplasia* the "beads" are usually less numerous and are smaller in diameter than those in the proximal unaffected part of the artery (see Fig. 5B). In histologic examinations, perimedial fibroplasia exhibits marked fibroplasia of the outer half of the media, and the external elastic membrane often is effaced. This fibroplasia is almost exclusively seen in young women

320

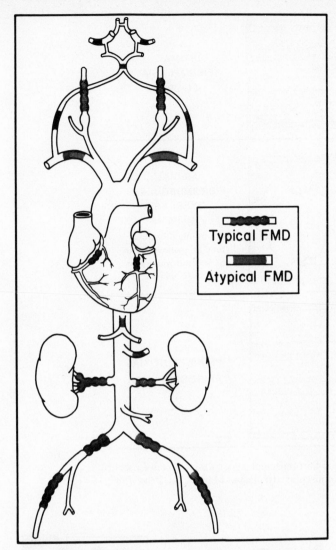

Figure 1 Anatomic distribution of fibromuscular dysplasia in the arterial tree. About three-fourths of the patients with FMD have renovascular disease and about one-fourth have cerebrovascular disease. Other locations are less frequently seen. In some vascular beds classical "string of beads" stenoses are more common (typical FMD), while in other circulations, variants of the disease appear to predominate (atypical FMD). (From Lüscher TF, Lie JT, Stanson EW, et al. Arterial fibromuscular dysplasia. Mayo Clin Proc 1987; 62:931–952; with permission.)

with rightsided renal artery stenosis, marked collateral circulation, and hypertension.

Medial hyperplasia is characterized by focal concentric stenosis that is caused by excessive medial smooth muscle proliferation without associated fibrosis (see Fig. 6). The stenosis is usually smooth, severe, and sometimes tubular in shape. As in other forms of FMD, medial hyperplasia typically involves the middle or distal part of the affected artery (see Fig. 7). This is an unusual type of FMD, probably accounting for less than 5 percent of fibroplastic stenoses.

Intimal hyperplasia is angiographically indistinguish-

able from medial hyperplasia. Histologically, however, it is characterized by a circumferential or eccentric accumulation of fibrous tissue in the intima (see Fig. 4B). The internal elastic lamina can always be identified. In contrast to features of atherosclerosis, no inflammatory changes and no lipid accumulation occurs. The lesion is rare and accounts for only 1 to 5 percent of all fibromuscular arterial lesions. In young patients, long tubular stenoses are common, while smooth focal stenoses predominate in elderly patients.

Periarterial fibroplasia is the rarest form of FMD. Here, fibroplasia with collagen encompasses the adventitia and extends into the surrounding tissue.

The differential diagnosis of FMD includes arteriosclerosis, inflammatory vascular diseases such as Takayasu's arteritis, and vascular lesions of neurofibromatosis. True idiopathic intimal hyperplasia is very rare and structurally indistinguishable from atherosclerotic intimal fibrosis. On an angiogram, intimal and medial hyperplasia can be distinguished from atherosclerotic plaques by their anatomic location. Atherosclerotic stenoses usually occur within 1 cm of the orifice of the main renal or internal carotid artery, are often eccentric, and are associated with atherosclerotic changes in the abdominal aorta. FMD almost always involves the middle or distal parts of the renal or carotid artery; the focal stenoses are concentric and typically have a smooth appearance. Classic "string of bead" stenoses are easily recognized and consistent with FMD (see Fig. 5A).

Takayasu's arteritis almost always involves the aorta and its major branch arteries at or near their origin and in its active stage usually is accompanied by laboratory evidence of inflammation. Ehlers-Danlos syndrome sometimes leads to aneurysms of major arteries similar to those seen in patients with FMD. Patients with the syndrome have characteristic clinical signs such as joint laxity and increased skin elasticity. In neurofibromatosis, stenoses at the orifices of the renal, celiac, and superior mesenteric arteries can occur, as can narrowing of the abdominal aorta, although this happens less frequently. The proximal site of arterial involvement along with stigmata of neurofibromatosis of the skin and bones usually is diagnostic in these patients with this disorder. Congenital abdominal coarctation also may be associated with proximal renal artery stenosis.

NATURAL HISTORY

Progression of FMD has been documented on repeated angiograms as well as through the course of clinical symptoms. In normotensive potential kidney donors in whom renal FMD was documented angiographically, hypertension developed in about one-fourth within 4 years, suggesting that the disease progressed with time (Cragg and co-workers, 1989). In contrast, in cerebrovascular FMD, subsequent cerebral ischemic events occur in less than 5 percent of the patients within 5 years after the initial angiogram, indicating a slow progression of the disease process (Youngberg and

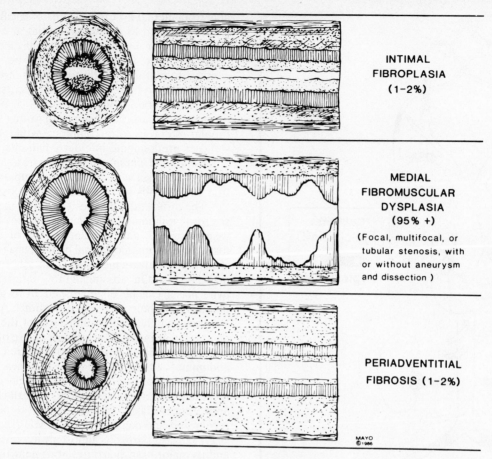

INTIMAL
FIBROPLASIA
(1-2%)

MEDIAL
FIBROMUSCULAR
DYSPLASIA
(95% +)

(Focal, multifocal, or
tubular stenosis, with
or without aneurysm
and dissection)

PERIADVENTITIAL
FIBROSIS (1-2%)

Figure 2 Histopathologic classification of arterial fibromuscular hyperplasia. (From Lüscher TF, Lie JT, Stanson AW, et al. Arterial fibromuscular dysplasia. Mayo Clin Proc 1987; 62:931–952; with permission.)

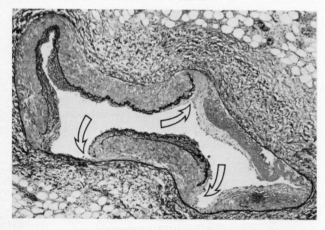

Figure 3 Cross-sectional view of fibromuscular dysplasia in a coronary artery with medial dissection at multiple sites (*arrows;* Elastin stain, ×40).

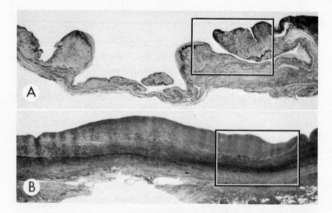

Figure 4 Two different histologic types of arterial fibromuscular dysplasia. *A,* Medial fibromuscular dysplasia. *B,* Intimal fibroplasia (Elastin stain, ×16).

co-workers, 1977). Meany et al reported angiographic progression of FMD in 16 percent of patients, as compared with 36 percent in those who had had atherosclerotic renovascular hypertension for 0.5 to 10 years. Others observed progression of renovascular FMD in about one-third of the patients over several years (Sheps and co-workers, 1972; Kincaid and co-workers, 1968; Pohl and Novick, 1985; Felts and co-workers, 1979). Progression was more common in older patients with focal or tubular stenoses than in those with medial fibroplasia, but it did not lead to total occlusion.

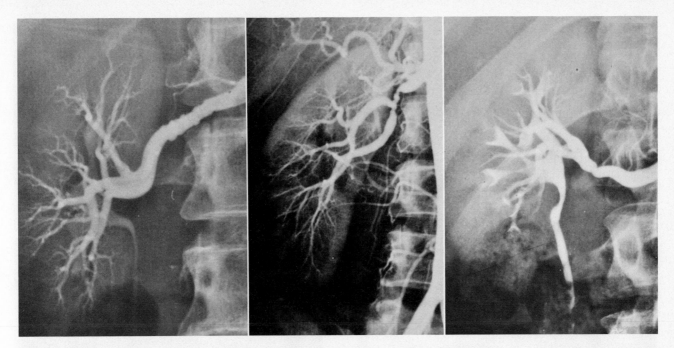

Figure 5 Angiographic aspects of fibromuscular dysplasia of the renal artery; medial fibroplasia gives rise to the typical "string of beads" stenosis *(A)*. In perimedial fibroplasia the "beads" are smaller than the proximal part of the artery and they are less regular in appearance *(B)*. Medial hyperplasia gives rise to smooth and concentric stenoses of the distal part of the main renal artery *(C)*.

Rarely, spontaneous reversal of FMD with reversal of hypertension may occur. In patients with renovascular hypertension the natural history of FMD is influenced by superimposed arteriosclerotic changes, particularly in smokers, who make up a large percentage of patients with renovascular FMD.

PATHOGENESIS

The cause of FMD remains unknown, but humoral, mechanical, and genetic factors as well as smoking and ischemia of the blood vessel wall have been suspected. FMD is much more frequent in females (particularly in the child-bearing age) than in males. In a series of patients with cerebrovascular incidents who took oral contraceptives, radiologic features consistent with FMD were found in 18 percent of the patients (Hardy-Gordon and co-workers, 1979). Oral contraceptives can cause intimal hyperplasia, and pregnancy is associated with alterations of the media and elastic tissue. In vitro, smooth muscle cells and fibroblasts have been shown to increase collagen production after exposure to estrogen. However, in patients with FMD, gravidity and parity rates are not different from those found in the general population and pregnancy does not worsen the natural history of fibromuscular vascular lesions. Moreover, in a recent study by Sang and co-workers, no evidence for an association of FMD with prior oral contraceptive use or endogenous sex hormone abnormality could be found.

Although nephroptosis is frequently associated with FMD of the right renal artery an increased renal mobility is not associated with a higher risk for FMD. In line with this clinical finding, experimental studies by Leung and co-workers and Rothfield revealed only minor histologic changes in response to stretching of the renal artery. Trivial traumas of the blood vessel wall, however, might be an important triggering factor of medial dissection in the internal carotid artery. Major traumas may cause occlusion of diseased arterial segments in previously asymptomatic patients.

The importance of genetic factors in the pathogenesis of FMD is supported by a high incidence in some families and in Caucasians. The inheritance pattern appears to be consistent with an autosomal dominant trait, with variable penetrance in about two-thirds of the cases. Renovascular hypertension is much less frequent in adult blacks than in Caucasians and, if present, usually can be attributed to atherosclerotic lesions. Furthermore, the HLA-DRW6 antigen is associated with an increased risk for FMD.

Experimental occlusion of arterial vasa vasorum causes distinct vascular changes. In the media the amount of extracellular connective tissue increases and myofibroblasts appear. Thus, a decreased blood supply to the vascular wall due to functional or morphologic obstruction of the vasa vasorum might lead to proliferative responses. The extracranial internal carotid artery and the external iliac artery (which are frequently involved in FMD) have relatively few branches, a site at which in most instances the vasa vasorum of muscular arteries originate. This could make them more susceptible to mural ischemia and might explain why, in perimedial fibroplasia, the outermost part of the media is involved and why fibroplasia exclusively involving the inner

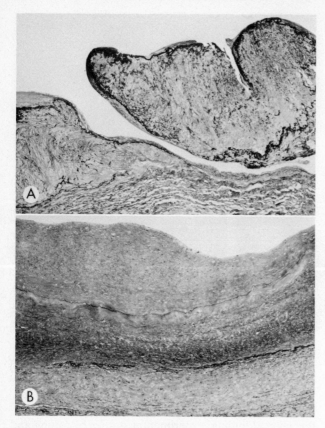

Figure 6 *A,* Close-up view of the boxed area in Figure 4*A* showing the alternating smooth muscle proliferation and deficiency in medial fibromuscular dysplasia. *B,* Close-up view of the boxed area in Figure 4*B* showing a thick band of bland intimal fibrosis (Elastic stain, ×64).

media does not occur. Some patients with pheochromo-cytoma show "string-of-beads"–like stenoses. The high catecholamine levels associated with this endocrine tumor may cause or precipitate functional stenoses of larger arteries and possibly of vasa vasorum. In some patients in one study, stenotic lesions of the renal artery disappeared after the tumor was removed. Vascular lesions resembling those in FMD also occur in ergotamine intoxication and chronic methysergide use. As in FMD, most patients with vascular complications during ergotamine therapy are women.

Smoking is strongly associated with FMD in a dose-dependent manner (Fig. 9). The way in which smoking is related to the pathogenesis of the disease process, however, remains uncertain.

Finally, FMD has been considered to be the endstage of some form of vasculitis or an immunologic process. Vascular changes ascribed to the rubella syndrome show similarities with FMD.

CLINICAL PRESENTATION AND MANAGEMENT OF FIBROMUSCULAR VASCULAR DISEASE IN VASCULAR BEDS

The clinical presentation of FMD depends on the arteries involved, the degree of vascular obstruction, and

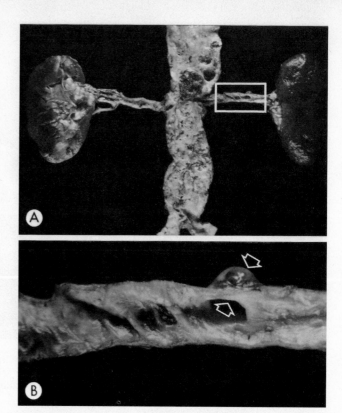

Figure 7 *A,* Bilateral renal artery fibromuscular dysplasia co-existing with aortic atherosclerosis (aorta opened posteriorally). *B,* Close-up view of boxed area in part *A* showing an aneurysm *(arrows)* of the right renal artery.

the presence or absence of a collateral circulation. Thus, patients may be asymptomatic or may have signs and symptoms of occlusive vascular disease.

Renovascular Disease

As compared with patients with renal arteriosclerosis, patients with renovascular FMD are younger, typically female, and have a shorter duration of hypertension (Lüscher and co-workers, 1987). In some series, a family history of hypertension was less common in FMD (Simon and co-workers, 1972), while others reported a high incidence of hypertension, stroke, or other cardiovascular disease in relatives of these patients (Lüscher and co-workers, 1986, 1987; Sang and co-workers, 1989; Rushton, 1980). Impaired kidney function is rare in renovascular FMD, even in the presence of bilateral disease.

Renal arterial aneurysms can cause hypertension as a result of concomitant stenosis, dissection, compression of arteries or renal tissue, or peripheral emboli (Fig. 10). The rupture of FMD aneurysms occurs very rarely, even in the presence of hypertension. The rupture of fibromuscular aneurysms into a renal vein, however, may cause renal arteriovenous fistulas (Fig. 11). Dissection of the renal artery in patients with FMD (see Fig. 3) seems to occur much less frequently than in the cerebrovascular circulation. Renal infarction is a potential complica-

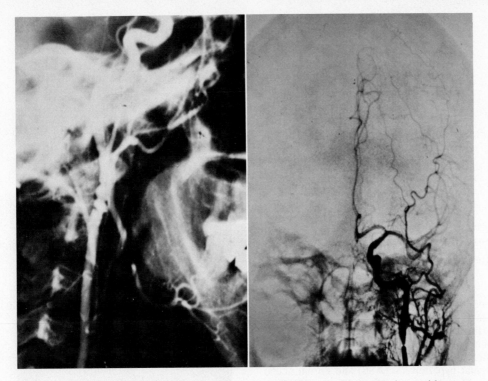

Figure 8 Angiographic aspect of fibromuscular dysplasia in the internal carotid artery: medial fibroplasia gives rise to typical "string of beads" stenoses, which are typically located at the level of the C_1 and C_2 vertebrae *(A)*. Medial or intimal hyperplasia results in smooth and concentric stenoses at the same anatomic site *(B)*.

tion of renovascular FMD, particularly in the presence of a dissection or large aneurysm. The emboli may cause abdominal or flank pain and hypertension in some patients. Selective renal venous renin samplings in the branches of the renal vein may be useful to collect to detect local renin oversecretion in hypertensive patients with renal embolization.

The treatment of renovascular disease with either surgery, percutaneous transluminal renal angioplasty (PTRA), or antihypertensive drugs may be indicated to normalize blood pressure or to preserve renal function. In contrast to patients with atherosclerotic renovascular disease, drugs are rarely used as a first-line measure in the treatment of FMD.

The cure rates from vascular reconstructive surgery are higher and the mortality rates are lower in patients with FMD treated surgically as compared with those in patients treated surgically for atherosclerotic renovascular disease, and range from 43 percent to 75 percent. Twenty-two to forty percent of the patients improve after surgery. In the Cooperative Study of Renovascular Hypertension the complication rate was 13 percent and the surgical mortality rate was 2.4 percent (Franklin and co-workers, 1975). In recent years the surgical mortality rate and morbidity have decreased, particularly in older patients. Surgical mortality is closely related to the presence of coronary artery disease and impaired kidney function, both of which are infrequent findings in FMD. Extracorporeal or ex vivo surgical techniques permit repair of FMD involving the branches and segmental arteries, which is particularly common in medial and perimedial fibroplasia (Fig. 12).

PTRA is the treatment of choice for renovascular FMD. About one-half to two-thirds of the patients are cured after the intervention. Because the long-lasting effects of PTRA have been documented and the cure rates are similar to those from surgical techniques, PTRA is being used more and more. The results of both surgery and PTRA are best in patients with unilateral FMD, poorer in those with bilateral FMD, and poorest in those with systemic FMD.

To date, no controlled randomized trial comparing surgery, PTRA, and antihypertensive drug regimens in the treatment of renovascular hypertension has been performed. The advantages of PTRA are its relative noninvasiveness, avoidance of general anesthesia, very low mortality and complication rates and short hospital stay, and similar cure rates to those obtained with surgery. In addition, an unsuccessful PTRA does not preclude later renovascular surgery. With the advent of modern antihypertensive drugs, the blood pressure lowering effect of medical therapy in patients with renovascular FMD is excellent, although drug side effects and low patient compliance may be a problem in certain patients. In bilateral renovascular FMD, angiotensin-converting enzyme inhibitors should be used with caution because dramatic increases in creatinine levels have been reported. A potential risk to the use of medical therapy is progression of the arterial disease with reduction in renal function, as was discussed earlier.

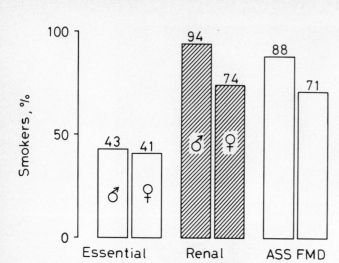

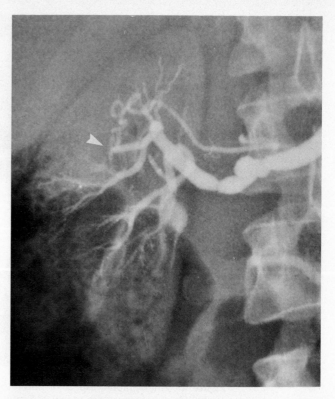

Figure 9 Percentage of patients with essential hypertension who smoke *(left two columns)* given separately for males (♂) and females (♀). In patients with renal artery stenosis *(shaded bars)*, the number of smokers is markedly higher. This prevalence of smoking applies both for patients with atherosclerotic renovascular hypertension (ASS) and fibromuscular dysplasia ([FMD]; *right two columns*). (From Lüscher TF, Jäger K, Müller FB, Bühler FR. Renovascular hypertension: update on diagnosis and treatment. In: Bühler FR, Laragh JH, eds. The management of hypertension. Amsterdam: Elsevier, 1990:90; data from Nicholson JP, Alderman MH, Pickering TG, et al. Cigarette smoking and renovascular hypertension. Lancet 1983; ii:765–766; with permission.)

Figure 10 Embolic occlusion *(arrowhead)* of peripheral intrarenal artery, most probably caused by an embolus originating from an aneurysm of the main right renal artery in a patient with meidal fibroplasia and renovascular hypertension. (From Lüscher TF, Vetter H, Tenschert W, et al. Problem cases in renovascular hypertension. Clin Nephrol 1983; 19:299–308; with permission.)

Cerebrovascular Fibromuscular Dysplasia

Cerebrovascular FMD may be an incidental finding or it may be related to clinical symptoms such as ischemic or hemorrhagic stroke, transient ischemic attacks, amaurosis fugax, or syncope (see Fig. 8). Symptoms are related to stenotic lesions or occlusions of major cephalic arteries, rupture of intracerebral aneurysms, or cerebral emboli originating from small intravascular thrombi. The presence of cerebral emboli may in part explain why, in symptomatic patients, the fibromuscular changes at angiography may be less pronounced than clinically suspected and why occlusions are relatively rare except in patients with spontaneous dissections. Bilateral lesions and fibromuscular changes involving multiple cephalic arteries are common.

Minor symptoms include headache, tinnitus, vertigo, bruits, and fatigue. Major symptoms such as transient ischemic attacks, strokes, or subarachnoidal bleedings occur in about one-third of the patients. The prognosis in symptomatic patients with cerebrovascular FMD appears to be excellent, because only a few of the patients show progression of the disease or symptoms over several years.

A potentially serious complication of cerebrovascular FMD is spontaneous dissection of the internal carotid artery or, less commonly, of the vertebral artery

or superior cerebellar artery. Rarely, dissections are associated with carotid-cavernous fistulas. Patients with spontaneous internal carotid artery dissection may experience headache, neck pain, hemiplegia, aphasia, blurred vision, or Horner's syndrome. In some patients, dissection occurred during physical exercise, after abrupt head movements, or after neck trauma. In patients with multiple vessel involvement the mortality is high. In contrast, spontaneous dissections of the vertebral artery seem to have a favorable outcome. The diagnosis of spontaneous carotid artery dissection is made by angiography, which shows long irregular filling defects ("string sign"). The lesions typically extend up to the carotid siphon, thus making a surgical approach difficult. Usually FMD vascular stenoses characteristic of FMD are present in other arteries.

The incidence of single or multiple intracranial aneurysms in patients with cerebrovascular FMD averages about 25 percent. Most aneurysms are located in the intracranial portion of the internal carotid artery and the middle cerebral artery. In contrast, in necropsy series the incidence of intracranial aneurysms in patients without FMD was found to be less than 5 percent.

Because of the relatively benign natural history of cerebrovascular FMD, surgical interventions should be

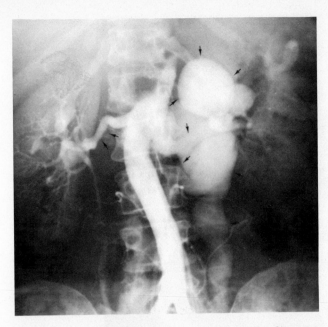

Figure 11 Arteriovenous fistula in a patient with fibromuscular dysplasia of the right renal artery *(arrows)*.

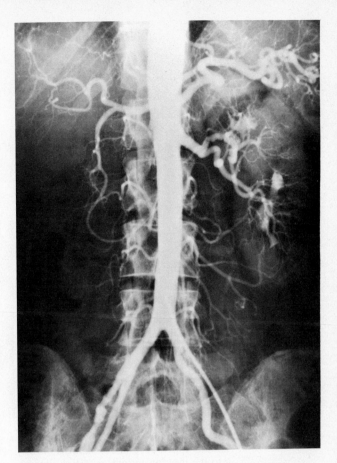

Figure 12 Intrarenal extension of medial hyperplasia of the left renal artery. Note that particularly the branches of the main left artery are involved and show typical "string of beads" stenoses. The right renal artery is occluded. Typical "string of beads" stenoses are also present in the external iliac artery.

reserved for patients with evidence of progressive cerebral ischemia. The mortality associated with surgery is almost zero, the postoperative morbidity is low, and recurrence of symptoms is rare. When FMD lesions are not surgically accessible (i.e., extending into the intracranial portions of the carotid artery), external carotid artery to middle cerebral artery bypass has been used. Percutaneous transluminal angioplasty (PTA) has been successfully performed in a limited number of patients with FMD of the internal carotid artery. In most patients the angiographic and clinical results were excellent. Neurologic complications may occur as a result of intimal dissection following PTA. Another concern against the use of PTA in these patients is the potential danger of cerebral microembolism during and after the intervention. This has led to the use of intraoperative PTA of carotid artery lesions so as to control carotid flow and thus prevent embolism. Antiplatelet agents have been used as medical therapy for cerebrovascular FMD. In a series of 19 patients with a mean follow-up period of almost 2 years, only 2 had recurrent symptoms during antiplatelet therapy (Wessen and Elliott, 1986). During surgery, patients with spontaneous carotid artery dissection have been treated with anticoagulants or with antiplatelet drugs. Recanalization of the dissected area was reported in a considerable number of patients treated with heparin, while acetylsalicylic acid appeared to be less successful.

Fibromuscular Dysplasia of the Visceral Arteries

FMD may be observed in the visceral arteries (the celiac, superior mesenteric, inferior mesenteric, hepatic, and splenic arteries). Tubular stenoses are more common than "string of beads" stenoses (Fig. 13A). Symp-

tomatic patients may have the classical triad of occlusive intestinal arterial disease such as postprandial abdominal pain, weight loss, and an epigastric bruit. Because of the development of collateral circulation through the inferior mesenteric artery (Riolan's anastomosis; Fig. 13B) or between the celiac branches and the superior mesenteric artery, the intestine is relatively resistant to ischemia unless at least two of the major arteries are obstructed. Single-vessel FMD with clinical symptoms is very rare, but may be successfully treated surgically. Mesenteric infarction due to FMD is extremely rare. Rupture of FMD aneurysms of visceral arteries have led to massive bleeding and even death in a few patients. FMD of the superior rectal artery can cause ischemic proctitis. In symptomatic patients, surgical revascularization or PTA may be required.

Fibromuscular Dysplasia of the Limb Arteries

Subclavian FMD seems particularly common in patients with systemic FMD (Fig. 14). Subclavian FMD may be associated with blood pressure difference between the right and the left arm, weakness, paresthe-

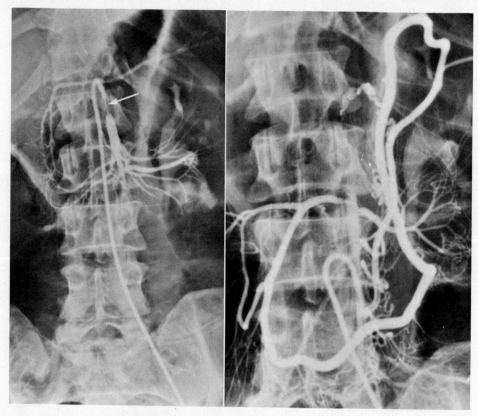

Figure 13 Fibromuscular dysplasia of the superior mesenteric artery *(A)*. Note the tubular smooth appearance of the stenosis *(arrow)*, which spares the orifice of the artery. Injection into the inferior mesenteric artery shows retrograde filling of the distal superior mesenteric artery through the marginal artery of the colon (Riolan's collateral) *(B)*. (From Lüscher TF, Lie JT, Stanson EW, et al. Arterial fibromuscular dyplasia. Mayo Clin Proc 1987; 62:931–952; with permission.)

sias, and, eventually, claudication during exercise. If the proximal part of the artery is occluded or severely obstructed, a subclavian steal syndrome with dizziness and other symptoms of cerebrovascular insufficiency during arm exercise may develop. Most patients with subclavian FMD have surprisingly few symptoms even in the presence of bilateral stenoses or occlusions. Symptomatic FMD of the axillary and brachial artery is extremely rare. Vascular surgery or PTA should be considered only in symptomatic patients.

In the lower extremities the external iliac arteries are predominantly involved. Rarely, FMD occurs in the common iliac, deep femoral, popliteal, tibial, and peroneal arteries. The lesions may be of several subtypes of FMD, such as perimedial or medial fibroplasia, or intimal fibroplasia. The majority of the published cases were in symptomatic patients with intermittent claudication, coldness of the lower extremities, or pain and cyanosis of the toes due to peripheral microembolisms. Dissecting aneurysms of the external iliac artery with acute severe pain in the inguinal region was reported to be rare.

Revascularization surgery, which may be required in symptomatic patients, has been very successful. As judged from the limited number of cases published, PTA of FMD of the iliac arteries appears to yield excellent angiographic and clinical results.

Fibromuscular Dysplasia of Coronary Arteries

Coronary artery FMD is extremely rare. FMD of epicardial coronary arteries with or without dissection and, eventually, myocardial infarction and death have been reported, however. In addition, histologic changes similar to those seen in FMD of large conduit arteries have also been found in the sinus node artery and the AV nodal artery of certain patients who have succumbed to sudden death. Hill and Antonius in 1965 reported morphologically questionable examples of coronary FMD in two patients, both women, aged 73 and 26 years. Later, James and Marshall reported cases in two patients who died suddenly and who had had multifocal narrowing of the sinus node artery with histologic changes that were classified as intimal hyperplasia. Whether or not these vascular changes represent the same entity as initial hyperplasia in other vascular beds remains a controversial question.

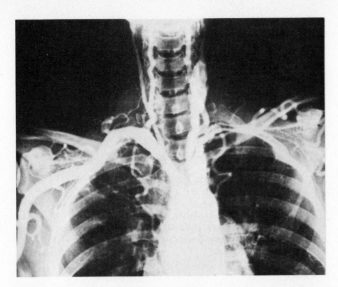

Figure 14 Fibromuscular dysplasia of the branches of the aortic arch in a patient with bilateral renal artery stenosis. Note the slight fibroplastic changes in the innominate artery and the occlusion of the left subclavian artery. In addition, an aneurysm of the left carotid artery is visualized. (From Lüscher TF, Vetter H, Studer A, et al. Extrarenaler Gefässbefall bei fibromuskulär bedingter renovaskulärer Hypertonie. Klin Wochenschr 1980; 58:493–500; with permission.)

Coarctation of the Aorta

Coarctation of the abdominal aorta occasionally is associated with FMD of the renal arteries or internal carotid arteries. In patients with abdominal coarctation, the diagnosis of neurofibromatosis should be carefully excluded. Abdominal coarctation may be either infrarenal or suprarenal or both, but the infrarenal location is more common.

SUGGESTED READING

Cragg AH, Smith TP, Thompson BH, et al. Incidental fibromuscular dysplasia in potential renal donors: long-term clinical follow-up. Radiology 1989; 172:145–147.

Felts JH, Whitley NO, Johnston FR. Progression of medial fibroplasia of the renal artery and the development of renovascular hypertension. Nephron 1979; 24:89–90.

Foster JH, Maxwell MH, Franklin SS, et al. Renovascular occlusive disease: results of operative treatment. JAMA 1975; 231:1043–1048.

Franklin SS, Young JD, Maxwell MH, et al. Operative morbidity and mortality in renovascular disease. JAMA 1975; 231:1148–1153.

Gruentzig A, Kuhlmann U, Vetter W, et al. Treatment of renovascular hypertension with percutaneous transluminal dilatation of a renal artery stenosis. Lancet 1978; i:801–802.

Hardy-Gordon S, Fredy D, Chodkiewicz JP, et al. Aspects angiographiques des accidents vasculaires cerebraux sous oestroprogestatifs. J Neuroradiol 1979; 6:239–254.

Harrison EG, McCormack LJ. Pathologic classification of renal arterial disease in renovascular hypertension. Mayo Clin Proc 1971; 46:161–167.

Heffelfinger MJ, Holley KE, Harrison EG. Arterial fibromuscular dysplasia studied at autopsy (abstract). Am J Clin Pathol 1970; 54:274.

Hill LD, Antonius JI. Arterial dysplasia: an important surgical lesion. Arch Surg 1965; 90:585–595.

James TN, Marshall TK. Multifocal stenoses due to fibromuscular dysplasia of the sinus node artery. Circulation 1976; 53:736–742.

Kincaid OW, Davis GD, Hallermann FJ, Hunt JC. Fibromuscular dysplasia of the renal arteries. AJR 1968; 104:271–282.

Leung DYM, Glagov S, Mathews MB. Cyclic stretching stimulates synthesis of matrix components by arterial smooth muscle cells in vitro. Science 1976; 191:475–477.

Lie JT, Berg KK. Isolated fibromuscular dysplasia of the coronary arteries with spontaneous dissection and myocardial infarction. Hum Pathol 1987; 18:654–656.

Lüscher TF, Jäger K, Müller FB, Bühler FR. Renovascular hypertension: update on diagnosis and treatment. In: Buhler FR, Laragh JH, eds. Handbook of hypertension. Vol 13. The Management of Hypertension. Amsterdam: Elsevier, 1990:90.

Lüscher TF, Keller HM, Imhof HG, et al. Fibromuscular hyperplasia: extension of the disease and therapeutic outcome. Nephron 1986; 44(suppl 1):109–114.

Lüscher TF, Lie JT, Stanson AW, et al. Arterial fibromuscular dysplasia. Mayo Clin Proc 1987; 62:931–952.

Meany TF, Dustan HP, McCormack LJ. Natural history of renal arterial disease. Radiology 1968; 91:881–887.

Mettinger KL. Fibromuscular dysplasia and the brain: II. Current concepts of the disease. Stroke 1982; 13:53–58.

Mettinger KL, Ericson K. Fibromuscular dysplasia and the brain: I. Observations on angiographic, clinical and genetic characteristics. Stroke 1982; 13:46–52.

Pohl MA, Novick AC. Natural history of atherosclerotic and fibrous renal artery disease: clinical implications. Am J Kidney Dis 1985; 5:A120–A130.

Rothfield NJH. Fibromuscular arterial disease: experimental studies. Aust Radiol 1970; 14:294–297.

Rushton AR. The genetics of fibromuscular dysplasia. Arch Intern Med 1980; 140:233–236.

Sang CN, Whelton PK, Hamper UM, et al. Etiologic factors in renovascular fibromuscular dysplasia. Hypertension 1989; 14:472–479.

Sheps SG, Kincaid OW, Hunt JC. Serial renal function and angiographic observations in idiopathic fibrous and fibromuscular stenoses of the renal arteries. Am J Cardiol 1972; 30:55–60.

Simon N, Franklin SS, Bleifer KH, Maxwell MH. Clinical characteristics of renovascular hypertension. JAMA 1972; 220:1209–1218.

Sos TA, Pickering TG, Sniderman K, et al. Percutaneous transluminal renal angioplasty in renovascular hypertension due to atheroma or fibromuscular dysplasia. N Engl J Med 1983; 309:274–279.

Wesen CA, Elliott BM. Fibromuscular dysplasia of the carotid arteries. Am J Surg 1986; 151:448–451.

Youngberg SP, Sheps SG, Strong CG. Fibromuscular disease of the renal arteries. Med Clin North Am 1977; 61:623–640.

THE MARFAN SYNDROME

REED E. PYERITZ, M.D., Ph.D.

The Marfan syndrome was one of the first of a small group of conditions to be classified as a heritable disorder of connective tissue by Victor McKusick more than 35 years ago. Since then, more than 150 separate conditions have been described for which the cause is likely to be an alteration in a single gene that specifies a component of the extracellular matrix. Some of these conditions share manifestations, while others are quite distinct. Only recently have the basic biochemical and genetic defects begun to be described, and few laboratory tests are available to assist in definitive diagnosis. Thus, the primary physician, the clinical geneticist, and clinical specialists for each of the organ systems affected in these disorders rely on the clinical presentation (the phenotype) to establish the diagnosis, guide genetic counseling, and indicate appropriate management.

DIAGNOSIS

Progress is being made on defining the biochemical abnormalities of the extracellular matrix that underlie the Marfan syndrome. After years of focusing on collagen, elastin, and proteoglycans, attention was directed to the microfibrils, filaments 10-12 mm in width, that are ubiquitous throughout the body. Recently, defects in the gene that encodes the major protein of microfibrils, fibrillin, were discovered to cause the Marfan syndrome. At this time, it is not possible to screen rapidly this entire large gene for mutations, so the diagnosis of the Marfan syndrome remains, in most instances, based on phenotype, with particular attention to the family history and findings in the eye, skeleton, heart, and aorta (Table 1).

If a patient has a negative family history (confirmed if possible by evaluation of close relatives such as parents, siblings, and children), more manifestations need to be present to establish the Marfan diagnosis than when a relative definitely has the condition. Some manifestations are of greater diagnostic importance because they occur infrequently in other conditions; included in this category are aortic dilatation, ectopia lentis, and dural ectasia. Signs such as mitral valve prolapse (MVP), myopia, and tall stature are less reliable as diagnostic criteria because of their frequency in the general population. The central role of echocardiography must be emphasized. The cardinal cardiovascular manifestations of the Marfan syndrome may be present, and even at an advanced clinical stage, yet may be undetected on careful physical examination. The diagnosis of the Marfan syndrome should not be *excluded* until echocardiography is performed, with the caveat that a small percentage of children with the Marfan

Table 1 Diagnostic Criteria for the Marfan Syndrome

1. If the family history is negative or unknown:
   Manifestations should be present in three organ systems and should include at least 1 hard criterion (*)
2. If the family history is positive:
   Manifestations should be present in at least two organ systems
3. A negative urine amino acid screen for homocystinuria
4. Manifestations in the cardinal organ systems:

Skeletal
   Stature > mean + 2 SD for age
   Arachnodactyly
   Dolichostenomelia (arm span > 1.03 × height)
   Anterior chest deformity
   Scoliosis
   Abnormal lordosis, kyphosis, or both
   Joint hypermobility, congenital contractures, or both
   Pes planus, calcaneoplanovalgus, or both
   Highly arched palate

Ocular
   Ectopia lentis*
   Myopia
   Retinal detachment

Cardiovascular
   Aortic root dilatation*
   Aortic dissection*
   Aortic regurgitation
   Mitral valve prolapse
   Mitral regurgitation

syndrome, and even fewer adults, may have neither MVP nor an aortic root diameter that exceeds the "upper limit of normal."

The diagnosis of the Marfan syndrome is relatively straightforward when cardinal manifestations are present in the skeletal, ocular, and cardiovascular systems. The Marfan phenotype is highly variable, even within a single family. Unfortunately, even classically affected patients continue to be undiagnosed well into adulthood, and often the pathologist is the one who establishes the presence of the condition at autopsy.

The diagnosis of the Marfan syndrome need not rely solely on the manifestations in the classic triad of organ systems. A variety of changes in other systems have been described and can be used to indicate the presence of a systemic connective tissue abnormality (Table 2).

Each of the clinical manifestations occurs in people in the general population who do not have the Marfan syndrome; some of these individuals may have other connective tissue disorders or may be variants of normal. As the biochemistry and the molecular genetics of the extracellular matrix are better defined over the coming decade, it will be possible to examine the patients who do not warrant a diagnosis of the Marfan syndrome to understand the cause of their manifestations. It is likely that some will have a defect in fibrillin, the same protein defective in the Marfan syndrome, while others will have alterations in different connective tissue elements. Understanding basic defects will clarify inheritance and enable more accurate genetic counseling.

Table 2 Manifestations of the Marfan Syndrome in
Diverse Organ Systems

Central Nervous System
  Dural ectasia
  Anterior lumbosacral meningocele
  Learning disability, attention deficit disorder, or both

Dental
  Malocclusion

Lung
  Apical bleb
  Spontaneous pneumothorax
  Reduced lung volume (due to thoracic cage deformity)

Skin and Integument
  Striae atrophicae
  Inguinal hernia
  Ventral hernia (after abdominal surgery)

Several heritable disorders of connective tissue are closely related to the Marfan syndrome. Familial MVP syndrome, which has been called the MASS phenotype (*m*itral valve, *a*orta, *s*kin, *s*keletal), is a group of heritable conditions that may cause mild aortic enlargement and predispose to progressive myxomatous deterioration of the mitral apparatus. On the other hand, there are autosomal dominant conditions that affect primarily the aorta, without the ocular or striking skeletal changes of the Marfan syndrome. Included in the grouping are disorders that produce progressive aortic root dilatation typical of the Marfan syndrome; bicuspid aortic valve, medial degeneration with supravalvular aneurysm formation, and coarctation; and familial aortic dissection without pre-existing aortic dilatation. To a large degree, these conditions that overlap with the Marfan syndrome should have their cardiovascular manifestations diagnosed and treated as in the more familiar disorder.

CARDIOVASCULAR MANIFESTATIONS AND THEIR NATURAL HISTORIES

The Heart

All the cardiac valves may undergo myxomatous degeneration. The mitral valve is most often and most severely affected. Mitral regurgitation is the most frequent serious cardiovascular manifestation of the Marfan syndrome in childhood and the most common cause of death before age 20.

Mitral valve prolapse in the Marfan syndrome shows some of the same characteristics as it does in the general population. It is age dependent, with only a few infants showing true prolapse, and the prevalence increases through young adulthood. Females are more frequently affected than males. There is an increased risk of endocarditis over the general population. Ruptured chordae may occur and cause rapid worsening of mitral regurgitation. The clinical signs of a midsystolic click and a late-systolic murmur, both of which move earlier in

systole with maneuvers that either decrease left ventricular filling or increase afterload, are characteristic. Aside from the clinical examination, cross-sectional echocardiography is the diagnostic procedure of choice. Patients with redundant, apparently thickened leaflets seen on echocardiography appear to be most prone to progressive valvular dysfunction. The mitral annulus dilates in the Marfan syndrome and in a few patients becomes heavily calcified. About 25 percent of Marfan patients show progressive mitral valvular disease; most require medical therapy directed specifically at the mitral valve, and eventually surgery.

The tricuspid valve is usually redundant and shows prolapse, especially in patients with flagrant mitral valve dysfunction. However, tricuspid regurgitation is rarely an important clinical problem.

The aortic and pulmonic valve cusps become thinned, primarily because of stretching of the commisures, although histologic studies show myxomatous change. Aortic regurgitation is generally due to progressive dilatation of the sinuses of Valsalva, rather than to intrinsic valvular deterioration.

It remains an open question whether a primary cardiomyopathy occurs in the Marfan syndrome. Some patients do seem to develop dilated ventricles out of proportion to any valvular disease that is present, but other phenotypic characteristics can not identify these patients.

Dysrhythmia is relatively common and often, but not exclusively, occurs in association with flagrant mitral valve disease. Both supraventricular and ventricular dysrhythmia occur and are potentially life-threatening.

The Aorta

Dilatation generally begins in the sinuses of Valsalva and is symmetric. Infants with Marfan syndrome often have an aortic diameter beyond what is predicted for their body size. The rate of progression is unpredictable, both in childhood and later in life. The vast majority of patients, however, show progressive dilatation leading to the major causes of morbidity and mortality in the Marfan syndrome: chronic aortic regurgitation progressing to congestive heart failure; aortic dissection; and aortic dissection with rupture. Without treatment, life expectancy for men is until the early thirties and for women until the forties. Patients in whom the diagnosis has not been suspected often are completely asymptomatic until the time of sudden death. Aortic dilatation of major degree (60 mm or more) is occasionally limited to the sinuses, but generally extends above the sinotubular junction. Stretching of the upper commissures of the aortic valve leads to aortic regurgitation of progressive severity. The dilatation rarely extends as far as the innominate artery. Life-threatening complications are uncommon before dilatation of the sinuses reaches 50 mm, but by the time the diameter is 55 mm, aortic regurgitation is usually present, at least as seen on Doppler imaging. As the sinotubular ridge expands further, the aortic regurgitation worsens, and the natural history of this valvular lesion is accelerated in the Marfan syndrome compared with, for example, rheumatic aortic valve disease. Dissection usually begins in the ascending aorta (type A) with an intimal tear just above the coronary ostia. Such dissections usually progress along the entire length of the aorta. About 10 percent of dissections are limited to the descending aorta. Dissection may be clinically silent and be discovered during routine evaluation. More often, patients have some complaints that bring them to medical attention, but the symptoms do not necessarily include tearing chest pain radiating to the back, and health professionals may not consider acute dissection seriously enough despite the patient's history and habitus suggesting the Marfan syndrome.

Whether patients with the Marfan syndrome are more prone to developing abdominal aneurysms later in life is an open question that will only be answered as patients live longer as a result of aggressive and successful management of the proximal aorta.

Other Cardiovascular Manifestations

The main pulmonary artery frequently dilates but rarely presents any clinical problem. Numerous complications of peripheral arteries, including aneurysms and dissections, have been described in patients with the Marfan syndrome, and there may be some mild predisposition to such events, which are nonetheless infrequent. Some patients seem predisposed to venous varicosities. Septal defects and other congenital heart abnormalities and hypertension are no more prevalent than in the general population.

MANAGEMENT

Routine Follow-up

Patients with the Marfan syndrome require comprehensive evaluation at least annually. This should be coordinated by a generalist who understands the condition in all its manifestations. In most cases, a cardiologist should also be involved on a regular basis. Regular ophthalmologic care is essential, especially for children. Orthopedic evaluation and management should be initiated in children at the first signs of abnormal vertebral column curvature; early bracing and occasionally surgery can prevent severe thoracic cage deformity and secondary cardiopulmonary compromise.

Mitral Valve Dysfunction

Virtually every person with the Marfan syndrome is at risk for progressive mitral valve dysfunction, aortic valve dysfunction, aortic root dilatation, and aortic dissection. It is never too early in a patient's life to begin regular follow-up for these possibilites. The timing of more aggressive interventions can be individualized.

The clinical examination and echocardiography are generally satisfactory for systematic evaluation of mitral valve function. Doppler interrogation has a role in following mitral regurgitation, but there is sufficient variation from examination to examination that the history and bedside examination should generally carry more weight. Catheterization of both the right and left sides of the heart can be reserved for patients with symptoms of heart failure, or for the occasional patient who is about to undergo aortic surgery and requires a thorough evaluation of the mitral apparatus to ensure that the mitral valve does not need repair.

Chronic mitral regurgitation can be managed medically as in similar problems of other etiology. Attention must be paid to avoid increasing stress on the dilated aorta, but afterload reduction and beta-blockade can generally be combined to improve forward flow. Furthermore, ventricular dilatation caused by beta-blockade can reduce prolapse by increasing tension on the chordae.

Mitral valve repair is successful in many patients with the Marfan syndrome. Most often a mitral annuloplasty ring is sufficient. Occasionally, plastic repair of the valve is also required. Repair is less successful when the apparatus has been damaged by endocarditis, when chordae have ruptured, or when the annulus is heavily calcified. Isolated mitral valve surgery is necessary in some patients, especially children, but most often the issue arises in conjunction with prophylactic repair of the ascending aorta. I recommend an elective mitral valve annuloplasty if even mild mitral regurgitation is present, because the procedure does not greatly increase cardioplegic or cross-clamp time, and future surgery may be avoided.

The Ascending Aorta

Dilatation of the sinuses of Valsalva is progressive, but unpredictably so. The diameter can be followed relative to the patient's body surface area during childhood and adolescence; I use either a standard curve or a regression equation to give the predicted value. The equation to calculate the predicted aortic root diameter is

$$= 24.0 \ (\text{BSA})^{1/3} + 0.1 \ (\text{age}) - 4.3 \pm 18\%$$
(in which BSA is the body surface area in square meters and the age is in years.)

The measured diameter is then divided by the predicted value to yield a ratio. Any value over 1.18 is clearly abnormal, and this ratio can be followed to give perspective on further enlargement. For ratios less than 1.2, echocardiography should be performed annually; as the ratio gets progressively larger, more frequent assessment is required, and should be performed every 3 months as the time for prophylactic repair nears.

The dilated aorta can be managed medically in all patients, beginning early in life. One cornerstone is activity restriction, both to prevent chronic stress that tends to dilate the aorta and to reduce sudden stress that might cause dissection. Accordingly, I recommend that parents of children with the Marfan syndrome encourage them to participate in noncompetitive athletics. Isometric exertion should be avoided because of its more pronounced effect on raising blood pressure and heart rate than that of isokinetic exercise. In most cases, affected children can participate in the usual playground activities through elementary school. Adolescents and adults should avoid all strenous activities, whether at work or play. Exertion at a moderate aerobic level is probably not detrimental except for patients with large aneurysms (aortic ratio >1.5) or chronic dissections.

Chronic beta-adrenergic blockade has long been a cornerstone of the medical management of acute and chronic aortic dissections. Several studies have now largely been completed that point to a beneficial effect of beta-blockade in protecting the aorta in Marfan patients. The beneficial effect pertains both to prevention of aortic dissection and to reduction in the rate of aortic root dilatation in children and adults. Atenolol (Tenormin) has several advantages as the drug of choice: its relatively long half-life (although twice-daily dosing clearly provides a more even therapeutic effect); its beta$_2$-selectivity; and its decreased cerebral side effects compared with propranolol. The dosage must be individualized in order to keep the resting heart rate in adults under 60 and the heart rate after moderate exertion (such as in running up and down two flights of stairs) under 100. The dose required for this effect varies tremendously among individuals. Children can be started on beta-blockade quite early in life if the aorta is dilated. Atenolol is easy to administer to children who can take pills; otherwise propranolol suspension can be given.

During the past two decades the techniques of surgical repair of the ascending aorta have evolved to the point that prophylactic surgical management of the Marfan aorta is warranted. The major breakthrough was the development by Bentall of a composite graft involving a prosthetic valve sewn to the end of a woven conduit. The coronary arteries are anastomosed to side holes cut in the conduit. About 15 years ago we at the Johns Hopkins Hospital began advocating prophylactic repair of the Marfan aorta when the diameter reached 60 mm in adolescents and adults. Since then, more than 100 elective repairs have been performed there with no perioperative deaths. Emergency repairs, primarily for acute dissection, can also be managed by this technique with better perioperative mortality rates than by any other technique. Equally important have been the long-term results. Follow-up with magnetic resonance imaging (MRI) has shown only slight dilatation of the distal ascending aorta and aortic arch over an average of 5 years in all but two cases. The principal long-term complication is endocarditis, and patients must be carefully instructed about aggressive prophylaxis and management of minor wounds.

I prefer the St. Jude composite graft and do not use porcine valves except in elderly patients. For patients who cannot tolerate warfarin (Coumadin) or those who require repeat surgery because of endocarditis, cryopreserved aortic homografts offer an attractive alternative, although their longevity is uncertain at this time.

Aortic dissection in the Marfan syndrome usually involves the entire aorta, with the initial intimal tear in the aortic root. For both acute and chronic dissections of the ascending aorta, regardless of how far the dissection extends, composite graft repair is generally the first step in surgical management. In some instances of extensive dissection, repair of the intimal tear is all that is necessary. If branch occlusion has occurred elsewhere along the course of the aorta, if there is aneurysmal dilatation more than 60 mm in diameter, or if signs and symptoms of acute dissection persist or recur, other regions of the aorta must be repaired. A staged sequential approach can be employed, and in some patients the entire aorta has been replaced successfully.

Chronic dissections of the aorta in Marfan patients must be monitored carefully because of an increased predisposition to dilatation and further dissection. Until the aorta stabilizes, MRI should be performed every 3 to 4 months. Even if there has been no apparent change for several years, it is still prudent to evaluate the entire length of the aorta noninvasively every 6 months. Patients with chronic dissection should be kept on negative-inotropic doses of beta-blockade regardless of their blood pressure readings; systolic blood pressure should be maintained at less than 110 mm Hg.

Cardiac Transplantation

There is little experience with cardiac transplantation in adults and children with the Marfan syndrome. End-stage cardiac failure does occur in a minority of patients as a result of severe valvular dysfunction or an intrinsic cardiomyopathy. One attractive aspect of cardiac transplantation is the opportunity to provide a normal ascending aorta, provided that the donor organ is free of disease and can be harvested appropriately. One potential, but largely unexplored, disadvantage is the effect of cyclosporine on the already abnormal connective tissue in the Marfan patient. Because of the current marked disparity between the number of patients requiring transplantation and the supply of donor organs, most programs restrict access to patients who do not have chronic, systemic illnesses. Many programs classify the Marfan syndrome accordingly, and restrict eligibility.

Pregnancy

Two issues confront the woman with the Marfan syndrome when she considers pregnancy. The first is the 50-50 risk that any child will have the syndrome; prenatal diagnosis is now possible in selected cases. The second issue concerns the risk of damage to the maternal aorta. Numerous case reports attest to the increased risk of dissection during pregnancy and in the weeks just after parturition. The increased risk of dissection is largely, but not totally, restricted to women with pre-existing aortic dilatation. A woman whose aortic root measures less than 40 mm when she conceives appears to have little risk of dissection, although there have been some instances of type B dissection. I have selected a limit of 40 mm; women with aortic root diameters larger than that are advised not to undertake pregnancy. I do not use beta-blockade during the first trimester, but reinstitute medication at the first sign of blood pressure elevation or dysrhythmia. Echocardiography throughout pregnancy seems warranted.

Delivery should be by whatever method will produce the least hemodynamic stress. This obstetric decision must be individualized and often may not be made until the final stages of the pregnancy.

DISCUSSION

The natural history of the Marfan syndrome is dismal indeed. Fortunately, the clinical history has deviated strikingly from the natural history as a result of advances made in the past several decades. With aggressive, prophylactic management, many patients with the Marfan syndrome should live relatively normal life spans. However, a minority of patients have such severe cardiovascular involvement from an early age that even the most aggressive medical and surgical therapy will not produce entirely satifactory results.

SUGGESTED READING

Dietz HC, Cutting GR, Pyeritz RE, et al. Marfan syndrome caused by a recurrent de novo missense mutation in the fibrillin gene. Nature 1991; 352:337–339.
Glesby MJ, Pyeritz RE. Association of mitral valve prolapse and systemic abnormalities of connective tissue: a phenotypic continuum. JAMA 1989; 262:523–518.
Gott VL, Pyeritz RE, Magovern GJ Jr., et al. Surgical treatment of aneurysm of the ascending aorta in the Marfan syndrome: results of composite-graft repair in 50 patients. N Engl J Med 1986; 314:1070.
Hollister DW, Godfrey M, Sakai LY, Pyeritz RE. Marfan syndrome: immunohistologic abnormalities of the elastin-associated microfibrillar fiber system. N Engl J Med; in press.
Pyeritz RE, Fishman EK, Bernhardt BA, Siegelmann SS. Dural ectasia is a common feature of the Marfan syndrome. Am J Hum Genet 1988; 43:726–732.
Pyeritz RE, Wappel MA. Mitral valve dysfunction in the Marfan syndrome. Am J Med 1983; 74:797–807.

VASCULAR TUMORS, ANGIODYSPLASIA, AND ARTERIOVENOUS MALFORMATION

WAYNE L. MILLER, M.D., Ph.D.
J. T. LIE, M.D.

VASCULAR TUMORS

Types and Incidence

The generic designation *vascular tumors* includes all those tumors occurring in the soft tissue, skin, bone, or viscera that are composed of cells with an endothelial phenotype and, more restrictively, a second category of neoplasms that occur within an anatomically intact blood vessel.

Tumors in major blood vessels are distinctly uncommon; fewer than 300 cases of primary benign and malignant tumors of major blood vessels have been documented in the world literature since the first description of a myoma of the ulnar vein by Boettcher in 1869. The overall incidence of these primary vascular tumors is about 20 percent of that of primary tumors of the heart and pericardium. Approximately two-thirds of all primary tumors of major blood vessels occur in large veins, and about two-thirds of all primary tumors of the large arteries arise in the pulmonary artery—only one-third occur in the aorta.

Although sarcomas of the major blood vessels typically show myogenic differentiation, they are in fact a heterogenous collection of tumors with diverse histopathologic features. Polyphenotypic expression of several mesenchymal lineages suggests that the progenitor cell has many potential properties, and more than one-third of the tumors are histologically undifferentiated (Table 1). The generally poor prognosis in patients with tumors of major blood vessels is attributable to the critical anatomic location of the neoplasm rather than its metastatic potential, which is low.

Diagnosis and Management

The clinical manifestations of tumors of the major blood vessels are attributable to the general effects of a space-occupying lesion and obstruction of arterial or venous circulation. The symptoms may be insidious, however, with nonspecific cough, dyspnea, chest pain, and progressive heart failure predominating. Distension of neck, abdominal, and peripheral veins or an audible thrill or precordial systolic murmur may be detected in a physical examination.

Before the advent of two-dimensional echocardiography, Doppler ultrasound examination, gallium scans, and sophisticated imaging techniques, angiography was the standard diagnostic modality. Currently, computed

Table 1 Histologic Types and Frequency of Tumors Arising in Major Blood Vessels

Histologic Type	Estimated	Percentage
Undifferentiated sarcoma		34
Undifferentiated	15	
Spindle cell	8	
Pleomorphic	6	
Anaplastic	2	
Spindle angiosarcoma	2	
Round cell	1	
Myogenic Sarcoma		26
Leiomyosarcoma	20	
Rhabdomyosarcoma	6	
Fibrocystic sarcoma		21
Fibromyxosarcoma	11	
Fibrosarcoma	10	
Chondrosarcoma		4
Osteogenic sarcoma		3
Vascular sarcoma		4
Angiosarcoma	2	
Hemangioendothelioma	1	
Hemangiosarcoma	1	
Malignant fibrous histiocytoma		2
Mesenchymoma		6
Malignant mesenchymoma	3	
Mesenchymoma	2	
Mixed mesenchymal sarcoma	1	
Total		100

tomography and magnetic resonance imaging are the diagnostic methods of choice. Despite this improvement in diagnostic technique, only about 50 percent of all cases of tumors of the major blood vessels are diagnosed.

The prognosis in patients with these tumors is generally poor, with death occurring within 12 to 24 months of diagnosis. Successful surgical resection is possible in a few cases; the use of adjuvant chemotherapy, radiation therapy, or both has achieved only modest or negligible additional benefits. Intractable heart failure with or without metastases is the most common cause of death. Pulmonary metastases occur in about two-thirds of patients and systemic metastases, in about one-third. Direct extension of the sarcoma to the adjacent heart occurs not infrequently and may limit the feasibility of a successful surgical resection.

ANGIODYSPLASIA AND ARTERIOVENOUS MALFORMATIONS

Angiodysplasia refers to a developmental abnormality with alterations in size, shape, organization, and function of blood or lymph vessels. The cause of congenital angiodysplasias is not known but does not appear to be an inherited condition. The lesions are commonly found in the gastrointestinal tract but may also occur in the extremities and visceral vessels (Figs. 1 and 2). Arteriovenous malformation has been considered synonomous with angiodysplasia but more appropriately represents a subgrouping. A considerable amount of confusion exists in this area of medicine with regard to the terms used and their definitions. This is fueled by an abundance of disparate classifications of limited application and acceptance. The basic focus and most important distinctions to be made among angiodysplasias are the presence or absence of shunting and the quantity of shunting produced, which may range from inconsequential to massive and hemodynamically compromising.

Malan and Puglionisi provided a detailed discussion and classification of congenital arterial, venous, and arterovenous dysplasias of the extremities. Two types of primary lesions were distinguished: 1) dysplasias and hamartias (developmental defects in the combining of tissues) of the arterial and venous trunks, and 2) capillary hamartias, from which angiomas (flat cutaneous, hyperplastic, and cavernous) are derived. In the congenital angiodysplastic syndromes, these elements are present singly or in combination and in various stages of maturation. In the category of arteriovenous lesions are the forms that involve arteriovenous short circuits (trunk arteriovenous fistulas and arteriovenous angiomas) and all the possible hemodynamic and clinical associations. Clinically, these lesions may be silent (i.e., hemodynamically insignificant) and may only become evident when arteriovenous shunt flow exceeds a threshold level relative to the capacity of the normal vessel. In the category of venous angiodysplasias the hemodynamic pathogenic component is venous stasis (Fig. 3).

The congenital angiodysplastic lesions that cause arteriovenous shunts in general have two morphologic appearances: 1) arteriovenous communications caused by fusion of arterial and venous conductance vessels or abnormal channels between the conductance vessels, and 2) angiomas that result in arteriovenous shunts because of their structure and anatomic close association with arterial and venous vessels. The terminology often applied to this group of angiodysplasias is *congenital arteriovenous fistulas;* this term, however, may be considered too broad and does not permit appropriate anatomic and pathologic distinction of the various forms. Clinically, it becomes important to distinguish forms with large shunts from those with small or moderate shunts because symptoms, prognosis, and therapy depend on the size of the shunt. Arteriovenous fistulas may also be acquired (most commonly traumatic) (Table 2) in addition to being of congenital origin; the focus of this discussion, however, is on congenital anomalies, and data on acquired disease are presented only for comparisons.

Clinical Findings

Common presentations with extremity involvement include pain, swelling, and disfigurement in the affected area. Symptoms associated with angiodysplasias, particularly those with dominant arteriovenous shunts, may be a feeling of heaviness in the extremity due to hypertrophy, increased circulating blood volume in the limb, edema or venous stasis, and often a sensation of intense heat. Fifty percent of patients complain of pain that is often intermittent and related to muscular activity or

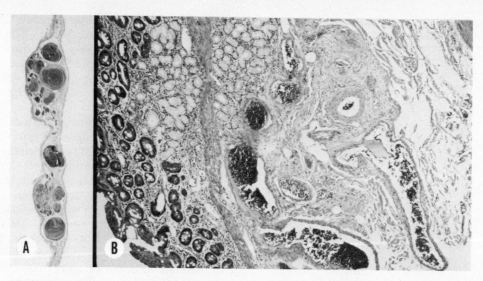

Figure 1 Angiodysplasia of the gastrointestinal tract, shown here involving the small bowel. *A,* Gross appearance of the bowel wall distended with engorged large and small vascular spaces. *B,* Close-up view of thick- and thin-walled dysplastic submucosal blood vessels. (Hematoxylin and eosin, *A* × 4; *B* × 160.)

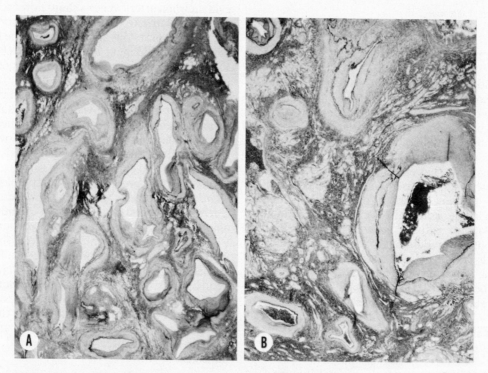

Figure 2 *A* and *B* are variations of the true arteriovenous fistula type malformation with a maze of thick-walled blood vessels, some of which are structurally well-defined small arteries and veins while others are hybrid nonartery, nonvein vascular spaces. (Hematoxylin and eosin, *A* and *B,* ×160).

ambient temperature—factors that influence shunt flow. Lower extremity pain can also be similar to pain from intermittent claudication but, unlike in typical claudication, resolves slowly when the patient stops walking. The appearance of an extremity affected by angiodysplasia with arteriovenous shunting is characterized in some

situations (e.g., Klippel-Trenaunay syndrome) by hypertrophy of the limb (soft tissue and bone), varices, and angiomas. A palpatory thrill is often present at the site of the shunt, and an increase in cutaneous temperature of the affected limb is commonly noted. Figure 4 angiographically demonstrates shunts that have pro-

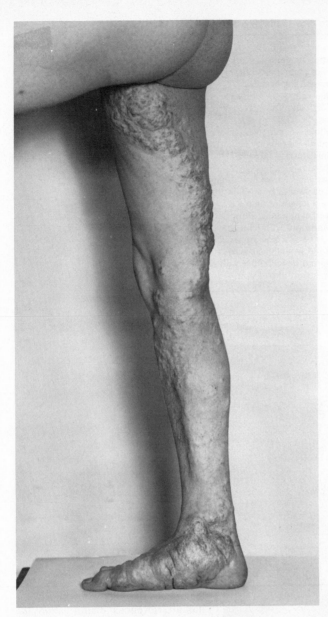

Figure 3 A 38-year-old man with asymptomatic congenital venous hemangioma of the right saphenous vein system with distal extremity stasis changes.

duced findings and symptoms such as those described above.

Arteriovenous fistulas and malformations can occur virtually anywhere in the body (Table 3); lesions involving the lower extremities, however, are very common (Fig. 5). Other common sites include the lungs (Rendu-Osler-Weber syndrome) (Fig. 6) and the head and neck regions. The clinical presentation of arteriovenous malformations in the head and neck area depends on the location of the lesion. Malformations of the spinal cord and occipital dura may have serious complications, with associated headache and seizure activity. Spinal arteriovenous malformations can also produce symptoms of neurogenic claudication (pseudoclaudication) that are

virtually indistinguishable from those of lumbar spondylosis (spinal stenosis). Deterioration of function after decompressive surgery (laminectomy) for supposed spinal stenosis should suggest the possibility of underlying arteriovenous malformation. Hypertrophy of soft tissue and bone, with disproportionate growth of the ipsilateral extremity in association with hemangioma (port-wine stain) and varicose veins has been described (the triad of features in the Klippel-Trenaunay syndrome) (Fig. 7). Venous fibromuscular dysplasia is a prominent vascular lesion in this setting in association with venous stasis. Unilateral involvement is the rule, usually affecting a lower extremity. Overgrowth of a limb can occur in the setting of extensive or mild arteriovenous shunting (Fig. 8), but the mechanism is not understood. Tissue growth factor or a developmental anomaly of mesenchymal tissue have been considered as possible explanations.

Visceral involvement of angiodysplasias and arteriovenous malformation is not uncommon and may cause life-threatening complications. Angiodysplasia has been cited as the most common cause of covert gastrointestinal bleeding in elderly persons and may account for up to 8 percent of all cases of gastrointestinal bleeding. Although the cause is uncertain, it has been proposed that angiodysplasia represents a degenerative condition related to aging and repeated partial obstruction of submucosal veins, which results in dilation of submucosal veins, incompetence of sphincters, and development of small arteriovenous communications. This and other similar theories, however, do not explain the occurrence of angiodysplasia in younger people with gastrointestinal bleeding. Therefore, the implications of both congenital and acquired factors must be considered. Acquired submucosal arteriovenous malformations develop in the terminal ileum, cecum, or ascending colon in elderly persons and are in some instances associated with severe aortic stenosis (Heyde's syndrome) or atherosclerosis. The incidence of idiopathic gastrointestinal bleeding has been reported to be 100 times greater in the subset of patients with aortic stenosis than in the general hospital population (2.6 versus 0.025 percent). Most cases of angiodysplasia, however, occur in patients without any cardiac disorder. Congenital arteriovenous malformations occur most commonly in the small bowel and in younger patients. Angiomas of the gastrointestinal tract may also occur as a manifestation of the hereditary Rendu-Osler-Weber syndrome. Histologic differences have been shown between capillary hemangiomas, which usually involute as part of their natural history, and other arteriovenous malformations that grow from birth and may rapidly increase in size at puberty or with pregnancy. In the assessment of a possible arteriovenous malformation a differential diagnosis must be considered and includes malignant vascular tumors and false aneurysms.

Assessment

Depending on location, the diagnosis of arteriovenous malformation can most often be made from the

Table 2 Classification of Arteriovenous (A-V) Fistulas and Malformations

I.	Acquired	Penetrating wound
II.	Iatrogenic	Hemodialysis shunts; arterial punctures
III.	Congenital	Failure of embryonic differentiation and dysplastic angiogenesis
	A. Types:	Hemangioma
		Micro- or macrofistulous A-V communication
	B. Location:	Extremities—commonly, femoral artery
		Pulmonary—hereditary hemorrhagic telangiectasia (Rendu-Osler-Weber syndrome)
	C. Findings:	Varicose veins common
		Increased sweating and hair growth
		Increased length of limb
		Increased skin temperature
		Thrill and bruit with large AVM
		Bradycardic sign less pronounced than acquired fistula or absent
		High output heart failure with cardiac enlargement uncommon

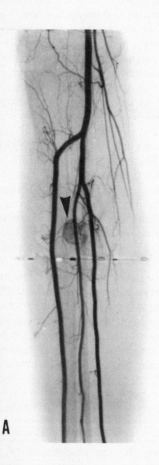

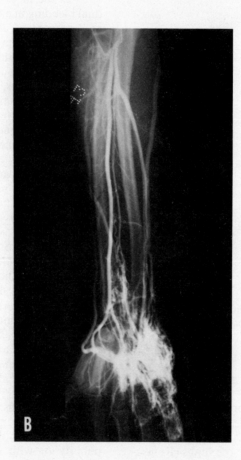

Figure 4 *A;* Angiogram of the right leg of a 49-year-old man with congenital arteriovenous malformation *(arrowhead).* Patient presented with a 30-year history of right lower extremity pain, heaviness, and swelling. *B;* Arteriogram in a 17-year-old man with congenital arteriovenous malformation of the right hand and distal arm with slight elongation of the right forearm (1.5 cm), a thrill over the dorsum of the right hand, and machinery-like bruit in the right hand and forearm.

history and physical examination. Angiography is commonly used to confirm the impression but noninvasive testing, such as hand-held Doppler ultrasound imaging, may be very useful in detecting the presence of significant arteriovenous shunting. The sound provides a clue as to the dominant component present: high-pitched arterial or low-frequency venous. Contrast echocardiography has also been reported to be helpful in the diagnosis of pulmonary arteriovenous fistulas and in the detection of residual shunts after surgery. Magnetic

Table 3 Number of Arteriovenous (A-V) Fistulas Found in 10 Years at the Mayo Clinic

Location	Acquired	Congenital
A-V fistulas of the extremities	17	80
A-V fistulas of the neck and face	4	11
Aorto-inferior vena caval fistulas	7	–
A-V fistulas of the mammary vessels	2	–
Pulmonary A-V fistulas	–	47
Renal A-V fistulas	6	–
A-V fistulas of the portal system	1	–
Pelvic A-V fistulas	5	1
Total	42	139

Modified from Fairbairn JF II, Juergens JL, Spittell JA Jr, eds. Peripheral Vascular Diseases, 5th ed. Philadelphia: WB Saunders, 1981.

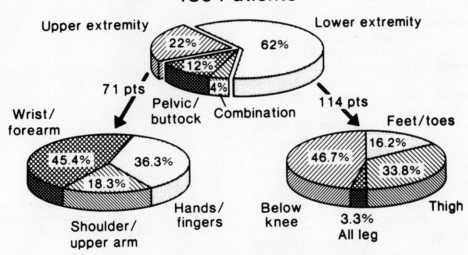

Figure 5 Anatomic sites of involvement of congenital arteriovenous malformations in 185 patients. (From Schwartz RS, et al: Phlebology 1:171, 1986; with permission.)

resonance imaging has the advantage of not requiring contrast agents and gives accurate, detailed information for flow assessment and for the possibility of surgical resection in both sagittal and longitudinal planes. Computed tomography (CT), however, remains an important diagnostic tool but requires contrast enhancement for optimal delineation of the lesion from surrounding tissue. Nevertheless, CT may be unable to distinguish hypervascular tumors from arteriovenous malformations. Magnetic resonance imaging provides an advantage in this circumstance.

Radionuclide scanning of technetium-labelled microsphere or human albumin can be used to estimate shunt flow quantitatively. The labelled substance is injected first into the artery proximal to the lesion and then later into a peripheral vein. The lungs are then scanned and an estimate of shunt to total limb flow is calculated. With venous injection all of the isotope is caught in the lungs, but with arterial injection the percentage of radioactivity in the lungs will depend on the shunt flow; normally, it should not exceed 3 to 5 percent. This technique can only be used, however, if the arteriovenous fistula is peripherally located.

Angiography should be considered only for lesions with high flows and for lesions in which there is a significant shunt that will require surgical or embolization treatment (Fig. 9). With the current advances in technique, selective and superselective catheterization

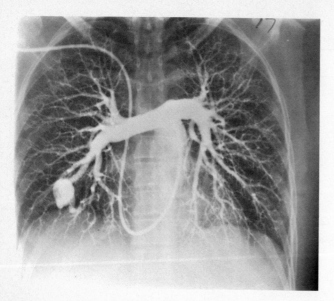

Figure 6 Pulmonary angiogram showing arteriovenous fistula in patient with Rendu-Osler-Weber syndrome (hereditary hemorrhagic telangiectasia).

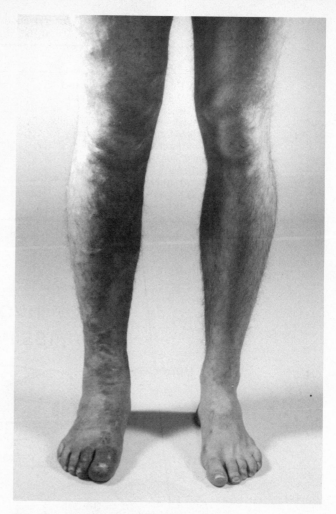

Figure 7 Klippel-Trenaunay syndrome in a 29-year-old man with history of chronic venous insufficiency since early childhood with discomfort and a sensation of heaviness of the right leg. No history of deep venous thrombosis or lymphedema. Right foot and leg are larger than left.

and injection can be performed routinely. Angiography can demonstrate the major supplying arteries and the study should evaluate all possible sources. The size of shunt (shunt volume) can be estimated by the appearance time of contrast material in the vein. There are many lesions, however, in which angiography gives only indirect evidence of shunting—e.g., early venous filling, reduced opacification of distal vessels, or abnormally elevated arterial flow to the lesion with tortuosity and dilation of the artery. An estimated 30 to 40 percent of congenital arteriovenous malformations cannot be localized by angiography alone.

Therapy

The therapy for specific lesions is based on vascular origin and clinical significance. Many angiodysplastic anomalies are asymptomatic and uncomplicated and, therefore, require observation only. Cure of these lesions is often not possible unless complete excision can be done, which generally implies the presence of a small lesion. Large lesions that are compromising to the patient (disfigurement or progressive overgrowth of an extremity) are difficult to manage. Also, complications such as pain, ulceration, infection, and bleeding can provide additional management problems.

Invasive, nonsurgical approaches such as embolization by catheterization techniques are important treatment options for arteriovenous malformations with significant shunts. The goal of embolization is to occlude the communications at the precapillary level. Blocking the main arterial supply is of minimal benefit because the communications remain intact and new distal collateral vessels open. Also, access for future treatment is precluded. Congenital arteriovenous malformations are often supplied by several arteries; there-

fore, repeated superselective angiography may be necessary.

The selection of embolization material depends on the site and size of shunt vessels. The material needs to be small enough to reach the precapillary level but large enough to avoid pulmonary embolization. Stainless steel coils are adequate for large vessels but the reopening of capillaries may refill the arteriovenous shunt. Silicon and polyvinyl particles are permanent materials, whereas gelatin foam sponge and microfibrillar collagen are temporary and usually dissolve within days to a few weeks. The process may also require several staged procedures and still not be of long-term benefit. Embolization of distal arteries of extremities is contraindicated because gangrene and tissue loss can easily occur. In general, this procedure should be undertaken only if amputation is the final alternative.

Laser therapy is possible in some low-shunt-flow situations. Argon lasers are used for port-wine stains (intradermal capillary anomalies) and at times in pa-

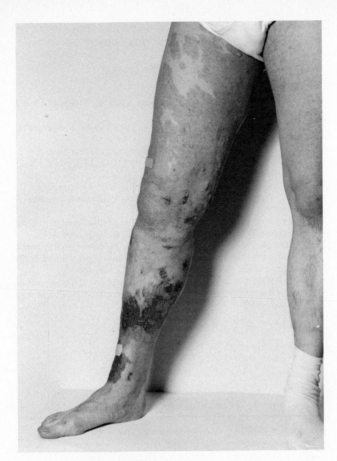

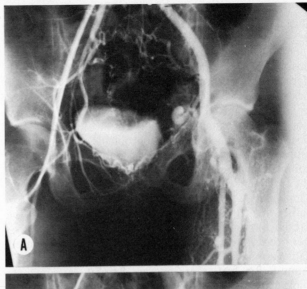

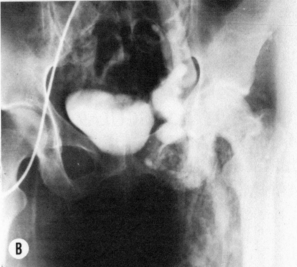

Figure 8 A 30-year-old man with congenital arteriovenous malformation of the right leg with limb lengthening and chronic venous insufficiency with stasis changes.

Figure 9 Arteriogram in a symptomatic 25-year-old woman with marked congenital arteriovenous malformation of the pelvic and left femoral area and resultant severe degenerative joint disease of the left hip. *A,* Arterial phase showing markedly enlarged left iliac artery. *B,* Venous phase showing large left iliac and femoral veins. (From Fairbairn JF II, Juergens JL, Spittell JA Jr, eds. Peripheral vascular diseases, 5th ed. Philadelphia: WB Saunders, 1981; by permission of Mayo Foundation.)

tients with Klippel-Trenaunay syndrome. Unavoidable scarring, however, may occur in up to 25 percent of patients so treated.

Venous malformations contain small shunts but in general do not require investigation and treatment. In some instances a "skeletonization" technique may be used by tying off the microshunts from the artery to the affected vein. Venous dilatations caused by localized aneurysm formation can cause disfigurement and complications such as thrombosis and pulmonary embolism. Thrombocytopenia with giant venous hemangioma is believed to be caused by platelet trapping and shorter platelet survival. In arteriovenous malformations coagulant abnormalities occur most often in large venous lesions, are of a consumptive nature, and can be precipitated by surgery. Heparinization is necessary to prevent perioperative disseminated intravascular coagulation. Elastic stocking support is very beneficial in providing compression in legs and feet with hemanigomas or dilated superficial veins and will substantially reduce shunt and cardiac output in very large arteriovenous malformations. In addition, such garments provide some protection from trauma to these vulnerable vascular lesions.

The surgical approaches to the elimination of angiodysplastic lesions that cause arteriovenous shunts

are not always sufficient to restore normal vascular integrity. Extensive but indiscriminate removal of abnormal vascular structures usually leads to incomplete results and possibly stimulates further vascular overgrowth. Ligation of proximal feeding vessels alone is inappropriate because, as a result, more collateral vessels develop and access for future catheterization procedures is compromised. An additional problem for a surgical approach to deep arteriovenous malformations of the extremities is that these malformations may extend intraosseously. These are particular concerns at the wrist and knee joint areas, and therefore, embolization may be the only alternative to amputation.

Results of studies from surgery and embolization suggest the best results in lesions with exclusively arterial or venous components. If en-bloc excision is considered, then one should resect the lesion as completely as possible using a one-stage procedure. Multiple procedures should be avoided. Unfortunately, only about 20 percent of all arteriovenous malformations can be cured by excision. Mixed extensive arteriovenous malformations are best managed by embolization alone; surgery is reserved for specific clinical problems. The need for biopsy should be considered if doubt exists as to the complete character of the lesion or lesions. In general, the treatment of angiodysplastic lesions with or without significant arteriovenous shunts is aimed at control rather than cure. Also, it should be recognized that the presence of an arteriovenous malformation alone does not necessitate aggressive treatment and that a conservative approach is prudent in the majority of situations. Amputation may represent an extreme outcome for some patients but may limit long-term morbidity associated with complications of the vascular lesion itself or serial surgical and nonsurgical procedures.

SUGGESTED READING

Hemingway AP. Angiodysplasias: current concepts. Postgrad Med J 1988; 64:259–263.

Lie JT. Pathology of angiodysplasia in Klippel-Trenaunay syndrome. Pathol Res Pract 1988; 183:747–755.

Malan E, Puglionisi A. Congenital angiodysplasia of the extremities. I. Generalities and classification: venous dysplasia. J Cardiovasc Surg 1964; 5:87–130.

Malan E, Puglionisi A. Congenital angiodysplasia of the extremities. II. Arterial, arterial and venous, and haemolymphatic dysplasia. J Cardiovasc Surg 1965; 6:255–345.

McAllister HA, Fenoglio JJ. Tumors of the cardiovascular system. Washington, D.C.: Armed Forces Institute of Pathology, 1978.

McGlennen RC, Manivel JC, Stanley SJ, et al. Pulmonary artery trunk sarcoma: a clinicopathologic, ultrastructure, and immunohistochemical study of four cases. Mod Pathol 1989; 2:486–494.

Schwartz RS, Osmundson PF, Hollier LH. Treatment and prognosis in congenital arteriovenous malformation of the extremity. Phlebology 1986; 1:171–180.

CONGENITAL VASCULAR MALFORMATIONS OF THE UPPER EXTREMITY: SURGICAL MANAGEMENT

FRANCISCO L. CANALES, M.D.
JOSEPH UPTON, M.D.

Until recently the field of congenital vascular anomalies was plagued by a confusing terminology that muddled the differences between hemangiomas and vascular malformations. Currently, vascular birthmarks are best differentiated by a biologic classification that relies on the endothelial characteristics of the particular lesion (Table 1). *Vascular malformations* have a normal rate of endothelial turnover, a normal mast cell count, and a normal growth cycle. In contrast, *hemangiomas* exhibit increased endothelial turnover and mast cell counts, and have a rapid postnatal growth followed by spontaneous involution (see Fig. 1).

Vascular malformations arise from defects in embryogenesis. By definition, they are present at birth but may not manifest themselves until later in life. They occur with equal frequency in males and females. Although they are usually sporadic, there are a few familial syndromes. Malformations are best categorized as capillary, arterial, venous, and lymphatic. These cell types may occur in isolation, but frequently there are two or more types within one lesion. The most common malformation is the venous type (see Figs. 2 to 5) followed by lymphatic (see Figs. 6 and 7), lymphaticovenous, and arteriovenous lesions (see Figs. 8 and 9). The flow characteristics of the latter allow further subdivision into high-flow and low-flow lesions (Table 2).

Approximately 10 to 15 percent of all vascular anomalies affect the upper extremity. Previously published data from The Children's Hospital in Boston revealed that hemangiomas outnumbered vascular malformations in a ratio of 1.5:1. However, from the standpoint of the upper extremity surgeon, vascular malformations can be much more disabling than hemangiomas. Bone deformity, nerve compression syndromes, and severe functional impairment can all result from vascular malformations.

INITIAL EVALUATION

Careful history taking and physical examination is essential. In most cases, this simple step will help the

Table 1 Terminology for Vascular Birthmarks

Old Terminology	New Terminology
Capillary	Hemangioma
Strawberry	Hemangioma
Port-wine	Capillary malformation
Capillary-cavernous	Hemangioma
Cavernous	Venous malformation
Venous	Venous malformation
Hemangiolymphangioma	Lymphatic malformation
Lymphangioma	Lymphatic malformation
Arteriovenous	Arteriovenous malformation

Table 2 Characteristics of Vascular Birthmarks

Hemangioma	*Malformation*
Clinical	
Usually nothing seen at birth; 30% present as red macule	All present at birth; may not be evident
Rapid postnatal proliferation and slow involution	Commensurate growth; may expand as a result of trauma, sepsis, hormonal modulation
Female:male ratio 1:1	Female:male ratio 1:1
Cellular	
Plump endothelium, increased turnover	Flat endothelium, slow turnover
Increased mast cells	Normal mast cell count
Multilaminated basement membrane	Normal thin basement membrane
Capillary tubule formation in vitro	Poor endothelial growth in vitro
Hematologic	
Primary platelet trapping; thrombocytopenia (Kasabach-Merritt syndrome)	Primary stasis (venous); localized consumptive coagulopathy
Radiologic	
Angiographic findings: well-circumscribed, intense lobular-parenchymal staining with equatorial vessels	Angiographic findings: diffuse, no parenchyma
	Low-flow: phleboliths, ectatic channels
	High-flow: enlarged, tortuous arteries with arteriovenous shunting
Skeletal	
Infrequent "mass effect" on adjacent bone; hypertrophy rare	Low-flow: distortion, hypertrophy, or hypoplasia
	High-flow: destruction, distortion, or hypertrophy

From Mulliken JB. Classification of vascular birthmarks. In: Mulliken JB, Young AE, eds. Vascular birthmarks: hemangiomas and malformations. Philadelphia: WB Saunders, 1988:35; with permission.

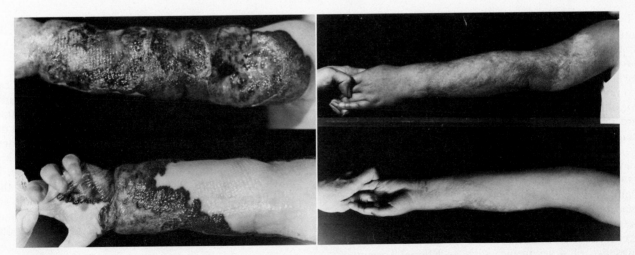

Figure 1 Hemangioma. *A,* Appearance of the dorsal and volar forearm and hand at age 1 year after a rapid postnatal growth phase. Central graying areas ("herald spots") are indicative of involution. Ulcerations were treated with local wound care. *B,* Appearance of the same area 6 years later. No surgery was performed. (From Upton J. Vascular malformations of the upper limb. In: Mulliken JB, Young AE, eds. Vascular birthmarks: hemangiomas and malformations. Philadelphia: WB Saunders, 1988:345; with permission.)

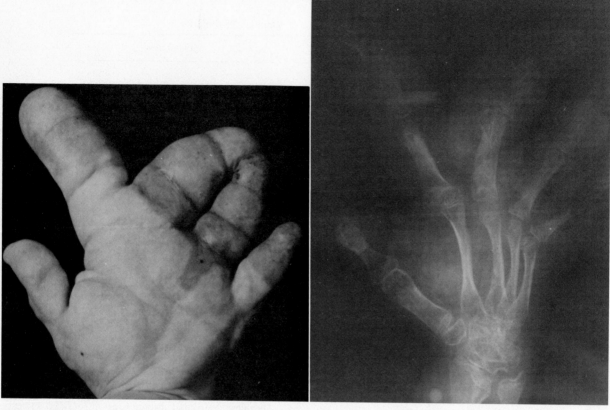

Figure 2 Malformation. *A,* Gigantism of the hand with macrodactyly is seen in a youngster with multiple, large, low-flow venous malformations. Note the areas of associated cutaneous capillary malformation (port-wine stain) involving the digits. Hand function was compromised by bulk and weight. *B,* Radiographic appearance demonstrates increased growth in both length and width of the skeleton. The mechanism of bone hypertrophy is unknown.

physician differentiate between a vascular malformation and a hemangioma. Hemangiomas are usually inconspicuous at birth, but subsequently have a characteristic proliferative phase that is usually followed by involution by ages 5 to 7 years (Fig. 1). In contrast, malformations do not involute and tend to grow commensurately with the child. They may be apparent at birth, but frequently are not and become obvious only with growth of the child.

During the initial evaluation, particular attention should be directed to the presenting signs and symptoms. Documentation of functional impairment of the upper limb, pain, weight, appearance, bleeding, ulceration, and maceration is essential in planning a rational course of treatment. Associated problems such as skeletal involvement should be noted, since they may denote the presence of a syndrome, such as Klippel-Trenaunay, Parkes-Weber, or Maffucci syndromes. Color photographs add an important element to the initial evaluation by serving as serial documentation of the growth and progression of the malformation.

The physical examination provides clues to the nature of the lesion. Venous malformations enlarge with dependency of the extremity and empty rapidly with elevation. Phleboliths can frequently be palpated within ectatic vascular channels.

Differentiation between low-flow and high-flow lesions should be readily apparent on examination. A thrill or bruit over the lesion indicates a high-flow arteriovenous malformation. The arteriovenous shunting that occurs in these high-flow lesions can lead to a "steal" syndrome of the distal extremity, with resultant neurologic symptoms, ischemia, and necrosis (see Figs. 8 and 9). Diagnostic occlusion of an extremity with a tourniquet, followed by reduction in the heart rate, is known as Branham's sign. This reflex, mediated by the vagus nerve, indicates hemodynamically significant arteriovenous shunting. It may be seen with proximal occlusion of either congenital or acquired arteriovenous malformations.

PRINCIPLES OF MANAGEMENT

The treatment of vascular anomalies of the upper limb should be directed toward maintenance and restoration of limb function. Aesthetic considerations, although important, are secondary. Initial management is usually supportive and nonoperative unless there is

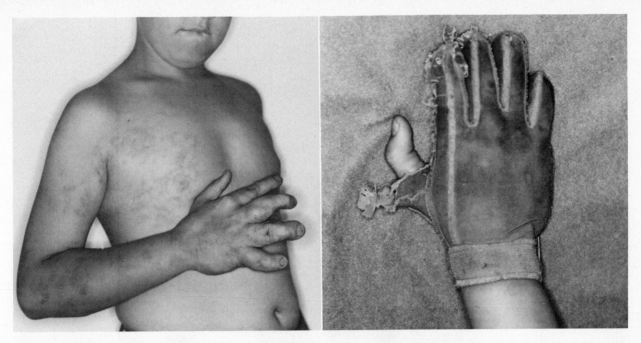

Figure 3 *A,* A large diffuse venous lesion involves the hand, arm, and ipsilateral chest wall. In the dependent position, the size of the hand and forearm circumference doubles. This lesion involves every skeletal and soft tissue structure in the hand. *B,* Although surgical debulkings can be performed, a compression garment provides a more practical method of treatment.

bleeding, infection, or cardiovascular compromise. Attention to local wound care is important. Lymphatic malformations are prone to frequent beta-streptococcal infections that respond to appropriate antibiotic management, local wound care, and meticulous hygiene. Splinting of the hand may help prevent contractures and preserve function.

Although it is tempting to proceed with early operative treatment, surgery should be considered only after conservative measures have failed. Treatment of asymptomatic lesions for cosmetic reasons should be performed only after careful consideration of the potential for anesthetic morbidity, loss of limb function, scarring, and disfigurement.

PREOPERATIVE EVALUATION

Before the decision is made to operate on an extensive lesion, a thorough diagnostic evaluation of the anatomy should be pursued. Plain radiographs should be obtained. Lymphatic malformations can be associated with skeletal hypertrophy, whereas high-flow lesions can lead to osseous destruction. If there is a suspicion that the malformation involves the bone itself, a computed tomographic (CT) or magnetic resonance imaging (MRI) scan should be obtained.

Although the above studies are important, contrast angiography forms the cornerstone of preoperative evaluation of large malformations. Digital subtraction angiography offers the opportunity to visualize the arterial system through an intravenous injection. When used as an initial diagnostic examination, this study provides a rough guide to the size and extent of the lesions and serves as a baseline for subsequent studies. The definitive study is properly performed selective arteriography that will provide more information in regard to the depth and three-dimensional characteristics of the vascular anomaly. Feeding vessels and abnormal communications between the venous and arterial systems can be visualized. The flow dynamics of the lesion can also be studied by selective catheterization, photographic subtraction, and proximal compression of the lesion. Recently, angiography has been combined with therapeutic embolization. Embolization can occasionally provide the definitive treatment, but usually it is performed to make the definitive surgical extirpation more manageable. Therapeutic embolization requires a highly skilled invasive radiologist, and its present use is restricted to head and neck, abdominal, and trunk lesions. Applications in the distal extremities are few because of the high probability of distal ischemia and gangrene.

Supplemental studies such as thermography, oxygen saturation, and plethysmography complete the preoperative evaluation but are not essential.

SURGICAL MANAGEMENT

Once a thorough preoperative evaluation is completed, a precise surgical plan is formulated. The use of loupe magnification or an operating microscope is imperative for preservation of neurovascular structures. The surgeon should be thoroughly familiar with the techniques of microsurgical reconstruction, because some radical resections necessitate re-establishing blood

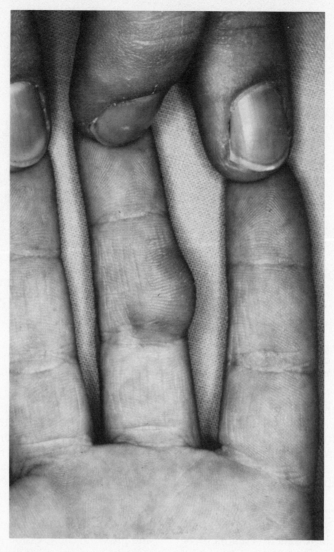

Figure 4 Venous malformation. A small compressible mass on a ring finger can be easily excised without extensive preoperative studies.

flow to an operated extremity once a major vascular lesion has been fully resected. Incisions should be planned to accommodate possible future operations. When a staged resection is necessary, the surgeon should undertake a complete resection of each area, so that reoperation in a previously scarred bed is avoided. Review of the principles outlined in Mulliken and Young's (1988) excellent text is recommended before extensive surgical ablation and reconstruction is undertaken.

CAPILLARY MALFORMATIONS

Popularly known as port-wine stains, capillary malformations occur alone infrequently in the upper extremity. Histologically, there is an increased number of ectatic vessels in the superficial dermis. As in other parts of the body, capillary malformations are present at birth and vary in color from pink to blue. With age, they develop a verrugated contour with a deep purple color.

In the past, conservative treatment was the mainstay of therapy. The application of cosmetics satisfactorily camouflages flat lesions, but make-up application is time-consuming and unacceptable to most children. The time required for daily treatment makes it an unpopular method even for adults. Excision of the lesion followed by skin grafting of the defect can also be performed, but the cosmetic result is not ideal. Excision and skin grafting should be considered primarily for thick, nodular port-wine stains.

The last 10 years have brought about an explosion of knowledge in the field of laser therapy. Initial encouraging results from the argon laser were tempered by

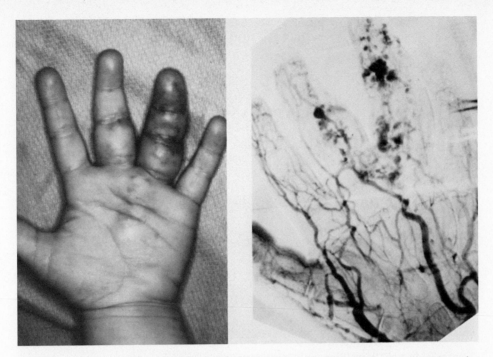

Figure 5 *A,* An extensive low-flow, predominantly venous malformation involves the palm and central two rays. *B,* The angiogram shows large tortuous vessels, varicosities, and saccular lakes. Arterial architecture is normal. The true extent of these lesions can never be completely visualized with these studies. Hand function and sensation approached normal.

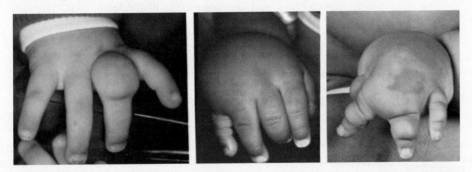

Figure 6 Lymphatic malformations in the hand may be localized to a single digit *(left),* the dorsal metacarpal portion of the hand *(center),* or the entire hand *(right).* The skin is hard, indurated, and minimally compressible. Cutaneous vesicles or blebs are common. Associated skeletal enlargement and cutaneous capillary malformations *(right)* may also be seen.

reports of hypertrophic scarring, especially in children, which was believed to be the result of nonselective damage to the epidermis and dermis. More recently, tunable dye lasers have yielded excellent results. With these lasers, the emitted wavelength can be varied to maximize absorption by the desired target, oxyhemoglobin. The most promising current therapy is photocoagulation with a pulsed dye laser, which has a very short burst of emitted energy. Light is emitted with a pulse duration shorter than the cooling time of oxyhemoglobin. Thus, the pulsed dye laser can create selective intravascular photocoagulation without allowing heat damage of adjacent structures. The initial results in the

treatment of flat port-wine stains with the pulsed dye laser have resulted in a greatly reduced incidence of hypertrophic scarring.

VENOUS MALFORMATIONS

These low-flow lesions are the most common vascular malformations of the upper limb. The spectrum ranges from congenital varicose veins to diffuse spongy malformations. Venous malformations may involve not only the epidermis and dermis, but any underlying structure, including bone (Fig. 2). They are found in

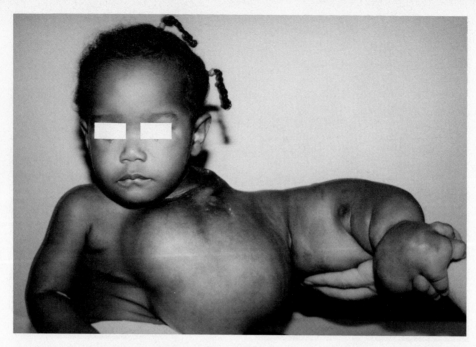

Figure 7 Lymphatic malformation. Massive enlargement of the entire extremity with chest wall, mediastinal, and neck involvement may be seen. The latter components have much larger cystic spaces, commonly called cystic hygromas. Extensive skeletal enlargement and weight of the extremity necessitated amputation despite initial attempts at debulking. (From Upton J. Vascular malformations of the upper limb. In: Mulliken JB, Young AE, eds. Vascular birthmarks: hemangiomas and malformations. Philadelphia: WB Saunders, 1988:363; with permission.)

several syndromes. Klippel-Trenaunay syndrome represents the concurrence of congenital varicose veins, capillary malformations, and limb hypertrophy. Maffucci's syndrome describes the association of dyschondroplasia and a vascular malformation, usually a complex venous or venous-lymphatic malformation.

Characteristic of venous malformations is tumescence with dependency of the extremity and rapid emptying with elevation. Symptoms may include pain and functional impairment. The size of the lesion and the presenting symptoms dictate treatment. A large, asymptomatic lesion that is problematic only with dependency of the extremity can be adequately managed with compressive garments (Fig. 3). Smaller lesions can usually be excised without much difficulty (Fig. 4). Treatment of symptomatic, extensive venous malformations should include preoperative angiographic investigation (Fig. 5), as well as a careful, staged operative plan. Often, it is not possible to radically excise a venous malformation owing to involvement of underlying vital structures. In this situation, subtotal resection in stages is preferable. Magnification, preferably using an operating microscope, and tourniquet ischemia are prerequisites for a meticulous dissection. Complications include hematoma, damage to underlying nerves and tendons, necrosis of the skin, and postoperative stiffness due to tendon adherence and joint contractures. With proper preparation and meticulous surgical technique,

these lesions can be safely excised. They are not hopeless problems.

LYMPHATIC MALFORMATIONS

Lymphatic malformations can present as diffuse swelling, focal lesions, or massive malformations involving the head and neck (Figs. 6 and 7). As with other types of malformations, the initial care is supportive and nonoperative. However, lymphatic malformations pose special problems. Superficial skin vesicles may result in open wounds that become the nidus for beta-streptococcal infections. Treatment consists of local wound care, antibiotics, immobilization of the affected extremity, and elevation. Recurrent infections may improve with long-term prophylactic antibiotic therapy.

Compression garments (Jobst) can control swelling, but in the upper extremity they are not as effective as with venous malformations. The use of sequential, intermittent pneumatic compression pumps sometimes has a dramatic effect, but requires time and strict adherence to the treatment. These pumps may be used during sleep.

Small, localized lymphatic malformations can be excised in one stage. Particular attention should be directed to the preservation of normal veins and the

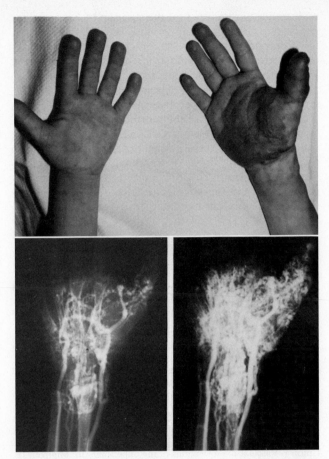

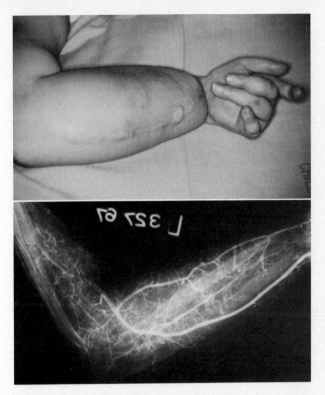

Figure 9 Arteriovenous fistula. *A,* This teenager presented with a Volkmann's ischemic contracture of the forearm caused by bleeding into an extensive malformation. Since childhood he had demonstrated pulsatile bruits over the volar forearm, which persisted despite aggressive attempts at individual ligations. *B,* Angiogram shows extensive fistulization. Below-elbow amputation was the eventual outcome.

Figure 8 Arteriovenous fistula. *A,* Appearance of the right hand in a 9-year-old girl. The hand is warm and has a pulsatile bruit throughout. Note the associated capillary malformation (port-wine stain). *B,* Angiographic views taken at 2 *(left)* and 3 *(right)* seconds after dye injection demonstrate extensive arteriovenous shunting in a 6-year-old girl who presented with a warm, swollen hand. This lesion is too extensive for adequate surgical ablation. She was treated with a compression garment.

excision of any redundant skin. Long-term results are excellent.

Large malformations of the upper extremity are often contiguous with axillary and chest wall abnormalities (Fig. 7). A single-stage procedure is a serious undertaking, but incontinuity resection may often be the procedure of choice. If anesthetic or hemodynamic considerations preclude a single-stage excision, removal of the upper extremity malformation can be followed by excision of the axillary and chest wall components. For removal of these large lesions, the incisions should be carefully planned to conserve as much normal skin as possible and to allow closure of the defect without tension. Liberal use of drains is recommended.

Generalized lymphedema is an entire subject in itself (see the chapter *Lymphedema*) and will be only briefly mentioned here. Serial debulkings have provided improvement in the bulk of massive extremities. These staged excisions should involve not more than one-half

of the circumference of the extremity at one time. The use of postoperative compression garments is recommended for maintenance of the achieved result. As with any lymphatic malformation, meticulous skin care and continued use of compression garments are essential in the long-term care of the patient.

ARTERIOVENOUS MALFORMATIONS

High-flow lesions constitute abnormal communications between the arterial and venous systems, bypassing a capillary bed. They can be extremely difficult to treat. The term "malformation" is usually reserved for congenital lesions, whereas acquired lesions are termed arteriovenous fistulas (Figs. 8 and 9). The pathophysiology is similar. There is arterial-to-venous shunting, dilatation of afferent arteries, reduced flow in the distal arteries, and increased venous pressure distal to the shunt. The reduced flow in the distal artery may lead to tissue ischemia, pain, ulceration, and soft tissue necrosis. Most congenital arteriovenous malformations have a multitude of arteries feeding into many veins, in contrast to one large channel as seen in post-traumatic or therapeutic (Brescia-type) fistulas.

The progression of size and symptoms should be carefully documented. Common presenting problems include pain, ulceration, paresthesias, hyperhidrosis, and increased warmth over the involved extremity. Cardiopulmonary compromise and consumption coagulopathies are rare, and limited to very large shunts. Associated limb hypertrophy is seen in Parkes-Weber syndrome.

Initial treatment consists of graduated elastic compression garments, which counteract the venous hypertension that accounts for the swelling and heaviness of the extremity. Invariably, growth of the child will lead to enlargement of the arteriovenous malformation. The severity and progression of symptoms dictate the timing of surgical intervention (Fig. 9).

The preoperative evaluation hinges on a detailed selective arteriogram. Owing to the high-flow shunting through a multitude of abnormal channels, the true extent of the lesion is difficult to determine. Intimate knowledge of normal and abnormal arterial anatomy is essential for the formulation of a careful preoperative plan.

Simple proximal ligation of feeding vessels is inadequate treatment. This procedure promotes further collateralization, decreases the distal arterial pressure, and may increase ischemia. Although selective embolization has been used successfully in the head and neck and abdomen, its use for high-flow arteriovenous malformations of the upper extremity is often accompanied by distal ischemia and gangrene. Complete resection of extensive arteriovenous malformations under tourniquet control and magnification is the preferred treatment. If total excision proves difficult or impossible, subtotal resections may need to be staged. The possibility of devascularization of the extremity with resection of the malformation requires that the surgeon be prepared for revascularization with autogenous vein grafts.

Complications from treatment of these difficult lesions are frequent. Infection, hematoma, persistent leaking through the wound, compromise of skin flaps, and ischemia of the distal extremity are potential pitfalls. Extreme care in preoperative planning and meticulous technique will minimize the morbidity of the procedure. The results of aggressive resection can be gratifying, but some extensive arteriovenous malformations may be recalcitrant to all forms of treatment and may necessitate amputation of the extremity. Extensive arteriovenous malformations challenge even the most experienced and confident hand surgeon.

SUGGESTED READING

Boyd JB, Mulliken JB, Kaban LB, et al. Skeletal changes associated with vascular malformations. Plast Reconstr Surg 1984; 74:789–795.

Mulliken JB, Glowacki J. Hemangiomas and vascular malformations in infants and children: a classification based on endothelial characteristics. Plast Reconstr Surg 1982; 69:412–420.

Mulliken JB, Young AE, eds. Vascular birthmarks. Philadelphia: WB Saunders, 1988.

Newmeyer WL. Vascular disorders. In: Green DP, ed. Operative hand surgery. 2nd ed. New York: Churchill Livingstone, 1988:2391.

Niechajev IA, Karlsson S. Vascular tumours of the hand. Scand J Plast Reconstr Surg 1982; 16:67–75.

Tan OT, Sherwood K, Gilchrest BA. Treatment of children with port-wine stains using the flashlamp-pulsed tunable dye laser. N Engl J Med 1989; 320:416–421.

Upton J. Vascular malformations of the upper limb. In: Mulliken JB, Young AE, eds. Vascular birthmarks. Philadelphia: WB Saunders, 1988:343.

Upton J, Mulliken JB, Murray JE. Classification and rationale for management of vascular anomalies in the upper extremity. J Hand Surg 1989; 10A:970–975.

HYPERCOAGULOPATHIES AND VASCULAR THROMBOSIS

ANDREW I. SCHAFER, M.D.

Although the concept of hypercoagulability was clearly recognized by Rudolf Virchow over 130 years ago, it has only been in recent years that specific disorders of coagulation have been causally associated with a thrombotic tendency. There is evidence that these hypercoagulable states are remarkably common, necessitating an understanding of their diagnosis and management by clinicians of many specialties.

PATHOPHYSIOLOGY AND CLINICAL MANIFESTATIONS

Patients who are unusually predisposed to thrombosis can be categorized as those with secondary and those with primary hypercoagulable states. The secondary hypercoagulable states generally involve acquired systemic conditions that are associated with an increased risk of thromboembolic complications. Cancer, the myeloproliferative disorders, pregnancy, the use of oral contraceptives, and the postoperative state are common examples of secondary hypercoagulable states. The pathogenesis of thrombosis in these patients is usually complex and multifactorial.

The primary hypercoagulable states are abnormalities of specific coagulation factors that generally cause a lifelong thrombotic diathesis. Many of these are inherited disorders. It is now recognized that the human body is normally endowed with an array of physiologic antithrombotic mechanisms. These operate to prevent thrombosis in the absence of vascular damage and, when vascular injury does occur, to localize the hemostatic plug precisely to the site of injury. Prostacyclin (PGI_2) is a product of vascular endothelial cells that is a potent inhibitor of platelet activation and a vasodilator. Lipoprotein-associated coagulation inhibitor (LACI), also referred to as extrinsic pathway inhibitor, blocks the extrinsic pathway of coagulation by forming a complex with factor X_a, tissue factor, and factor VII_a. As yet no specific PGI_2 or LACI deficiency states have been described that cause a hereditary predisposition to thrombosis. Antithrombin III (ATIII) is the major serine protease inhibitor that neutralizes the actions of thrombin and several other activated coagulation factors. Inherited heterozygous ATIII deficiency, due to either an absolute quantitative deficiency or a functional abnormality of the protein, leads to a lifelong thrombotic tendency. Protein C is a vitamin K–dependent factor that is activated to protein C_a when thrombin is bound to specific endothelial cell surface sites (termed "thrombomodulin"). Protein C_a acts as an anticoagulant with its cofactor protein S, another vitamin K–dependent protein, by destroying activated factors VIII and V and possibly also by stimulating the fibrinolytic system. Inherited heterozygous protein C or protein S deficiency is associated in some patients with a lifelong predisposition to thrombosis. Homozygous protein C deficiency causes fatal neonatal purpura fulminans. Both quantitative and functional variants of these protein deficiency states have been described. Finally, the fibrinolytic system functions to generate the active lytic enzyme plasmin from its inactive plasma precursor plasminogen by endothelium-derived tissue plasminogen activator (tPA). Fibrinolytic defects, including quantitative deficiency and qualitative abnormalities of plasminogen and deficiency of tPA, have been considered to cause a thrombotic diathesis.

The most common types of thrombotic complications that occur in patients with primary hypercoagulable states are deep vein thrombosis (DVT) and pulmonary embolism (PE). Other, more unusual sites of venous thrombosis are occasionally encountered, but arterial thrombosis is distinctly unusual. The first thrombotic event can occur at any age, but there is a peculiar clustering of initial episodes in young adulthood. In most cases a precipitating event can be identified. These inciting factors include many of the secondary hypercoagulable states such as pregnancy, surgery, immobilization, or the use of oral contraceptives. An unknown percentage, perhaps the majority, of patients with inherited primary hypercoagulable states remain asymptomatic throughout much of their lives and are detected only in the course of family studies or screening tests for research purposes. Lifelong prophylactic anticoagulation is usually recommended for patients who have had one or more clinical thromboembolic events, but the role of prophylactic anticoagulation for asymptomatic individuals with primary hypercoagulable states remains unsettled.

DIAGNOSIS

The diagnostic search for an underlying hypercoagulable state in patients who have suffered thromboembolic events must be strictly individualized. Clearly, a young and otherwise healthy patient with recurrent thrombosis merits a more vigorous and comprehensive diagnostic approach than does a patient who has developed a thrombotic complication associated with terminal metastatic cancer.

Evaluation for a secondary hypercoagulable state should be guided by the clinical presentation of previous thrombotic events. For example, patients who develop hepatic vein (Budd-Chiari) or portal vein thrombosis should be worked up for a myeloproliferative disorder (including polycythemia vera "masked" by concomitant iron deficiency) and paroxysmal nocturnal hemoglobinuria (PNH). An underlying malignancy should be suspected in patients presenting with migratory superficial thrombosis (Trousseau's syndrome) or nonbacterial thrombotic endocarditis (NBTE). There are conflicting data in the literature about whether deep vein thrombosis (DVT) and PE are harbingers of an occult malignancy. Unless symptoms or physical signs suggest a specific site of cancer in such previously healthy patients with DVT or PE, evaluation beyond a thorough physical examination, testing of stool for occult blood, and routine chest radiography is not generally recommended. Women with habitual spontaneous abortions should be tested for the presence of a lupus anticoagulant. Finally, in patients with recurrent arterial thrombosis, secondary hypercoagulable states such as a myeloproliferative disorder, diabetes mellitus, hypercholesterolemia, or homocystinuria should be considered. In some cases, routine laboratory test abnormalities may suggest the cause of hypercoagulability: e.g., a prolonged partial thromboplastin time (PTT) with the lupus anticoagulant or thrombocytopenia with thrombotic thrombocytopenic purpura (TTP).

After secondary hypercoagulable states have been ruled out, many patients with a history of thrombosis should be evaluated for primary hypercoagulable states. A particularly high index of suspicion for such disorders should be entertained in patients without other risk factors who develop thromboembolism as young adults, and in those with positive family histories of thrombotic problems.

The methods and timing of laboratory testing for primary hypercoagulable states are crucial. Both immunologic (antigenic) and functional (biologic) assays are available for quantitating ATIII, protein C, protein S, and plasminogen. In classic cases, there is a quantitative deficiency of a biologically normal protein, and these disorders can be detected by conventional immunologic assays (Laurell rocket electrophoresis, enzyme-linked immunoabsorbent assay, radioimmunoassay, and others). However, many patients with deficiencies of these proteins have qualitative variants that cause a functional defect in anticoagulant activity even though antigenic levels are normal. Therefore, whenever possible, functional rather than immunologic assays should be used to screen for these disorders. The laboratory testing for protein S deficiency is more complicated, since 60 to 65 percent of the plasma protein S is normally bound to C4b-binding protein, and the functionally active protein S resides in the free form. In patients with heterozygous deficiency states, the decreased level of ATIII, protein C, or protein S may be sufficiently high to overlap with the lower limits of the normal range. In these cases, repeat assays or family studies may be required to make the diagnosis. These not infrequently encountered borderline situations also highlight the need to consider carefully the circumstances under which the tests are taken, since the levels of these proteins can be significantly influenced by several variables.

Transient decreases in levels of ATIII, protein C, and protein S can be found during active thrombosis even in patients without congenital deficiencies of these proteins. Therefore, it generally is not advisable to obtain these tests around the time of acute thromboembolism, even though it could be argued that the finding of a normal level of a protein in these situations essentially rules out a deficiency state. Since the approach to anticoagulation for a patient with DVT or PE (beginning with full-dose heparin or a thrombolytic agent, and followed by at least a 3-month course of warfarin or adjusted-dose subcutaneous heparin) is the same regardless of whether the patient has an underlying primary hypercoagulable state, there is no urgency in making the diagnosis of a hereditary deficiency. It is only after the 3-month course of prophylactic anticoagulation following DVT or PE that the clinician has to consider whether anticoagulation should be continued indefinitely (if a hereditary hypercoagulable state is found) or discontinued.

Concurrent use of anticoagulants complicates the measurements of ATIII, protein C, and protein S. Oral anticoagulants can raise the level of ATIII. In patients with ATIII deficiency, therefore, warfarin occasionally raises levels of the protein into the normal range, thereby masking the deficiency state. ATIII levels return to baseline approximately 3 to 6 days after discontinuation of warfarin. Systemic heparin administration can decrease ATIII levels by as much as 30 percent, an effect that disappears 2 to 3 days after stopping the anticoagulant.

Both immunologic and functional levels of proteins C and S are decreased during warfarin therapy, along with levels of the other vitamin K–dependent coagulation factors. Under these conditions, therefore, detection of protein C or protein S deficiency can be difficult. If temporary discontinuation of warfarin therapy is not deemed to be clinically safe for the purpose of determining levels of proteins C and S, an alternative approach is to simultaneously measure antigenic levels of another vitamin K–dependent factor (e.g., prothrombin or factor X). In patients on warfarin therapy who are not congenitally protein C or protein S deficient, levels of all vitamin K–dependent factors should be proportionately decreased. In these cases, therefore, the ratios of protein C or S antigen to prothrombin antigen or protein C or S antigen to factor X antigen should remain near unity. In patients with a congenital deficiency state who are on warfarin therapy, however, a disproportionately low level of protein C or S antigen will be found. Measurements of these ratios are valid only during fully stabilized warfarin therapy. Severe liver disease and other vitamin K deficiency states likewise decrease the levels of all vitamin K–dependent plasma proteins, including proteins C and S.

Levels of ATIII, protein C, and protein S may also be transiently suppressed during the third trimester of pregnancy, with oral contraceptive therapy, and with disseminated intravascular coagulation, or, as noted above, with active thrombosis. Therefore, blood tests for these proteins are most reliably determined in patients who are not acutely ill, not pregnant, and not on anticoagulant therapy.

ANTICOAGULANT THERAPY

The indications for and contraindications to the use of thrombolytic agents in the treatment of acute thrombosis are generally not modified by the presence of an underlying primary hypercoagulable state. However, some special considerations apply to the use of heparin and oral anticoagulants in these patients.

The traditional treatment of patients with proximal DVT or PE is initial therapy with intravenous heparin for several days, followed by prophylactic anticoagulant therapy (with warfarin or adjusted-dose subcutaneous heparin) for 3 months or more. In patients with an underlying primary hypercoagulable state who have had a thrombotic event, oral anticoagulant therapy should be continued indefinitely, probably for life.

The treatment of choice for acute thrombosis is continuous intravenous heparin. This is initially given as an intravenous bolus of 5,000 U, followed by a continuous dose of 20,000 to 40,000 U per 24 hours. The activated PTT should be checked 4 to 6 hours after the initial bolus, and the continuous heparin dose should be titrated to maintain the PTT above 1.5 times the control level. If the PTT exceeds 2.5 times control, the continuous infusion should be interrupted for 1 hour and then restarted at a total daily heparin dose reduced by 2,000 to 4,000 U. Once the heparin dose has been stabilized, the PTT can be checked once daily for the duration of full-dose heparin therapy. Increased doses of heparin are generally required for a short period immediately after a thrombotic event. However, subsequent variations in apparent anticoagulant effect are usually caused by technical problems with the intravenous infusion or in laboratory monitoring, rather than changes in heparin clearance.

Heparin acts as an anticoagulant by binding to ATIII and thereby greatly accelerating the ability of ATIII to neutralize thrombin and other coagulation enzymes. Since the action of heparin is mediated by ATIII, deficiency of ATIII would be expected to cause a state of heparin resistance. Although this phenomenon has been observed in some patients with ATIII deficiency, it tends to occur only in patients with very severe reductions in ATIII levels, and is usually managed by administering increased amounts of heparin with careful monitoring of the PTT.

Long-term prophylactic anticoagulant therapy for DVT or PE is directed toward preventing recurrent thromboembolism. The usual regimen is warfarin at doses adjusted to maintain a prothrombin time (PT) between 1.3 to 1.5 times control, using rabbit brain thromboplastin. This guideline represents a recently revised recommendation for warfarin usage, based on the recognition that American physicians have been for many years erroneously monitoring the PT according to a therapeutic range established for the more sensitive human brain thromboplastin reagents used in Europe.

It has been common practice to begin anticoagulant treatment of DVT or PE with a 10-day course of full-dose continuous heparin, with warfarin added on days 5 to 10 to ensure a crossover period of 4 to 5 days before heparin is discontinued. It has been recently demonstrated, however, that a shorter course of heparin administered by continuous intravenous infusion (5 days), in which warfarin is instituted on the first day, is equally effective and safe in preventing recurrent thromboembolism.

An alternative to warfarin is adjusted-dose subcutaneous heparin. The starting dose is determined from the patient's initial intravenous heparin dose requirement; one-third of the 24-hour intravenous heparin dose is initially injected every 12 hours, and then adjusted to achieve a PTT above 1.5 times the control value at the halfway mark (at 6 hours) between injections. This approach is as effective as warfarin, and may be safer than warfarin in pregnant women (see below), patients with liver disease, and those whose anticoagulation cannot be reliably monitored over the long-term. Low-dose subcutaneous heparin (5,000 U every 12 hours) may be effective in preventing thromboembolism in some general surgical patients who have not had previous thrombotic problems, but not preventing recurrent thromboembolism in patients with established DVT or PE. The transvenous insertion of a Greenfield filter or other methods of interrupting the inferior vena cava should be considered to prevent PE in patients with DVT in whom anticoagulation is absolutely contraindicated, or in those who suffer recurrent thromboembolism while therapeutically anticoagulated.

In contrast to heparin, the anticoagulant effect of warfarin is influenced by many factors that can alter an individual patient's response. Diet and some drugs can alter absorption, while other drugs and various diseases can modify the metabolism and excretion of warfarin. Therefore, changes in the medical condition of the patient require special precautions in monitoring warfarin anticoagulation.

A major concern with warfarin therapy is the risk of warfarin skin necrosis. This rare complication is characterized by the sudden development of a localized, painful skin lesion, initially erythematous or hemorrhagic in appearance, which then becomes bullous and eventually culminates in gangrenous necrosis. Although the site of involvement is unpredictable, there is a striking predilection for areas of increased subcutaneous fat content such as the breasts, thighs, and buttocks. Pathology testing of the skin lesions typically shows thrombosis of the dermal capillaries and venules. In most cases, the skin necrosis appears between the third and sixth days of initiation of warfarin. It has been particularly noted that it tends to occur when large loading doses of warfarin are administered, and even in the presence of simultaneous heparin anticoagulation. Approximately one-third of patients who develop this potentially serious complication of warfarin have underlying protein C deficiency. Since protein C has a shorter half-life than factor IX, factor X, and prothrombin, it has been proposed that this unusual form of thrombosis is due to a transiently increased hypercoagulability of congenitally protein C–deficient patients, because warfarin-induced suppression of an already reduced protein C level occurs before the drug can exert its effect on the longer-lived procoagulant factors. In protein C–deficient patients, it is possible to avoid this complication by covering patients with heparin and initiating warfarin therapy at a low dose (2 mg per day). The rare occurrence of skin necrosis should certainly not be considered to contraindicate warfarin therapy for these patients, since long-term oral anticoagulation has been clearly demonstrated to be effective in preventing recurrent thrombosis.

Purified concentrates of ATIII have recently been licensed in the United States for management of congenitally deficient patients. ATIII concentrates should be effective in preventing thrombosis in these patients during periods of increased risk such as the peripartum period (see below) and the postoperative state. Rare ATIII-deficient patients with recurrent thrombosis that is refractory to anticoagulation may also respond to infusions of ATIII concentrates. The risk of viral transmission by use of this blood product should be negligible, since heat treatment or other viral inactivating methods are routinely used in the manufacturing process. It has been demonstrated that the intravenous infusion of 1 ATIII IU per kg body weight leads to a rise in ATIII activity of about 2 percent, with a half-life of about 2 to 3 days. The in vivo recovery of ATIII may be significantly lower, however, in acutely ill patients.

SPECIAL THERAPEUTIC CONSIDERATIONS

Pregnancy

There is a strikingly increased risk of thrombosis during pregnancy, particularly in the peripartum period, in women with underlying primary hypercoagulable states. Prophylactic anticoagulation is clearly indicated during pregnancy in these patients.

Warfarin and other coumarin derivatives cross the placenta. When administered during the first trimester, these oral anticoagulants can cause spontaneous abortions in up to about 40 percent of patients and can produce a characteristic embryopathy, including nasal hypoplasia and stippled epiphyses, in up to 30 percent. The teratogenic effects of warfarin have been specifically noted between the sixth and 12th weeks of gestation. It has also been suggested that the use of coumarin derivatives during the last two trimesters of pregnancy may result in central nervous system or eye abnormalities, although these complications have not been observed in other studies. The use of warfarin at the time of delivery has been associated with an increased incidence of stillbirths and neonatal deaths due to hemorrhage, as well as an increased risk of maternal bleeding.

In view of these considerations, women with primary hypercoagulable states who are on prophylactic warfarin therapy should discontinue this drug as soon as pregnancy is diagnosed, and should be switched to subcutaneous adjusted-dose heparin (see above) for the remainder of the pregnancy and the immediate postpartum period. Heparin does not cross the placenta; it has been considered to be safe for the fetus and associated with an acceptable risk of bleeding in the mother. It has been suggested by others that this strategy of heparin throughout pregnancy be also used in women who have had previous DVT or PE even in the absence of a clearly defined underlying hypercoagulable state. Heparin causes cumulative dose-related osteoporosis, but clinically important effects of heparin on bone density are not usually observed with prophylactic heparin use throughout pregnancy. The administration of ATIII concentrates for women with ATIII deficiency during labor and delivery should be considered.

Cancer

Both the diagnosis and management of thrombosis in cancer patients involve some special considerations. The diagnosis of DVT in patients with pelvic tumors may be complicated. Neither impedance plethysmography (IPG) nor Doppler ultrasonography can differentiate between thrombosis and extrinsic compression of the veins in the lower extremities. Even the venogram can be difficult to interpret under these circumstances. CT of the iliac veins or inferior vena cava can be helpful in this situation. One approach in cancer patients with suspected acute DVT is to use the IPG as a screening test; proximal DVT is highly unlikely if this study is negative, but if it is positive, a venogram with or without CT scan is required to establish the diagnosis.

In some patients with lung cancer or pulmonary metastases, the clinical diagnosis of PE and interpretation of a ventilation-perfusion lung scan may be equivocal. Because of the increased bleeding risks of long-term anticoagulation (especially in patients with brain metastases or pericardial involvement), pulmonary angiography should be performed when the diagnosis of PE is uncertain.

The initial therapy for cancer patients with acute thromboembolism is generally the same as for those without cancer. The presence of brain or pericardial metastases and recent surgery are relative contraindications to anticoagulation. Therefore, in these patients, the insertion of a Greenfield filter to interrupt the inferior vena cava should be performed electively after initiating therapy with heparin; this approach avoids the need for long-term anticoagulation in these patients. A relative state of heparin resistance is encountered in some patients with malignancies. A dissociation between plasma levels of circulating heparin (measured by protamine titration) and the PTT is sometimes found in such situations. Some experts have advocated following the heparin levels in these cases, rather than aiming for a therapeutic PTT. However, it is also reasonable to cautiously administer heparin doses that are sufficient to raise the PTT into the therapeutic range, while carefully monitoring the patient for signs of bleeding.

The duration of warfarin or adjusted-dose subcutaneous heparin treatment in cancer patients who have had a thrombotic event may have to be extended beyond the usually recommended 3 months, since they are at continued high risk for recurrence as long as there is persistent tumor. It may be reasonable to continue prophylactic anticoagulation indefinitely in these patients, although the increased risk of bleeding must be recognized.

When recurrent thromboembolism occurs in a cancer patient on warfarin maintenance while the PT is subtherapeutic, another course of full-dose heparin should be administered and the subsequent warfarin dose increased. If recurrent thromboembolism occurs while the patient is therapeutically anticoagulated with warfarin, another course of full-dose heparin should be given, followed by adjusted-dose subcutaneous heparin. Consideration should also be given to placement of a Greenfield filter.

Indwelling central venous catheters in cancer patients are prone to thrombotic occlusion. It has been suggested that very-low-dose warfarin (1 mg daily), which is insufficient to change the PT, is effective in maintaining catheter patency.

SUGGESTED READING

Comp PC. Hereditary disorders predisposing to thrombosis. Prog Hemostas Thromb 1986; 8:71–102.

Ginsberg JS, Kowalchuk G, Hirsh J, et al. Heparin therapy during pregnancy. Risks to the fetus and mother. Arch Intern Med 1989; 149:2233–2236.

Levine M, Hirsh J. The diagnosis and treatment of thrombosis in the cancer patient. Semin Oncol 1990; 17:160–171.

Luzzatto G, Schafer AI. The prethrombotic states in cancer. Semin Oncol 1990; 17:147–159.

Raskob GE, Carter CJ, Hull RD. Anticoagulant therapy for venous thromboembolism. Prog Hemostas Thromb 1989; 9:1–27.

Schafer AI. Focusing the clot: normal and pathologic mechanisms. Annu Rev Med 1987; 38:211–220.

LUPUS ANTICOAGULANT, ANTICARDIOLIPIN ANTIBODIES, AND THE ANTIPHOSPHOLIPID SYNDROMES

J. MICHAEL BACHARACH, M.D., M.P.H.
J. T. LIE, M.D.

In recent years, there has been a growing awareness of autoimmune phenomena and immune-mediated mechanisms in the pathogenesis of vascular diseases. This chapter briefly reviews the known association between a family of autoantibodies directed against anionic phospholipids and their clinical manifestations, together with a rational approach toward diagnosis and treatment of the antiphospholipid syndromes.

BRIEF HISTORICAL PERSPECTIVE

Antiphospholipid antibodies represent a heterogeneous group of autoantibodies to anionic phospholipids. These antibodies were first recognized with the phenomenon of the so-called biologically false-positive VDRL (venereal disease research laboratory) test in serologic testing for syphilis, and then later identified as immunoglobulins that interfere with phospholipid-dependent clotting tests. Their association with systemic lupus erythematosus (SLE) resulted in the term "lupus anticoagulant." Subsequently, an associated increased inci-

Table 1 Clinical Manifestations of Antiphospholipid Syndromes

Venous thrombosis
    Recurrent deep vein and vena cava thrombosis
    Cerebral and retinal vein thrombosis
    Budd-Chiari syndrome
    Visceral/splanchnic vein thrombosis
    Adrenal vein thrombosis (Addison's disease)

Arterial thrombosis
    Peripheral arterial thrombosis
    Carotid and retinal artery thrombosis
    Coronary thrombosis; cardiac chamber thrombosis; marantic endocarditis
    Pulmonary hypertension/recurrent pulmonary thromboembolism
    Visceral/splanchnic arterial thrombosis

Obstetric complications
    Recurrent fetal loss
    Fetal distress in utero
    Preeclampsia
    Postpartum syndrome

Neurologic disorders
    Ischemic infarction
    Transient ischemic attacks
    Postinfarction dementia
    Cerebral venous thrombosis

Hematologic abnormalities
    Thrombocytopenia
    Positive Coombs test with or without hemolytic anemia

Miscellaneous
    Livedo reticularis and stroke (Sneddon's syndrome)
    Chorea
    Lupoid sclerosis/myelopathy
    Guillain-Barré syndrome
    Degos' disease

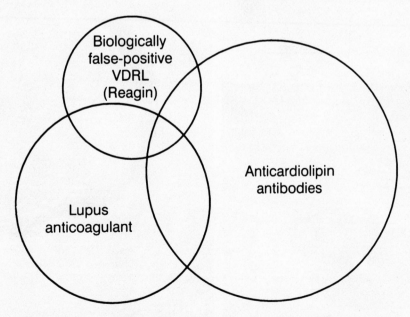

Figure 1 A hypothetical relationship of the prevalence of the three major antiphospholipid antibodies in various diseases.

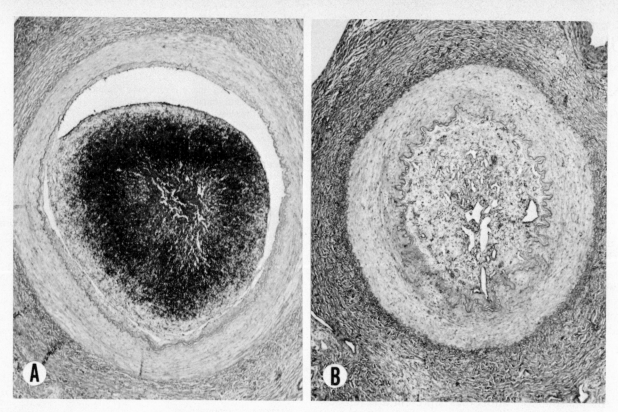

Figure 2 Large-vessel, recent *(A)* and old *(B)* arterial thrombosis in primary antiphospholipid syndrome. (H & E: ×40.)

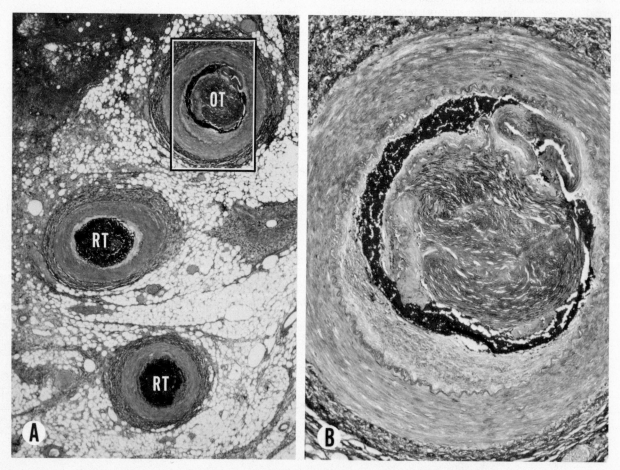

Figure 3 *A,* Small-vessel, recent (RT) and old (OT) arterial and venous thrombosis. *B,* Close-up view of the boxed area of old (OT) arterial thrombosis in *A.* (H & E: *A,* ×16; *B,* ×64.)

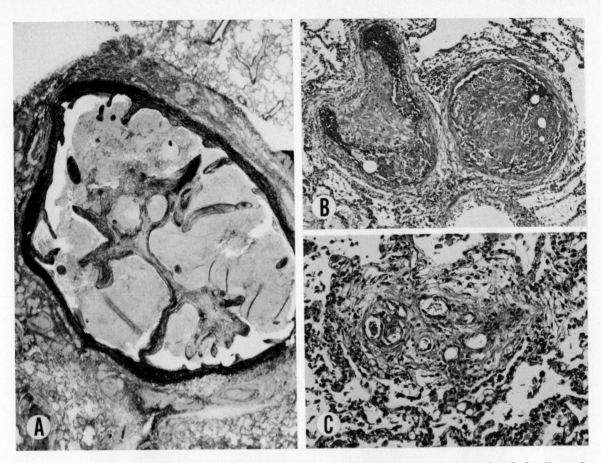

Figure 4 Recurrent pulmonary thromboembolism: *A,* Large vessel with old, organized embolus. *B,* Small vessels with recurrent emboli. *C,* Small vessel with organizing embolus. (H & E: *A,* ×40; *B* and *C,* ×160.)

dence of venous and arterial thrombosis was described in patients with lupus anticoagulant activity. The development of a radioimmunoassay for anticardiolipin antibodies has been instrumental in furthering the study of antiphospholipid antibodies and their role in various forms of vascular disease. Figure 1 shows schematically the presumed relationship between the major antiphospholipid antibodies.

The association of antiphospholipid antibodies and arterial and venous thrombosis was initially described in patients with SLE. Subsequently, it has been recognized that antiphospholipid antibodies and their associated vascular problems can occur in patients without SLE or evidence of any of the other connective tissue diseases. These findings support the concept of a primary antiphospholipid syndrome in distinction to the similar vascular occlusive disease associated with SLE, a lupus-like disease, or another connective tissue disease (secondary antiphospholipid syndrome).

CLINICAL MANIFESTATIONS

The clinical spectrum associated with antiphospholipid syndromes is broad, and a detailed review of these syndromes is beyond the scope of this chapter. The best

known and most extensively studied clinical manifestation associated with antiphospholipid antibodies is venous thrombosis; however, arterial occlusive disease involving multiple sites has also been well documented. Other clinical manifestations include recurrent fetal loss presumed to be on the basis of placental thrombosis with infarction; stroke; transient ischemic attacks; and a variety of less common disorders including thrombocytopenia, livedo reticularis, migraine, and chorea. Table 1 summarizes the known clinical manifestations associated with antiphospholipid antibodies.

POSSIBLE PATHOGENIC MECHANISMS

The specific role of antiphospholipid antibodies in the development of vascular occlusive disease remains obscure. The proposed pathogenesis implicates cellular-humoral interactions involving the platelets, endothelial cells, prostacyclin production, and thrombomodulin-mediated activation of protein C. The exact mechanism is unknown, but evidence points to a complex interplay between the antiphospholipid immunoglobulins and the activation of coagulation cascade that results in thrombophilia. Although vasculitis may be an independent, albeit uncommon, manifestation of the underlying dis-

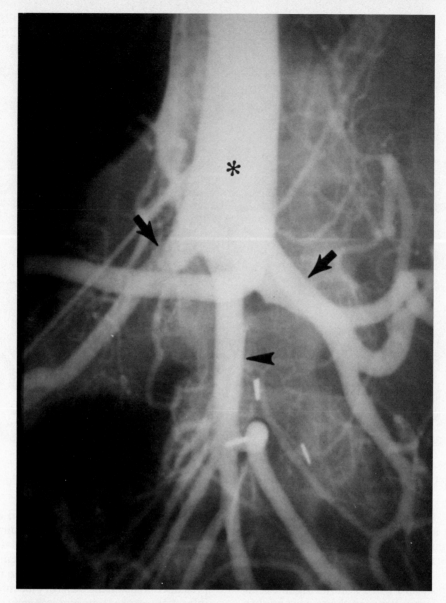

Figure 5 Abdominal aortogram showing thrombotic occlusion of the abdominal aorta (*) below level of renal arteries *(arrows)*. Note that the superior mesenteric artery *(arrowhead)* is projected over the course of the occluded aorta.

ease, the histologic hallmarks of vascular disease in antiphospholipid syndromes are almost exclusively large- and small-vessel recurrent arterial and venous thrombosis (Figs. 2 to 4).

DIAGNOSIS AND MANAGEMENT CONSIDERATIONS

Once suspected, the location and extent of vascular occlusive disease should be systematically evaluated. In addition to the routine physical examination and laboratory studies, noninvasive vascular evaluations, including duplex ultrasonography, are often necessary. Selective angiographic studies should be performed to localize

and characterize the nature of arterial and venous thrombosis (Figs. 5 and 6).

Rapidly accumulating clinical experience suggests that detection of lupus anticoagulant and anticardiolipin antibodies provides useful information for the diagnosis and management of patients with unexplained vascular occlusive disease. However, the available data indicate that indiscriminative screening for these antibodies in the general population is ineffective in identifying those at risk for the development of vascular occlusive disease. On the other hand, prospective testing for cardiolipin antibodies in a target population, such as pregnant SLE patients, has been shown to be of benefit in the management of unexplained recurrent fetal loss.

In patients with unexplained vascular occlusive

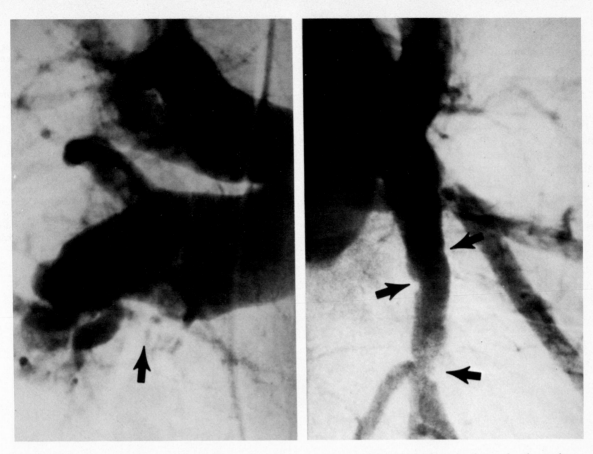

Figure 6 Recurrent pulmonary emboli: *A,* Pulmonary arteriogram of the right lung in the early phase shows occlusion of the lower lobe artery *(arrow). B,* Left lower lobe artery shows evidence of old emboli that have partially recanalized, as noted by luminal irregularities *(arrows).*

Table 2 Prevalence and Types of Unexplained Vascular Occlusive Disease in 102 Patients with Anticardiolipin Antibodies

Clinical Manifestations	No. of Patients	No. Without CTD
Arterial occlusive disease	11	7
Venous occlusive disease	17	14
Cerebrovascular occlusive disease	27	22
Coronary thrombosis	3	3
Visceral arterial/venous thrombosis	5	5
Fetal loss	17	14
	80	65

CTD, connective tissue disease.

disease, testing for antiphospholipid antibodies is important in establishing the diagnosis of recurrent thrombosis. In a recently completed study at the Mayo Clinic, we analyzed clinical and serologic findings in a series of 102 consecutive patients tested positively for antiphospholipid antibodies as detected by an enzyme-linked immunosorbent assay (ELISA) for anticardiolipin antibodies. The prevalence of associated unexplained vascular occlusive disease in this cohort was 80 patients, or 78 percent. Of these 80 with unexplained vascular occlusive disease, 65 (81 percent) showed no evidence of an underlying connective tissue disease. Our observations thus provide further support for the concept of primary or secondary antiphospholipid syndromes, and underscore the importance of testing patients with unexplained vascular occlusive disease (Table 2).

THERAPY

The mainstay of treatment for patients with recurrent thrombosis and elevated antiphospholipid antibodies is long-term anticoagulation and antiplatelet therapy. Preliminary data suggest that a combination of corticosteroid and aspirin (prednisone, 40 to 60 mg per day and aspirin, 75 mg per day) may prevent recurrent fetal loss in pregnant women who have lupus anticoagulant. There are ongoing trials attempting to confirm the efficacy of immunosuppression with corticosteroids. There is as yet no conclusive evidence of the beneficial role of corticosteroids in patients with recurrent venous or arterial occlusive disease. Long-term anticoagulation with warfarin (Coumadin) is important in all patients who have vascular occlusive disease associated with antiphospholipid syndromes. According to our own experience, and several reports in the literature, discontinuation of anticoagulation has often resulted in recurrent thrombotic episodes with disastrous outcomes.

DISCUSSION

Testing for the presence of antiphospholipid antibodies provides a prognostic indicator and some guidance in the management of vascular occlusive disease, but additional information is required. Prospective controlled clinical trials are needed to provide such information and identify other variables or risk factors that will improve the diagnosis and management of these patients.

SUGGESTED READING

Asherson RA. A "primary" antiphospholipid syndrome? J Rheumatol 1988; 15:1742–1746.

Asherson RA, Harris EN. Anticardiolipin antibodies: clinical associations. Postgrad Med J 1986; 62:1081–1087.

Asherson RA, Khamashta MA, Gil A, et al. Cerebrovascular disease and antiphospholipid antibodies in systemic lupus erythematosus, lupus-like disease, and the primary antiphospholipid syndrome. Am J Med 1989; 86:391–399.

Chartash EK, Lans DM, Paget SA, et al. Aortic insufficiency and mitral regurgitation in patients with systemic lupus erythematosus and the antiphospholipid syndrome. Am J Med 1989; 86:407–412.

Harris EN, Asherson RA, Hughes GRN. Antiphospholipid antibodies: autoantibodies with a difference. Annu Rev Med 1988; 39:261–271.

Lie JT. Vasculopathy in the antiphospholipid syndrome: thrombosis or vasculitis, or both? J Rheumatol 1989; 16:713–715.

Love PE, Santoro SA. Antiphospholipid antibodies: anticardiolipin and the lupus anticoagulant in systemic lupus erythematosus (SLE) and in non-SLE disorders. Ann Intern Med 1990; 112:682–698.

Macleworth-Young CG, Loizou S, Walport MJ. Primary antiphospholipid syndrome: features of patients with raised anticardiolipin antibodies and no other disorder. Ann Rheum Dis 1989; 48:362–367.

Note: Page numbers followed by (f) indicate figures; page numbers followed by (t) indicate tables.

A

Abdominal aortic aneurysm, 168–170, 170–171, 219–220, 241(f)

Abdominal aortic occlusion, antiphospholipid antibodies and, 358(f)

Abdominal vascular compression, 281, 281(f)

Abortion, spontaneous, antiphospholipid antibody syndromes and, 357, 358, 360

Acebutolol, for hypertension, 10, 21(t)

Acetaminophen, for migraine, 149

Acetazolamide, for hypertension, in children, 21(t)

Acetylated plasminogen:streptokinase complex, for acute arterial occlusion of extremities, 236

Acromegaly, hypertension and, 75

ACTH, in Cushing's syndrome, 69

Activated partial thromboplastin time, in heparin therapy, for pulmonary embolism, 304–305, 306(t), 307, 308(t)

Acute coronary syndromes, antithrombotic therapy for, 112–116

Adenoma
adrenal. See Adrenal tumors
pituitary, resection of, in Cushing's syndrome, 70

Adrenalectomy
bilateral, in Cushing's syndrome, 70
in hyperaldosteronism, 66
indications for, 73
in pheochromocytoma, 72

Adrenal hyperplasia
bilateral, vs. primary hyperaldosteronism, 64–66
congenital, hypertension in, 67

Adrenal tumors
aldosterone-producing, vs. primary hyperaldosteronism, 64–66
Cushing's syndrome and, 69, 70
deoxycorticosterone-secreting, hypertension and, 67
incidentally discovered, hypertension and, 72–73
surgery of. See Adrenalectomy

Adrenergic inhibitors. See also Alpha-adrenergic blocking agents; Beta-blockers
for hypertension
centrally acting, 11
in elderly, 15, 16(t)
peripherally acting, 10–11

Adrenocorticotropic hormone, in Cushing's syndrome, 69

Adventitial cystic disease, 230–231, 231(f), 232(f)

Aerobic capacity, functional, 209, 221

African-Americans, hypertension in, 24–25, 25(t)

Alcohol intake, restriction of, in hypertension, 3

Aldosterone, plasma, in primary hyperaldosteronism, 64

Aldosterone-producing adenoma, vs. primary hyperaldosteronism, 64–66

Allen's test, 249, 266

Allergic angiitis and granulomatosis, 256

Alpha-adrenergic blocking agents. See also specific agents
for hypertension, in subarachnoid hemorrhage, 155
for Raynaud's phenomenon, 245, 246(t)

Amiloride
for hyperaldosteronism, 66
for hypertension, in children, 21(t)

Amitryptiline, for migraine prophylaxis, 152

Amputation, in Buerger's disease, 270, 270(f)

Aneurysm
aortic. See Aortic aneurysm
axillary artery, 243, 243(f)
coronary artery, in Kawasaki disease, 260–261, 261(f), 263–264
definition of, 166
dissecting, 166
aortic. See Aortic dissection
of cervical internal carotid artery, 140–141, 142(t)
false, 166
post-traumatic, 275, 275(f)
femoral artery, 240–242, 241(f)
fibromuscular, renal arteriovenous fistula and, 324, 327(f)
intracranial
cerebrovascular fibromuscular dysplasia and, 326
complications of, 153–156
pathogenesis and natural history of, 166
popliteal, 237–239, 238(f), 238(t), 239(t)
subclavian artery, 241(t), 242(f), 242–243
true, 166
vascular compression by, 282

Aneurysmal subarachnoid hemorrhage, 153–156, 154(f)

Angiitis, allergic, with granulomatosis, 256

Angina, intestinal, in mesenteric ischemia, 188, 192

Angina pectoris
in aortoiliac occlusive disease, 177
coronary angioplasty for, 93–103. See also Coronary angioplasty
medical management of, 87–92, 108
stable, myocardial ischemia and, 119–120
surgery for, 106–111. See also Coronary artery bypass grafting
unstable
antithrombotic therapy for, 112–116
coronary angioplasty for, 99, 118
management of, 117–118, 118(f)
variant, 122–127. See also Coronary vasospasm

Angiodysplasia, 335–342
classification of, 335, 336(f), 338(t)
clinical findings in, 335–337, 337(f)
diagnosis of, 337–340
treatment of, 340–342
visceral, 337

Angiography
in acute mesenteric ischemia, 189, 190, 190(f)
in aortic dissection, 159, 160(f)
in aortoiliac occlusive disease, 174(f), 174–175, 175(f), 176(t)
in arterial injuries, 272(f), 273, 273(f), 275(f)
in arteriovenous malformations, 339–340, 340(f)
in Buerger's disease, 268(f), 269, 269(f)
in celiac artery compression syndrome, 193, 193(f)
in coarctation of aorta, 183
coronary
in Kawasaki disease, 260–261, 261(f)
preoperative, 223
digital subtraction, in carotid artery disease, 130–131, 133(f), 133(t)
limitations of, 132
preoperative, 146
exercise radionuclide, 221. See also Exercise testing
in fibromuscular dysplasia, 320–321, 322(f)-325(f)
magnetic resonance, in carotid artery disease, 129(t), 130, 132, 132(f)
in mesenteric ischemia
acute, 190, 190(f)

superior vena cava thrombosis and, 295

Page-Schroetter syndrome, 293–294

Pain. *See also* Angina
in abdominal aortic aneurysm, 166
in aortic dissection, 158
in intermittent claudication. *See* Intermittent claudication
ischemic rest, 203, 227
in pulmonary embolism, 301, 306
in thoracic aortic aneurysm, 168

Palma-Dale cross-pubic bypass, 313(f), 314

Papaverine
for acute mesenteric ischemia, 189
in impotence
for diagnosis, 195
for treatment, 196

Paradoxical embolus, acute arterial occlusion of extremities and, 234

Parathyroidectomy, for hyperparathyroidism, 74

Partial thromboplastin time, in heparin therapy, for pulmonary embolism, 304–305, 306(t), 307, 308(t)

Patch aortoplasty, for coarctation of aorta, 184, 184(f)

Pavlovian conditioning, for Raynaud's phenomenon, 245

Penetrating aortic ulceration, 170, 171(f), 172(f)

Penile-brachial index, 194

Penile plethysmography, 194

Penile prosthesis, 197

Penis, intracavernous injection of
in impotence evaluation, 195
in impotence treatment, 196

Pentoxifylline
for chronic mesenteric ischemia, 193
for peripheral arterial disease, 207, 209
for upper extremity ischemia, 250

Percutaneous transluminal angioplasty. *See* Angioplasty, percutaneous transluminal

Perfusion scan, in pulmonary embolism, 301–302, 302(t)

Periarterial fibroplasia, 321. *See also* Fibromuscular dysplasia

Perimedial fibroplasia, 320. *See also* Fibromuscular dysplasia

Periorbital directional Doppler signals, in carotid artery disease, 128–129, 129(t)

Peripheral arterial aneurysm, 237–243

Peripheral arterial disease
adventitial cystic disease and, 230–231, 231(f), 232(f)
angioplasty for
indications for, 217–218
methods of, 214

morphologic changes with, 213–214, 214(t)
results of, 214–216, 215(t)-217(t)
angioscopy in, 216–217
antiplatelet therapy for, 207
atherectomy for, 214, 217–218
coronary artery disease and, 219–226
diabetic, 206–207, 227
evaluation of, 203–206
exercise rehabilitation in, 206, 208–212
foot care in, 206
functional capacity in, assessment of, 210–211
hemodynamic assessment in, 210
hemorrheologic therapy for, 207
intermittent claudication in, 203–206
intra-arterial ultrasonography in, 216–217
medical management of, 203–208, 209
noninvasive tests for, 199–202, 200(f)-202(f), 205–206
classification of, 199–200
preoperative, 220–226, 228
percutaneous interventional treatment for, 212–218
popliteal arterial entrapment and, 231
progression of, 213, 213(t)
risk factor modification in, 206–207
surgery for, 227–233, 308–310
cardiac risk assessment for, 219–226
choice of procedure for, 228–2298
complications in, 231–232, 232(f)
graft failure after, 233
hemodynamic monitoring for, 224
in high-risk patients, 223–225
indications for, 208–209, 227
late incidence of, 213, 213(t)
perioperative myocardial ischemia/infarction in, 224–225
postoperative care in, 231
preoperative evaluation for, 219–226, 227–228
for high-risk patients, 223(t), 223–225, 224(f)
for intermediate-risk patients, 223(t), 223–225, 224(f), 225(f)
for low-risk patients, 223(t), 225–226, 226(f)
tests in, 220–222
results of, coronary artery disease and, 219–220
risk stratification for, 223(t), 223–226, 224(f)-226(f)
technique of, 229(f), 229–230, 230(f)
vasodilator therapy for, 207

Peripheral circulation, evaluation of, 210–211

Peritoneal dialysis patients. *See* Dialysis patients

Peroneal artery, fibromuscular dysplasia of, 328

Phenelzine, for migraine prophylaxis, 152

Phenoxybenzamine
for hypertension, in children, 21(t)
preoperative, for pheochromocytoma, 72
for Raynaud's phenomenon, 246t, 247

Phentolamine
for hypertensive crisis, 45
for pheochromocytoma crisis, 41

Pheochromocytoma, hypertension and, 70–72

Pheochromocytoma crisis, 41
labetalol for, 42(t), 45
phentolamine for, 45

Phlebography
in deep venous thrombosis, 288
in thoracic outlet syndrome, 279

Phrenic nerve injury, in coronary artery bypass grafting, 111

Pindolol
for hypertension, 10
in children, 21(t)
in elderly, 15
in renal parenchymal disease, 79
for orthostatic hypotension, 85

Pituitary adenoma, Cushing's syndrome and, 69, 70

Plaque embolus. *See* Embolus, atheromatous

Plaque rupture, thrombosis and, 112, 112(f)

Plasma aldosterone, in primary hyperaldosteronism, 64

Plasma renin activity
in blacks, 24
in elderly, 28
in malignant hypertension, 36
in primary hyperaldosteronism, 64
in renovascular hypertension, 58, 59–60

Plasminogen activator, for deep venous thrombosis, 290

Plethysmography
impedance
in deep venous thrombosis, 287–288
in pulmonary embolism, 301, 302
penile, 194

Pneumatic compression, for deep venous thrombosis, 291, 291(f)

Polyarteritis nodosa, 255–256

Polytetrafluoroethylene graft
for aortic coarctation, 184, 184(f)
for femoral aneurysm, 241–242
for peripheral arterial disease, 228–229